Issues in Clinical Child Psychology

Series Editor

Michael C. Roberts
Clinical Child Psychology Program
University of Kansas
Lawrence, KS, USA

The *Issues in Clinical Child Psychology* book series represents a broad spectrum of professional psychology books, integrating clinical psychology with the development of children, adolescents, and their families and developmental psychopathology. The age coverage ranges from infancy to childhood to adolescence. Populations of interest include normally developing children and those exhibiting problems in developmental, behavioral, psychological, health, and academic realms. Settings include schools, mental health clinics, independent practice, pediatric offices and centers, and juvenile facilities. Topics of interest include developmental psychopathology, externalizing and internalizing disorders, assessment and diagnosis, interventions and treatments, consultation, prevention, school mental health, normal and abnormal development, family psychology, service delivery, diversity and cultural differences, and ethical and legal issues in clinical practice and research.

More information about this series at http://www.springer.com/series/6082

Bryan D. Carter • Kristin A. Kullgren
Editors

Clinical Handbook of Psychological Consultation in Pediatric Medical Settings

Springer

Editors
Bryan D. Carter
Pediatric Consultation-Liaison Service
Norton Children's Hospital
Louisville, KY, USA

Department of Pediatrics
University of Louisville
School of Medicine
Louisville, KY, USA

Kristin A. Kullgren
Department of Pediatrics
C.S. Mott Children's Hospital
Michigan Medicine
Ann Arbor, MI, USA

ISSN 1574-0471
Issues in Clinical Child Psychology
ISBN 978-3-030-35597-5 ISBN 978-3-030-35598-2 (eBook)
https://doi.org/10.1007/978-3-030-35598-2

This Springer imprint is published by the registered company Springer Nature Switzerland AG
The registered company address is: Gewerbestrasse 11, 6330 Cham, Switzerland

This book is dedicated to our dear friend and colleague, Dennis Drotar, Ph.D., a true pioneer in pediatric psychology who mentored and influenced so many students and early career psychologists and opened doors for our collaboration with our pediatric colleagues to the benefit of the children and families coping with challenges to their health and welfare.

BCD and KAK

Acknowledgments

We are indebted to each of the talented clinician-authors who contributed to this book and our numerous student reviewers who provided feedback on each of the chapters: Kristina Brookshire, Shannon Brothers, Kirsten Drucker, Allison Gornik, Lauren Harrison, Rachel Kentor, Sharon Lo, Isabelle Oh, Chris Poitevien, Kate Price, Samantha Schires, Erin Van Seeters, Kristina Suorsa, and Chelsea VanderWoude.

–KAK and BDC

My deepest appreciation to my wife, Amy, for her support and encouragement for not just this project, but for being my source of inspiration for Life. And to my valued colleagues, especially Bill Kronenberger, the many pediatricians, residents, interns, children and families who have taught me so much about how genuine caring relationships can sustain us through the greatest challenges. Finally, to my co-editor, Kris.... you Rock!

–BDC

Many thanks to my family, Bryan, Lydia, and Dean, who have been my biggest cheerleaders through this process...yes, you will get an autographed copy! In memory of my mom, Bonnie Kullgren, who always believed in my professional pursuits and would have loved to have a copy of this on her shelf. To my CL family for protecting my writing and editing days even when the service was busy. Final thanks to my partner-in-crime and mentor, Bryan Carter, for the inspiration to think critically and creatively about CL practice. Go Blue!

–KAK

Contents

Contributors

Ariel M. Aballay Department of Surgery, West Penn Hospital Burn Center, Allegheny Health Network, Pittsburgh, PA, USA

Temple University, Philadelphia, PA, USA

Dana Albright Department of Pediatrics, C.S. Mott Children's Hospital, University of Michigan School of Medicine, Ann Arbor, MI, USA

Anthony Alioto Department of Pediatrics, Nemours/AIDHC, Wilmington, DE, USA

Thomas Jefferson University, Sidney Kimmel College of Medicine, Philadelphia, PA, USA

Melissa N. Andersen Department of Pediatrics, C.S. Mott Children's Hospital, University of Michigan School of Medicine, Ann Arbor, MI, USA

Amy E. Baughcum Nationwide Children's Hospital, Columbus, OH, USA

Department of Pediatrics, The Ohio State University College of Medicine, Columbus, OH, USA

Katherine K. Bedard-Thomas Behavioral Medicine and Clinical Psychology, Cincinnati Children's Hospital Medical Center, Cincinnati, OH, USA

Behavioral Medicine and Clinical Psychology, Cincinnati Children's Hospital Medical Center, Cincinnati, OH, USA

Laura M. Bennett Murphy Department of Pediatrics, University of Utah School of Medicine, Primary Children's Hospital, Salt Lake City, UT, USA

Ethan Benore Center for Pediatric Behavioral Health, Cleveland Clinic Children's, Cleveland, OH, USA

Clinical Assistant Professor at Cleveland Clinic Lerner College of Medicine, Cleveland, OH, USA

Hillary S. Blake Department of Psychiatry, Riley Hospital for Children, Indiana University School of Medicine, Indianapolis, IN, USA

Adrienne P. Borschuk Cincinnati Children's Hospital Medical Center, Cincinnati, OH, USA

Behavioral Medicine and Clinical Psychology, Cincinnati Children's Hospital Medical Center, Cincinnati, OH, USA

University of Cincinnati College of Medicine, Cincinnati, OH, USA

Christine E. Brady Kaiser Permanente, Santa Clara, California, United States

Child Psychiatry, Kaiser Permanente, Santa Clara, California, United States

Kira S. Branch Department of Pediatrics, Nemours/AIDHC, Wilmington, DE, USA

Thomas Jefferson University, Sidney Kimmel College of Medicine, Philadelphia, PA, USA

Michelle R. Brown Lucile Packard Children's Hospital Stanford, Palo Alto, CA, USA

Department of Psychiatry, Stanford University School of Medicine, Stanford, CA, USA

Teryn Bruni Department of Pediatrics, C.S. Mott Children's Hospital, University of Michigan School of Medicine, Ann Arbor, MI, USA

Simona Bujoreanu Boston Children's Hospital, Boston, MA, USA

Department of Psychiatry, Boston Children's Hospital, Harvard Medical School, Boston, MA, USA

Kimberly Burkhart UH Rainbow Babies and Children's Hospital, Cleveland, OH, USA

Pediatrics and Psychiatry, Case Western Reserve University, Cleveland, OH, USA

Brenda Bursch UCLA Mattel Children's Hospital, Los Angeles, CA, USA

Jane and Terry Semel Institute for Neuroscience and Human Behavior, Los Angeles, CA, USA

Department of Psychiatry and Biobehavioral Sciences, David Geffen School of Medicine at UCLA, Los Angeles, CA, USA

Department of Pediatrics, David Geffen School of Medicine at UCLA, Los Angeles, CA, USA

Jennifer Butcher Department of Pediatrics, C.S. Mott Children's Hospital, University of Michigan Medical School, Ann Arbor, MI, USA

Chrissy Cammarata Division of Behavioral Health, Department of Pediatrics, Nemours/A.I. DuPont Hospital for Children, Sidney Kimmel Medical College, Thomas Jefferson University, Wilmington, DE, USA

Deirdre A. L. Caplin Department of Pediatrics, University of Utah School of Medicine, Primary Children's Hospital, Salt Lake City, UT, USA

Bryan D. Carter Pediatric Consultation-Liaison Service Norton Children's Hospital, Louisville, KY, USA

Department of Pediatrics, University of Louisville School of Medicine, Louisville, KY, USA

Crystal L. Cederna-Meko Department of Pediatrics and Human Development, Michigan State University College of Human Medicine, Hurley Children's Hospital, East Lansing, MI, USA

Christine T. Chambers Department of Psychology and Neuroscience, Centre for Pediatric Pain Research, IWK Health Centre, Dalhousie University, Halifax, NS, Canada

Department of Pediatrics, Centre for Pediatric Pain Research, IWK Health Centre, Dalhousie University, Halifax, NS, Canada

Jennifer M. Colombo Department of Pediatrics, Children's Mercy Kansas City, University of Missouri-Kansas City, Kansas City, MO, USA

Megan E. Connolly Department of Pediatrics, Children's National Health System, George Washington University School of Medicine and Health Sciences, Washington, DC, USA

Department of Psychiatry and Behavioral Science, Children's National Health System, George Washington University School of Medicine and Health Sciences, Washington, DC, USA

Melissa K. Cousino C.S. Mott Children's Hospital, Ann Arbor, MI, USA

University of Michigan Transplant Center, Ann Arbor, MI, USA

Department of Pediatrics, University of Michigan Medical School, Ann Arbor, MI, USA

Lori E. Crosby Cincinnati Children's Hospital and Medical Center, Cincinnati, OH, USA

Department of Pediatrics, University of Cincinnati College of Medicine, Cincinnati, OH, USA

Allyson L. Davis Division of Behavioral Health, Nemours/Alfred I. duPont Hospital for Children, Wilmington, DE, USA

Division of Behavioral Health, Swank Autism Center, Wilmington, DE, USA

Amanda D. Deacy Department of Pediatrics, Children's Mercy Kansas City, University of Missouri-Kansas City, Kansas City, MO, USA

Robert Dempster Department of Pediatric Psychology and Neuropsychology, Nationwide Children's Hospital, Columbus, OH, USA

Department of Pediatrics, The Ohio State University, Columbus, OH, USA

Dawn Dore-Stites Department of Pediatrics, C.S. Mott Children's Hospital, University of Michigan Medical School, Ann Arbor, MI, USA

Amy Drayton Department of Pediatrics, C.S. Mott Children's Hospital, University of Michigan School of Medicine, Ann Arbor, MI, USA

Christina L. Duncan Department of Psychology, West Virginia University, Morgantown, WV, USA

Department of Pediatrics, West Virginia University School of Medicine, Morgantown, WV, USA

Rebecca E. H. Ellens Department of Pediatrics and Human Development, Michigan State University College of Human Medicine, Hurley Children's Hospital, East Lansing, MI, USA

Natacha D. Emerson UCLA Mattel Children's Hospital, Los Angeles, CA, USA

Jane and Terry Semel Institute for Neuroscience and Human Behavior, Los Angeles, CA, USA

Department of Psychiatry and Biobehavioral Sciences, David Geffen School of Medicine at UCLA, Los Angeles, CA, USA

Michelle M. Ernst Cincinnati Children's Hospital Medical Center, Cincinnati, OH, USA

Division of Behavioral Medicine and Clinical Psychology, University of Cincinnati School of Medicine, Cincinnati, OH, USA

Stephanie Spear Filigno Cincinnati Children's Hospital Medical Center, Cincinnati, OH, USA

Division of Behavioral Medicine and Clinical Psychology, Cincinnati Children's Hospital Medical Center, Cincinnati, OH, USA

University of Cincinnati College of Medicine, Cincinnati, OH, USA

Courtney Landau Fleisher Departments of Psychiatry and Pediatrics, Robert Larner MD College of Medicine, Burlington, VT, USA

University of Vermont Medical Center, Burlington, VT, USA

Stacy R. Flowers Family Medicine Residency, Dayton, OH, USA

Department of Family Medicine, Boonshoft School of Medicine, Dayton, OH, USA

Wright State University, Dayton, OH, USA

Emily Foxen-Craft Department of Pediatrics, C.S. Mott Children's Hospital, University of Michigan Medical School, Ann Arbor, MI, USA

Emily M. Fredericks C.S. Mott Children's Hospital, Ann Arbor, MI, USA

University of Michigan Transplant Center, Ann Arbor, MI, USA

Department of Pediatrics, University of Michigan Medical School, Ann Arbor, MI, USA

Lauren L. Garbacz Department of Pediatric Psychology and Neuropsychology, Nationwide Children's Hospital, Columbus, OH, USA

Department of Pediatrics, The Ohio State University, Columbus, OH, USA

Elaine A. T. Gilbert Departments of Psychiatry and Pediatrics, Riley Hospital for Children, Indiana University School of Medicine, Indianapolis, IN, USA

Julianne Giust Department of Psychiatry, Riley Hospital for Children, Indiana University School of Medicine, Indianapolis, IN, USA

Michelle M. Greene Rush University Children's Hospital, Chicago, IL, USA

Department of Pediatrics, Rush University Medical Center, Chicago, IL, USA

Jennifer A. Hansen-Moore Department of Pediatric Psychology and Neuropsychology, Nationwide Children's Hospital, Columbus, OH, USA

Department of Pediatrics, The Ohio State University College of Medicine, Columbus, OH, USA

Lillian C. Hayes Department of Psychiatry, Boston Children's Hospital, Harvard Medical School, Boston, MA, USA

Aimee K. Hildenbrand Nemours/AI duPont Hospital for Children, Wilmington, DE, USA

Division of Behavioral Health, Center for Healthcare Delivery Science, New York, NY, USA

Casey Hoffman The Children's Hospital of Philadelphia, Philadelphia, PA, USA

Department of Child and Adolescent Psychiatry and Behavioral Sciences, The Children's Hospital of Philadelphia, Philadelphia, PA, USA

Christina E. Holbein Children's Hospital of Philadelphia, Philadelphia, PA, USA

Department of Child and Adolescent Psychiatry and Behavioral Sciences, Children's Hospital of Philadelphia, Philadelphia, PA, USA

Anna M. Hood Developmental Neurosciences, UCL Great Ormond Street Institute of Child Health, London, UK

Naomi E. Joffe Cincinnati Children's Hospital and Medical Center, Cincinnati, OH, USA

Department of Pediatrics, University of Cincinnati College of Medicine, Cincinnati, OH, USA

Laura Judd-Glossy Departments of Psychiatry and Pediatric Surgery, University of Colorado School of Medicine, Aurora, CO, USA

Children's Hospital Colorado, Aurora, CO, USA

Jacqueline N. Kaufman Department of Physical Medicine and Rehabilitation, University of Michigan Medical School, Ann Arbor, MI, USA

Anne E. Kazak Center for Healthcare Delivery Science, Nemours Children's Health System, Wilmington, DE, USA

Department of Pediatrics, Sidney Kimmel Medical School of Thomas Jefferson University, Philadelphia, PA, USA

Jessica C. Kichler Behavioral Medicine and Clinical Psychology, Cincinnati Children's Hospital Medical Center, Cincinnati, OH, USA

Department of Pediatrics, University of Cincinnati School of Medicine, Cincinnati, OH, USA

Christine Kindler Department of Pediatrics, Kentucky Children's Hospital, University of Kentucky School of Medicine, Lexington, KY, USA

Rachel M. Knight Department of Pediatrics, C.S. Mott Children's Hospital, University of Michigan School of Medicine, Ann Arbor, MI, USA

Michele Knox Department of Psychiatry, University of Toledo College of Medicine and Health Sciences, Toledo, OH, USA

William G. Kronenberger Department of Psychiatry, Riley Hospital for Children, Indiana University School of Medicine, Indianapolis, IN, USA

Kristin A. Kullgren Department of Pediatrics, C.S. Mott Children's Hospital, Michigan Medicine, Ann Arbor, MI, USA

Ann M. Lagges Department of Psychiatry, Riley Hospital for Children, Indiana University School of Medicine, Indianapolis, IN, USA

Sarah Lahey Clinical Neuropsychologist, Brain Injury and Pediatric Programs, Brooks Rehabilitation, Jacksonville, FL, USA

Nicole E. MacKenzie Department of Psychology and Neuroscience, Centre for Pediatric Pain Research, IWK Health Centre, Dalhousie University, Halifax, NS, Canada

Michele H. Maddux Department of Pediatrics, Children's Mercy Kansas City, University of Missouri-Kansas City, Kansas City, MO, USA

Meghan L. Marsac Department of Pediatrics, Kentucky Children's Hospital, UK Health Care, University of Kentucky College of Medicine, Lexington, KY, USA

Ashley McGar Department of Pediatrics, Kentucky Children's Hospital, University of Kentucky School of Medicine, Lexington, KY, USA

Emily A. McTate Cincinnati Children's Hospital and Medical Center, Cincinnati, OH, USA

Department of Pediatrics, University of Cincinnati College of Medicine, Cincinnati, OH, USA

Amy Meadows Department of Pediatrics, Kentucky Children's Hospital, UK Health Care, University of Kentucky College of Medicine, Lexington, KY, USA

Department of Psychiatry, Kentucky Children's Hospital, UK Health Care, University of Kentucky College of Medicine, Lexington, KY, USA

Susan B. Meister Child Health Evaluation and Research (CHEAR) Center, Ann Arbor, MI, USA

Janelle M. Mentrikoski Children's Mercy Kansas City, Kansas City, MO, USA

Department of Pediatrics, University of Missouri-Kansas City, Kansas City, MO, USA

Emily Mudd Cleveland Clinic, Cleveland, OH, USA

Cleveland Clinic Lerner College of Medicine of Case Western Reserve University, Cleveland, OH, USA

Sara Multerer Department of Pediatrics, Norton Children's Hospital, University of Louisville School of Medicine, Louisville, KY, USA

Brittany R. Myers Department of Psychiatry, MetroHealth Medical Center, Case Western Reserve University School of Medicine, Cleveland, OH, USA

Maia M. Noeder Division of Behavioral Health, Nemours/Alfred I. duPont Hospital for Children, Wilmington, DE, USA

Pediatrics, Sidney Kimmel Medical College - Thomas Jefferson University, Philadelphia, PA, USA

Carisa Parrish Johns Hopkins Medicine, Baltimore, MD, USA

Department of Psychiatry and Behavioral Sciences, Johns Hopkins School of Medicine, Baltimore, MD, USA

Sara Golden Pell Boston Children's Hospital, Boston, MA, USA

Department of Psychiatry, Harvard Medical School, Boston, MA, USA

Lisa Y. Ramirez Department of Psychiatry, MetroHealth Medical Center, Case Western Reserve University School of Medicine, Cleveland, OH, USA

Rachelle R. Ramsey Cincinnati Children's Hospital Medical Center, Cincinnati, OH, USA

Division of Behavioral Medicine and Clinical Psychology, Department of Pediatrics, University of Cincinnati College of Medicine, Cincinnati, OH, USA

Anne Reagan Golisano Children's Hospital, Syracuse, NY, USA

Department of Pediatrics, SUNY Upstate Medical University, Syracuse, NY, USA

Kelly E. Rea Department of Psychology, University of Georgia, Athens, GA, USA

Monique Ribeiro Boston Children's Hospital, Boston, MA, USA

Department of Psychiatry, Harvard Medical School, Boston, MA, USA

Laura Sayers Department of Pediatrics, C.S. Mott Children's Hospital, University of Michigan School of Medicine, Ann Arbor, MI, USA

Kristie V. Schultz Department of Pediatrics, Norton Children's Hospital, University of Louisville School of Medicine, Louisville, KY, USA

Eric L. Scott Department of Pediatrics, C.S. Mott Children's Hospital, University of Michigan Medical School, Ann Arbor, MI, USA

Department of Anesthesiology, C.S. Mott Children's Hospital, University of Michigan School of Medicine, Ann Arbor, MI, USA

Heather Shepard Department of Pediatrics, C.S. Mott Children's Hospital University of Michigan School of Medicine, Ann Arbor, MI, USA

Barbara Sourkes Lucile Packard Children's Hospital Stanford, Palo Alto, CA, USA

Department of Pediatrics, Stanford University School of Medicine, Stanford, CA, USA

Michael K. Sowell Department of Neurology, Norton Children's Hospital, University of Louisville School of Medicine, Louisville, KY, USA

Terry Stancin Department of Psychiatry, Pediatrics and Psychological Sciences, MetroHealth Medical Center, Case Western Reserve University School of Medicine, Cleveland, OH, USA

Amanda L. Thompson Department of Pediatrics, Children's National Health System, George Washington University School of Medicine and Health Sciences, Washington, DC, USA

Department of Psychiatry and Behavioral Science, Children's National Health System, George Washington University School of Medicine and Health Sciences, Washington, DC, USA

Brooke Threlkeld Department of Pediatrics, Norton Children's Hospital, University of Louisville School of Medicine, Louisville, KY, USA

Kevin K. Tsang Department of Psychiatry, Boston Children's Hospital, Harvard Medical School, Boston, MA, USA

Perri R. Tutelman Department of Psychology and Neuroscience, Centre for Pediatric Pain Research, IWK Health Centre, Dalhousie University, Halifax, NS, Canada

Eileen Twohy Department of Psychiatry and Behavioral Medicine, University of Washington School of Medicine, Seattle, WA, USA

Seattle Children's Hospital, Seattle, WA, USA

Erin Webster Department of Psychology, Dayton Children's Hospital, Dayton, OH, USA

Amy E. Williams Department of Psychiatry, Riley Hospital for Children, Indiana University School of Medicine, Indianapolis, IN, USA

Sara E. Williams Department of Pediatrics, University of Cincinnati College of Medicine, Cincinnati, OH, USA

Division of Behavioral Medicine and Clinical Psychology, Cincinnati Children's Hospital Medical Center, Cincinnati, OH, USA

Karen Wohlheiter Department of Pediatrics, Nemours/A.I. DuPont Hospital for Children, Sidney Kimmel Medical College, Thomas Jefferson University, Wilmington, DE, USA

Nicole E. Zahka Division of Behavioral Medicine and Clinical Psychology, Cincinnati Children's Hospital Medical Center, Cincinnati, OH, USA

About the Editors

Bryan D. Carter, Ph.D. is a Professor in the Department of Pediatrics, Division of Child and Adolescent Psychiatry and Psychology, University of Louisville School of Medicine. He is the Service Chief of the Pediatric Consultation-Liaison Service to Norton Children's Hospital (formerly Kosair Children's Hospital) and Director of Training for the Postdoctoral Fellowship in Pediatric Psychology with the University of Louisville SOM. Dr. Carter received his Ph.D. in Clinical Child Psychology from the University of Virginia, predoctoral residency at Wilford Hall USAF Medical Center in San Antonio, and postdoctoral fellowship in Pediatric Psychology at the University of Oklahoma School of Medicine. He is a recipient of the Carolyn D. Schroeder Clinical Practice Award given by American Psychological Association Division 54 (Society of Pediatric Psychology) for nationally recognized excellence, innovation, and leadership in the clinical practice of pediatric psychology and was co-founder of the Consultation-Liaison Special Interest Group for Division 54. He is the developer of the Children's Health and Illness Recovery Program (CHIRP) and senior author of the *CHIRP Clinician Handbook* and *CHIRP Teen and Family Workbook* (Oxford University Press Treatments That Work series), a manualized treatment program for maximizing functional independence in adolescents coping with the challenges of chronic illness. Dr. Carter has published numerous scientific articles and book chapters related to his interests in pediatric psychology, CL, and chronic pediatric illness and injury.

Kristin A. Kullgren, Ph.D. is an Associate Professor in the Department of Pediatrics at the University of Michigan School of Medicine and C.S. Mott Children's Hospital. Dr. Kullgren is also a faculty member in the University of Michigan Center for Human Growth and Development. She completed her Ph.D. in Clinical Psychology at Georgia State University, her predoctoral internship in Pediatric Psychology at the University of Maryland School of Medicine, and postdoctoral fellowship in Pediatric Psychology at Emory University School of Medicine. Dr. Kullgren is the director of the pediatric psychology consultation-liaison service at C.S. Mott Children's Hospital. Dr. Kullgren is the past co-chair of the Consultation-Liaison Special Interest Group for Division 54. She has published numerous scientific articles and book chapters on consultation-liaison practice and the impact of chronic illness on youth and families.

Part I

Pediatric Consultation-Liaison Psychology: Models, Roles, Settings, and Practice

Introduction to the Clinical Handbook of Psychological Consultation in Pediatric Medical Settings

Kristin A. Kullgren and Bryan D. Carter

In recent years, there has been increased demand for pediatric mental health consultation services in the context of changes in the current health-care environment, increasing recognition of bio-psychosocial factors impacting health, and the challenge of highly complex pediatric patients and medical conditions (Shaw, Pao, Holland, & DeMaso, 2016). Consultation-liaison (CL) in pediatric psychology is a core practice when interfacing with medical colleagues in pediatric settings. Specifically, *consultation* refers to the direct clinical activities provided to children and families at the request of medical colleagues with the goal of identifying and addressing the impact of psychosocial factors on the child's medical condition or functioning (Carter et al., 2017; Ernst et al., 2014). Consultation can occur in a variety of pediatric settings (e.g., inpatient hospital, outpatient subspecialty clinic, primary care clinic) via many different models of practice that vary by setting, team composition, scope of practice, and the psychologist's function within the team (Ernst et al., 2014; see chapter "Pediatric Consultation-Liaison: Models and Roles in Pediatric Psychology", this volume). Typically, the act of consultation starts with a medical provider identifying a clinical need with a patient or family and initiating a referral for the psychologist to conduct an evaluation, provide brief interventions and referrals, and communicate feedback and recommendations to the medical team. Consultants in medical settings are often seen as the "mediators" or "interpreters" between physician and psychology toward a more integrated, holistic point of view of patient care (Lipowski, 1971).

The *liaison* functions of the CL psychologist are broader and primarily relate to indirect patient care activities and systems-level interventions reflective of the psychologist's integration into the medical team (Carter et al., 2017; Carter, Kroenenberger, Scott, & Ernst, 2009; Ernst et al., 2014). These activities vary by the psychologists' role within the medical team and can range from participating in bedside rounds and care conferences to representing psychology on hospital committees, to educating medical learners through didactics, to conducting staff in-services and advocacy work (Carter et al., 2009; Ernst et al., 2014). The impact of liaison work cannot be understated as it allows the psychologist to promote our subspecialty, increases knowledge about psychosocial factors impacting youth

K. A. Kullgren (✉)
Department of Pediatrics, C.S. Mott Children's Hospital, Michigan Medicine, Ann Arbor, MI, USA
e-mail: kullgren@med.umich.edu

B. D. Carter
Department of Pediatrics, University of Louisville School of Medicine, Louisville, KY, USA

B. D. Carter, K. A. Kullgren (eds.), *Clinical Handbook of Psychological Consultation in Pediatric Medical Settings*, Issues in Clinical Child Psychology, https://doi.org/10.1007/978-3-030-35598-2_1

experiencing medical illness or injury, and models for the medical community how to sensitively and empathically communicate with and about pediatric patients (Carter, Thompson, & Townsend, 2014). It is important to keep in mind that the above consultation and liaison activities are not mutually exclusive and that consultants often function best when these roles are intertwined (Drotar, 1995; Lipowski, 1971).

Distinguishing Aspects of CL Practice Within Pediatric Psychology

While the practice of CL psychology has more in common with other forms of pediatric psychology clinical practice than not, there are unique aspects of pediatric psychology CL that distinguish it from other forms of pediatric psychology practice (Table 1). The expectation for the pediatric psychologist is to adhere to the competency practice parameters set forth by the Society of Pediatric Psychology (Palermo et al., 2014). However, CL practice represents a unique application of pediatric psychology in that the psychologist is a consultant and adviser to the medical team rather than functioning as an independent practitioner. As such, the psychologist is not the primary provider with patients remaining the primary responsibility of the medical team. Additionally, the focus of the CL psychologist's activities often extends beyond the individual patient to address more broad systems-level issues that impact care. In CL practice, the referral source is almost always the medical team, making relationships between the psychologist and the medical team a crucial aspect of care. While CL treatment time may vary, it is often brief relative to more traditional therapy practice (Rodrigue et al., 1995). The CL psychologist is more often integrated into the practice setting, and the liaison functions are integrated into practice.

Table 1 Comparison between consultation-liaison and traditional pediatric psychology practice

	Traditional practice	Consultation-liaison
Focus of intervention	• Individual and/or family	• Individual and/or family • Medical system • Medical team
Source of referral	• Variable—often initiated by family	• Medical team • Less often family initiated • Protocol driven
Responsibility for patient	• Psychologist	• Physician maintains (Olson et al., 1988)
Timing	• Collaborative with family and psychologist schedule	• Dependent on accessibility of patient within the setting • Typically same day
Intervention targets	• Variable to psychologist practice	• Focused on a specific target
Length of treatment	• Variable to psychologist practice and intervention • More likely to be brief therapy at regular intervals with some long-term therapy	• Brief evaluation and intervention, often 1–2 sessions • Referral to outpatient therapist to continue treatment • Intermittent contact with patients who have frequent contacts in setting
Integration	• Independent • May be referral source for a specific hospital group, but not as likely to be integrated	• More likely to be integrated into setting of practice
Liaison	• May be limited based on degree of integration and psychologist interest	• Integrated into CL practice

Key Competencies in CL Practice

Being an effective CL psychologist is not without significant challenges (Table 2). A strong set of clinical skills for the practice of pediatric psychology forms the foundation for all CL practice, regardless of setting (Palermo et al., 2014). Other necessary qualities include tolerating the uncertainty and fast pace of the consult setting and an ability to move within and across multiple systems in a respectful, empathic way. This will ensure that the psychologist is able to meet the competing needs of the referring medical provider, patient/family, and medical system. Working in collaboration with our pediatric health-care colleagues is one of the core concepts of consultation (Carter et al., 2009; Drotar, 1995). Strong communication skills will help the CL psychologist serve as a "mediator" or "interpreter" between the family and medical providers (Carter et al., 2014; DeMaso, 2009; Lipowski, 1971). The CL psychologist must have strong skills in written communication/documentation and the ability to respond to the medical team's requests in an expeditious manner. Diplomacy and awareness of differences in professional and personal perspectives are essential to facilitate the joining process with patients and medical providers alike, in order to demonstrate and model sensitivity to all concerns (Carter et al., 2014). For example, the CL psychologist can play an important role as a facilitator of staff communication, particularly in stressful or dysfunctional situations (Drotar, 1975). Finally, the CL psychologist has the opportunity to significantly impact medical provider understanding and appreciation of the biopsychosocial factors impacting health and the roles that psychologist can play toward improving health and mental health outcomes. By attending to these competencies necessary for effective CL practice, the pediatric psychologist is more likely to increase referrals and medical provider satisfaction with psychology care (Shaw et al., 2016).

Table 2 Characteristics of the effective consultation-liaison (CL) pediatric psychologist

Characteristic	Description
Strong core pediatric psychology skills	Per pediatric psychology professional competencies outlined in 2014 Task Force report (Palermo et al., 2014)
Flexibility	Ability to cope with unpredictable schedule, flow of consults, and consult requests. Tolerance of uncertainty. Calm response in crisis. Ability to modify practice based on nature of setting, CL service makeup, nature of referral question, etc. (Olson et al., 1988)
Empathy	Ability to empathically respond to both patient and provider concerns, being understanding of the differential roles of colleagues and a shared willingness to enhance their skills
Respect	Understanding the unique contribution of all providers and willingness to interact across disciplines for the benefit of enhancing patient care. Appreciation of the culture within which you practice along with the culture of the families you are working with
Multisystem perspective	Being able to understand and operate across and within the multiple systems within which the child exists
Customer driven	Relationships with customers (i.e., physicians, nurses, etc.) determine referrals. Providing timely response and practical management strategies which match setting demands (Shaw et al., 2016)
Communication skills	Able to communicate across range of patients, families, and medical providers as the "interpreter" or "mediator" (Lipowski, 1971). Ability to communicate with diplomacy while respecting multiple viewpoints. Excellent oral and written communication skills
Acceptance of limitations of consultant role	Appreciating that the consultant role is to evaluate and give advice that may or may not be accepted or implemented
Role advocacy	Ability to educate in a nonhierarchical way about psychology's contribution to improving patient care and the benefit of a biopsychosocial perspective to care

From Collaboration to Consultation: CL in History

Mental health consultation was defined in the 1950s and was focused on the interactional, interpersonal relationship between two professional workers, one (the consultant, typically a psychiatrist or psychologist) aiming to assist the other (the consultee, typically a medical provider) by providing recommendations toward solving mental health concerns of a particular client (Bindman, 1959). In medicine, the development of CL psychology and psychiatry evolved from trends in medicine shifting toward prevention, patient-oriented, and community practice (Lipowski, 1971). Early discussions of the role of pediatric psychologists highlighted the consultant role and the importance of the "liaison between pediatric and psychological inquiry" even before these roles were more clearly defined (Kagan, 1965; Wright, 1967). There are references to pediatric psychological consultation services being established within hospitals and medical centers as early as the 1960s (Olson et al., 1988). The 1970s brought an increased focus on the consultation roles that pediatric psychologists can play in the hospital setting. Dennis Drotar, PhD, in whose memory this book is dedicated, was a pioneer in developing and promoting CL practice in the 1970s (see Drotar, 1975). His book *Consulting with Pediatricians* remains relevant to CL practice to this day and provides detailed description of consultation models and practices across pediatric settings (Drotar, 1995). It is notable that, while rather common for pediatric psychologists to work in primary care and subspecialty pediatric clinics today, Drotar described similar practices existing over three decades prior to the current time (Katon et al., 1995). One early conceptual model is that of the psychologist working independently from the pediatrician (referral with post-consultation information exchange), providing indirect consultation (psychologist providing the pediatrician with advice, instruction, protocols, etc.), and more integrated team collaboration (shared decision-making and treatment responsibility). This was followed shortly by the proposal of a systems model that broadened the scope of consultation to addressing family and multilevel systemic factors.

Training in CL Practice

Historically, training in consultation has been identified as a primary component in training to become a pediatric psychologist (La Greca, Stone, Drotar, & Maddux, 1988). CL roles have been one of the core pediatric psychology competencies since the development of the SPP Task Force on Recommendations for the Training of Pediatric Psychologists was published in 2003 (Spirito, 2003). The 2003 Task Force addressed the growing need for psychologists to develop competencies in consultation skills in ambulatory care settings in addition to more traditional hospital services (Spirito, 2003). With the revision of the training guidelines in 2014, competencies in consultation were subsumed under the category of application, addressing those evidence-based skills pertinent to the clinical practice of pediatric psychology (Palermo et al., 2014). These revised guidelines provide specific recommendations for the developmental progression of consultation skills from *readiness for practicum* (understanding of the pediatric psychology consultant's role relative to other health-care professionals), *internship* (knowledge of the consultant's role unique from other roles, communicating findings to other professionals with supervision), and *independent practice* (ability to identify and shift roles to match referrals, provide effective feedback and recommendations to referring providers) (Palermo et al., 2014). In creating this current volume, it is the editors' intent to complement these training and competency guidelines by providing a rich resource of applied practice information for pediatric psychologists at every level of training and practice.

Structure of this Pediatric CL Handbook

Thus far, the literature on pediatric CL psychology, particularly addressing the hospital inpatient setting, has largely focused on practice patterns and program evaluation (Brosig & Zahrt, 2006; Kullgren et al., 2015; Kullgren, Bravender, & Sullivan, 2018; Piazza-Waggoner, Roddenberry, Yeomans-Maldonado, Noll, & Ernst, 2013; Shaw et al., 2016; Shaw, Walmboldt, Bursch, & Stuber, 2006; Tunick, Gavin, DeMaso, & Meyer, 2013) with limited treatment of clinical practice strategies or guidelines for evidence-based practice (Ernst et al., 2010; Gallagher, McKenna, & Ibeziko, 2014; Victor, Hesham, & Tsang, 2018). As a result, education and training in CL psychology has relied heavily on the skills of experienced providers to pass on their clinical practice wisdom and experiences, as well as requiring the novice practitioner to translate and adapt clinical tools from the extant evidence-based literature to meet the needs of any particular clinical referral. In response, this volume was created to provide CL psychology practitioners with an accessible go-to, clinician-friendly handbook reference providing concise coverage of the major areas of CL psychology practice across pediatric medical settings. Each chapter is written by authors with clinical expertise in real-world pediatric medical settings. In areas of consultation practice lacking a direct evidence base or supporting literature, chapter authors were encouraged to share their rich clinical and professional experience to inform the reader of the current accepted best practices in their topic area. Our intent is that this sharing of expertise will encourage others to expand the clinical and research literature supporting these adapted interventions.

Section one, Pediatric Consultation-Liaison Psychology: Models, Roles, Settings, and Practice, provides an overview of roles, models, and configurations of pediatric psychology CL practice that one might encounter across diverse pediatric settings. The chapters in this section address the unique issues a CL psychologist faces that are impacted by practice setting, with chapters addressing inpatient, outpatient specialty clinic, and primary care environments. Other chapters address issues that are globally relevant and reflect the systemic nature of pediatric psychology CL work from the understanding of systems and organizational factors in practice, collaboration with our psychosocial colleagues in the medical setting (social workers, child life, psychiatry, etc.), and the basic medical information needed to become a medically informed psychologist. The important role that the CL psychologist plays in the education of medical learners (medical interns, residents, fellows, etc.) is highlighted, given the importance of educating the new generation of physicians on biopsychosocial factors in pediatric health and illness and the role that psychology can play in pediatric care. This section ends with a discussion of screening and assessment approaches and tools for addressing psychosocial concerns critical to CL practice across settings.

Section two, Clinical Conditions and Interventions, provides a structured overview of the most frequently seen major pediatric conditions encountered in consultation practice, with each subsection written by practicing clinician experts in the evaluation and intervention/treatment of the condition. Chapters in this section provide pediatric psychologists of all levels of training and practice (graduate students, practicum students, interns/residents, fellows, and practicing CL psychologists) with the basics needed to approach a referral, conduct a problem-focused assessment, and plan an intervention strategy targeting the referral question as applied in all the major medical settings (inpatient/hospitalization, integrated primary care, and subspecialty care clinic settings). For ease of reader access, authors were requested to conform to a consistent structure including brief topic background; concise review of the available research and adaptation to the relevant clinical populations; clinical formulation; consideration of relevant patient, provider, and system factors; and discussion of adaptation of interventions to the major medical settings (Spring & Hitchcock, 2009). Where applicable, authors have provided treatment protocols, handouts, digital resources, and educational materials which can be found in the Springer online Electronic Supplemental Material (ESM).

Section three, Crosscutting Issues in Consultation-Liaison Practice, addresses issues that are relevant across patient populations and settings. A wide range of general medical concerns are addressed (e.g., non-accidental injury, medical child abuse, palliative care), issues that present challenges to medical care (e.g., distressed parents and families, psychiatric emergencies) and practice factors (e.g., technological innovations, advocacy). The practice of psychological consultation in medical settings has expanded considerably, with the growing need to provide our profession with the guidance, tools, and systemic perspectives necessary for practicing in ever-changing medical environments. Our goal is for the *Clinician's Handbook of Pediatric Psychological Consultation in Medical Settings* to serve as a ready resource and reference for the busy pediatric psychologist consultant in furthering the important work we do for the benefit of the children and families coping with the challenges of pediatric illness/injury.

References

Bindman, A. (1959). Mental health consultation: Theory and practice. *Journal of Consulting Psychology, 23*, 473–482.

Brosig, C., & Zahrt, D. (2006). Evolution of an inpatient pediatric psychology consultation service: Issues related to reimbursement and the use of health and behavior codes. *Journal of Clinical Psychology in Medical Settings, 13*, 420–424.

Carter, B., Kroenenberger, W., Scott, E., & Ernst, M. (2009). Inpatient pediatric consultation-liaison. In M. Roberts & R. Steele (Eds.), *Handbook of pediatric psychology* (4th ed., pp. 114–129). New York, NY: The Guilford Press.

Carter, B., Thompson, S., & Townsend, A. (2014). Pediatric consultation-liaison in the children's hospital: The psychological hospitalist. In M. Roberts, B. Aylward, & Y. Wu (Eds.), *Clinical practice of pediatric psychology* (pp. 63–77). New York, NY: The Guilford Press.

Carter, B. D., Kronenberger, W. G., Scott, E. L., Kullgren, K. A., Piazza-Waggoner, C., & Brady, C. E. (2017). Inpatient pediatric consultation-liaison. In M. G. Roberts & R. G. Steele (Eds.), *Handbook of pediatric psychology* (5th ed., pp. 105–118). New York, NY: The Guilford Press.

DeMaso, D. M. (2009). Practice parameter for the psychiatric assessment and management of physically ill children and adolescents. *American Academy of Child and Adolescent Psychiatry, 48*, 213–233.

Drotar, D. (1975). Death in the pediatric hospital: Psychological consultation with medical and nursing staff. *Journal of Clinical Child & Adolescent Psychology, 4*, 33–35.

Drotar, D. (1995). *Consulting with pediatricians psychological perspectives*. New York, NY: Plenum.

Ernst, M., Piazza-Waggoner, C., Chabon, B., Murphy, M., Carey, J., & Roddenberry, A. (2014). The hospital-based consultation and liaison service. In C. Hunter, C. Hunter, & R. Kessler (Eds.), *Handbook of clinical psychology in medical settings* (pp. 369–416). New York, NY: Springer.

Ernst, M., Wooldridge, J., Conway, E., Dressman, K., Weiland, J., Tucker, K., & Seid, M. (2010). Using quality improvement science to implement a multidisciplinary behavioral intervention targeting pediatric inpatient airway clearance. *Journal of Pediatric Psychology, 35*, 14–24.

Gallagher, K., McKenna, K., & Ibeziko, P. (2014). Feasibility and impact of a multidisciplinary training of an evidence-based intervention within a pediatric psychiatry consultation service. *Academic Psychiatry, 38*, 445–450.

Kagan, J. (1965). The new marriage: Pediatrics and psychology. *American Journal of Diseases in Childhood, 110*, 272–278.

Katon, W., Von Korff, M., Lin, E., Walker, E., Simon, G. E., Bush, T., ... & Russo, J. (1995). Collaborative management to achieve treatment guidelines: impact on depression in primary care. Jama, 273(13), 1026–1031.

Kullgren, K., Bravender, T., & Sullivan, S. (2018). Understanding the unique needs of hospitalized adolescents and young adults referred for psychology consults. *Clinical Pediatrics, 57*, 1–8.

Kullgren, K., Tsang, K., Ernst, M., Carter, B., Scott, E., & Sullivan, S. (2015). Inpatient pediatric psychology consultation-liaison practice survey: Corrected version. *Clinical Practice in Pediatric Psychology, 3*, 37–47.

La Greca, A., Stone, W., Drotar, D., & Maddux, J. (1988). Training in pediatric psychology: Survey results and recommendations. *Journal of Pediatric Psychology, 13*, 121–139.

Lipowski, Z. (1971). Consultation-liasion psychiatry in the general hospital. *Comprehensive Psychiatry, 12*, 461–465.

Olson, R., Holden, E. W., Friedman, A., Faust, J., Kenning, M., & Mason, P. (1988). Psychological consultation in a children's hospital: An evaluation of services. *Journal of Pediatric Psychology, 13*, 479–492.

Palermo, T., Janicke, D., McQuaid, E., Mullins, L., Robins, P., & Wu, Y. (2014). Recommendations for training in pediatric psychology: Defining core competencies across training levels. *Journal of Pediatric Psychology, 39*, 965–984.

Piazza-Waggoner, C., Roddenberry, A., Yeomans-Maldonado, G., Noll, J., & Ernst, M. (2013). Inpatient pediatric psychology consultation-liaison program development: 5-year practice patterns and implications for trends in health care. *Clinical Practice in Pediatric Psychology, 1*, 28–41.

Rodrigue, J., Hoffmann, R., Rayfield, A., Lescano, C., Kubar, W., Streisand, R., & Banko, C. (1995). Evaluating pediatric psychology consultation services in a medical setting: An example. *Journal of Clinical Psychology in Medical Settings, 2*, 89–107.

Shaw, R., Pao, M., Holland, J., & DeMaso, D. (2016). Practice patterns revisited in pediatric psychosomatic medicine. *Psychosomatics, 57*, 576–585.

Shaw, R., Walmboldt, M., Bursch, B., & Stuber, M. (2006). Practice patterns in pediatric consultation-liaison psychiatry. *Psychosomatics, 47*, 43–49.

Spirito, A. B. (2003). Society of pediatric psychology task force report: Recommendations for the training of pediatric psychologists. *Journal of Pediatric Psychology, 28*, 85–98.

Spring, B., & Hitchcock, K. (2009). Evidence-based practice in psychology. In I. B. Weiner (Ed.), *Corsini's encyclopedia of psychology* (4th ed., pp. 603–607). New York, NY: Wiley.

Tunick, R., Gavin, J., DeMaso, D., & Meyer, E. (2013). Pediatric psychology critical care consultation: An emerging subspecialty. *Clinical Practice in Pediatric Psychology, 1*, 42–54.

Victor, E., Hesham, H., & Tsang, K. (2018). Implementation of a behavioral intervention in consultation-liaison with an international family. *Clinical Practice in Pediatric Psychology, 6*, 42–50.

Wright, L. (1967). The pediatric psychologist: A role model. *American Psychologist, 22*, 323–325.

Pediatric Consultation-Liaison: Models and Roles in Pediatric Psychology

Bryan D. Carter, Kevin K. Tsang, Christine E. Brady, and Kristin A. Kullgren

Consultation-Liaison Defined

Consultation is defined as the action or process of formally consulting or discussing and a meeting with an expert, such as a medical doctor, in order to seek advice (Oxford's Lexico Online Dictionary, n.d.). The process of *consulting* involves the act of engagement in the business or activity of giving expert advice to people working in a professional or technical field. For pediatric psychologists, this typically involves the provision of some form of direct patient care via a referral from a physician, subspecialty service, or other health-care team member (nursing, social work, child life, etc.) in order to address a specific clinical problem or concern. *Liaison* involves the establishment of a relationship wherein two parties or organizations are involved in the exchange of information or ideas, with a goal of developing mutual understanding and cooperation (Oxford's Lexico Online Dictionary, n.d.). The liaison role of the consultation-liaison (CL) psychologist addresses the integration of the psychologist in the health-care team and is often dictated by the model of consultation adopted by the hosting medical organization. In the liaison role, the psychologist may have formally dedicated time to address the broader systemic and mental health concerns of a service that may directly or indirectly affect the adjustment and coping of individual patients and families. When applied to the practice of pediatric psychologists and child mental health professionals working in medical settings, the recipients of consultation-liaison (CL) services may be the pediatric patient and/or their family, those professionals providing direct clinical care to a population, those providing administration of health-care services, or those at the level of designing systems and executing policies and procedures impacting the overall health-care services or even the general socio-environmental conditions in which the population lives.

An important aspect in defining and considering the adoption of models of psychological consultation involves the realization that CL services typically evolve out of the unique characteristics of the parent institutions in which they reside (Ernst et al., 2014). Each institution has a unique

B. D. Carter (✉) · C. E. Brady
Pediatric Consultation-Liaison Service, Norton Children's Hospital, Louisville, KY, USA

Department of Pediatrics, University of Louisville School of Medicine, Louisville, KY, USA
e-mail: bryan.carter@louisville.edu

K. K. Tsang
Department of Psychiatry, Boston Children's Hospital, Harvard Medical School, Boston, MA, USA

K. A. Kullgren
Department of Pediatrics, C.S. Mott Children's Hospital, Michigan Medicine, Ann Arbor, MI, USA

B. D. Carter, K. A. Kullgren (eds.), *Clinical Handbook of Psychological Consultation in Pediatric Medical Settings*, Issues in Clinical Child Psychology, https://doi.org/10.1007/978-3-030-35598-2_2

culture and history that variously shape the nature and range of the services provided. Factors such as patient demographics, institutional subcultures, financial resources, and the impact of local, regional, state, and national government policies all have an influence on the evolution of any given CL service. However, in considering the development and maintenance of any consultation service or program, it is important to acknowledge the contexts in which various models of psychological consultation services have evolved before trying to fit that model to one's own unique health-care setting.

Models

A *model* is defined as a representation of a person or thing or of a proposed structure, typically on a smaller scale than the original, and a thing used as an example to follow or imitate (Oxford's Lexico Online Dictionary, n.d.). A model is an attempt to construct a representation of a particular phenomenon in the world and can be employed merely to conceptualize a construct or more actively to operationalize the processes necessary to make the model work. Ideally, the validity of a model can be determined by its utility and effectiveness in a given setting.

Traditional Models

Armstrong (2009) has posited a theoretical model for understanding the different levels of multispecialty collaboration in clinical care: *unidisciplinary*, *multidisciplinary*, *interdisciplinary*, and *transdisciplinary*. *Unidisciplinary* collaboration, akin to indirect consultation (and almost a vanishing model in modern medical systems), is that system in which a pediatrician/specialist practices in relative isolation from other disciplines. This model has been made virtually obsolete by a number of factors including the technology connectivity in today's health-care world (e.g., telehealth (Doarn et al., 2014)), provisions under the Affordable Care Act for the "medical home" (Bachrach, Anthony, & Detty, 2014), increased emphasis on multidisciplinary care (Conroy & Logan, 2014), interprofessional education (Ward, Shaffer, & Getzoff, 2018), and the increased recognition of the biopsychosocial model in health care (Bolton & Gillett, 2019).

According to Armstrong (2009), the distinguishing feature between the *multidisciplinary* and *interdisciplinary* models of care is the degree of coordination and integration of the providers from different disciplines (with unique areas of knowledge and skill) working in conjunction to benefit patient health and functioning. Within the *multidisciplinary* model, while there may be an agreed-upon common problem, there is a relatively low level of integration and an often poorly formulated or loosely agreed-upon case conceptualization. This can lead to a failure in addressing complex interactions of physical and psychological factors contributing to symptom and illness management. For example, within the *multidisciplinary* model, the physician may make a referral to a psychologist colleague who applies evidence-based interventions to address the patient's presenting symptoms, e.g., cognitive-behavioral therapy and biofeedback for chronic headaches, while the neurologist manages medications. However, when the patient has a pain flare, the lack of closely coordinated and ongoing communication within a shared conceptual framework makes it difficult to determine whether the patient needs a change in medication, help with treatment adherence, different behavioral and coping skills, or some combination of medical and psychosocial interventions.

Integrative Models

Armstrong (2009) posits that the degree of coordination and integration of the providers from different disciplines employed in *interdisciplinary* and *transdisciplinary* models can reduce the risk of the types of diagnostic and treatment errors in the above example. Efforts to conceptualize the varied processes of psychological consultation in medical settings have led to the creation of visual models such as the *Integrated Comprehensive Consultation-Liaison Model* (ICCLM; Carter, Kronenberger, Kullgren, Piazza-Waggoner, & Brady, 2017; Carter,

Kronenberger, Scott, & Ernst, 2009; Carter & Von Weiss, 2005) (see Fig. 1). This model attempts to integrate the perspectives of three conceptual biopsychosocial models that view the prevention and maintenance of health and welfare from the individual to the population level.

First, *Bronfenbrenner's bioecological systems model* (BSM) addresses the complex layers (systems environments) in which the child's development takes place (Bronfenbrenner, 1979). These layers interact in a way that influences the overall system, and interactions between layers influence the child's outcomes. In this model, the CL psychologist may facilitate the child's adjustment and development by improving functioning and integration from the level of individual systems (e.g., providing behavioral interventions to address adherence to type 1 diabetes regimen) and/or at a exosystems level (e.g., advocating with the local school board for increased in-school specialized diabetes nursing training).

Second, Kazak's *Pediatric Psychosocial Preventative Health Model* (PPPHM; Kazak, 2006) of assessment and intervention addresses the health-related stressors faced by families with acutely and chronically ill children. Preventive and intervention services are stratified in response to such factors as family adaptation and coping styles, family dynamics (e.g., distress provoking versus resilience promoting), and targeted support of adaptive functioning all within the context of broader systems (e.g., school, health-care system). Kazak employs a family-risk model in screening and providing services for all families and children entering the health-care system at three levels: *universal*, *targeted*, and *clinical/ treatment*. *Universal*-level intervention would be providing family education on the known stressors associated with chronic illness and treatments while facilitating service access and availability. *Targeted*-level consultation would provide families at risk with specific education and short-term intervention around illness-related demands and transitions. *Clinical-/treatment*-level services would involve patients and families being referred to traditional mental health services.

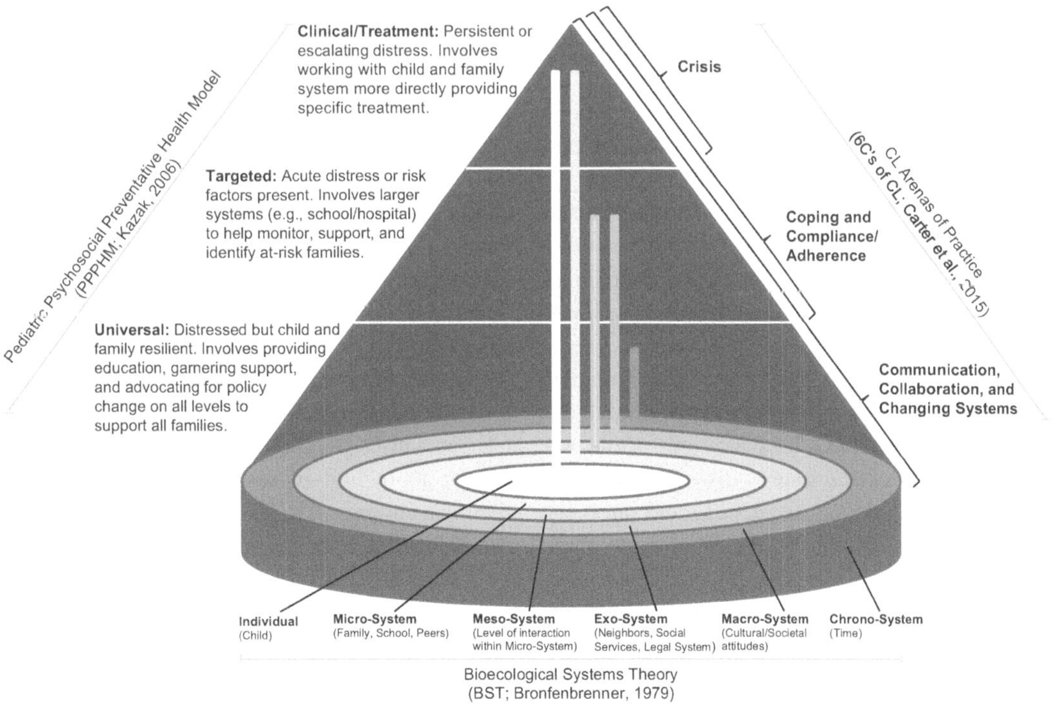

Fig. 1 Integrated comprehensive CL model (ICCLM)

Third, the *ICCLM* identifies arenas in the practice of psychological consultation (see Fig. 2, the C's of consultation: *crisis*, *coping*, *compliance*, *communication*, *collaboration*, and *changing systems*), which may be conceptualized from the micro- to the macrosystems levels (Carter et al., 2017). The C's represent often overlapping areas in which patients and families struggle in their efforts to address the child's medical condition and in which the consulting pediatric psychologist has the potential to intervene and impact on multiple levels, as represented by the *BSM* and *PPPHM*. From the *ICCLM* perspective, the psychologist may assist via direct psychological intervention with a patient and family in *crisis* over a new diagnosis, assess, and address styles of and risks associated with their *coping* with the demands of the medical condition and treatments, which can further facilitate patient and family *compliance/adherence* to treatments/interventions and lifestyle management while joining with the family and serving as a liaison between the patient/family and the medical team in addressing the *communication* challenges that can impact care provision and disease management. More systems-level involvement and administrative skills are often required of the psychologist in facilitating *collaboration* among disciplines in integrating the psychosocial perspective into comprehensive care on both the patient/family level and the broader medical setting and ideally allowing for *changing systems* via impacting institutional policies and practices at the local, state, and national health-care levels (Carter et al., 2017).

From the *ICCLM* perspective, psychological consultation is seen as having the potential to target interventions that alter conditions prior to or early in the onset of a state of dis-ease in an individual or a population, to identify and intervene with at-risk populations in the more acute phase of dis-ease, and to provide evidence-based services for those manifesting clinical levels of disease and distress. More recently, Gilbert and Schultz (see chapter "Advocacy in Pediatric Psychological Consultation", this volume) have identified the role of the pediatric psychologist in providing *advocacy* at the clinical and systems levels to improve patient and family health and quality of life, particularly with highly vulnerable populations. To fit in with the alliterative "C's of consultation," they have suggested *championing* (advocacy) be adopted as the seventh "C" of pediatric psychological consultation.

Roles of the Consultation-Liaison Pediatric Psychologist

A *role* is defined as a part or function taken or assumed by a person, the part played by a person in a particular social setting (Merriam-Webster Online Dictionary, n.d.). Understanding, defining, and expanding one's role as a psychologist within a medical system/setting is the first step in building a successful model for the practice of CL psychology. Variables that can further impact the CL psychologist's role include the composition of the CL team, one's work assignment, the job setting, and the extent to which the psychologist has the opportunity for involvement in shaping system factors impacting psychosocial aspects of pediatric illness and medical care.

Multidisciplinary CL Team Composition

The members of a CL service can vary significantly depending on the setting. These differences often have to do with larger intuitional factors, including the history of psychology as a department, division, or section, the relationship of psychology with pediatrics and psychiatry, and the history of how the CL service came into existence. For example, in a recent practice survey of CL pediatric psychologists (Kullgren et al., 2015), about half of respondents reported that their psychology CL and psychiatry CL teams functioned as separate services within the hospital setting. Typically, within this model, psychiatry will be tasked with management of patients presenting after suicide attempts, with medical-psychiatric presentations such as delirium or autoimmune encephalopathies, and for psychopharmacologic management (Shaw & DeMaso, 2006). A pediatric psychologist may be consulted to assist with patient coping with hos-

THE 7 C'S OF CONSULTATION (Carter et al., 2017; Gilbert & Schultz, this volume)	**Consultation Practice Arena Description**
CRISIS	Providing rapid assessment and guidance to patients and families in the midst of acute health-related stressors; addressing systemic policies and practices that can minimize the stress for children and families engaged with the health care system.
COPING	Assessing and intervening to strengthen the adoption of more effective coping skills and strategies in pediatric patients and families under the stress of medical evaluation and treatment.
COMPLIANCE (ADHERENCE)	Assessing and engaging patients and families in removing barriers, increasing illness/treatment understanding, and improving life-style management strategies; assessing and intervening in health care systemic issues that contribute to poor adherence; all directed to improving health outcomes and quality of life.
COMMUNICATION	Facilitating communication, understanding and integration of behavioral health principles between various parties: patient/family and health care providers; primary and specialist providers and other involved providers and community supports.
COLLABORATION	Team building and facilitating the integration of multiple professionals in providing coordinated and comprehensive care, quality improvement procedures, and research projects that increase the evidence base for behavioral health integration in medical settings.
CHANGING SYSTEMS	Activities in this arena involve researching, designing and advocating for health care delivery systems that integrate mental/behavioral and physical health interventions at the population level, while equally emphasizing effective and efficient prevention and targeted interventions with diagnosed health conditions both in and beyond the inpatient environment.
CHAMPIONING (ADVOCACY)	Activities within a health care facility or system to improve availability and access to resources; at the larger community, regional, state or even national level to create resources, procedures and/or policies that address the health and welfare of in-need and vulnerable populations. Championing can occur at multiple levels: on behalf of an individual patient or family; community; population.

Fig. 2 The 7 C's of consultation

pitalization, adjustment to new diagnosis, psychological assessment screening/testing, and specific psychological needs with services embedded in or primarily assigned to specific subspecialties (Carter et al., 2003, 2014). Separate CL services may allow more tightly defined differences in what types of cases are seen by each service, allowing the services to vary depth, specialization, and time demands to meet staffing and care provision needs of their specific setting. There is inherent overlap in what these two services would provide, though not entirely, and providers from both services may be requested for any given case. The challenges inherent in this model are within this overlap and in how services coordinate with each other and where variance can be problematic. Where providers overlap or feel like they are competing for credibility or justification of one service over the other is where egos and beliefs (the natural propensity of us versus them) about care negatively impact the quality of care provided to patients.

Combined or multidisciplinary CL services are often housed in a common department such as psychiatry, behavioral/developmental pediatrics and behavioral pediatrics, psychiatry/psychology, or pediatrics. Within these combined services, psychologists, psychiatrists, and sometimes additional providers such as psychiatric nurse practitioners and social workers collaborate in coverage of CL services to all referrals. This model has the advantage of reducing redundancy of provider skills and playing to the strengths of each provider's training and background while allowing the service providers to work collaboratively as part of a well-defined team for the service of their patients. The obvious downside is that combined services require providers to learn to work together, across disciplines, respecting the strengths and weaknesses and overlap between various service providers in a manner that enhances versus diminishes the quality of care. Though the history of a given institution, including funding, can shape the working relationship between psychology and psychiatry providers, developing these relationships and finding invested partners to develop a combined CL program can also serve as a model for effective collaboration. While combined CL programs may be more common in institutions with a history of positive engagement between psychologists and psychiatrists, these programs also generally demonstrate the strength of these relationships and enhanced care effect of working together.

In the process of establishing one's unique identity in the provision of CL services, it is essential to identify those other specialties and services within one's health-care organization that may have significant overlap in role and responsibility (social work, child life, palliative care, etc.), to formulate patterns of interdisciplinary communication, and to establish collaborative networks with these colleagues in order to provide streamlined coordinated care (Ernst et al., 2014; see chapters "Collaborating with Psychosocial Colleagues in the Hospital Setting" and "Collaborating with Child Psychiatry", this volume). Additionally, delineating one's unique contributions/services as a pediatric psychologist is essential to the success and sustainability of psychological CL practice. Finally, in the course of a career focused on providing psychological CL to our health-care colleagues and in an ever-changing health-care environment, a critical consideration is how to maintain high-level expectations and productivity while simultaneously avoiding professional burnout.

Negotiating Roles and Work Assignment

Traditionally, the historical role of a pediatric psychologist has been to provide direct clinical services to a group of identified patients in one or more medical settings. However, CL psychologists working within medical settings, particularly academically affiliated medical centers, typically have a multitude of roles included in their work assignments (Drotar, 1995). These duties most often involve the provision of clinical services to pediatric patients and their families in one or more settings (inpatient, outpatient primary and specialty care), the teaching/training of psychology and medical residents and fellows, clinical supervision, program development, and, for some, research. Indeed, the ideal overarching goal of establishing a CL service should not only be to provide behavioral and mental health services to medical populations but also to inform and educate our physician and other health-care provider colleagues on the psychosocial aspects involved in the comprehensive management of children's health and welfare, to contribute to the evidence-based support for our services, and to advance existing programs via quality improvement initiatives and research regardless of practice setting.

Survey data of practicing pediatric psychologists suggests that the distribution of these duties will vary from psychologist to psychologist depending on the identified needs of the organization, often driven by the unique interests, skills, and career goals of the individual psychologist (Kullgren et al., 2015). Ernst and colleagues (2014) describe four dimensions on which psychological CL services vary: (1) team makeup (sole consulting psychologist versus multidisciplinary including psychiatry, social worker, and trainees); (2) the scope of issues and populations targeted by the CL service (general service seeing all referrals versus focused on specific medical conditions or hospital units); (3) function (assessment and recommendations versus direct intervention); and (4) conceptualization (primarily psychodiagnostic versus focusing assessment on specific referral questions and problem-focused formulations that drive intervention).

Institutional variables shaping the roles of the CL psychologist include such factors as the system's dependence on purely clinically generated revenue versus internal funding to partially or fully cover salary and benefits and the institution's priority for and availability of support for unfunded research (particularly critical to early career psychologists who are unlikely to bring their own research funding to their position). Some institutions allow for little or no internal support for psychologist research involvement, with increased research time requiring the psychologist to obtain grant funding. Of course, a key career decision for the CL psychologist will be the extent to which they desire increased research/academic/teaching time versus primarily focusing on more direct clinical service. Within most institutions, defining the CL psychologist's role is formally negotiated in creating a work assignment which involves balancing the needs and goals of the organization and individual career aspirations.

Determinants of CL Scope of Practice

Setting Factors

Beyond the basic distribution of time spent between clinical care, teaching, research, etc., a main determinant of one's role and function is the actual setting in which the CL psychologist practices. The three major arenas of medical setting practice for pediatric CL psychologists typically include inpatient/hospitalization, integrated primary care, and specialty care. As illustrated in Figs. 1 and 2, the clinical tasks of the inpatient CL psychologist may mainly revolve around providing care to patients in the *clinical* or *targeted* range (top two tiers of the triangle), for example, working with the patient and family in safety planning (*crisis*), pill swallowing (*compliance/adherence*), and facilitating adjustment to a new diagnosis (*coping*). In an inpatient setting, CL psychologists are unlikely to provide care at the *universal* level due to limited access to resources, short medical stays, and billing restrictions unless seeing every patient admitted for a certain medical condition (i.e., bone marrow transplant).

In outpatient specialty and primary care settings, providers will still provide services to patients in the *clinical* range but are less likely to be providing crisis management services, with more focus on *targeted* treatments. By way of example, a CL psychologist embedded within a specialty pediatric neurology service would focus on providing behavioral intervention to headache patients to improve their compliance with medical recommendations, conduct clinical biofeedback and psychological pain management, assist the patient in managing lifestyle habits that may contribute to their symptom presentation and level of functional disability, and facilitate their functioning in the presence of ongoing chronic pain/headaches, e.g., providing 504 Plan recommendations to the school to decrease absences. Finally, a pediatric psychologist in an integrated primary care setting will likely be engaged in providing more short-term and problem-focused services to a larger volume of patients. In this model, the CL psychologist may focus on providing preventative care, education with patients and parents around a new diagnosis, and referral for more comprehensive services to patients (e.g., discussing with families the early signs of autism or ADHD and making referrals for more in-depth evaluations) while still providing *targeted-* and potentially *clinical*-level services.

CL Systemic Meta-Roles

CL pediatric psychologists, regardless of their work assignment, setting, etc., are likely to be engaged in activities addressing systemic issues related to optimizing *communication* and *collaboration*. These are not only patient-directed arenas and tasks but physician/health-care colleague directed as well. One practice role of the CL psychologist is to improve communication within and between systems (e.g., patient and medical team); this is often subsumed under the liaison component of CL and best facilitated when the psychologist is functionally embedded within the medical team. Often, CL psychologists are tasked with the role of contacting schools, writing and coordinating the implementation of 504 Plans, providing physicians with mental health referrals, and/or communicating with Child Protective Services. These communications are critical to creating bridges toward collaboration. Collaborations can be clinical in nature (e.g., streamlining referrals to reputable services in the community/region) or quality improvement/ research oriented.

Carter and colleagues (2017) described another practice role as one of *changing systems*, i.e., "researching, designing, and advocating for health-care delivery systems that integrate mental/behavioral and physical health interventions at the population level, while equally emphasizing effective and efficient prevention and targeted interventions" (p. 108). While CL psychologists can often address this arena as part of engaging in their daily activities, efforts are likely to be more impactful when they become active members of planning/steering committees within the hospital, serve on local and state councils, and/or run for office in professional organizations to maximize their influence. In this way, psychologists can effect change and impact patients beyond an individual reach and potentially for years or decades to come (see chapter "Systems Issues and Considerations", this volume).

CL Service Sustainability: Maintaining your Role

Regardless of the model, the health and viability of a CL service can only exist with competent and committed psychologists to deliver services. However, maintaining the high level of engagement across all of the roles that a CL psychologist is responsible for can be daunting and contribute a high level of burnout, such as that described by Kullgren and colleagues (2015) in their survey of inpatient CL psychologists. Burnout has been commonly defined by three core components: emotional exhaustion, depersonalization, and reduced personal accomplishment (Maslach, 1982). In their review of the literature on burnout in professional psychologists, Simionato and Simpson (2018) found a majority experienced low to moderate levels of burnout, with over half reporting moderate to high levels. Identified risk factors for burnout included younger age, less work experience, and boundary issues, such as becoming overinvolved with patient problems. Knowing that psychologists who provide clinical services experience high levels of burnout due to the demanding and emotional nature of our work, when combined with the unique and complex challenges of working in a multidisciplinary medical setting, likely compound the already high risk of burnout.

Simionato and Simpson (2018) highlighted trainees and early career psychologists as populations who may be particularly at risk for burnout. Several theories on the relationship between age/experience and vulnerability to burnout have been posited, including lack of resources/coping skills and having strong idealistic expectations. Given this phenomenon, early career psychologists, and the systems in which they work, should take special care to not only monitor for signs of burnout and respond appropriately but also implement preventative measures to keep burnout from occurring. One strategy for preventing burnout is clearly defining and negotiating one's role, as discussed previously, and advocating for reasonable time allocation for one's various work activities. In order to sustain a long-term career in CL psychology, the psychologist must have access to adequate and responsive resources, build a professional and personal support system, and develop coping strategies to help build resiliency. It is recommended that early career psychologists form support systems within and outside of their practicing institutions. Consultants need consultants, and having an ongoing relationship with more experienced mentors to discuss difficult and demanding cases and professional/ethical dilemmas, to problem-solve and generate new ideas, or to just commiserate with and provide support and validation can prove invaluable in minimizing burnout (Carter, 2014). Pediatric psychologists can join local-, state-, and national-level organizations such as APA Division 54 (Society of Pediatric Psychology), including involvement in CL-specific special interest groups, to provide another network of support and professional stimulation. Finally, it is always important to engage in regular self-care, as we routinely encourage our patients to embrace, including engaging in pleasurable activities and hobbies, socializing outside of work, and taking care of our dietary and sleep needs.

Another avenue for increasing psychologist career sustainability is through interdisciplinary collaborations that potentially benefit patient care, workflow, and outcomes. Psychologists within pediatric medical settings can offer their skills in operationalizing research questions to support quality improvement processes. Clinical pathway development (such as somatic symptom and related disorders for inpatients (see Ibeziako et al., 2019), diabetes clinic patients (see Gellfand et al., 2004), and autism in primary care (see McGuire et al., 2016) as setting-relevant examples) can provide the chance to collaborate with and model interdisciplinary work for our pediatric colleagues while simultaneously planting the seeds for institution-wide change. Establishing clinical pathways and other quality improvement projects that positively impact patient care and outcomes, decrease provider burden, and/or reduce length of medical admissions, also increases recognition of the value-added nature of the consultation-liaison approach and provides the psychologist with stimulating diversity in their professional development (Lawal et al., 2016; Rotter et al., 2010).

Integration and Differentiation of Roles

Effective psychological CL work is dependent upon fostering effective *communication* and *collaboration* with multidisciplinary providers, including medical and other psychosocial disciplines. The same skills of clinical assessment, formulation, and communication that are utilized to effectively liaison with multidisciplinary providers, reduce stigma associated with psychiatric presentations and treatment, and provide care in the medical setting are also vital to the viability and development of any CL psychology service. As providers are able to demonstrate the utility and improved quality of care associated with CL services, the recognized need and benefit of growing and maintaining these services becomes self-evident. Thus, professional relationships are key to integration within medical setting.

In early phases of developing an integrated CL service, it is important for the psychologist to be aware of common misunderstandings/misconceptions about psychologist training and scope of practice. Pediatric psychologists inherently share some clinical overlap with the activities of child and adolescent psychiatrists, social workers, child life specialists, etc. Physicians and even administrative decision-makers within the medical setting are more likely to be familiar with the training and recognize the expertise of psychiatrists due to their shared medical background.

Social workers and child life specialist are more likely to be preexisting, more familiar, and simply more numerous in most medical settings. Just as in navigating any clinical change within a milieu, the addition or growth of a CL psychology position may cause a shift in the homeostasis of a group, and these dynamics will need to be anticipated and addressed.

One strategy to allow other subspecialty providers or disciplines to better understand the added value of a consulting pediatric psychologist can include lending time of psychology trainees to various services that have the potential to become a future a referral resource. For example, a psychology practicum student, predoctoral intern, or psychology fellow may be assigned to spend part of their clinical experience within the Pediatric Gastroenterology Clinic under the supervision of an established psychologist operating within the same clinic or hospital structure. This trainee would be essentially cost-free for a predefined period of time for the GI service, allowing a "test drive" to more directly understand how psychologists might operate as a unique addition to the GI clinical team. With the increased availability and visibility of a well-skilled and closely supervised psychology trainee, CL psychologists cannot only increase consultation referral rates but also increase the recognized need to fund additional licensed psychologist positions, particularly as training needs continue to evolve.

Another skill specific to most pediatric psychologists, and of value in fostering increased collaboration with our medical colleagues, is that of research. Many physicians have limited research training, and partnering with a psychologist on investigative projects, quality improvement programs, and grants can lead to mutually productive experiences that nurture long-term relationships and mutual cooperation in the provision of clinical care. Additionally, in academic medical centers, the scientific presentations and publications that can be produced from collaborative research serves to support promotion in academic rank and tenure, benefitting all the professionals involved in the collaborative research (Carter, 2014).

As mentioned previously, clinical skills specific to pediatric psychologists should support differentiation from related disciplines. For example, the provision of clinical biofeedback, use of technology-based assessment and intervention strategies (see chapter "Technological Innovations in Pediatric Psychological Consultation", this volume), strong skills in health psychology, and psychological assessment (see chapter "Assessment in Pediatric Psychology Consultation-Liaison", this volume) can serve as distinguishing aspects of clinical care. Obviously, the provision of these services may not be appropriate for all settings or job roles, but emphasizing these unique skills increases the value of psychology to the medical setting.

Financial Factors

Perhaps one of the most challenging factors impacting the development of psychological consultation services, whether inhospital, integrated specialty, or primary care settings, is financial, particularly the issue of reimbursement for services consistent with the level of care provided (Bruns, Kessler, & Dorsten, 2014; Shaw & DeMaso, 2006). With a changing and uncertain health-care system, psychologists may be faced with changes from fee-for-service to alternate payment models that may require either demonstration of quality or advocacy in advance of payment (McGrady, 2018; Tynan, 2016). To be successful at developing and maintaining effective CL services in the face of health-care changes, it is essential that both administrators and clinicians within the medical setting strongly support the integration of psychological CL services in their health-care delivery system. Administrators and business managers should assertively negotiate for flexible and favorable rates of reimbursement with insurance carriers (e.g., making rates relatively commensurate with those negotiated for physical medicine services, including such factors as health and behavior code reimbursement) while closely monitoring billing and collection processes and underwriting those services (including liaison time) where time allocation and ability to bill insurance are limited or nonexistent (Bierenbaum, Katsikas, Furr, & Carter, 2013).

While there is often significant job description overlap with other psychosocial disciplines in medical settings, the salary/compensation rate for doctoral psychologists is understandably greater than that for a master's degree-level social worker or child life specialist, requiring an even higher burden of justification for the creation and retention of psychologist positions. And in the provision of CL services, particularly inpatient hospitalization-based services, studies have shown an average of 25–35% of psychologists' time is spent in nonreimbursable activities (Bierenbaum et al., 2013). Although it may be the rare pediatric psychologist who can manage to fully excel as a "triple threat," a strong grounding in empirically based approaches to clinical care, facility at applied research methodology, and talents for teaching/training/supervision can lead to career stability and the ability to accumulate salary support from diverse sources. Whether related to billing tracking, quality improvement, or development/adoption of a new clinical pathway, psychologists can demonstrate their value and garner support due to their unique roles in diverse medical settings. As an example, being able to demonstrate that earlier psychological consultation leads to shorter length of stay and hospital charges can help the CL psychologist advocate with the hospital for increased support or hiring (Bujoreanu, White, Gerber, & Ibeziako, 2015).

Increasing Involvement with Administration and Leadership

In the course of a career as a CL pediatric psychologist, one needs to look for opportunities to establish relationships and cultivate to assume leadership roles within their medical system setting or institution. This can be highly contingent on gaining the support of champions at various levels within the pediatric care system. Whether a primary care physician who can attest to the quality of work produced by the psychologist, the hospitalist or nurse manager recognizing improvements in care coordination or decreased length of stay, or visibility and collaborative partnerships with other psychosocial providers, creating opportunities to work with others allows for more champions who can recognize and speak to the work of the CL psychologist. Developing these competencies and the confidence of our pediatric colleagues can provide the psychologist with opportunities to assume leadership roles where one has the opportunity to shape policies and practices that positively affect the integration of psychosocial factors into overall health care.

Case Example

Tanya, a 14-year-old Latina female with a psychiatric history significant for generalized anxiety disorder diagnosed at age 10, presented to the Children's Hospital ED with symptoms of bradycardia, orthostatic blood pressure and heart rate instability, and hypothermia. She was admitted to the floor under the care of a pediatric hospitalist team, for medical stabilization. She disclosed to one of her nurses that she had been restricting her caloric intake since the start of summer, noting a previous history of being marginally overweight and trying to "eat healthy." Tanya reported that a number of her peers, as well as her mother and girlfriend, had complimented her about looking "healthier." She continued her restrictive intake into the fall (though concealing this from her family and friends), with reported increased stress at school and associated increasing social avoidance. She denied purging or use of laxatives.

Tanya's admitting medical team diagnosed her with anorexia nervosa (AN) and presented this to the patient and parents at a multidisciplinary care conference. The parents were quite tearful and immediately questioned whether or not the medical team had missed a possible underlying gastrointestinal disorder in their medical workup. Culturally, the family was somewhat aversive to considering that the patient might have a psychiatric condition and in their state of *crisis* was reluctant to agree to Tanya being started on the medical team's AN protocol. Later that afternoon, a multidisciplinary team meeting was held (hospitalist, psychiatry, psychology, social work, nutritionist, child life) to discuss strategies for helping the patient and family with the "buy in" to accepting her diagnosis and treatment plan. The social worker at the team meeting, who was quite familiar with cultural stereotypes in the Latina community regarding mental health issues, suggested strategies for meeting with the parents to help them gradually become more comfortable and accepting of the diagnosis, including involving another family member of the patient, a cousin, who was a nurse. After meeting with the family with the nurse cousin, explaining the symptoms of AN, the health risks, and the larger cultural influences on adolescent body image issues, the parents agreed for the patient to be placed on the AN protocol (*communication, compliance*).

Upon starting the AN protocol, Tanya minimized the impact of her restrictive diet and dramatic weight loss and struggled with meeting her meal goals, citing intense intrusive ideation specifically related to meal volume and fears of "getting fat" and not being able to control her intake once she started eating regular meals again. She subsequently refused supplementation with liquid nutrition orally, requiring supplemental nasogastric tube (NGT) feeds after every meal. The medical team and nursing reported that Tanya became increasingly distressed around NGT placements, occasionally requiring hands-on to keep her from pulling out the tube during bolus NG feeds.

In the model of separate psychiatry and psychology CL services with their Children's Hospital, both services were consulted by the primary medical team. Psychiatry CL was specifically tasked with addressing the patient's anxiety and medical management around NG placement. The CL psychiatrist contacted the CL psychologist, who under the hospital's protocol for AN was to provide cognitive-behavioral treatment of anxiety and evidence-based individual and family therapy to address the patient's eating disorder, with both working out a daily schedule for patient and family contact (*collaboration*). Both the CL psychologist and psychiatrist attended the team meeting to discuss the case with the primary team, nursing, and the dietician and to arrange a "warm hand off" after the social worker had met with the family.

Over the next 10 days, the CL psychologist continued to work with Tanya and her family, listening to their stories about the patient's past struggles with anxiety, reviewing past effective therapeutic strategies for the management of GAD, and helping them better understand the diagnosis of anorexia nervosa and the parental role for managing meals after discharge. Daily therapy sessions were held with Tanya on the unit directed at helping her therapeutically "externalize" her eating disorder via cognitive therapy techniques and adopting more effective *coping* strategies for dealing with peer-related stressors and body image issues. Relaxation strategies, behavioral activation, and elements of family-based treatment were utilized. Meanwhile, the CL psychiatrist made medication recommendations to assist with Tanya's anxiety and worked with the pediatric hospitalist to address Tanya's low weight, vital sign instability, and distress around NG feeds. Every-other-day 30-minute team meetings were held to allow all providers to discuss their impressions, review Tanya's progress, and modify care as indicated.

By the time of discharge, Tanya had made significant improvement in her ability to tolerate oral meals, which she was able to do without liquid nutritional supplementation via NG feeds or orally. Tanya and her family were considerably more accepting of her diagnosis and demonstrated reasonable skills at implementing effective strategies to limit her eating disorder behaviors that interfered with meal completion; Tanya's anxiety was also much better controlled. At the multidisciplinary discharge care conference with Tanya and her parents, it was communicated that it was the opinion of the team that Tanya would be appropriate for step-down to an eating disorder day treatment program for continued care with close medical monitoring and follow-up but with the caution that a relapse leading to further medical hospitalization would necessitate more lengthy and comprehensive residential eating disorder intervention.

Over the course of reviewing the outcomes of several eating disordered patients seen over the prior year, the CL psychologist on the multidisciplinary team made several recommendations to improve patient care (*changing systems*): implement a more formal assessment process at admission to better target individual patient clinical needs; more formally assess patient and family readiness to change; and, in collaboration with the case manager/discharge planner, initiate the process of finding appropriate programs and facilities for patients earlier in their hospital admission to minimize the gap between their discharge and starting outpatient, partial hospitalization, or residential treatment. These were accepted by the medical team and eventually formalized in the AN protocol and hospital order set.

Conclusions

Consultation-liaison pediatric psychology has a rich history as an area of subspecialty practice and represents one of the most integrated applications of our psychological skills in multiple medical settings. As has been pointed out previously (Carter et al., 2017), due to the considerable diversity of applications and setting factors, research on CL interventions and outcomes remains challenging yet essential to sustaining these services in the rapidly changing health-care system. This current volume represents one effort to provide busy CL pediatric psychologists with the resources needed to support our valuable work. We want to express our gratitude to the many highly skilled professionals who have generously shared their expertise in the development of this clinician handbook.

References

Armstrong, F. D. (2009). Individual and organizational collaborations: A roadmap for effective advocacy. In M. C. Roberts & R. G. Steele (Eds.), *Handbook of pediatric psychology* (3rd ed., pp. 774–784). New York, NY: The Guilford Press.

Bachrach, D., Anthony, S., & Detty, A. (2014). *State strategies for integrating physical and behavioural health services in a changing medicaid environment.* New York, NY: The Commonwealth Fund.

Bierenbaum, M. L., Katsikas, S., Furr, A., & Carter, B. D. (2013). Factors associated with non-reimbursable activity on an inpatient pediatric consultation-liaison service. *Journal of Clinical Psychology in Medical Settings, 20*(4), 464–472.

Bolton, D., & Gillett, G. (2019). The biopsychosocial model 40 years on. In *The biopsychosocial model of health and disease* (pp. 1–43). Cham: Palgrave Pivot.

Bronfenbrenner, U. (1979). *The ecology of human development: Experiments by nature and design.* Cambridge, MA: Harvard University Press.

Bruns, D., Kessler, R., & Dorsten, V. (2014). The practice of psychology in medical settings: Financially sustainable models. In M. C. Roberts, B. S. Aylward, & Y. P. Wu (Eds.), *Clinical practice of pediatric psychology* (pp. 199–218). New York, NY: The Guilford Press.

Bujoreanu, S., White, M. T., Gerber, B., & Ibeziako, P. (2015). Effect of timing of psychiatry consultation on length of pediatric hospitalization and hospital charges. *Hospital Pediatrics, 5*(5), 269–275.

Carter, B. D. (2014). Carolyn S. Schroeder award for outstanding clinical practice: Creativity and innovation in the practice of pediatric psychology. *Clinical Practice in Pediatric Psychology, 2*(4), 378–383.

Carter, B. D., Kronenberger, W. G., Baker, J., Grimes, L. M., Crabtree, V. M., Smith, C., & McGraw, K. (2003). Inpatient pediatric consultation-liaison: A case-controlled study. *Journal of Pediatric Psychology, 28*(6), 425–432.

Carter, B. D., Kronenberger, W. G., Kullgren, K., Piazza-Waggoner, C., & Brady, C. E. (2017). Inpatient pediatric consultation-liaison. In M. Roberts & R. Steele (Eds.), *Handbook of pediatric psychology* (5th ed., pp. 105–118). New York, NY: The Guilford Press.

Carter, B. D., Kronenberger, W. G., Scott, E., & Ernst, M. M. (2009). Pediatric consultation-liaison. In M. Roberts & R. Steele (Eds.), *Handbook of pediatric psychology* (4th ed., pp. 114–129). New York, NY: The Guilford Press.

Carter, B. D., Thompson, S. M., & Townsend, A. N. (2014). Pediatric consultation-liaison in the children's hospital: The psychological hospitalist. In M. C. Roberts, B. S. Aylward, & Y. P. Wu (Eds.), *Clinical practice of pediatric psychology: Cases and service delivery* (pp. 63–77). New York, NY: The Guilford Press.

Carter, B. D., & Von Weiss, R. (2005). Pediatric consultation-liaison. In M. Roberts & R. Steele (Eds.), *Handbook of mental health services for children and adolescents* (pp. 63–82). New York, NY: Kluwer.

Conroy, C., & Logan, D. E. (2014). Pediatric multidisciplinary and interdisciplinary teams. In M. C. Roberts, B. S. Aylward, & Y. P. Wu (Eds.), *Clinical practice of pediatric psychology* (pp. 93–108). New York, NY: The Guilford Press.

Consultation. (n.d.). Oxford's Lexico Online Dictionary. Retrieved from https://www.lexico.com/en/definition/consultation

Doarn, C. R., Pruitt, S., Jacobs, J., Harris, Y., Bott, D. M., Riley, W., … Oliver, A. L. (2014). Federal efforts to define and advance telehealth—A work in progress. *Telemedicine and e-Health, 20*(5), 409–418.

Drotar, D. (1995). *Consulting with pediatricians psychological perspectives*. New York, NY: Plenum.

Ernst, M., Piazza-Waggoner, C., Chabon, B., Murphy, M., Carey, J., & Roddenberry, A. (2014). The hospital-based consultation and liaison service. In C. Hunter, C. Hunter, & R. Kessler (Eds.), *Handbook of clinical psychology in medical settings* (pp. 369–416). New York, NY: Springer.

Gellfand, K., Geffken, G., Lewin, S., Heidgerken, A., Grove, M. J., Malasanos, T., & Silverstein, J. (2004). An initial evaluation of the design of pediatric psychology consultation service with children with diabetes. *Journal of Child Health Care, 8*(2), 113–123.

Ibeziako, P., Brahmbhatt, K., Chapman, A., De Souza, C., Giles, L., Gooden, S., … Steinbuchel, P. (2019). Developing a clinical pathway for somatic symptom and related disorders in pediatric hospital settings. *Hospital Pediatrics, 9*(3), 147–155.

Kazak, A. (2006). Pediatric psychosocial preventative health model (PPPHM): Research, practice, and collaboration in pediatric family systems medicine. *Families, Systems, and Health, 24*(4), 381–395.

Kullgren, K. A., Tsang, K. K., Ernst, M. M., Carter, B. D., Scott, E. L., & Sullivan, S. K. (2015). Inpatient pediatric psychology consultation-liaison practice survey: Corrected version. *Clinical Practice in Pediatric Psychology, 3*(4), 340–351.

Lawal, A. K., Rotter, T., Kinsman, L., Machotta, A., Ronellenfitsch, U., Scott, S. D., … Groot, G. (2016). What is a clinical pathway? Refinement of an operational definition to identify clinical pathway studies for a cochrane systematic review. *BMC Medicine, 14*(1), 35.

Liaison. (n.d.). Oxford's Lexico Online Dictionary. Retrieved from https://www.lexico.com/en/definition/liaison

Maslach, C. (1982). *Burnout: The cost of caring*. Englewood Cliffs, NJ: Prentice Hall.

McGrady, M. E. (2018). Introduction to the CPPP special issue: Building the economic evidence base for pediatric psychology services. *Clinical Practice in Pediatric Psychology, 6*(2), 101–106.

McGuire, K., Fung, L. K., Hagopian, L., Vasa, R. A., Mahajan, R., Bernal, P., … Veenstra-VanderWeele, J. (2016). Irritability and problem behavior in autism spectrum disorder: A practice pathway for pediatric primary care. *Pediatrics, 137*(Supplement 2), S136–S148.

Model. (n.d.). Oxford's Lexico Online Dictionary. Retrieved from https://www.lexico.com/en/definition/model

Role. (n.d.). Merriam-Webster Online Dictionary. Retrieved from http://www.m-w.com/dictionary/

Rotter, T., Kinsman, L., James, E., Machotta, A., Gothe, H., Willis, J., … Kugler, J. (2010). Clinical pathways: Effects on professional practice, patient outcomes, length of stay and hospital costs. *Cochrane Database of Systematic Reviews*, (3), CD006632.

Shaw, R. J., & DeMaso, D. R. (2006). *Clinical manual of pediatric psychosomatic medicine: Mental health consultation with physically ill children and adolescents*. Washington, DC: American Psychiatric Publishing.

Simionato, G. K., & Simpson, S. (2018). Personal risk factors associated with burnout among psychotherapist: A review of the literature. *Journal of Clinical Psychology, 74*(9), 1431–1456.

Tynan, W. D. (2016). Commentary: Integrated primary care psychology evolving with the affordable care act. *Journal of Pediatric Psychology, 41*(10), 1165–1167.

Ward, W. L., Shaffer, L. A., & Getzoff, E. A. (2018). Pediatric psychologists' collaboration in a national pediatric obesity initiative: A case study in interprofessional collaboration. *Journal of Clinical Psychology in Medical Settings, 25*(3), 367–369.

Systems Issues and Considerations

Deirdre A. L. Caplin, Laura M. Bennett-Murphy, and Anne E. Kazak

The Affordable Care Act (ACA) and associated advancements in healthcare policy are rapidly shifting the focus of healthcare toward interprofessional, integrative approaches. These models of care are enriched by psychological and systems theory that informs our understanding of the integrative and reciprocal nature of physical and behavioral health (Brown et al., 2002; Rozensky & Janicke, 2012). In addition, the majority of health risk factors, illness management activities, and medical decisions are influenced by behavioral processes. Thus, pediatric psychologists' expertise in interpersonal relationships and processes, analysis of individuals in context, and clinical outcomes research may promote the development of more effective and efficient healthcare systems (Janicke, Fritz, & Rozensky, 2015; Ward, Zagoloff, Rieck, & Robiner, 2018). Consultation-liaison (CL) psychologists are increasingly present in myriad medical settings: medical hospitals, inpatient subspecialty treatment teams, medical subspecialty clinics, primary care clinics, and traditional psychological clinics. CL may represent the most active collaboration between medical providers and psychologists (Carter et al., 2009). Understanding the ways in which embedded systems affect patients and patient care is critical for providing quality care. This chapter presents some of the ways in which psychologists may affect the systems in which we work and how systems routinely affect the nature of a pediatric psychologist's work.

The major activities of CL psychology within medical systems include the following:

Screening, assessment, and diagnosis. A majority of primary care visits involve psychological concerns that typically go unaddressed or untreated (Wissow, van Ginneken, Chandna, & Rahman, 2016). Improving partnerships among key collaborators—providers, patients, families, and psychologists—promotes access to standardized screening, formal assessment, and diagnosis. This may result in earlier identification of mental and behavioral health disorders, saving significant costs and human suffering.

Health promotion. Health behaviors, beliefs about illness, and access to preventative care are strongly related to health outcomes.

D. A. L. Caplin (✉) · L. M. Bennett-Murphy
Department of Pediatrics, University of Utah School of Medicine, Primary Children's Hospital, Salt Lake City, UT, USA
e-mail: Deirdre.Caplin@hsc.utah.edu

A. E. Kazak
Center for Healthcare Delivery Science, Nemours Children's Health System, Wilmington, DE, USA

Department of Pediatrics, Sidney Kimmel Medical School of Thomas Jefferson University, Philadelphia, PA, USA

B. D. Carter, K. A. Kullgren (eds.), *Clinical Handbook of Psychological Consultation in Pediatric Medical Settings*, Issues in Clinical Child Psychology, https://doi.org/10.1007/978-3-030-35598-2_3

Psychologists have demonstrated the utility of evidence-based programs (Weisz, Doss, & Hawley, 2005) in promoting school achievement, abstinence from drug use, reducing teen pregnancy, curbing bullying, and fostering resilience in the face of adversity. In healthcare settings, prevention strategies also include parent training, psychoeducation, and changes in systems (e.g., advocating for healthy school lunches, later start times, or recess).

Behavior change. Understanding the barriers that exist for implementation of change, where patients are in the change process, and working with resistance are skills psychologists bring to our work. Often, the patients that medical providers find most difficult are the very patients with whom psychologists are trained to work (Gordon-Elliott & Muskin, 2010; Mack, Ilowite, & Taddei, 2017). Physicians often feel ill-equipped when working with difficult patients or recognize that they have little time to address the array of medical and psychosocial concerns of patients (Gordon-Elliott & Muskin, 2010; Johansen et al., 2014; Mack et al., 2017). Psychologists integrated into the healthcare team are able to provide the much-needed behavioral interventions to improve quality of care at the time and place patients present.

Quality improvement, systems design, access, and education. Psychologists' clinical and research skills allow for evaluation of treatment efficacy, with a view toward improving the healthcare delivery systems. With the advent of medical homes and strides toward greater integration of physical and behavioral health, psychologists have the opportunity to reach a larger audience. Further, they have the opportunity to educate and supervise other disciplines (medicine, social work, physical and occupational therapies (PT/OT), education, nursing) promoting the role of biopsychosocial factors in health and illness (Rosen et al., 2018; Wissow et al., 2016). Finally, psychologists have a strong knowledge base in teams and group behavior that can be used to promote better teamwork and safer, high-quality care (Kazak, Nash, Hiroto, & Kaslow, 2017; Rosen et al., 2018).

One's professional practice and identity as a CL psychologist is shaped over time by a network of systems, both directly and indirectly. Bronfenbrenner's social ecological theory helps explain development of an individual within a series of layered, nested, interacting systems and is a model for medical adherence, health promotion, and healthcare disparities (Bronfenbrenner, 1994; Carter et al., 2018; Kazak, 1989; Seid, Opipari-Arrigan, Gelhard, Varni, & Driscoll, 2009). For the CL psychologist, the social ecological model also provides a frame for how our professional practice and identity develop as a function of our interactions with various nested systems in healthcare (Fig. 1). Delineating the ways in which these interacting systems affect the pediatric patient is necessary for providing care as well as identifying barriers that may interfere with care (Seid et al., 2009). Locating oneself within nested systems is also necessary to maximize interventions, strengthen the healthcare system, and promote professional development.

Working in the Microsystem

At the microsystem level, individual relationships with those with whom one interacts on a daily basis (patients, parents, colleagues, and trainees) collectively shape the environment within which you work.

Relating to Patients and Families

The CL psychologist has a core relationship to the individual patient that influences what occurs at all levels of the system. In pediatrics, patient-provider and parent-provider relationships can be unique and distinct from one another. In part, the psychologist is tasked with creating awareness and understanding of the core influences of parents on children and children on parents in the context of healthcare encounters, as these relationships may facilitate or interfere with care. Advising the patient and family on the psychological determinants and sequelae of disease and

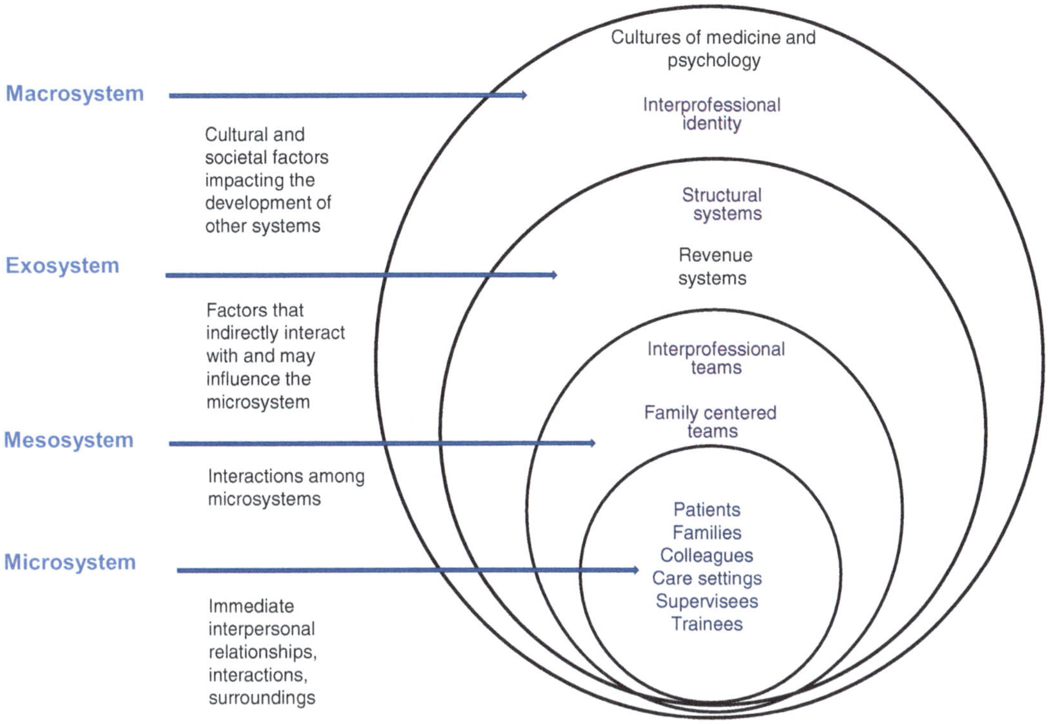

Fig. 1 A social ecological approach to systems in pediatric consultation liaison psychology

the potential benefits of behavioral health interventions, for example, can improve physical and mental health (Brown et al., 2002; Klein & Hostetter, 2014). However, for the message to be heard, it needs to be salient and credible and address patient and family concerns. Psychologists are poised to use their relational skills, active listening, reflecting, and reframing to encourage rapport and positive communication within the family and between the family and their care providers.

The potential benefit of behavioral health integration in pediatric care is unknown to most patients and their families. Although 70–80% of pediatric subspecialty visits involve a behavioral health component, patients and families are usually highly focused on the health issue at hand, rather than thinking about broader biopsychosocial aspects of health, illness, and healthcare (Sulik & Sarvet, 2016). They may not anticipate nor are they explicitly seeking psychological treatment, especially for concerns related to medical symptoms (e.g., pain, fatigue) or illness management (e.g., diabetes, asthma, IBS). The majority of families leave subspecialty visits without an understanding of how behavioral issues may be impacting their child's health and without a referral for psychological treatment to promote health and decrease distress (Klein & Hostetter, 2014). Parents often have mixed feelings and some discomfort about addressing mental health concerns with their pediatrician. Psychologists have a role to play in fostering relationships with patient and providers to reduce the variability that exists in acceptance of behavioral healthcare, independent of where services are located (Wissow et al., 2016).

Relating to Colleagues

In medical settings, a psychologist relies on their professional relationships with other healthcare professionals to facilitate integration of behavioral health practices. Working side by side with physicians, nurses, and therapists in other disciplines, interpersonal interactions are critically important to how one is recognized individually and how well one represents his or her profession.

Like patients and families, physician expectations and attitudes about mental health can challenge the CL psychologist. For instance, interviews conducted with subspecialty physicians in hospital settings indicate that many are skeptical of the effectiveness of integrated behavioral health services (Johansen et al., 2014). Even for those physicians who agree that psychological health is an important aspect of medicine, there is often a gap between awareness and clinical practice (Johansen et al., 2014). A large survey of physicians in a variety of outpatient specialties found that the vast majority of physicians (68% of pediatric, 70% of family medicine) recognized psychosocial health techniques in medicine would enhance overall treatment outcomes for their patients. However, analysis also suggested actual practice and use of behavioral health services was less positive for mind-body methods such as therapy and relaxation techniques (Astin, Soeken, Sierpina, & Clarridge, 2006).

In relationships with our medical colleagues, psychologists must focus liaison work on increasing exposure to the evidence base for integration of behavioral health. It isn't enough to provide good clinical interventions; we must work to address misinformation and to promote integrated care. Often, this occurs through informal conversations with colleagues. Psychologists may share articles, information, or suggestions for clinical practices. This may also occur through structured interdisciplinary meetings, round, or care conferences. Participation in medical education (medical school classrooms, resident didactics, institutional grand rounds, etc.) encourages wider dissemination of ideas. Ultimately, the involvement of psychologists at an administrative and policy-making level may provide the greatest push for integration.

Relating to Care Settings

The successful CL psychologist is expected to wear many different hats. For example, in hospital and medical clinical settings, the psychologist is simultaneously a liaison between physical and behavioral health, an expert consultant to care team, a supervisor to various trainees, and a provider of patient care. There are times in practice where individual obligations to these roles are cooperative and smooth. At other times, competing needs in one role may interfere with successful performance in another.

When it works well, the psychologist's involvement can improve access, reduce stigma, and lead to early recognition and treatment of mental health concerns. In primary care, for example, where a majority of visits involve a psychological or behavioral concern, the physician's office is an ideal setting for providing mental healthcare (APA Center for Psychology and Health, 2014). However, across medical settings, practices differ significantly from a traditional mental health environment and require adaptation in care delivery.

Successful implementation of behavioral health services requires that the CL psychologist be explicitly aware of what can realistically be accomplished in a specific clinical environment. As an example, the average outpatient pediatrics practice is a fast-paced environment that thrives on targeted diagnosis and treatment in brief bursts of interaction. Contrary to this, the average mental health practice thrives on longer-term, continuous intervention with a focus on process (Pidano, Arora, Gipson, Hudson, & Schellinger, 2018). As an adjunct provider, the CL psychologist typically does not control or manage time allocation, patient flow, or workload. Thus, some treatment protocols may require adaptation to respond to the demands of the environment. Other concerns, like major depressive disorder, may continue to require referral and treatment in more traditional psychological settings.

Relating to Supervisees and Trainees

In academic medicine, clinical supervision is often "on the fly" while rounding, in the hallway, or at the patient bedside. In medicine, timing is an important teaching tool. When information is provided at a time when it is salient, in small chunks, and by a credible source (i.e., evidence based), the information is better absorbed by the learner. Supervision models for psychologists, in contrast, often involve dedicated time away from patient care duties, focusing on deeper process issues to guide learning.

The CL psychologist, in their role as teacher, needs to be flexible in their teaching approach, adapting methods to an interprofessional audience that supports integration (Rozensky & Janicke, 2012). Our role in medical education is twofold. First, teaching learners at all levels about the overlapping areas of physical and mental health is paramount to cohesive practice between disciplines. Second, teaching trainees strategies for communicating with patients, families, and each other increases our value and creates an environment for shared responsibility and decision-making (Rosen et al., 2018). The value of learning how to provide and receive a "warm handoff" is often understated in teaching but imperative to collaboration (Buche et al., 2017).

In the fast pace of a medical subspecialty clinic or hospital ward, we must also prepare our trainees to understand their role as a member of a team. Speaking succinctly, responding to a consultation question, teaching medicine trainees of the subtleties that can influence patients and families, and the care they receive are refined skills in CL work. Poor role definition or "turf issues" can be a barrier to integrated mental health and also an opportunity for teaching the next generation of psychologists to focus on shared values and combined competencies in team-teaching environments (Rozensky & Janicke, 2012).

Working in the Mesosystem

The influence of larger teams lies beyond the direct interpersonal impact of practicing in a medical system. Team dynamics and structure are powerful forces that control the relative effect of providers across disciplines.

Interprofessional Team Dynamics

Being part of a team is necessary in healthcare, demanding appropriate skills to function as a team member and interact effectively with others. Teams allow access to a broad pool of perspectives, conceptualizations, capabilities, skills, and shared workload (Bell, Brown, Colaneri, & Outland, 2018). However, teams are neither inherently beneficial nor cohesive. Fostered by cultural training and practice differences between medicine and psychology, colleagues are likely to view you differently than you see yourself (Astin et al., 2006; Pidano et al., 2018). For example, in the context of chronic disease management, there exists a frequent misconception that psychological problems are secondary to medical concerns which neglects the complexities of the biopsychosocial framework (Johansen et al., 2014). Psychology is also at fault for holding a narrow view of professional responsibility. Maintaining this protectionist approach interferes with integration efforts and can thwart the cooperation of any team. Further, fragmented delivery of healthcare services contributes to medical errors and diffusion of responsibility (Young, Olsen, & McGinnis, 2010). Creating a cohesive, integrated team with shared goals takes work and intentionality.

Cultivating collaboration does not have to mean letting go of your diverse knowledge and skills. Teams that are diverse provide the prospect of greater results through exploration of differences in care approach or disagreements in diagnostic formulations. Ward and her colleagues suggest that we can foster collaborative, effective interprofessional teams by exploring and resolving misconceptions, enhancing respect, and recognizing respective skill sets of each other (Ward et al., 2018). Familiarity through regular communication, interest in others' profession, and shared settings (clinical and didactic) are all strategies to improve team communication (Pidano et al., 2018). Openness to adapting intervention strategies to the structure of the team is another effective strategy to promote integration that also meets the goals of a more efficient and cost-effective approach to care (Rozensky & Janicke, 2012). Attending to the ABCs of teams (affective and motivational states, behavioral processes, and cognitive states) leads to greater interdependence and effectiveness (Bell et al., 2018).

At times, communication can be hindered if not in close proximity. Services that are not integrated or even colocated may require virtual collaboration. It is a common complaint among pediatricians that they do not receive follow-up communication from psychologists to whom they refer, despite having expressed interest in knowing about diagnosis and treatment progress (Pidano et al., 2018). Using standardized communications, developing individual relationships, and simply reaching out are all ways of improving relationships with extended team members that have some efficacy (Pidano et al., 2018).

Family-Centered Team Dynamics

The patient (and family) is at the center of any team and is often the most important factor in determining the dynamic of a team. Low motivation, perceived stigma, and lack of insight have all been cited as perceived barriers to communicating with families about psychological concerns (Astin et al., 2006; Johansen et al., 2014). Physicians are often reluctant to engage families in conversations about psychological factors if they feel they do not have the time, expertise, or resources to address them. The CL psychologist has an opportunity to be a source for mental health interventions but is also critical in promoting understanding of all team members of the value added by behavioral health methods. Facilitating partnerships with families around a cohesive plan is difficult if team members are not acting as a single unit. Practically speaking, a parent may have a healthcare agenda that is different from what the patient presents and may influence how care is initiated and received.

A well-developed team is focused on complementing skills of other team members, treating the whole child, and engaging families in assessment and development of a plan of care (Kazak et al., 2017). Effective teams provide all team members with an active role in patient care and management, considering expertise and input from all members. Patients and families are encouraged and expected to participate and partner in care.

Working in the Exosystem

Effective mental healthcare improves medical outcomes and reduces healthcare costs; patients with comorbid mental health concerns add significantly to the cost of healthcare and contribute to poorer outcomes (Klein & Hostetter, 2014). It is also well-known that despite the evidence for integration, it has been difficult to achieve at the practice level, primarily because of how institutions and revenue systems are designed.

Institutional Systems

The majority of pediatric psychologists practice in hospital systems, either children's hospitals or academic medical centers, and are housed in departments of pediatrics or psychiatry (Carter et al., 2018; Rozensky & Janicke, 2012). Institutional policies may promote or interfere with coordinated care. The best practices identified for an integrated care environment are those who practice in organizations where collaboration is a cultural norm (Buche et al., 2017). Communication across disciplines, interdisciplinary training and orientation, and a patient-centered rather than clinician-centered approach are key to alignment in values across disciplines. Organizations are less likely to be integrated if disagreements about provider roles, workflows, and restrictions on patient information sharing exist or logistical problems with reimbursement or adequate staffing persist (Buche et al., 2017).

Traditional clinical workflows and payment structures prohibit rather than promote cooperation in healthcare. Fragmentation of services is common and can affect when and how patients have access to psychological services (Miller et al., 2017). It is possible, for example, to have a patient receive integrated mental healthcare during a medical hospitalization only to find out that same service is not available to them when they discharge. Outpatient clinics may have different financial contracts with insurers than the tertiary care hospital. With carve outs, separate payment practices, competing funding streams, and variable reimbursement policies, a psychologist's practice may be pushed outside the medical setting (Bachrach, Anthony, & Detty, 2014; Klein & Hostetter, 2014).

State regulatory rules can also impede care provision in some settings. For instance, licensing rules can interfere with cross-discipline supervision, create redundancy in practice, and put constraints on information sharing between providers (Bachrach et al., 2014).

Revenue Systems

CL psychology, like other psychology services, requires tangible institutional support. There are several systems factors that limit a CL psychology service from being completely self-sustaining. These include the business model and priorities of an institution, as well as state and federal policies around reimbursement. First, most reimbursement models only compensate face-to-face time spent with patients. However, it is well-known that a significant portion, as much as 38% of psychologist's time, is spent in non-billable activities (Bierenbaum, Katsikas, Furr, & Carter, 2013; Carter et al., 2018; Kullgren et al., 2015). Direct service to patients does not account for the many tasks psychologists complete in providing quality care, such as work with family members, health record review, consultation with other providers, patient conferences, care coordination, and disposition planning.

Second, reimbursement may be complicated by the emergent and unpredictable nature of CL consult work. Psychologists respond to concerns before prior authorization for services may occur, increasing the likelihood of denial or loss of revenue (Bierenbaum et al., 2013). And while a medical system, i.e., the children's hospital, may be part of the patient's medical insurance network, the individual psychologist providing inpatient services may not be on the mental health panel, again leading to denial of payment.

The billing codes available to psychologists create another revenue challenge. Health and behavior (H&B) codes were designed to better capture the services psychologist provides in medical settings. However, they are not well-utilized by psychologists (Kullgren et al., 2015) and have higher denial rates than psychotherapy codes. Insurance companies may deny payment for psychological services when a patient has only a medical diagnosis (Tynen, Woods, & Carpenter, 2009). This is often due to (1) limits set on the number of units allowed to be billed under H&B codes by insurers or (2) disagreements due to "carve outs." The boundary between physical and mental is variable for insurers; some payors only allow medical personnel to bill for medical diagnoses, limiting reimbursement for psychologists providing health and behavior assessments or interventions. Those same companies may not allow for billing of mental healthcare if no psychological diagnosis is present. So, with payors using separate billing and coding practices, provider networks, and record-keeping requirements, supporting the integration of behavioral health and CL services remains difficult to achieve (Klein & Hostetter, 2014).

In short, most CL services cannot be sustained by traditional collection/fee-for-service models (Bierenbaum et al., 2013; Kullgren et al., 2015). "Behavioral health integration is still rare … in part because there is no financial incentive or administrative advantage to bringing … stand-alone operations together" (Klein & Hostetter, 2014, p. 4). That being said, many systems and states across the country are finding creative ways to embrace integrated care delivery for behavioral and physical comorbidities (Bachrach et al., 2014; Buche et al., 2017; Klein & Hostetter, 2014; Miller et al., 2017). In Colorado, for example, Rocky Mountain Health Plans partnered with the University of Colorado Denver and the Collaborative Family Healthcare Association and developed a global payment system for team-based care. This pilot program charges a global fee that accounts for staffing resources and patient complexity. It allows for flexibility in practices, including between visit follow-ups, to lead to greater health. Bachrach et al. (2014) note that after the ACA, more states are reassessing the complex needs of Medicaid beneficiaries. States are providing financial incentives for providers to integrate behavioral healthcare and consolidate billing. Further, some states are moving to "behavioral health carve ins" to promote greater integration and collaboration and to set up specific treatment programs for individuals with serious mental illness.

Healthcare systems continue to move away from fee-for-service models to care models that demonstrate that they are cost-effective *and* that they are providing effective treatment. Psychologists' expertise in the measurement of outcomes may allow healthcare systems, including behavioral health services, to demonstrate efficacy and "value added."

Working in the Macrosystem

Despite the Institute of Medicine's (IOM) conclusions almost two decades ago that lack of integration results in inferior care, behavioral healthcare continues to be invisible and typically separates from medical care (Klein & Hostetter, 2014). In spite of strong evidence that psychological interventions improve outcomes for disease, reduce morbidity and healthcare costs, and improve health promotion, these data are poorly disseminated to patients as well as policy-makers. As a result, the disconnect between healthcare policy and healthcare practice persists (Brown et al., 2002; Klein & Hostetter, 2014).

Cultures of Medicine and Psychology

As implementation of integrative care continues across the healthcare system (tertiary care centers, hospitals, medical subspecialty clinics, and primary care clinics), ways to enhance collaborative practice are sought (Pidano et al., 2018). One of the greatest barriers to integrative, interprofessional practice may be working across cultures. Medical practice has historically been hierarchical, with the attending physician the ultimate decision-maker at the head of a team. Most decision-making is communicated orally. Further, specialization is rewarded. Physicians have been trained to "stay in your own lane," taking responsibility for medical decision-making within a defined set of parameters (Groopman, 2007). This model has some strengths and also accounts for adverse events (i.e., miscommunication of medication name or dose, loss of critical information.). It is a system that operates primarily on a division of labor and unequal power (Rosen et al., 2018). Integration challenges that model, asking providers to take a broad view of the patient, work interdependently, and share responsibility for treatment and care planning. Again, psychologists' training in culturally informed practice may serve us well as we navigate the medical culture of the healthcare system.

With this new model, everyone has something to learn. Hierarchy can inhibit assertive communication that may prevent errors trainees and allied health providers must learn how to challenge and communicate what they observe. Physicians benefit from a renewed emphasis on cultivating relationships with patients and team members and thinking holistically (Pidano et al., 2018). Psychologists working in a medical environment are expected to learn how to communicate their conceptualization of patients orally in 2–3 min. They also need greater familiarity with medical tests, procedures, language, and acronyms (Schmaling, Giardino, Korslund, Roberts, & Sweeny, 2002). Finally, all may benefit from collaborating clinically and also in research, documenting successes and pitfalls in the care of complex patients. Surface-level diversity (race, gender, profession) is important in the effectiveness of teams, but deep-level factors (personality, conscientiousness, agreeableness, attitudes) significantly affect team processes. These are often discovered only after interacting with someone over time.

Novel educational approaches are emerging to address cultural differences and promote interprofessional care models (see Ward et al., 2018). At the behest of the IOM and then the Institute for Healthcare Improvement (Institute of Medicine, 2010; Ward et al., 2018), more academic medical centers are creating opportunities for trainees from different health practices to share didactics and training materials, learning activities, and clinical training experiences, in the hopes of fostering appreciation for one another's skills and knowledge. These shared experiences may range from one workshop to a fully developed curriculum (Ward et al., 2018). Best practices for interprofessional education (IPE) continue to emerge. Roles for psychologists in these programs include curriculum design, faculty development, supervising faculty member, and program assessment. Interprofessional education is also emerging in psychology graduate training (Rozensky & Janicke, 2012; Ward et al., 2018). In 2017, the APA Commission on Accreditation expanded prior competencies to include *consultation and interprofessional/interdisciplinary skills* as a core competency. Psychology trainees must now demonstrate knowledge and respect for the roles and perspectives of other professions, as well as engage with healthcare professionals or interprofessional groups and systems.

Psychology's Interprofessional Identity

A CL psychologist is responsible not only for themselves but also for the reputation and understanding of their profession in the healthcare system. Janicke and his colleagues have underscored the incredible opportunity available to psychologists in the changing landscape of healthcare if we are willing to take ownership of our identity as a profession (Janicke et al., 2015). It is clear that the medical profession perceives us differently than we see ourselves (Astin et al., 2006; Johansen et al., 2014; Pidano et al., 2018). While physicians may be comfortable making a referral to a psychologist for a crisis or clearly identified psychological disorder, they may be less certain how to create space for integrative and collaborative, interprofessional practices within the medical setting. This is in part the fault of our struggles to promote ourselves effectively. Psychologists must take the lead on defining our value in medicine, our role in the patient-centered medical home, and our role in providing high-quality medical care in a value-driven system (Janicke et al., 2015). Our role as educators, advocates, and policymakers is already woven into current healthcare policy (Institute of Medicine, 2010; National Academy of Engineering and Institute of Medicine Committee on Engineering and the Health Care System, 2005). While these roles are not new, psychologists continue to need to function as ambassadors of the field. Through this process, we may also serve to destigmatize working with a psychologist.

The processes described in this chapter highlight the many roles of the CL psychologist: *Clinician, Collaborator, Educator, Scholar, Leader, Agent of Change.* These roles demand a broad and integrated identity. If CL providers were once called "the guardian of the holistic approach to the patient" (Ajiboye, 2007), we may also be guardians of a holistic approach in healthcare. Psychologists work within the system, but we also work to change the system. Perhaps, the next challenge for the field of CL psychology is to demonstrate the value added by psychologists' participation in healthcare (reduced costs, improved outcomes, reduced morbidity, etc.). Janicke et al. (2015) argue that child and adolescent psychologists must take the lead in advocating for our patients and our profession. APA continues to produce advocacy tool kits to assist providers. While the complexity of the current healthcare system is overwhelming and the future of the ACA is uncertain, psychologists must not be discouraged from presenting how evidence-based interventions improve patient health, reduce costs, and improve quality (APA Center for Psychology and Health, 2014; Brown et al., 2002; Janicke et al., 2015; Pidano et al., 2018). Partnering with our medical colleagues to both advocate and to collect data demonstrating cost-benefits may further strengthen relationships, with positive benefit reverberating throughout the levels of the bioecological system. Thus, our identity shifts from a partner in change with the patient to an agent of change within the system.

Conclusions

As articulated a decade ago, *there is no health without mental health* (Prince et al., 2007). Psychologists are uniquely situated to improve patient care, develop models of interprofessional care, affect current education practices in medicine and psychology, and alter the healthcare systems in which we work. The profound political and social shifts of the last 20 years have led us to a place where psychologists are increasingly present and integrated into medical systems. The biopsychosocial model of health is widely recognized. Nonetheless, a gap remains between knowledge and implementation of best educational, clinical, and structural practices. Data clearly document the economic and health burden of those suffering from psychological disorders (Klein & Hostetter, 2014). The efficacy of psychological interventions in treating these disorders is equally well-documented (Weisz et al., 2005). While the case for the effectiveness of psychological interventions is well-made, more is needed than skilled practitioners implementing empirically supported interventions. We affect and are affected by factors at all system levels. Psychologists must forge the way for greater co-coordination and comprehensive management of patients at all levels of the medical system. Addressing issues of equity, access, ethics, efficacy, accountability, education, and teamwork in a patient-centered system requires that psychologists embrace leadership roles in myriad settings.

References

Ajiboye, P. O. (2007). Consultation-liaison psychiatry: The past and the present. *African Journal of Medicine and Medical Sciences, 36*(3), 201–205.

APA Center for Psychology and Health. (2014). *Integrated health care*. Washington, DC: Author.

Astin, J. A., Soeken, K., Sierpina, V. S., & Clarridge, B. R. (2006). Barriers to the integration of psychosocial factors in medicine: Results of a national survey of physicians. *Journal of the American Board of Family Medicine, 19*, 557. https://doi.org/10.3122/jabfm.19.6.557

Bachrach, D., Anthony, S., & Detty, A. (2014). *State strategies for integrating physical and behavioural health services in a changing medicaid environment*. New York, NY: The Commonwealth Fund. https://www.commonwealthfund.org/sites/default/files/documents/___media_files_publications_fund_report_2014_aug_1767_bachrach_state_strategies_integrating_phys_behavioral_hlt_827.pdf

Bell, S. T., Brown, S. G., Colaneri, A., & Outland, N. (2018). Team composition and the ABCs of teamwork. *American Psychologist, 73*, 349. https://doi.org/10.1037/amp0000305

Bierenbaum, M. L., Katsikas, S., Furr, A., & Carter, B. D. (2013). Factors associated with non-reimbursable activity on an inpatient pediatric consultation-liaison service. *Journal of Clinical Psychology in Medical Settings, 20*, 464. https://doi.org/10.1007/s10880-013-9371-2

Bronfenbrenner, U. (1994). Ecological models of human development. *Readings on the Development of Children, 2*, 37–43. Retrieved from http://www.psy.cmu.edu/~siegler/35bronfebrenner94.pdf.

Brown, R. T., Freeman, W. S., Brown, R. A., Belar, C., Hersch, L., Hornyak, L. M., … Reed, G. (2002). The role of psychology in health care delivery. *Professional Psychology: Research and Practice, 33*, 536. https://doi.org/10.1037/0735-7028.33.6.536

Buche, J., Singer, P. A., Grazier, K., King, E., Maniere, E., & Beck, A. J. (2017). *Primary care and behavioral health workforce integration: Barriers and best practices*. Ann Arbor, MI: University of Michigan Behavioral Health Workforce Research Center. Retrieved from http://www.behavioralhealthworkforce.org.

Carter, B. D., Kronenberger, W. G., Scott, E., & Ernst, M. M. (2009). Inpatient Pediatric Consultation—Liaison. In M.C. Roberts & R. G. Steele (Eds.) Handbook of pediatric psychology (4th ed., pp. 114–129)

Carter, B. D., Kronenberger, W. G., Scott, E. L., Kullgren, K. A., Piazza-Waggoner, C., & Brady, C. E. (2018). Inpatient pediatric consultation-liaison. In M. C. Roberts & R. G. Steele (Eds.), *Handbook of pediatric psychology* (5th ed.). New York, NY: The Guilford Press.

Gordon-Elliott, J. S., & Muskin, P. R. (2010). An approach to the patient with multiple physical symptoms or chronic disease. *Medical Clinics of North America, 94*(6), 1207–1216. https://doi.org/10.1016/j.mcna.2010.08.007

Groopman, J. (2007). *How doctors think* (pp. 33–34). Boston, MA: Houghton Miffin.

Institute of Medicine. (2010). The healthcare imperative: Lowering costs and improving outcomes*:* Workshop series summary. https://doi.org/10.17226/12750

Janicke, D. M., Fritz, A. M., & Rozensky, R. H. (2015). Healthcare reform and preparing the future clinical child and adolescent psychology workforce. *Journal of Clinical Child and Adolescent Psychology, 53*, 1030. https://doi.org/10.1080/15374416.2015.1050725

Johansen, C., Torenholt, R., Hommel, E., Wittrup, M., Cleal, B., & Willaing, I. (2014). Psychology &

psychotherapy barriers to addressing psychological problems in diabetes: Perspectives of diabetologists on routine diabetes consultations in Denmark. *Journal of Psychology and Psychotherapy, 4*, 141. https://doi.org/10.4172/2161-0487.1000141

Kazak, A. E. (1989). Families of chronically ill children: A systems and social-ecological model of adaptation and challenge. *Journal of Consulting and Clinical Psychology, 57*, 25. https://doi.org/10.1037/0022-006X.57.1.25

Kazak, A. E., Nash, J. M., Hiroto, K., & Kaslow, N. J. (2017). Psychologists in patient-centered medical homes (PCMHs): Roles, evidence, opportunities, and challenges. *American Psychologist, 72*, 1. https://doi.org/10.1037/a0040382

Klein, S., & Hostetter, M. (2014). In focus: Integrating behavioral health and primary care. *Quality Matters Archive*. New York, NY: The Commonwealth Fund.

Kullgren, K. A., Tsang, K. K., Ernst, M. M., Carter, B. D., Scott, E. L., & Sullivan, S. K. (2015). Inpatient pediatric psychology consultation-liaison practice survey. *Clinical Practice in Pediatric Psychology, 3*, 37. https://doi.org/10.1037/cpp0000089

Mack, J. W., Ilowite, M., & Taddei, S. (2017). Difficult relationships between parents and physicians of children with cancer: A qualitative study of parent and physician perspectives. *Cancer, 123*, 675. https://doi.org/10.1002/cncr.30395

Miller, B. F., Ross, K. M., Melek, S. P., Davis, M. M., Kathol, R., & Gordon, P. (2017). Payment reform in the patient-centered medical home: Enabling and sustaining integrated behavioral health care. *American Psychologist, 72*, 55. https://doi.org/10.1037/a0040448

National Academy of Engineering and Institute of Medicine Committee on Engineering and the Health Care System. (2005). A framework for a systems approach to health care delivery. In P. Reid, W. Compton, J. Grossman, & G. Fanjiang (Eds.), *Building a better delivery system: A news engineering/health care partnership*. Washington, DC: National Academies Press. Retrieved from ncbi.nlm.nih.gov.

Pidano, A. E., Arora, P., Gipson, P. Y., Hudson, B. O., & Schellinger, K. B. (2018). Psychologists and pediatricians in the primary care sandbox: Communication is key to cooperative play. *Journal of Clinical Psychology in Medical Settings, 25*, 32. https://doi.org/10.1007/s10880-017-9522-y

Prince, M., Patel, V., Saxena, S., Maj, M., Maselko, J., Phillips, M. R., & Rahman, A. (2007). No health without mental health. *The Lancet, 370*, 859. https://doi.org/10.1016/S0140-6736(07)61238-0

Rosen, M. A., DiazGranados, D., Dietz, A. S., Benishek, L. E., Thompson, D., Pronovost, P. J., & Weaver, S. J. (2018). Teamwork in healthcare: Key discoveries enabling safer, high-quality care. *American Psychologist, 73*, 433. https://doi.org/10.1037/amp0000298

Rozensky, R. H., & Janicke, D. M. (2012). Commentary: Healthcare reform and psychology's workforce: Preparing for the future of pediatric psychology. *Journal of Pediatric Psychology, 37*, 359. https://doi.org/10.1093/jpepsy/jsr111

Schmaling, K. B., Giardino, N. D., Korslund, K. E., Roberts, L. J., & Sweeny, S. (2002). The utility of interdisciplinary training and service: Psychology training on a psychiatry consultation-liaison service. *Professional Psychology: Research and Practice, 33*, 413. https://doi.org/10.1037/0735-7028.33.4.413

Seid, M., Opipari-Arrigan, L., Gelhard, L. R., Varni, J. W., & Driscoll, K. (2009). Barriers to care questionnaire: Reliability, validity, and responsiveness to change among parents of children with asthma. *Academic Pediatrics, 9*, 106. https://doi.org/10.1016/j.acap.2008.12.003

Sulik, L. R., & Sarvet, B. (2016). Collaborating with primary care. In M. K. Dulcan (Ed.), *Dulcan's textbook of child and adolescent psychiatry* (2nd ed., pp. 1075–1087). Arlington, VA: American Psychiatric Association.

Tynen, W. D., Woods, K., & Carpenter, J. (2009). Integrating child psychology services in primary care. Retrieved from https://www.apa.org/pi/families/resources/primary-care/integrating-services.aspx

Ward, W., Zagoloff, A., Rieck, C., & Robiner, W. (2018). Interprofessional education: Opportunities and challenges for psychology. *Journal of Clinical Psychology in Medical Settings, 25*, 250. https://doi.org/10.1007/s10880-017-9538-3

Weisz, J. R., Doss, A. J., & Hawley, K. M. (2005). Youth psychotherapy outcome research: A review and critique of the evidence base. *Annual Review of Psychology, 56*, 337. https://doi.org/10.1146/annurev.psych.55.090902.141449

Wissow, L. S., van Ginneken, N., Chandna, J., & Rahman, A. (2016). Integrating children's mental health into primary care. *Pediatric Clinics of North America, 63*, 97. https://doi.org/10.1016/j.pcl.2015.08.005

Young, P. L., Olsen, L., & McGinnis, J. M. (2010). *Value in health care: Accounting for cost, quality, safety, outcomes, and intervention: Workshop summary*. Washington, DC: National Academies Press.

Hospitalization and Its Impact: Stressors Associated with Inpatient Hospitalization for the Child and Family

Chrissy Cammarata, Simona Bujoreanu, and Karen Wohlheiter

Overview of the Hospital Experience

Each year, between 3 and 6 million children are hospitalized in the United States (Witt, Weiss, & Elixhauser, 2014), and although hospitalizations overall are declining, nearly one out of every six discharges from US hospitals was for children aged 17 years and younger (Witt et al., 2014). With the increase in outpatient and ambulatory treatments, hospitalizations tend to occur for more serious conditions, such as traumatic injuries and chronic physical illnesses, rather than minor events (Berry et al., 2013; Perrin & Shipman, 2009).

Most healthcare professionals would agree that hospitalizations are disruptive events for youth and their families, regardless of whether they are planned or unplanned and recurring or single events (Rennick, Johnston, Dougherty, et al., 2002; Vessey, 2003; Wilson, Megel, Enenbach, & Carlson, 2010). A hospital stay requires children (and their families) to adapt to a variety of changes, such as new medical diagnoses, new routines and environments, other children with medical concerns, new adult caregivers, strange and scary equipment, and unusual experiences involving and invading their bodies. The most basic everyday tasks become disruptive and different. Eating and sleeping are no longer within the child or parents' control. The most challenging aspect is often the pain or discomfort related to disease/injury or procedures. Almost all children have to experience some amount of "pokes," dietary changes, mobility and activity limits, and, sometimes, even isolation while in the hospital (Coyne, 2006; Lindeke, Nakai, & Johnson, 2006; Perrin & Shipman, 2009).

Even though most families are resilient and do not experience any lasting stress post discharge, estimates suggest that as many as 20–30% of families may experience negative psychological reactions at levels significant enough to interfere with their daily lives or impact their functioning (National Center for Traumatic Stress/NCTS, 2018; Rennick et al., 2014; Vernon & Thompson, 1993). This may be an underestimate of the actual

C. Cammarata (✉)
Division of Behavioral Health, Department of Pediatrics, Nemours/A.I. DuPont Hospital for Children, Sidney Kimmel Medical College, Thomas Jefferson University, Wilmington, DE, USA
e-mail: cc0077@nemours.org

S. Bujoreanu
Department of Psychiatry, Boston Children's Hospital, Harvard Medical School, Boston, MA, USA

K. Wohlheiter
Department of Pediatrics, Nemours/A.I. DuPont Hospital for Children, Sidney Kimmel Medical College, Thomas Jefferson University, Wilmington, DE, USA

B. D. Carter, K. A. Kullgren (eds.), *Clinical Handbook of Psychological Consultation in Pediatric Medical Settings*, Issues in Clinical Child Psychology, https://doi.org/10.1007/978-3-030-35598-2_4

impact due to the tendency for research to exclude very young children and due to the limitations of using formal diagnostic criteria, such as posttraumatic stress disorder (PTSD), to determine impairment (Rennick et al., 2014).

In this chapter, we will discuss the range of typical responses to the stress of hospitalization and factors that may exacerbate stress. Our discussion will be guided by two models, the Pediatric Psychosocial Preventative Health Model (PPPHM) and the Integrative Model of Pediatric Medical Traumatic Stress (PMTS), which have been found to be helpful for predicting families at risk for greater levels of distress during and following hospitalization and for guiding intervention plans. Finally, we will discuss recommendations for the Consultation/Liaison (CL) psychologist in order to reduce stress and facilitate resilience in families undergoing medical care during and after hospitalization.

Models of Screening and Intervention for Families Undergoing Hospitalization

The Pediatric Psychosocial Preventative Health Model (Kazak, 2006) and the Integrative Model of Pediatric Medical Traumatic Stress (Bruce, 2006; Kazak et al., 2006; Stuber, Shemesh, & Saxe, 2003) are two competency-based frameworks that have been applied to families undergoing a medical event. These models have been studied with children facing cancer diagnoses, accidental injury, cardiac surgery, transplant, and new-onset diabetes and children in the intensive care units or pediatric gastroenterology inpatient unit (Kazak et al., 2006; see Price, Kassam-Adams, Alderfer, Christofferson, & Kazak, 2016 for review). Core assumptions of both of these models are that families undergoing medical care are resilient and do not necessarily have any elevated risk for pathology or require formal and ongoing intervention simply because of their medical needs (Kazak et al., 2007). Instead of applying focused intervention to all families, these models suggest using population-based principles of screening and tailoring interventions for providing care to the vulnerable groups of youth and families experiencing a medical event.

The Pediatric Psychosocial Preventative Health Model (PPPHM)

Based on Social Ecological Theory (Bronfenbrenner, 1979), this model assumes that children receiving medical care should be viewed within the context of multiple systems, all of which interact to influence their functioning (e.g., family, school, other medical providers, extending to broader systems such as culture, community, religion, socioeconomic status). Therefore, it is important to assess a family's strengths and risk factors within this broader context while also considering expectations for normative stress reactions of youth and families facing a medical event. Since medical teams tend to see only the brief, situational experience of a family in front of the backdrop of acute distress, this may not accurately reflect the family's full capabilities, as positive coping can coexist along with distress. By integrating in the formulation the larger family and their life context, CL psychologists can understand how these systems can either act as protective or risk factors or can foster resilience in children and families. Through assessment and with the use of screening tools, families can be identified to belong to one of three categories based on their risks and strengths.

Most families who are participating in hospital-based care will fall in the *universal* category. These families are seen to be functioning normally prior to and during the medical event but may exhibit distress related to the medical experience. While other psychosocial stressors may be present, these stressors do not impede coping and these families continue to be functioning well. The next, smaller group of families is the *targeted* group who may present with factors that are associated with risk for adjustment or continued stress related to the medical experience. These families may have preexisting psychosocial concerns (e.g., financial stress, family conflict), comorbid mental health diagnoses, or lack of effective social support. These families may experience greater challenges if more medical stressors are present, such as intense medical diagnoses, longer hospitalization, and ongoing needs for medical care. Finally, the smallest group of families, but most often referred to CL psychologists for consultation, is the *clinical/treatment* group. These children and families often have preexisting factors which put them at greatest risk for ongoing difficulties and potential medical traumatic stress (Kazak, 2006), such as a history of clinically significant anxiety, depression, behavior problems, substance abuse, and/or legal troubles. These families will need more ongoing support during the child's hospitalization and may also need support after discharge from the hospital.

The Integrative Model of Pediatric Medical Traumatic Stress (PMTS)

According to this model, "pain, injury, serious illness, medical procedures, and invasive or frightening experiences" are seen as potentially traumatic events (PTE), and children and families' responses to the PTE, such as irritability, avoidance of situational reminders of the hospital, anxiety, and depression, are defined as Pediatric Medical Traumatic Stress (PMTS) (NCTSN, 2018). PMTS may be associated with stress disorders (e.g., PTSD, acute stress disorder) and should be conceptualized on a continuum of post-traumatic stress symptoms (PTSS; Kazak, 2005) that unfold in three potential phases:

Phase I: Peritrauma consists of the time during and immediately following the PTE. This may include events related to an accident scene, transport to the hospital, invasive medical procedures, and communication of the diagnosis of a life-threatening disorder (Price et al., 2016; Rennick et al., 2014).

Phase II: Early, ongoing, and evolving responses include active medical treatments and the hospital stay and related demands and may involve up to 6 weeks posthospital discharge.

Phase III: Longer-term PMTS may include the time past the end of active medical treatment, involving years after treatment or the PTE concludes.

Figure 1 details this model, highlights the factors that may exacerbate and moderate stress reactions in hospitalized youth, and suggests recommendations for intervention at each of these phases.

Stress Reactions to Hospitalization

While most children report fears and anxiety about unknown events, both real and imagined (Carney et al., 2003), children's emotional expressions of stress can range from simple verbalizations or expressions of discomfort (e.g., crying, withdrawal) to more disruptive reactions (e.g., regression such as bed-wetting, tantrums, refusal to comply with procedures/medical regimens; changes in eating and sleeping; and increased dependency on caregivers/parents) (DeMaso & Snell, 2013; Perrin & Shipman, 2009; Vernon & Thompson, 1993). The most frequently occurring psychological reactions observed in medically ill children during their medical admission are internalizing struggles, such as depressed mood, anxiety, and somatic complaints (DeMaso & Bujoreanu, 2013; Justus et al., 2006), likely due to a loss of control over one's life, restrictions on positive and age normative activities, isolation from peers, and/or adverse medical experiences (Justus et al., 2006). Externalizing "acting out" behaviors may also be present around medical procedures and medical stress (Maneta & DeMaso, 2017), especially for younger children (9–11%; Van Horn et al., 2001), and these negative reactions generally occur as a result of the effort to avoid unpleasant and scary situations (DeMaso & Snell, 2013).

Additionally, in the assessment and management of physically ill children presenting with significant psychological reactions, it is important to be mindful that co-occurring/preexisting mental disorders can impact the management of

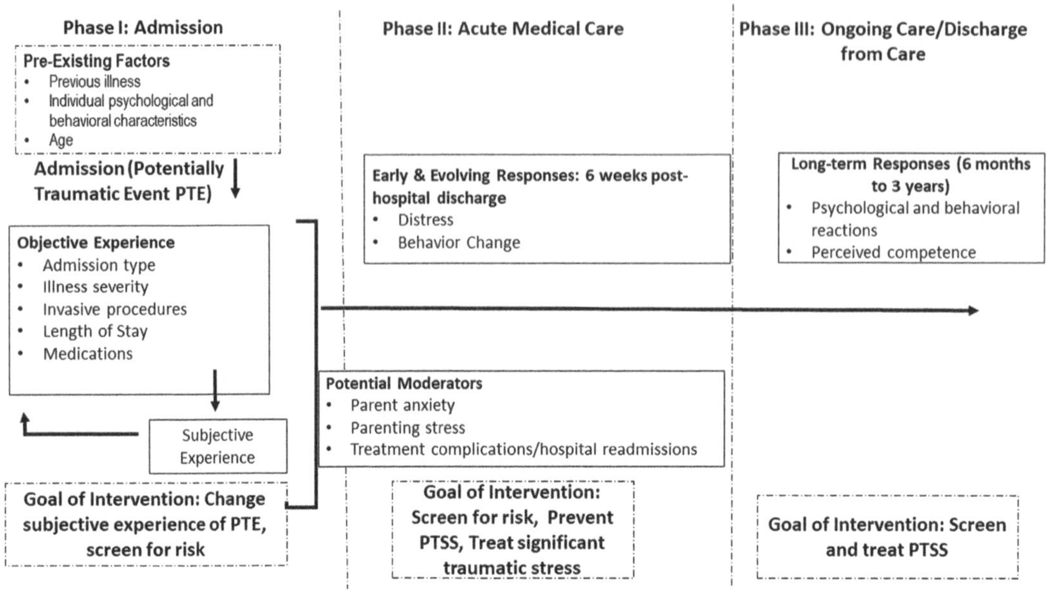

Fig. 1 An integrated model of pediatric medical traumatic stress. This work has been adapted from the original article "Children's psychological and behavioral responses following pediatric intensive care unit hospitalization: the caring intensively study" by Rennick, Dougherty, Chambers, Stremler, et al. BMC Pediatrics 2014, 276 (https://doi.org/10.1186/1471-2431-14-276). The original article is an open-access article distributed under the terms of the Creative Commons Attribution License (http://creativecommons.org/licenses/by/2.0), which permits unrestricted use, distribution, and reproduction in any medium, provided the original work is properly cited

the medical condition (DeMaso & Bujoreanu, 2013). Similarly, it is possible that psychiatric illness, such as depression, is often underdiagnosed in the face of medical illness due to attributions of irritable mood and somatic symptoms to medical treatments/condition or due to avoidance of stigma associated with mental illness (Maneta & DeMaso, 2017).

Factors Associated with Stress During Hospitalization

Factors such as younger age, preexisting psychosocial stressors, previous medical experiences, illness severity, length of hospital stay, and extent of invasive procedures are associated with greater PTSS and medical fears in children following discharge (Rennick et al., 2014; Rennick, Johnston, Dougherty, Platt, & Ritchie, 2002). Potential moderators may include parental stress and anxiety and treatment complications/readmissions (Rennick et al., 2014).

Regarding the child's chronological age and developmental level, many studies have found that children between the ages of 6 months and 6 years have the most emotional distress and risk for ongoing PTSS (Perrin & Shipman, 2009), as children at this age are more likely to have an external locus of control, have fewer coping skills, and rely on adults for coping and coaching through procedures (Cohen, Bernard, Greco, & McClellan, 2002). In addition, they are the least likely to understand their illness and treatments and may view their treatments as punishment (Lerwick, 2013). Younger children tend to be most affected by fears about pain and separation from families (Coyne, 2006). Similarly, children 7–14 years of age also report fears about pain, separation from family and friends, being alone, being in an unfamiliar environment, disruption of routine, and loss of control due to the interference of hospitalization with the developmental task of achieving increased independence (Coyne, 2006; DeMaso & Snell, 2013; Wilson et al., 2010). Older children are also more likely to worry about things like mutilation or the effects of surgery on their body (Coyne, 2006). Finally, while adolescents have the cognitive resources to understand their medical condition and treatment at a more sophisticated abstract level, they might struggle emotionally during their hospitalization due to impact of illness on self-image, peer interactions, normal exploration, and achievement of independence (DeMaso & Snell, 2013).

Coping Style

Coping can be defined as specific behaviors and thoughts (coping strategies) used to allow a person to go through a situation that is perceived as stressful, such as a medical procedure (Lazarus & Folkman, 1984). Coping strategies can be voluntary (e.g., actions taken or avoided) or involuntary (e.g., physiological reactions such as increased heart rate); emotion focused (e.g., "this makes me very sad") or problem-solving (e.g., "I can handle this"); and active (e.g., engaging in activities, using distraction) or passive coping (e.g., resting, taking medication) (Blount et al., 2008). Research has shown that when medically involved children use active coping skills they have better outcomes, such as better quality of life and less psychological distress than children that use passive ones (Vervoort, Goubert, Eccleston, Bijttebier, & Crombez, 2006). Helping children adapt to medical interventions does not only impact the reactions immediately before, during, and after procedures but also may improve coping with future medical procedures. For example, children who avoid any medical information before a procedure display greater distress during the encounter phase of the medical intervention (Hubert, Jay, Saltoun, & Hayes, 1988), while an active coping style during the anticipation phase is associated with internal locus of control (Lamontagne, 1984). Finally, youth who are information-seeking about their medical experience appear to be less stressed after medical encounters than information-avoiding youth (Peterson & Toler, 1986).

Caregiver Distress and Presence

Supportive parental presence is associated with reduced child distress, shorter stays, and improved health outcomes (Perrin & Shipman, 2009; Shields, 2001). Families who were able to be present, lived closer to the hospital, and who were able to also balance outside responsibilities report the least stress related to hospitalization (Lam, Chang, & Morrissey, 2006; Stremler, Haddad, Pullenayegum, & Parshuram, 2017). Parental emotional experiences and attitudes about their child's treatment and condition are related to the child's level of stress (DeMaso & Snell, 2013; Foster, Young, Mitchell, Van, & Curtis, 2017; Maneta & DeMaso, 2017). Maternal anxiety is significantly related to a child's negative emotional and behavioral reactions. Children are calmed by families who themselves are calm (Glasper & Haggarty, 2005; Small & Melnyk, 2006), and research has shown that the amount of pain and distress children experience during medical procedures is directly related to parents' and staff's behaviors during the procedure (Cohen et al., 2002). Distress reactions in parents and children tend to increase if hospitalization is repeated (two or more admissions) or is 2 weeks or longer (Perrin & Shipman, 2009; Tsironi & Koulierakis, 2018).

Type of Admission

The type and extent of the hospitalization are important variables in their impact on children and their families. Generally, outpatient procedures are the least disruptive and stressful, even when the care is the same, and so are recommended when possible (Perrin & Shipman, 2009). At the opposite spectrum of medical involvement, the PICU is one of the most stressful experiences for youth and families compared to the general inpatient unit (Board & Ryan-Wenger, 2003; Rees, Gledhill, Garralda, & Nadel, 2004), as this experience is often accompanied by ongoing, intensive monitoring and invasive diagnostic procedures which are required to overcome an acute and frequently life-threatening health change. There can be long-term impacts from PICU stays on parents, including distress, anxiety, and depression lasting for months post discharge (Board & Ryan-Wenger, 2003; Colville & Cream, 2009). Parental report of their children's behavior following PICU hospitalization indicated reduced self-esteem and sense of well-being, social isolation, sleep disturbances, changes in friendships, medical fears, and even clinically significant post-traumatic stress and depression (Rennick & Rashotte, 2009).

Some medical hospitalizations are planned events, such as for a specialized test, surgical procedure, or ongoing treatment for a chronic illness. In these cases, parents can adequately prepare themselves and their children for the time away from home, gather information about the procedures and their medical team, and sort out other factors. However, many times, hospitalizations are the result of sudden illness or injuries sustained in an accident or traumatic event. The less prepared a family is for the hospitalization and the more uncertainty about the environment, their roles, and their child's condition, the more stress they are likely to experience (Hagstrom, 2017; Moorey, 2010).

Severity of Illness or Procedure

As one might expect, the perceived severity of the youth's condition is related to the family's level of distress as they may be associated with more invasive procedures and longer hospital stays, all of which contribute to the child's and family's distress (Foster et al., 2017; Tomlinson & Harbaugh, 2004). Ongoing PTSS and PTSD are associated with situations where families fear for their child's life (e.g., traumatic injuries, cancer diagnoses, cardiac conditions, children admitted to the PICU/NICU) (Muscara et al., 2018). However, family perception of severity is more important in predicting distress than the actual objective severity (Price et al., 2016).

Minimizing Stress

During inpatient medical admissions, it is important to focus on maintaining a sense of normalcy and assure that the developmentally appropriate psychological needs, in addition to the medical needs of the youth, are considered. As described above, social support, especially parent presence, is a significant protective factor. Rooming in for parents, visits from family/friends, time out of the medical bed/room, and involvement of child life services for diversional activities can make youth feel safe and secure in the hospital. Maintaining as much of a familiar routine as possible, such as respecting the usual family rules and limits, can help.

Supporting parents' preparation and adjustment for the hospitalization is as important an intervention as preparing the youth (DeMaso & Snell, 2013). There is a plethora of web-based and video education materials that families can access or that the medical team can provide to help youth and families better understand what to expect (Kassam-Adams et al., 2016; Kullgren, 2012). CL psychologists can help families better support their child by helping parents ask questions and get clarification from medical providers to foster their sense of control and partnership with the medical teams. This, in turn, can help families talk to their child about the medical interventions in a simple, honest, straightforward manner, therefore allowing children to ask questions, express worries, and get support. Parents can also be encouraged to "trade off" with other caregivers if possible, to allow time for self-care during longer hospital stays (DeMaso & Snell, 2013). They can also be encouraged to utilize hospital supports such as exercise rooms, chapels, and sleep resources, for example.

CL psychologists can help families be mindful of their child's developmental stage when discussing medical care with their child. For example, telling the child 1 or 2 days in advance of the hospital visit is more appropriate for a preschool-age child; school-aged children can be told about a week ahead of time, while teenagers usually do best when involved in treatment planning as it happens. Medical play with parents or with the child life specialists in the preadmission appointments are good mediums for children to learn information about medical procedures and the hospital stay. Touching and playing with medical tools can have a desensitizing effect, and providing education about the roles of the various medical care providers can have great outcomes in the child adjusting to potentially traumatic experiences. Children can also be encouraged to learn more about the members of their medical team and to communicate things about themselves to their team (e.g., favorite color, pets, and favorite foods) and to tell stories about themselves.

For medical procedure support, finding ways in which the youth can be involved (e.g., hold bandages or remove tape) can help control fears and feelings of helplessness. It helps youth to let them know what their "job" is during a procedure: being told what they can or should do, rather than what they should not do (e.g., "it is your job to try to be as still as you can," vs. "don't move"). Also, giving youth choices when possible can make them feel part of the experience. CL psychologists can help providers and families understand how to give control to the youth and formulate the questions in a way in which the answer is constructive (e.g., "which arm do you want to have the blood pressure cuff placed on?" vs. "can I take your blood pressure?"). Several coping skills can be used during difficult procedures. Active distraction is one type of strategy that works by teaching youth to focus on non-anxiety-related content to reduce distress (Stinson et al., 2008). Common types of distraction include counting backward from 100 by 7's, blowing bubbles, or playing with an iPad or computer. Another strategy involves using self-talk, which includes teaching coping statements such as "I can get through this," (DeMaso & Snell, 2013). Several relaxation strategies such as diaphragmatic breathing, progressive muscle relaxation, and hypnosis have some supportive evidence for use with children (Abel & Rouleau, 2000; Blount, Piira, & Cohen, 2003).

CL Interventions for Youth and Families in the Hospital

Psychology involvement can promote patient- and family-centered pediatric care (Kitts et al., 2013), can minimize the length of hospital stay and healthcare utilization services (Bujoreanu, White, Gerber, & Ibeziako, 2015), and can enhance and maintain successful working relationships between parents and physicians (DeMaso & Bujoreanu, 2013). In the process of working with the youth and the family, it is important to prioritize the goals of psychological intervention in the hospital setting. Consultation work requires a short-term, problem-focused type of approach to assessment, management, and treatment planning. In collaboration with the medical team, patient, and family, psychologists should consider choosing specific and significant, measurable, attainable and agreed-upon, realistic, and time-bound (SMART) goals for their treatment interventions (Doran, 1981) which can yield the most desirable outcome, specifically in the inpatient medical setting, given the available resources at that particular point in time.

A wide variety of strategies can be included under the umbrella of intervention: from providing psychoeducation about the biopsychosocial formulation and diagnostic impressions to "planting seeds" for future behavioral change via further therapeutic work, to providing specific behavior modifications and skill-building opportunities. Treatment coordination with resources and supports in the community, based on the PPPHM and Integrative PMTS model, can be an extension of the supports created in the hospital; sharing clinical impressions and rallying the available resources can create the right settings for behavior change to be reinforced and expanded upon.

Both the PPPHM and PMTS model discussed earlier in the chapter can guide assessment and intervention for families undergoing medical care, following similar approaches from universal support to targeted interventions and specific clinical treatments based on the youth and families' risk for adjustment difficulties. For families that present with normative reactions and few preexisting risk factors to the potentially traumatic medical event, the consulting psychologist should aim to reduce the subjective experience of stress (Kazak, 2006). This can be done through providing general support and facilitating the youth and family's ability to draw on their own organic support systems from family members, community supports (e.g., school, religious communities), and additional illness-related resources (e.g., survivorship groups in the context of cancer, parent consultants, families and youth who have gone through the same situation). Support for these families should also include education and guidance about the range of emotional reactions to medical events in order to normalize their experience.

Collaboration and consultation between the psychologist, medical team, and support providers regarding delivery of care can help reduce the likelihood for potentially traumatic experiences during the hospitalization and may prevent the onset of ongoing PTSS. Specifically, medical teams can help with pharmacologic interventions by delivering maximum safe sedation and pain control at the time of initial procedures to help prevent conditioned maladaptive responses to subsequent procedures (Pardesi & Fuzaylov, 2017). Collaborating with child life specialists can allow an increase in the sense of safety and control through concrete involvement of both the youth and the caregiver in the hospital care such as during medical procedures (Kazak, 2006). The PMTS Toolkit for Healthcare Providers offers a collection of concrete tools for medical professions that can be used in assessing and treating both emotional and physical medical traumatic stress in both children and families (Stuber, Schneider, Kassam-Adams, Kazak, & Saxe, 2006). After the acute phase of the medical condition and of the hospitalization, CL psychologists may further facilitate support for such youth and families via connection with outpatient behavioral medicine and medical coping clinics, patient and family advisory, and support groups.

Targeted families may need ongoing support from the consulting psychologist and may benefit from briefer, problem-focused interventions not only during hospitalization but also after leaving the hospital, as assessed by the psychologist at the time of discharge. The targeted intervention might include focused cognitive-behavioral therapy (CBT) techniques (cognitive coping strategies and psychoeducation about the impact of stress on emotional and physical functioning; identifying cognitive distortions and challenging irrational beliefs; using cognitive reframing and problem-solving strategies that focus on muscle relaxation, deep breathing, guided imagery, progressive muscle relaxation, biofeedback-assisted relaxation techniques, mindfulness, etc.). Interventions may also focus on adherence to medical regimen (e.g., behavioral contracts, rewards and consequences, environmental modifications, systematic desensitization). Specific short-term interventions have been developed for some conditions, such as 3- to 5-session social learning and cognitive-behavioral therapy intervention for youth with abdominal pain (Levy et al., 2013).

For the small subsample of families who present with multiple serious psychosocial difficulties, the most intensive level of services will be needed on an ongoing intervention basis and across healthcare teams (Kazak, 2006). These families may have multiple preexisting psychosocial stressors; higher distress and behavior problems along with other multiple risk factors, such as longer hospital stay; and communication complications with the medical team (Carter et al., 2003). In these cases, the goal of the consulting psychologist is to provide safe medical care and reduce distress. Through a biopsychosocial, developmental, and cultural formulation of the child and family, the CL psychologist can collaborate closely with medical providers to encourage and implement interventions such as consistent treatment team members, strong team leadership, and regular team and team-family meetings and ensure that staff is supporting one another. One family-systems consultation model emphasizes acceptance, respect, curiosity, and honesty (ARCH) as a way of aligning with the family to meet the mutual goals of the family and medical team (Kazak, 2006). Similarly, DeMaso and Bujoreanu (2013) outline ways to enhance working relationships between physicians and families in the context of the child's hospitalization.

Case Study

Jane Smith was a typically developing 5-year-old female who was hospitalized due to new-onset type 1 diabetes. She initially presented with vomiting, polyuria, and polydipsia. After receiving a diagnosis of type 1 diabetes, a consult was placed to psychology to evaluate family adjustment to illness, coping strategies, and need for procedural supports.

Jane lived with her mother, her 2-year-old brother, and maternal grandparents in a rural area an hour away from the hospital. Her mother was the primary caregiver, but Jane's grandparents were highly involved. Jane's mother became pregnant when she was 17 years old and has a history of depression. She was employed part time and reported finances were a challenge. Her mother noted concerns regarding a history of temper tantrums as concerning but feels these were improving with Jane's age. Her mother also noted that Jane was a social and active child.

During the consultation, Ms. Smith reported feeling upset and scared about her daughter's diagnosis. She also indicated that she had a close friend with diabetes and so knows "a little bit about it." Ms. Smith noted that she was going to need to rely on her parents to help manage Jane's diabetes due to her variable work schedule. Due to distance and transportation issues, her parents could not attend teachings in the hospital, but Ms. Smith reported that she called them so they could listen to teaching via phone. Ms. Smith reported that Jane had been upset during finger sticks and injections. Nurses noted that Ms. Smith often waited until Jane was ready or chased Jane around the room to try to get her to test her blood sugar. Ms. Smith appeared distressed when this was happening and often cried afterwards.

Ms. Smith demonstrated a number of protective factors during the consultation, which included good social support, engaging in problem-solving distance barriers (e.g., calling her parents to receive education), seeking help from her nurse, and a maintaining a strong supportive relationship with Jane. Ms. Smith also experienced significant stressors including Jane's history of behavior problems and noncompliance during the hospitalization. The family presented with additional psychosocial challenges, including distance from home to the hospital, financial stressors, and Ms. Smith's history of depression. Despite the distance and unplanned hospitalization, Ms. Smith was able to be at Jane's bedside and remain with her during the stay.

The CL psychologist met with Ms. Smith to normalize her emotional experience, discuss potential challenges, and reduce any subjective distress. During the consultation, the CL psychologist provided a brief, problem-focused intervention to address medical adherence. Ms. Smith was open to hearing about behavioral strategies such as sticker charts for adherence behaviors; using calm, direct requests; and allowing Jane's choices when possible. These strategies were demonstrated by psychology and during follow-up visits throughout the stay. Given the challenges of managing a young child with type 1 diabetes and the above-discussed stressors, at discharge, it was recommended that Ms. Smith and Jane would benefit from ongoing support and were referred to meet with psychology during their follow-up endocrine outpatient visit. The CL psychology team collaborated with Jane's primary care pediatrician where the team discovered that integrated psychology support was available, and recommendations were made that outreach to her preschool providers be made, as well. The family agreed to biweekly sessions at this office to monitor adjustment and connect them with local community supports.

Summary and Conclusions

With the advances in technology and our understanding of how to reduce stress for these young patients, the hospital experience has changed dramatically. Today, most children's hospitals tend to be colorful places with recreational activity rooms, access to computers and internet, movies, and special supportive therapies such music, art, and pet therapies. Visitors and parent presence are typically actively encouraged. There is also high value placed on patient and family privacy, resulting in a move toward single-occupant rooms. Additionally, there is growing emphasis on patient-/family-centered care as it has been shown to lead to better health outcomes, allocation of health resources, and increased patient, staff, and parent satisfaction (Committee on Hospital Care and Institute for Patient- and Family-Centered Care, 2012).

Despite these positive developments, literature suggests that hospital admissions pose significant stress and can be traumatic for many children (Shields, 2001).

Models such as the PPPHM and the Integrative PMTS are helpful for guiding the CL psychologist's approach to screening, assessment, and intervention. These models suggest that there is a range of normative reactions. Major risk factors for stress and ongoing PTSS in response to hospitalization include younger age of child, more invasive procedures, and longer and/or more frequent admissions. Parent presence is one of the most significant protective factors, providing that parents are able to manage their own distress and assist with child coping. Families with preexisting psychosocial concerns may also be at risk for ongoing distress and may benefit from services by the CL psychology team. Recommendations for minimizing distress include brief therapeutic intervention following the initial hospitalization and coordination with medical services to help decrease stress of ongoing medical regimens in the case of new-onset diagnoses (e.g., diabetes, cancer, GI disorders). There are numerous books and web-based resources available for CL providers working with families who may be experiencing stress related to hospitalization.

Appendix: Resources

The following resources have useful information, including handouts, information for medical providers, training for CL psychologists, and worksheets for use with youth and families.

Organizations

- National Child Traumatic Stress Network—www.nctsn.org
- Society of Pediatric Psychology (SPP)—Consultation/Liaison Special Interest Group.
- Trauma-Focused CBT (TF-CBT)—www.TFCBT.org

Websites

- **After the Injury**—information for parents to understand how to help children cope with injuries.
  - www.aftertheinjury.org
- **Coping Club**—website created by pediatric psychologists with patient-generated videos to help other children coping with illness and hospitalizations.
  - http://copingclub.com/tools/
- **Healthcare Toolbox**—created by the Center for Pediatric Traumatic Stress; this website has information for providers and patients about trauma informed care.
  - https://www.healthcaretoolbox.org/
- **Helping Your Child with Medical Experiences**—parent handbook to help parents prepare themselves, their child, and families for hospitalizations.
  - http://www.childrenshospital.org/-/media/Centers-and-Services/Departments-and-Divisions/Department-of-Neurology/parent_guide2.ashx?la=en&hash=A5ADD98C4AAFB67A0F0C7F419FF67890D67A9E2D
- **Kids Health**—information for children and families on a variety of healthcare-related topics.
  - https://kidshealth.org/en/kids/hospital.html

References

Abel, C. G., & Rouleau, J. L. (2000). Behavioral therapy strategies for medical patients. In A. Stoudemire, B. S. Fogel, & D. B. Greenberg (Eds.), *Psychiatric care of the medical patient* (2nd ed., pp. 61–71). Oxford, UK: Oxford University Press.

Berry, J. G., Hall, M., Hall, D. E., Kuo, D. Z., Cohen, E., Agrawal, R., … Neff, J. (2013). Inpatient growth and resource use in 28 children's hospitals: A longitudinal, multi-institutional study. *JAMA Pediatric, 167*(2), 170–177. https://doi.org/10.1001/jamapediatrics.2013.432

Blount, R. L., Piira, T., & Cohen, L. L. (2003). Management of pediatric pain and distress due to medical procedures. In M. C. Roberts (Ed.), *Handbook of pediatric psychology* (3rd ed., pp. 216–233). New York, NY: Guilford Press.

Blount, R. L., Simons, L. E., Devine, K. A., Jaaniste, T., Cohen, L. L., Chambers, C. T., & Hayutin, L. G. (2008). Evidence-based assessment of coping and stress in pediatric psychology. *Journal of Pediatric Psychology, 33*(9), 1021–1045. https://doi.org/10.1093/jpepsy/jsm071

Board, R., & Ryan-Wenger, N. (2003). Stressors and stress symptoms of mothers with children in the PICU. *Journal of Pediatric Nursing, 18*(3), 195–202. https://doi.org/10.1053/jpdn.2003.38

Bronfenbrenner, U. (1979). *The ecology of human development*. Cambridge, MA: Harvard University Press.

Bruce, M. (2006). A systematic and conceptual review of posttraumatic stress in childhood cancer survivors and their parents. *Clinical Psychology Review, 26*, 223–256. https://doi.org/10.1016/j.cpr.2005.10.002

Bujoreanu, S., White, M. T., Gerber, B., & Ibeziako, P. (2015). Effect of timing of psychiatry consultation on length of pediatric hospitalization and hospital charges. *Hospital Pediatrics, 5*(5), 269–275. https://doi.org/10.1542/hpeds.2014-0079

Carney, T., Murphy, S., McClure, J., Bishop, E., Kerr, C., Parker, J., … Wilson, L. (2003). Children's views on hospitalization: An exploratory study of data collection. *Journal of Child Health Care, 7*, 27–40. https://doi.org/10.1177/1367493503007001674

Carter, B. D., Kronenberger, W. G., Baker, J., Grimes, L. M., Crabtree, V. M., Smith, C., & McGraw, K. (2003). Inpatient pediatric consultation-liaison: A case-controlled study. *Journal of Pediatric Psychology, 28*(6), 423–432. https://doi.org/10.1093/jpepsy/jsg032.

Cohen, L. L., Bernard, R. S., Greco, L. A., & McClellan, C. B. (2002). A child-focused intervention for coping with procedural pain: Are parent and nurse coaches necessary? *Journal of Pediatric Psychology, 27*(8), 749–757. https://doi.org/10.1093/jpepsy/27.8.749.

Colville, G., & Cream, P. (2009). Post-traumatic growth in parents after a child's admission to intensive care: Maybe Nietzsche was right? *Intensive Care Medicine, 35*(5), 919–923. https://doi.org/10.1007/s00134-009-1444-1

Committee on Hospital Care and Institute for Patient- and Family-Centered Care. (2012). Patient and family-centered care and the pediatrician's role. *Pediatrics, 129*(2), 394–404. https://doi.org/10.1542/peds.2011-3084

Coyne, I. (2006). Children's experiences of hospitalization. *Journal of Children's Health Care, 10*(4), 326–336. https://doi.org/10.1177/1367493506067884

DeMaso, D. R., & Bujoreanu, I. S. (2013). Enhancing working relationships between parents and surgeons. *Seminar Pediatric Surgery, 22*(3), 139–143. https://doi.org/10.1053/j.sempedsurg.2013.05.001

DeMaso, D. R., & Snell, C. (2013). Promoting coping in children facing pediatric surgery. *Seminar Pediatric Surgery, 22*(3), 134–138. https://doi.org/10.1053/j.sempedsurg.2013.04.004

Doran, G. T. (1981). There's a S.M.A.R.T. way to write management's goals and objectives. *Management Review, 70*(11), 35–36.

Foster, K., Young, A., Mitchell, R., Van, C., & Curtis, K. (2017). Experiences and needs of parents of critically injured children during the acute hospital phase: A qualitative investigation. *Injury, 48*(1), 114–120. https://doi.org/10.1016/j.injury.2016.09.034

Glasper, E. A., & Haggarty, R. E. (2005). The psychological preparation of children for hospitalization (Chapter 5). In E. A. Glasper & J. Richardson (Eds.), *A textbook of children's and young people's nursing* (pp. 61–76). Edinburgh, UK: Churchill and Livingstone.

Hagstrom, S. (2017). Family stress in pediatric critical care. *Journal of Pediatric Nursing, 32*, 32–40. https://doi.org/10.1016/j.pedn.2016.10.007

Hubert, N. C., Jay, S. M., Saltoun, M., & Hayes, M. (1988). Approach-avoidance and distress in children undergoing preparation for painful medical procedures. *Journal of Clinical Child Psychology, 17*(3), 194–202. https://doi.org/10.1207/s15374424jccp1703_1

Justus, R., Wyles, D., Wilson, J., Rode, D., Walther, V., & Lim-Sulit, N. (2006). Preparing children and families for surgery: Mount Sinai's multidisciplinary perspective. *Pediatric Nursing, 32*(1), 35–43.

Kassam-Adams, N., Marsac, M., Kohser, K., Kenardy, J., March, S., & Winston, F. (2016). Pilot randomized controlled trial of a novel web-based intervention to prevent posttraumatic stress in children following medical events. *Journal of Pediatric Psychology, 41*(1), 138–148. https://doi.org/10.1093/jpepsy/jsv057

Kazak, A. E. (2005). Evidence-based interventions for survivors of childhood cancer and their families. *Journal of Pediatric Psychology, 30*(1), 29–39. https://doi.org/10.1093/jpepsy/jsi013

Kazak, A. E. (2006). Pediatric psychosocial preventative health model (PPPHM): Research, practice, and collaboration in pediatric family systems medicine. *Families, Systems & Health, 24*(4), 381–395. https://doi.org/10.1037/1091-7527.24.4.381

Kazak, A. E., Kassam-Adams, N., Schneider, S., Zelikovsky, N., Alderfer, M. A., & Rourke, M. (2006). An integrative model of pediatric medical traumatic stress. *Journal of Pediatric Psychology, 31*(4), 343–355. https://doi.org/10.1093/jpepsy/jsj054

Kazak, A. E., Rourke, M. T., Alderfer, M. A., Pai, A., Reilly, A. F., & Meadows, A. T. (2007). Evidence-based assessment, intervention and psychosocial care in pediatric oncology: A blueprint for comprehensive services across treatment. *Journal of Pediatric Psychology, 32*(9), 1099–1110. https://doi.org/10.1093/jpepsy/jsm031

Kitts, R. L., Gallagher, K., Ibeziako, P., Bujoreanu, S., Garcia, G., & DeMaso, D. R. (2013). Parent and young adult satisfaction with psychiatry consultation services in a children's hospital. *Psychosomatics, 54*(6), 575–584. https://doi.org/10.1016/j.psym.2013.01.008

Kullgren, K. (2012). *Helping a child cope with a long hospitalization*. Ann Arbor, MI: University of Michigan CS Mott Children's Hospital. Retrieved from https://www.youtube.com/watch?v=NvDIdRZNJlg

Lam, L. W., Chang, A. M., & Morrissey, J. (2006). Parents' experiences of participation in the care of hospitalised children: A qualitative study. *International Journal of Nursing Studies, 43*(5), 535–545. https://doi.org/10.1016/j.ijnurstu.2005.07.009

Lamontagne, L. L. (1984). Children's locus of control beliefs as predictors of preoperative coping behavior. *Nursing Research, 33*(2), 76–79., 85. https://doi.org/10.1097/00006199-198403000-00004

Lazarus, R. S., & Folkman, S. (1984). *Stress, appraisal, and coping*. New York, NY: Springer.

Lerwick, J. L. (2013). Psychosocial implications of pediatric surgical hospitalization. *Seminars in Pediatric Surgery, 22*(3), 129–133. https://doi.org/10.1053/j.sempedsurg.2013.04.003

Levy, R. L., Langer, S. L., Walker, L. S., Romano, J. M., Christie, D. L., Youssef, N., … Whitehead, W. E. (2013). Twelve-month follow-up of cognitive behavioral therapy for children with functional abdominal pain. *JAMA Pediatrics, 167*(2), 178–184. https://doi.org/10.1001/2013.jamapediatrics.282

Lindeke, L., Nakai, M., & Johnson, L. (2006). Capturing children's voices for quality improvement. *MCN: The American Journal of Maternal Child Nursing, 31*(5), 290-295. https://doi.org/10.1097/00005721-200609000-00005

Maneta, E. K., & DeMaso, D. R. (2017). Depression in medically ill children. In D. S. Arthur & J. Barsky (Eds.), *Depression in medical illness* (p. 387). New York, NY: McGraw-Hill Education.

Moorey, S. (2010). Unplanned hospital admission: Supporting children, young people and their families. *Paediatric Nursing, 22*(10), 20–23. https://doi.org/10.7748/paed2010.12.22.10.20.c8133

Muscara, F., McCarthy, M. C., Hearps, S. J., Nicholson, J. M., Burke, K., … Anderson, V. A. (2018). Trajectories of posttraumatic stress symptoms in parents of children with a serious childhood illness or injury. *Journal of Pediatric Psychology, 43*, 1072–1082. https://doi.org/10.1093/jpepsy/jsy035

National Child Traumatic Stress Network (2018). National Child Traumatic Stress Network. Retrieved October 2, 2018, from https://www.nctsn.org/

Pardesi, O., & Fuzaylov, G. (2017). Pain management in pediatric burn patients: Review of recent literature and future directions. *Journal of Burn Care & Research, 38*(6), 335–347. https://doi.org/10.1097/BCR.0000000000000470

Perrin, E. C., & Shipman, D. (2009). Hospitalization, surgery, and medical and dental procedures. In W. B. Carey et al. (Eds.), *Developmental-behavioral pediatrics* (4th ed., pp. 329–336). Philadelphia, PA: Saunders/Elsevier.

Peterson, L., & Toler, S. M. (1986). An information seeking disposition in child surgery patients. *Health Psychology, 5*(4), 343–358. https://doi.org/10.1037/0278-6133.5.4.343

Price, J., Kassam-Adams, N., Alderfer, M. A., Christofferson, J., & Kazak, A. E. (2016). Systematic review: A reevaluation and update of the integrative (trajectory) model of pediatric medical traumatic stress. *Journal of Pediatric Psychology, 41*(1), 86–97. https://doi.org/10.1093/jpepsy/jsv074

Rees, G., Gledhill, J., Garralda, M. E., & Nadel, S. (2004). Psychiatric outcome following paediatric intensive care unit (PICU) admission: A cohort study. *Intensive Care Medicine, 30*(8), 1607–1614. https://doi.org/10.1007/s00134-004-2310-9

Rennick, J. E., Dougherty, G., Chambers, C., Stremler, R., Childerhose, J. E., Stack, D. M., … Hutchison, J. (2014). Children's psychological and behavioral responses following pediatric intensive care unit hospitalization: The caring intensively study. *BMC Pediatrics, 14*, 276. https://doi.org/10.1186/1471-2431-14-276.

Rennick, J. E., Johnston, C. C., Dougherty, G., Platt, R., & Ritchie, J. A. (2002). Children's psychological responses after critical illness and exposure to invasive technology. *Journal of Developmental & Behavioral Pediatrics, 23*(3), 133–144. https://doi.org/10.1097/00004703-200206000-00002

Rennick, J. E., & Rashotte, J. (2009). Psychological outcomes in children following pediatric intensive care unit hospitalization: A systematic review of the research. *Journal of Children's Health Care, 13*(2), 128–149. https://doi.org/10.1177/1367493509102472

Shields, L. (2001). A review of the literature from developed and developing countries relating to the effects of hospitalization on children and parents. *International Nursing Review, 48*(1), 29–37. https://doi.org/10.1046/j.1466-7657.2001.00032.x

Small, L., & Melnyk, B. M. (2006). Early predictors of post-hospital adjustment problems in critically ill young children. *Research in Nursing & Health, 29*(6), 622–635. https://doi.org/10.1002/nur.20169

Stinson, J., Yamada, J., Dickson, A., Lamba, J., & Stevens B. (2008). Review of systemic reviews on acute procedural pain in children in the hospital setting. *Pain Research and Management, 13*, 51–57.

Stremler, R., Haddad, S., Pullenayegum, E., & Parshuram, C. (2017). Psychological outcomes in parents of critically ill hospitalized children. *Journal of Pediatric Nursing, 34*, 36–43. https://doi.org/10.1016/j.pedn.2017.01.012

Stuber, M. L., Schneider, S., Kassam-Adams, N., Kazak, A. E., & Saxe, G. (2006). The medical traumatic stress toolkit. *CNS Spectrum, 11*(2), 137–142.

Stuber, M. L., Shemesh, E., & Saxe, G. N. (2003). Posttraumatic stress responses in children with life-threatening illnesses. *Child and Adolescent Psychiatric Clinics of North America, 12*(2), 195–209. https://doi.org/10.1016/S1056-4993(02)00100-1

Tomlinson, P. S., & Harbaugh, B. L. (2004). Assessing ambiguity at the family–nurse boundary interface in pediatric health crisis. *Journal of Pediatric Nursing, 19*(6), 399–410. https://doi.org/10.1016/j.pedn.2004.11.004

Tsironi, S., & Koulierakis, G. (2018). Factors associated with parents' levels of stress in pediatric wards. *Journal of Child Health Care, 22*(2), 175–185. https://doi.org/10.1177/1367493517749327

Van Horn, M., DeMaso, D.R., Gonzalez-Heydrich, J, Erickson, J.D. (2001). Illness-related concerns of mothers of children with congenital heart disease. *Journal of the American Academy of Child & Adolescent Psychiatry, 40*, 847–854. https://doi.org/10.1097/00004583-200107000-00020.

Vernon, D. T., & Thompson, R. H. (1993). Research on the effect of experimental interventions on children's behavior after hospitalization: A review and synthesis. *Journal of Developmental and Behavioral Pediatrics, 14*(1), 36-44.

Vervoort, T., Goubert, L., Eccleston, C., Bijttebier, P., & Crombez, G. (2006). Catastrophic thinking about pain is independently associated with pain severity, disability, and somatic complaints in school children and children with chronic pain. *Journal of Pediatric Psychology, 31*(7), 674–683.

Vessey, J. A. (2003). Children's psychological responses to hospitalization. *Annual Review of Nursing Research, 21*, 173–201. https://doi.org/10.1891/0739-6686.21.1.173

Wilson, M. E., Megel, M. E., Enenbach, L., & Carlson, K. L. (2010). The voices of children: Stories about hospitalization. *Journal of Pediatric Health Care, 24*(2), 95–102. https://doi.org/10.1016/j.pedhc.2009.02.008

Witt, W. P., Weiss, A. J., & Elixhauser, A. (2014). Overview of hospital stays for children in the United States, 2012: Statistical brief #187. In *Healthcare Cost and Utilization Project (HCUP) statistical briefs*. Rockville, MD: Agency for Healthcare Research and Quality.

Medical Subspecialty Clinic Consultation-Liaison

Dawn Dore-Stites and Jennifer Butcher

Advances in medicine expanded pediatric care to include management of both transient infectious disease and chronic illness (Shulman, 2004). While many children with chronic health conditions were once treated in acute care settings, the standard of care is now medical subspecialty clinics targeting individual diseases such as diabetes, cystic fibrosis, and inflammatory bowel disease or medical systems such as pulmonology, rheumatology, and cardiology. Along with this shift, pediatric specialists have recognized the value of a comprehensive holistic perspective to improve health outcomes and address patient adjustment/functioning. Attention has further broadened to include addressing the quality of life of children with chronic health conditions and their families, leading medical subspecialty clinics to integrate multidisciplinary providers with expertise beyond treating core medical symptoms.

Pediatric psychology as a subspecialty in clinical psychology has emerged and grown to a great degree in response to this shift in perspective. With expertise in understanding the biopsychosocial factors contributing to child health and wellness, an applied understanding of child development and family systems, as well as training in program development and evaluation, pediatric psychologists are uniquely poised to contribute to the optimal care of children served by medical subspecialty facilities. Relative to more acute care settings, pediatric psychologists integrated into subspecialty clinics have opportunities to provide in-depth and developmentally sensitive longitudinal care across the critical early life span transitioning into adulthood, responsive to both the shared and unique aspects of the child's chronic health condition.

The Chronic Care Model Applied to the Subspecialty Clinic Setting

Several models have been proposed that conceptualize the comprehensive management of pediatric chronic illness, ranging from those addressing individual health behavior change (Ng et al., 2018) to advocating for changes in the broader health-care delivery systems (Grover & Johsi, 2015; Wagner, 1998). One of the most researched models, the Chronic Care Model (CCM; Grover & Johsi, 2015), targets needs specific to patients with chronic illnesses including symptom management, addressing the emotional aspects of health conditions/treatments, and facilitating needed lifestyle modifications (Wagner et al., 2001). CCM posits several components that have

D. Dore-Stites (✉) · J. Butcher
Department of Pediatrics, C.S. Mott Children's Hospital, University of Michigan Medical School, Ann Arbor, MI, USA
e-mail: dawndore@med.umich.edu

B. D. Carter, K. A. Kullgren (eds.), *Clinical Handbook of Psychological Consultation in Pediatric Medical Settings*, Issues in Clinical Child Psychology, https://doi.org/10.1007/978-3-030-35598-2_5

been shown to improve health outcomes in patients with chronic illness including patient-oriented (e.g., self-management support), provider-oriented (e.g., decision support through continuing education and algorithms to standardize care), and system-oriented (e.g., managing patient flow; increased collaboration with community resources) components (Wagner et al., 2001). Elements of CCM have been widely researched and incorporated into patient-centered home models (Coleman, Austin, Brach, & Wagner, 2009). For subspecialty pediatric clinics, CCM supports a multidisciplinary approach to improving patient outcomes focusing on improving patient self-management, addressing systems-level factors that impact health outcomes, and fostering increased provider collaboration.

The following clinical scenario illustrates elements of the CCM that guide care for patients with chronic illness and outlines the skills needed by the consulting psychologist practicing within a pediatric subspecialty clinic: *A pediatric psychologist presents for a routine subspecialty clinic for pediatric patients with type I diabetes (T1D). The rest of the clinic multidisciplinary team consists of two pediatric endocrinologists, two certified diabetes educators (CDEs), a dietitian, and social worker. The team works together in a shared space when seeing patients and also has weekly team meetings for reviewing systems-related concerns (e.g., concerns in clinic flow). The clinic is housed within an academic medical center serving a large geographic area.* In the case of the above example diabetes clinic, a more traditional focus purely on medical disease management, minus the expanded focus advocated from the CCM approach (e.g., dietary, behavioral, social), would likely lead to diminished disease control and patient dissatisfaction with care (Wagner, 1998).

Multidisciplinary teams in pediatric subspecialty clinics. Multidisciplinary care involves collaboration among several different professions (e.g., pediatricians/pediatric subspecialists, psychologists, nursing, patient educators, speech/occupational/physical therapists, dietitians, social workers) ideally operating in concert toward specified health-related outcomes in a particular patient population (Conroy & Logan, 2014). In some medical settings, each discipline may conduct their own assessments and interventions within the scope of their individual practice while collaborating via team meetings and/or conferences where each shares their respective observations and recommendations. In other settings, professionals may see the patient in tandem (for at least a portion of the medical visit) so that each discipline can observe the same behaviors and interactions and collaborate on-site so that decisions and recommendations can be fully informed by the perspective of each contributing professional.

Conroy and Logan (2014) described the features of a successful multidisciplinary team as all members having a shared vision for their practice, the involvement of integration of all members of the team with frequent interaction, clear and effective communication skills, and competent leadership. Thus, it is important that each team member has a clear understanding of how their team functions, as well as the unique perspectives and roles and competencies of individual providers on the team.

In our example diabetes clinic embracing the CCM philosophy, team members find that operating in shared clinic space facilitates communication between providers and allows for more collaboration. The structure of weekly meetings also encourages strategic planning around organizational concerns that impact both patients and providers. Such logistical and structural considerations help provide opportunities to better communicate, hear one another's perspectives, and problem-solve in ways that improve and strengthen the team and improve patient care (Table 1).

Of the 24 patients on the afternoon schedule, 2 are new patients that have been diagnosed with T1D within the past 2 weeks. The remaining are established patients for return visits. During the start of clinic when all team members are in the shared space preparing to start their clinical responsibilities, the psychologist briefly consults with the larger team in order to identify those patients she needs to prioritize in her schedule.

Table 1 Characteristics of an effective team

Characteristic of effective MD team	Role of pediatric psychologist
Collaboration around vision for clinic and goals	Drafting proposals of statements capturing goals for clinic Identifying goals that are measurable Ensuring psychosocial goals are captured within broader vision for clinic
Integration into team	Seeking out consult from other providers to foster collaboration Identifying opportunities for further integration including in areas not necessarily recognized by other providers (e.g., research, QI projects)
Frequent interaction among team members	Being present in clinics and team meetings—even if not obligatory Sending copies of outpatient notes to other members of the team to ensure coordination of care
Strong communication and trust between team members	Modeling good communication skills and professionalism in all details of work from patient care to team dynamics Identifying ways to modify communication to address unique needs of patients and team members (e.g., education on communication around psychosocial stressors to team, modifications of patient handouts to address limited health literacy)
Appropriate structure	Assessing for problems with communication among team (e.g., decisions made without larger collaboration)
Competent leadership	Serving in a leadership capacity within the team Maintaining knowledge in new developments within scope of practice

Adapted from Conroy and Logan (2014)

From the CCM perspective, it is essential to incorporate nonbiologically driven factors that impact the course of care into assessment and management, a role well-suited to the team pediatric psychologist. While the complexity of self-management requirements varies widely between chronic health conditions, they often fall into the following broad categories: adherence to medical regimens (both taking medications and lifestyle modifications), recognizing and reporting symptom changes, responding to acute symptom developments appropriately, and skills at navigating the health-care system. Patient/family competence in addressing these situations is heavily influenced by factors such as developmental changes in the patient, overall functioning of the family, mental health concerns (both patient and caregivers), disease characteristics, and interactions with health-care providers (LaGreca & Mackey, 2009).

Prioritizing in Subspecialty Care

In order for the CL pediatric psychologist to best determine which of the 24 scheduled patients would best benefit from her services that day, she employs multiple methods including review of medical records and blood glucose logs while also approaching other team members, and even parents of the patients, for their input. Not every child or adolescent presenting to the subspecialty clinic will require direct services from the pediatric psychologist. In fact, some behavioral and psychosocial concerns that respond well to direct guidance and supportive counseling may be effectively addressed by other team members, particularly when the psychologist is available to "float" in the clinic and be available to consult with these providers. Thus, the diabetes clinic's model allows the consulting psychologist to prioritize seeing patients having more severe behavioral concerns/issues, e.g., those related to treatment adherence. Overall, the psychologist's prioritization involves identifying patients that may benefit from behavioral supports to increase self-management and assessing the urgency of each patient's behavioral support needs. Methods to achieve these goals can include both subjective review and systematic screening procedures.

Subjective review. The process of conducting a subjective review to prioritize patients to be seen entails surveying the schedule and medical record and/or communicating with team members to identify patients demonstrating factors associated with poor health or behavioral outcomes. Specific to T1D (see chapter "Diabetes", this volume), medical variables that present as red flags may include elevated HgbA1c (A1c; 3-month average of blood glucose), significant increase in A1c (regardless of value), weight loss and/or frequent ED visits, and/or hospitalizations for diabetes-related concerns. Poor adherence behaviors (e.g., infrequent blood glucose monitoring, failure to routinely perform carb counts) and/or psychosocial risk factors (e.g., family conflict, academic performance decline or difficulties) can be derived both from team communication and thorough review of other providers' notes.

Systematic screening. Universal screening has typically focused on the assessment of family psychosocial risks and adolescent mood/adjustment, which have both been associated with suboptimal health outcomes. One evidence-supported tool for assessing family functioning is the Psychosocial Assessment Tool (PAT), originally developed for use within a pediatric cancer setting (Kazak et al., 2001) and since adapted and validated with other chronic illness groups including solid organ transplant (Cousino et al., 2018; Pai, Tackett, Ittenbach, & Goebel, 2012) and acute, life-threatening pediatric illness (McCarthy et al., 2016). Adolescent depression screening using a variety of measures has been adopted in a number of health-care settings, including primary care (Zuckerbrot, Cheung, Jensen, Stein, & Laraque, 2018), and subspecialty settings (Corathers et al., 2013; Guilfoyle, Monahan, Wesolowski, & Modi, 2015).

Utilization of formalized screening instruments targeting known risk factors should be considered, particularly in high-volume clinical settings and/or where pediatric psychology may not be available to all patients due to patient volume/flow and time constraints. Screening programs can also target common clinic concerns and identify which providers will see which patients. Development of standardization in practice, including screening and intervention, is also a means to improve patient care (see chapter "Assessment in Pediatric Psychology Consultation-Liaison", this volume).

Logistical considerations. Variables including clinic flow and funding of pediatric psychology services should also be on the radar of the pediatric psychologist when determining which patients to prioritize. Many consulting psychologists operate within busy clinics serving high patient volumes necessitating brief assessment and intervention. This approach minimizes burden on the family due to lengthy appointment times and avoids interfering with care provided by other team members. Additionally, funding of pediatric psychology services within specialty clinics varies widely. Funding models range from medical centers underwriting/absorbing the costs of psychology services completely through provider requirements to fund programs with external sources (e.g., billing patients, grant funding). Funding models can impact clinical care delivery if the financial resources are tied to a particular patient population, i.e., if the pediatric psychology services are only covered by specific payors (e.g., Medicaid), thus excluding patients whose coverage does not include pediatric psychology.

Outside of the two patients newly diagnosed, the CDE notes concerns about adherence behaviors (decreased blood glucose checks, decreased insulin dosages) in one patient presenting for routine return visit. A second patient was prioritized by the psychologist to facilitate continuity of care around behavioral issues presenting in past visits. The clinic also uses the Patient Health Questionnaire-9 (PHQ-9) as a screener for depressive symptoms in patients aged 13–17. During the course of the afternoon clinic, two additional patients are identified as in need of prioritizing due to elevated scores in the clinical level. One of them endorses suicidal ideation.

Intervention in Pediatric Subspecialty Practice

Universal screening can be the sieve that identifies children needing further assessment and possible psychosocial intervention. Increasingly, standardized intervention programs targeting improved functional outcomes for children diagnosed with chronic health conditions have been developed. One such example is the Children's Health and Illness Recovery Program (CHIRP; Carter, Kronenberger, Scott, & Brady, 2020;

Carter, Kronenberger, Threlkeld, Townsend, & Pruitt, 2013), a 12-session manualized cognitive-behavioral/family systems intervention that has been shown to be an effective treatment for improving functioning and reducing symptoms of fatigue and pain in adolescent patients with chronic health conditions. Teens and parents completing CHIRP have reported highly favorable ratings of the helpfulness of the intervention in improving symptoms and overall daily functioning. The CHIRP intervention is not disease-specific, instead focusing on skill development in stress management, coping, communication and assertive behaviors, and family roles and parental support of increased teen independent functioning.

Other empirically supported interventions can be modified to the needs of the child with chronic illness. For instance, gradual exposure can be utilized for patients with needle anxiety requiring infusions. Aspects of parent training programs can be modified to address child cooperation with medical regimen tasks. As a third example, the Transtheoretical Stages of Change Model and associated motivational interviewing strategies have been translated from addiction research to chronic illness as a way to gauge and promote change in health behaviors (e.g., Gelfand et al., 2004).

Our example diabetes clinic is a 4-hour clinic, and six patients have been prioritized to be seen either by the consulting psychologist individually through systematic screening or by direct referral from other team members. Inevitably, this necessitates a focus on brief assessment and intervention strategies in order to maximize the impact of psychologist services with the prioritized patients within the time frame of the afternoon clinic. Therefore, the end decision is to determine whether the problem is amenable to brief contact in clinic or in need of more intensive outpatient services. Additional resources relevant to common presenting concerns seen in subspecialty pediatric clinics are illustrated in Table 2.

New-onset diagnosis. In our example diabetes clinic, a team decision was made that all providers meet all patients newly diagnosed with T1D. In preparation, patients are prepared for a longer first visit in order to accommodate this process. At one point in each newly diagnosed diabetes patient's visit, the psychologist conducts a structured interview that assesses areas associated with potential deleterious outcomes. The goal of the assessment is to identify risk and resiliency factors that guide the prioritization of specialty services over the next several visits. One of the two patients, a 10-year-old male, presents with minimal risk factors and several protective factors, including parents who are managing the stress of diagnosis well, limited behavioral concerns from the child that could impact adherence, and significant social support. In the case of this patient, the psychologist's recommendations are for a review of progress at a clinic visit in 6 months, allowing time to determine if psychosocial issues arise.

In contrast, the screening assessment of the newly diagnosed 4-year-old male reveals several risk factors, including sleep difficulties and dysregulated behaviors that have worsened since his T1D diagnosis. During the visit, the parents appear tense and express guilt that they had missed early signs of T1D. Finally, both parents mention that they are encountering difficulties navigating time off from work. The psychologist discusses meeting with them for a longer visit prior to their T1D education class (in approximately 2 weeks) for additional support. To address the parents' concerns related to their jobs, collaboration occurred with the clinic social worker who met with the parents separately to discuss documentation needed for the Family Medical Leave Act (FMLA).

Adherence concerns. At our example diabetes clinic, one of the CDEs identifies a 17-year-old male diagnosed 4 years prior as having significant changes in frequency of blood glucose checks relative to his last visit. The psychologist meets with the family to determine if there have been any new stressors or life changes since the last visit that may relate to his decreased adherence. The parents mention that the patient recently started an after-school job that has necessitated scheduling changes in which he returns home from school, grabs a quick snack, and then goes to work. He returns home after

Table 2 Brief assessment and intervention within subspecialty clinics

Presenting concern	Selected resources
Assessment: adherence	Duncan, Mentrikoski, Wu, and Fredericks (2014) Quittner et al. (2008)
Assessment: risk behaviors	Suicide: Columbia Suicide Severity Rating Scale (Kelly et al., 2011) Substance use: CRAFFT (Knight, Sherritt, Shrier, Harris, & Chang, 2002) General: HEEADSSS (Doukrou & Segal, 2018)
Assessment: other	The website of Division 54 (Society of Pediatric Psychology) of the American Psychological Association maintains resources around assessment of above areas as well as other domains. Website address is www.societyofpediatricpsychology.org
Intervention: adherence	Duncan et al. (2014) Pai and McGrady (2014)
Intervention: other presenting concerns	Duncan et al. (2014) outline approach to interventions delivered in clinic settings

dinner is served and retreats to his room to do homework. The father states "we don't see him at all" during the school week.

As this behavior is a relatively new change, and there appears to be a direct correlation between the start of the job and decreased blood glucose checking, the focus of the consultation is on increased problem-solving around adherence and increased parental monitoring. The patient agrees to set alarms on his phone after school and, upon his return home before heading to his job, to check his blood glucose. In addition, he agrees to having his parents review his meter readings 2–3 times per week to examine trends in his monitoring and discuss strategies to support increased checks. Agreement is made between the psychologist, the patient, and his family to review his blood glucose monitoring by phone in 1 month in order to determine if the intervention was effective. This plan is documented in the comprehensive summary of recommendations by all disciplines and reiterated to the family by the final provider (physician) seeing the patient.

Behavior problems. At our diabetes clinic, a 6-year-old female has been seen the CL psychologist several times since diagnosis at age four, due to repeated parent concerns with her "not wanting to listen." Standard assessment revealed behavioral concerns pre-diagnosis including difficulties complying with parent requests, bedtime problems, and selective eating. She is now 6 years old and compliance with parent requests and bedtime problems persists. She remains a selective eater; however, it has not negatively impacted her T1D care. Poor compliance with parental requests has intermittently adversely impacted her adherence. The family travels over 3 h to clinic from a rural community.

Previous referrals have been made for behavioral support in her local area with notable difficulties in finding providers using evidence-based approaches to her externalizing problems. Her parents attempted treatment on one occasion, but these services were more supportive in nature and the therapist did not involve the parents. The parents saw little change in patient behavior and terminated treatment. The CL psychologist decides to see the family to provide psychoeducation on principles of behaviorally based parent management training including child-directed play, differential attention, and giving effective commands. Each topic is distilled down to 10–15 min of instruction with modeling and handouts provided to the family at the end of the session.

Positive screen on PHQ-9. In our example diabetes clinic, during today's clinic, the psychologist consults with the team social worker to determine if follow-up is needed on a 15-year-old female patient whose PHQ-9 score was elevated. In the clinic, PHQ-9 scores ≥10 lead to same-day assessment by either social work or psychology, modeled after a published pathway (Corathers et al., 2013). The individual provider conducting the follow-up is determined by clinical availability, with decisions made at the time of the screening assessment in the clinic. For the 15-year-old female diabetes patient with an elevated score, but no suicidal ideation, it was decided that the clinic social worker would follow up on the elevated score as they had been in recent contact with the family due to the death of a parent.

A second positively screened patient, a 14-year-old male, endorses suicidal ideation. Determination was made when initiating the use of PHQ-9 in clinic that psychology would be the default provider to conduct a follow-up when suicidal ideation was reported. A semi-structured interview crafted by the consulting psychologist through review of the Columbia Suicide Severity Rating Scale (Kelly et al., 2011) and other resources identifying risk factors for suicide is administered to more thoroughly assess risk. Through this interview, it is determined that the patient is at low risk for suicide but does not currently have an outside mental health provider. State confidentiality laws mandate that child suicidal ideation be communicated to parents, and the psychologist does this in concert with the patient. Given the absence of a mental health provider for monitoring and follow-up, the parent is provided with a list of mental health resources in their local area. In addition, the psychologist maintains a portion of their schedule within an outpatient pediatric psychology clinic at the same academic medical center housing the T1D clinic. This allows the psychologist the flexibility of scheduling more intensive follow-up appointments with patients at risk on an as needed basis. The psychologist schedules the patient to be seen in that clinic setting in 1 week to follow up on recommendations and provide monitoring during the inevitable wait for services elsewhere.

Within the diabetes clinic, the pediatric endocrinologist is the last to see the patient in order to have all recommendations from the team integrated into one message. For a newly diagnosed patient, there are several pieces of information shared by the family including details of the mother's recent promotion leading to frequent travel, behavioral concerns of the child at preschool, problems with sleep, and the father's recent treatment for alcohol addiction.

In this fast-paced clinic setting, there may be only minutes to summarize the finding of a complex interview, formulate the case, and make pertinent recommendations to the team. For the CL pediatric psychologist, it is important to prioritize what information to share in this context. Competent clinical judgement is required in targeting those variables impacting care. Imagine two presentations of the information in the above case. In the first scenario, details known to more directly impact T1D care (child behavioral problems, disrupted routines due to new travel of mother) are summarized briefly. In the second scenario, intimate details of the mother's work, the father's addiction, and the patient's behavior in the consulting room are shared. While the details in the latter presentation may be interesting, they may not be the most relevant to medical decision-making at the time. It is important that the psychologist be skilled at clearly and concisely communicating the factors leading to their recommendations to the multidisciplinary team while striking a balance between respect for the family and understanding what the team needs to know to best inform care.

Documentation within the electronic medical record (EMR) is another method for capturing and communicating important information that can facilitate coordinated care between providers. With the integration of EMRs, most psychology notes are visible to all members of the medical team and even the larger medical community at that institution. One risk of this development is that psychologist clinical entries into the medical chart may not functionally have the protection that they had in the past. This raises questions about what is appropriate for a patient's note (Richards, 2009; see chapter "Advocacy in Pediatric Psychological Consultation", this volume). Questions to consider are numerous with the first being the amount of detail that should be provided. Whether stressors involving others outside of the patient (e.g. sibling behavior concerns) should be documented should take into account the possibility of the patient later requesting their medical record and becoming privy to such information.

Competencies and Skills Needed Within the Subspecialty Clinic

Regardless of setting, competencies provide a critical foundation for CL pediatric psychology practice (see Palermo et al., 2014). For providers within multidisciplinary settings, including those within subspecialty clinics, it is also helpful to review models outlined by professions outside of psychology, such as the Interprofessional Education Collaborative (Ward, Zagoloff, Rieck, & Robiner, 2018). It is important that the CL psychologist be attuned to the issues and competencies pertinent to their pediatric colleagues, such as trainee issues and shared goals important to the collaborative process (Ward, Shaffer, & Testa, 2018).

Significant overlap exists in the competencies required of pediatric psychologists in different medical settings. Specific to pediatric subspecialty practice, it is critical that the consulting psychologist become knowledgeable and skilled at addressing the multitude of psychosocial issues associated with the specific medical conditions seen in their practice group. This includes such factors as the pathophysiology of the condition, common treatment approaches, the cognitive-behavioral impact of medications and/or the disease process, symptoms warranting concern, and prognosis. Using our example diabetes clinic, the behaviors associated with the common presenting concern of "nonadherence" may appear similar (e.g., omitting insulin). However, one patient may skip insulin doses due to embarrassment at giving injections in front of peers, whereas another patient may engage in the same behavior in an effort to lose weight due to body image issues. Understandably, it is important for the consulting psychologist to acquire mastery of these factors in their chosen area of specialization in order to be optimally effective and their input be highly valued by the multidisciplinary team.

Table 3 presents a listing of competencies outlined by Conroy and Logan (2014) with links to additional resources and behavioral examples.

Table 3 Competencies in subspecialty care:associated resources and behavioral examples

Competency	Further information for pediatric psychologists	Behavioral examples: pediatric psychology
Expertise in discipline	Palermo et al. (2014) outline 10 crosscutting knowledge competencies in pediatric psychology	• Recognition of variant of normal child behavior vs. emerging psychopathology • Understanding of empirically supported treatments in child psychology and pediatric psychology • Describing basic behavioral principles that may be impacting child's actions
Understanding of medical condition of focus of team	*Handbook of Pediatric Psychology* (fourth edition) has several chapters detailing both medical and psychosocial factors related to chronic medical conditions	• Listing the basic physiological foundation of condition • Knowing the common lab values associated with optimal care • Understanding how the commonly used medications in the condition may impact behaviors or cognitive functioning
Strong communication and social skills	Ward et al. (2018) outline several behaviors associated with communication as proposed by the Interprofessional Education Collaborative Expert Panel (IECEP)	• Checking in with team members about an observed emotional response to a patient • Understanding when conversation may be better equipped to manage conflict rather than email exchanges • Running meetings among team members that are focused

Adapted from Conroy and Logan (2014)

Specific to pediatric subspecialty clinic practice, the consulting pediatric psychologist's skills can contribute to several elements critical to implementation of the CCM including promotion of patient self-management, identification of organizational changes leading to improved outcomes, and training other providers in behavioral health components.

Improving patient self-management. Improving patient self-management, as well as caregiver management, is understandably one of the more obvious expectations of CL psychologists involved in chronic illness subspecialty care. Skills critical to enhancing an individual patient's self-care behaviors include assessing the potential function of nonadherent behaviors, joining with and communicating effectively at an appropriate developmental level with children and adolescents and their parents, identifying potential "red flags" that predict suboptimal outcomes, and having access to state-of-the-art evidence-base information, resources, and peer consultation.

Identifying opportunities for organizational change. As a pediatric psychologist on a subspecialty team, there are multiple opportunities to actively collaborate on systems-related issues such as programmatic changes to clinic procedures and environment. While such opportunities are not exclusive to the subspecialty setting, features that differentiate subspecialty clinics include generally smaller patient populations (relative to primary care) and less heterogeneity medically (compared with inpatient medical settings). Psychologists are often skilled at developing screening programs, and the pediatric psychologist may be called on to identify appropriate measures, develop algorithms directing care in specific instances (e.g., if a patient reports elevated score on a screen for depression), consult on logistical issues related to measure administration (e.g., preserving confidentiality of measures), and collaborate on quality improvement projects centered around the screening. Consultation related to interventions also presents from development (e.g., identification of protocols) through implementation (e.g., who delivers treatment). Additional skills required include understanding funding and reimbursement mechanisms and developing collaborative relationships with administrative/billing personnel. Such skills are critical to sustaining programs and often to ensuring job security.

Training to other providers. Effective teaching skills are also beneficial to psychologists within subspecialty settings to promote more collaborative and comprehensive care among all providers. Some common techniques in behavioral change (e.g., prioritizing goals), patient communication (e.g., use of "teach back" to evaluate receipt of recommendations by patient), or assessment (e.g., phrasing of risk assessment questions) can be shared as a means of improving care across providers. Sharing assessment and/or intervention strategies that may enhance care while still preserving the unique scope of practice within pediatric psychology can enhance team dynamics as well as patient care.

Conclusion

Increasingly, CL pediatric psychologists are becoming involved as members of multidisciplinary teams in providing care for pediatric patients with chronic illness in medical subspecialty settings. Models of care such as CCM promote collaboration among providers from the level of individual patient care through systemwide changes. Consulting psychologists in pediatric specialty clinic settings are called upon to use a broad range of skills when collaborating on patient care initiatives—whether to enhance team functioning, collaboratively improve patient self-management, or address broader clinic initiatives. Future developments in this arena of consultation practice should focus on assessing and improving patient outcomes and enhancing the role and recognition of pediatric psychology as a valuable and essential component of multidisciplinary subspecialty clinic teams in the provision of pediatric care.

References

Carter, B. D., Kronenberger, W. H., Scott, E., & Brady, C. E. (2020). *Children's health and illness recovery program: Clinician handbook*. New York, NY: Oxford University Press.

Carter, B. D., Kronenberger, W. H., Threlkeld, B., Townsend, A., & Pruitt, A. (2013). The Children's Health & Illness Recovery Program (CHIRP): Feasibility and preliminary efficacy in a clinical sample of adolescents with chronic pain and fatigue. *Clinical Practice in Pediatric Psychology, 1*(2), 184–195. https://doi.org/10.1037/cpp0000012

Coleman, K., Austin, B. T., Brach, C., & Wagner, E. H. (2009). Evidence on the chronic care model in the new millennium. *Health Affairs, 28*(1), 75–85. https://doi.org/10.1377/hlthaff.28.1.75

Conroy, C., & Logan, D. E. (2014). Pediatric multidisciplinary and interdisciplinary teams and interventions. In M. C. Roberts, B. S. Aylward, & Y. P. Wu (Eds.), *Clinical practice of pediatric psychology* (pp. 93–107). New York, NY: The Guilford Press.

Corathers, S. D., Kichler, J., Jones, N.-H. Y., Houchen, A., Jolly, M., Morwessel, N., … Hood, K. K. (2013). Improving depression screening for adolescents with type 1 diabetes. *Pediatrics, 132*(5), e1395–e1402. https://doi.org/10.1542/peds.2013-0681

Cousino, M. K., Schumacher, K. R., Rea, K. E., Eder, S., Zamberlan, M., Jordan, J., & Fredericks, E. M. (2018). Psychosocial functioning in pediatric heart transplant recipients and their families. *Pediatric Transplantation, 22*(2). https://doi.org/10.1111/petr.13110

Doukrou, M., & Segal, T. (2018). Fifteen-minute consultation: Communicating with young people—how to use HEEADSSS, a psychosocial interview for adolescents. *Archives of Disease in Childhood: Education and Practice Edition, 103*, 15–19.

Duncan, C. L., Mentrikoski, J. M., Wu, Y. P., & Fredericks, E. M. (2014). Practice-based approach to assessing and treating nonadherence in pediatric regimens. *Clinical Practice in Pediatric Psychology, 2*(3), 322–336.

Gelfand, K., Geffken, G., Lewin, A., Heidgerken, A., Grove, M. J., Malasanos, T., & Silverstein, J. (2004). An initial evaluation of the design of pediatric psychology consultation service with children with diabetes. *Journal of Child Health Care, 8*(2), 113–123. https://doi.org/10.1177/1367493504041870

Grover, A., & Johsi, A. (2015). An overview of chronic disease models: A systematic literature review. *Global Journal of Health Science, 7*(2), 210–227.

Guilfoyle, S. M., Monahan, S., Wesolowski, C., & Modi, A. C. (2015). Depression screening in pediatric epilepsy: Evidence for the benefit of a behavioral medicine service in early detection. *Epilepsy and Behavior, 44*, 5–10. https://doi.org/10.1016/j.yebeh.2014.12.021

Kazak, A., Prusak, A., McSherry, M., Simms, S., Beele, D., Rourke, M., … Lange, B. (2001). The Psychosocial Assessment Tool (PAT): Pilot data on a brief screening instrument for identifying high risk families in pediatric oncology. *Families, Systems, & Health, 19*(3), 303–317.

Kelly, P., Gregory, K. B., Barbara, S., David, A. B., Kseniya, V. Y., Maria, A. O., … Mann, J. J. (2011). The Columbia–suicide severity rating scale: Initial validity and internal consistency findings from three multisite studies with adolescents and adults. *American Journal of Psychiatry, 168*(12), 1266–1277. https://doi.org/10.1176/appi.ajp.2011.10111704

Knight, J. R., Sherritt, L., Shrier, L. A., Harris, S. K., & Chang, G. (2002). Validity of the "CRAFFT" substance abuse screening test among general adolescent clinic outpatients [Abstract]. *Journal of Adolescent Health, 30*(2), 97.

LaGreca, A. M., & Mackey, E. R. (2009). Adherence to pediatric treatment regimens. In M. C. Roberts & R. G. Steele (Eds.), *Handbook of pediatric psychology* (4th ed., pp. 130–152). New York, NY: The Guilford Press.

McCarthy, M. C., Hearps, S. J. C., Muscara, F., Anderson, V. A., Burke, K., Hearps, S. J., & Kazak, A. E. (2016). Family psychosocial risk screening in infants and older children in the acute pediatric hospital setting using the psychosocial assessment tool. *Journal of Pediatric Psychology, 41*(7), 820–829. https://doi.org/10.1093/jpepsy/jsw055

Ng, C. Y., Thomas-Uribe, M., Yang, Y. A., Chu, M. C., Liu, S. D., Pulendran, U. P., … Wang, C. J. (2018). Theory-based health behavior interventions for pediatric chronic disease management. *JAMA Pediatrics, 172*(12), 1177–1186. https://doi.org/10.1001/jamapediatrics.2018.3039

Pai, A. L. H., & McGrady, M. (2014). Systematic review and meta-analysis of psychological interventions to promote treatment adherence in children, adolescents, and young adults with chronic illness. *Journal of Pediatric Psychology, 39*(8), 918–931. https://doi.org/10.1093/jpepsy/jsu038

Pai, A. L. H., Tackett, A., Ittenbach, R. F., & Goebel, J. (2012). Psychosocial Assessment Tool 2.0-General: Validity of a psychosocial risk screener in a pediatric kidney transplant sample. *Pediatric Transplantation, 16*(1), 92–98. https://doi.org/10.1111/j.1399-3046.2011.01620.x

Palermo, T. M., Janicke, D. M., McQuaid, E. L., Mullins, L. L., Robins, P. M., & Wu, Y. P. (2014). Recommendations for training in pediatric psychology: Defining core competencies across training levels. *Journal of Pediatric Psychology, 39*, 1–20. https://doi.org/10.1093/jpepsy/jsu015

Quittner, A. L., Modi, A. C., Lemanek, K. L., Ievers-Landis, C. E., & Rapoff, M. A. (2008). Evidence-based assessment of adherence to medical treatments in pediatric psychology. Journal of Pediatric Psychology, 33(9), 916–936. https://doi.org/10.1093/jpepsy/jsm064

Richards, M. M. (2009). Electronic medical records: Confidentiality issues in the time of HIPAA. *Professional Psychology: Research and Practice, 40*(6), 550–556. https://doi.org/10.1037/a0016853

Shulman, S. T. (2004). The history of pediatric infectious diseases. *Pediatric Research, 55*(1), 163–176. https://doi.org/10.1203/01.PDR.0000101756.93542.09

Wagner, E. H. (1998). Chronic disease management: What will it take to improve care for chronic illness? *Effective Clinical Practice, 1*, 2–4.

Wagner, E. H., Austin, B. T., Davis, C., Hindmarsh, M., Schaefer, J., & Bonomi, A. (2001). Improving chronic illness care: Translating evidence into action. *Health Affairs, 20*(6), 64–78. https://doi.org/10.1377/hlthaff.20.6.64

Ward, W., Zagoloff, A., Rieck, C., & Robiner, W. (2018). Interprofessional education: Opportunities and challenges for psychology. *Journal of Clinical Psychology in Medical Settings, 25*(3), 250–266. https://doi.org/10.1007/s10880-017-9538-3

Ward, W. L., Shaffer, L. A., & Testa, E. G. (2018). Pediatric psychologists' collaboration in a national pediatric obesity initiative: A case study in interprofessional collaboration. *Journal of Clinical Psychology in Medical Settings, 25*(4), 367–389. https://doi.org/10.1007/s10880-018-9540-4

Zuckerbrot, R. A., Cheung, A., Jensen, P. S., Stein, R. E. K., & Laraque, D. (2018). Guidelines for adolescent depression in primary care (GLAD-PC): Part I. Practice preparation, identification, assessment, and initial management. *Pediatrics, 141*(3), e20174081. https://doi.org/10.1542/peds.2017-4081

Models of Consultation in Primary Care Settings

Lisa Y. Ramirez, Brittany R. Myers, and Terry Stancin

Discussions about consultation models in pediatric psychology have historically focused on inpatient consultation-liaison work with children who have acute and chronic illnesses. Yet, less than 20% of pediatric patients have chronic health conditions, and most children will be seen by a medical provider at least annually in an *outpatient*—either primary care or specialty—clinic (Stancin & Perrin, 2014). Moreover, developmental, behavioral, and emotional problems in youth are common in primary care settings (as many as 25% have diagnosable conditions that cause functional impairment), but most do not receive effective specialty mental health services (Stancin & Perrin, 2014). As a result, outpatient primary care settings provide a unique opportunity for effective consultation, assessment, and intervention in a medical context that reaches beyond traditional inpatient-based models.

L. Y. Ramirez (✉) · B. R. Myers
Department of Psychiatry, MetroHealth Medical Center, Case Western Reserve University School of Medicine, Cleveland, OH, USA
e-mail: lramirez@metrohealth.org

T. Stancin
Department of Psychiatry, MetroHealth Medical Center, Case Western Reserve University School of Medicine, Cleveland, OH, USA

Departments Pediatrics and Psychological Sciences, Case Western Reserve University School of Medicine, Cleveland, OH, USA

A child born in the United States is expected to see a pediatric primary care provider (PPCP)[1] a minimum of 27 times by the time they turn 18, including annual visits after their third birthday (AAP, 2017). This affords an opportunity for longitudinal contacts that can promote and facilitate trust and open communication between the patient, family, and PPCP, and the medical provider can assess the child's development, health status, mood, and functioning over time. Unfortunately, there are many barriers that can impede the effectiveness of the PPCP's interventions. There are conflicting priorities in pediatric primary care, including pressure to increase visit volumes, expanding anticipatory guidance and developmental screening recommendations, and increasing demands for documentation. Many children will present to their pediatric visits with a psychosocial or behavioral health concern, yet inadequate preparation of PPCPs to address developmental and behavioral concerns of children is a well-known problem (McMillan et al., 2018).

Momentum for a central presence for behavioral health providers in primary care settings was advanced by recent changes in health-care

[1] We use "PPCP" to refer to a medical practitioner assuming the role of pediatric primary care provider, coordinating all the health care that the patient receives. In the United States, PPCPs are usually pediatricians, family medicine physicians, advance practice nurses, nurse practitioners, or physician assistants.

B. D. Carter, K. A. Kullgren (eds.), *Clinical Handbook of Psychological Consultation in Pediatric Medical Settings*, Issues in Clinical Child Psychology, https://doi.org/10.1007/978-3-030-35598-2_6

legislation, especially the passage of the Affordable Care Act (Patient Protection and Affordable Care Act, 2010) which recognized the importance of addressing behavioral health conditions for improving health outcomes of the US population and reducing overall costs. Healthcare redesign efforts have shifted the culture of [pediatric] health care to focus more on quality and health outcomes, emphasizing contributions of integrated, team-based care to facilitate real-time communication and an interdependence on complementing expertise in the treatment of primary care patients (Tynan, 2016).

Research has shown that at least half of adult mental health problems are present by the age of 14 years (Kessler et al., 2007), and there is often a gap of more than 10 years between onset of symptoms and treatment—especially for children, as most individuals did not have contact with mental health resources until early adulthood (Wang, Berglund, Olfson, & Kessler, 2004). This combination of systemic, logistical, and training issues creates an environment in which psychosocial concerns may be missed or ineffectively addressed during primary care visits, and thus, many of these issues will progress into significant mental health problems later in children's lives.

Consider the following case scenario:

An 11-year-old girl presents to her PPCP for routine well-child care and is accompanied by her father. During her annual visit, the PPCP notes that, since her last visit, her weight and body mass index (BMI) have increased significantly, and she is now within the range for pediatric obesity. It is also revealed that her parents divorced within the year, and they share custody of her and her younger brother. The PPCP is concerned that her weight for height growth curve is rising sharply and notes that her mood and affect appear flattened. The father appears irritable and overwhelmed, and the PPCP is unsure how best to make recommendations about the girl's weight and inquire about her mood.

Imagine the trajectories for the child above in each of the following scenarios. In one (and most typical) scenario, the PPCP would focus primarily on the medical issues presented in the visit and offer an outside community referral to the father for psychosocial or mental health services. In a second scenario, the family and PPCP has access to a behavioral health team member who can provide a curbside consult or even work directly with the family during the well-child visit to begin a therapeutic intervention. There is evidence that a family is twice as likely to initiate treatment and seven times more likely to complete treatment when services are provided onsite, as in the second scenario (Kolko et al., 2014).

Until very recently, conversations around integrated primary care have focused on the "why"—descriptions of the need and evidence that behavioral health practitioners in integrated primary care may be an effective way to address child behavioral health issues (Stancin & Perrin, 2014). "How" to best address issues by way of possible models to effectively integrate behavioral health specialists have also emerged (Stancin, 2016). In this chapter, we suggest that it may be time to shift conversations to "what" works—to determine what evidence-based or informed models can be best adapted to primary care settings and evaluated. Which developmental, behavioral, and social screening methods, assessment strategies, and behavioral interventions can be effective in integrated primary care? We will touch on the *why, how, and what* in this chapter as we explore models and current evidence in the field of pediatric integrated primary care.

Models of Application

More than half of primary care visits have primary or underlying psychosocial origins, which have compelled health-care systems and policymakers to consider ways to address these needs (Collins, Hewson, Munger, & Wade, 2010). Integrated primary care can be traced as far back as the 1970s to a health system in New York state and has steadily gained momentum since the early 1990s, especially in family medicine and military settings (Blount, 2015). There have been many advances since those first days of integrated practice, and the current models of integrated primary care exist along a continuum, from *coordinated care* to *fully integrated* practice (Stancin, Perrin, & Ramirez, 2009).

In practices relying on *coordinated* or consultation models of care, PPCPs seek consultation by mental health professionals and may share patients. Often, these two sets of professionals are in separate locations, and communication occurs via written, telephone, or electronic correspondence, usually following a visit with the patient/family. An example of coordinated care is the Massachusetts Child Psychiatry Access Project (MCPAP), which provides telephone hotline, staffed by a care coordinator who accepts the referral and assigns to either the dedicated child psychiatrist or psychotherapist (Collins et al., 2010; Sarvet et al., 2010). Education and resource support are also available. Practices without immediate or ready access to behavioral health providers (whether because of a lack of providers in a region or other factors) may find opportunities to improve care using coordinated model resources.

New videoconferencing/telehealth approaches have emerged as an effective means of delivering coordinated and collaborative care. Telehealth, or the practice of delivering health care via digital (e.g., telephone, Internet) mediums, is an approach that has been utilized in health care in some form for over 50 years but has more recently been formalized to include the direct delivery of medical, preventive, and public health interventions delivered remotely (Doarn et al., 2014). Within a primary care framework, the Extension for Community Healthcare Outcomes (ECHO) model uses a hub and spoke model, where a centralized training center ("superhub") aids in the creation of a regional hub made up of interprofessional team that provides remote simultaneous consultation and support to satellite sites ("spokes") around a particular issue or problem (Hager et al., 2018). This model has demonstrated a variety of valuable outcomes, especially in rural and underserved areas; some examples of positive outcomes include increases in specialized treatment around opioid use disorder and decreased emergency use utilization (Hager et al., 2018). Fleischman et al. (2016) demonstrated that when PPCPs in one rural setting added a telehealth visit with an obesity specialist, patient BMIs were reduced and maintained. Importantly, however, insurance providers may not reimburse for remote care delivery or time spent consulting with remote interprofessional team members, which may disincentivize institutions and practitioners with high revenue and clinical productivity expectations. However, payor networks may find that telehealth may have significant benefits once bundled payments and value-based care are the industry standard (Hager et al., 2018).

Colocated care practices involve closer collaboration among PPCPs and behavioral health providers and imply that professionals share a physical space. Often, the mental health professional occupies an office in the pediatric practice or close to it. There may be shared electronic health records and/or office staff. Key advantages of colocated models include familiarity of the setting and easier communication between providers. In addition, colocated models may also offer greater control over scheduling and therefore may be attractive if fiscal predictability is a priority to practices.

Finally, behavioral health integration is care resulting from a practice team of primary care and mental health professionals working together to care for the whole child in the context of the family, school, and community (Stancin & Perrin, 2014). *Integrated* care implies communication about treatment planning, and progress occurs in real time and face to face, often during the actual clinic visit (Stancin & Perrin, 2014). This allows for collaborative case conceptualization and treatment planning gears to turn quickly. Integrated care assumes that for any problem, patients have come to the right place—that there is no wrong door. Care may address mental health, developmental disorders, health behaviors that contribute to medical conditions, life stressors and crises, stress-related physical symptoms, or ineffective patterns of health-care utilization.

The MetroHealth Model is a mature pediatric integrated care practice within an academic medical center. Pediatric psychologists and psychology trainees (interns and postdoctoral fellows) are present to staff all primary care, specialty care, and urgent care clinic sessions and work collaboratively with attending pediatricians and pediatric resident physicians. Psychology staff provide "warm handoffs" (a transfer of care between the PPCP and psychologist that occurs in front of the patient and family), same-day and follow-up brief, problem-focused assessments and treatments, and risk/suicide assessments. The focus of attention varies greatly (e.g., developmental screening follow-up, ADHD, adjustment to medical conditions, family trauma, depression, sleep problems, self-harming behaviors, to name a few). Psychotropic medication consultation with a child and adolescent psychiatrist or developmental-behavioral pediatrician may be requested after a psychology provider and PPCP evaluate a child (Marwaha et al., 2017). Utilization data over a 6-month period indicated that 71% of psychology patient interactions resulted in billable encounters (Pereira, Wallace, Brown, & Stancin, 2016).

While not yet adapted for use with a pediatric population, a variation of the integrated care model has come be known as the "collaborative care model." The most well-known collaborative care model in adult primary care is the Improving Mood-Promoting Access to Collaborative Treatment (IMPACT) model (Collins et al., 2010; Unützer et al., 2001). The IMPACT model was borne out of a need to address depression in older patients with chronic medical problems who were not following through on psychiatry referrals and were not receiving mental health care. The IMPACT model uses a stepped approach to augment standard primary care with an embedded behavioral health-care manager who assists with screening, tracking, and guiding treatment toward an antidepressant medication and/or psychotherapy. An essential element to this model is availability of a psychiatrist to provide caseload consultation to the care manager who coordinates services with patients and the PCP (Hegel et al., 2002; Unützer et al., 2001).

Building on the collaborative care framework, Richardson et al. (2014) implemented the Reaching Out to Adolescents in Distress (ROAD) intervention to address depression in adolescent patients. Teenagers from pediatric primary care practices were telephone-screened for depression using the PHQ-2. Eligible participants who met depression criteria after further assessment were randomized to intervention or control groups. For the intervention condition, the adolescents and their families were empowered to engage in ongoing choices around treatment (e.g., medication alone, cognitive-behavioral therapy (CBT) alone, medication/CBT combination). Notably, all intervention participants' depression scores were monitored, and changes in intervention condition or dose were recommended based on these dynamic scores. In the control group, patients received care as usual along with a supplemental letter recommending treatment and summarizing the results of the telephone depression interview. Results indicated that the collaborative care intervention led to significant decreases in depression symptoms over 12 months compared to the control group (Richardson et al., 2014).

Strategies and Challenges in Implementation

Regardless of which integration model is selected for a primary care practice, appropriate and seamless introduction and application of a new care model is not always intuitive. Medical practices and hospital systems vary in their culture of integration and communication between medical and mental health professions. Irrespective of the setting, there are components that are crucial to integrated care and issues that can complicate implementation.

SAMHSA underscores four components that are critical to successful integration: leadership and organizational commitment, team development, team process, and team outcome (SAMHSA, 2014). Additionally, the Interprofessional Education Collaborative (IPEC, 2016) promotes four core values that are necessary in interprofessional collaboration: values/ethics for interprofessional practice, roles/responsibilities, interprofessional communication, and teams/teamwork. Each competency has several sub-competencies, and these competencies are grounded in family- and patient-centered care that is community- and population-oriented. In pediatric integrated primary care practice, each of these competencies has very real implications. Integrated care teams need to discuss common *values/ethics* considerations that may impact the team practices, e.g., how confidentiality will be maintained, how team members ensure they are practicing within the scope of their expertise, and how both provider and patient issues of diversity are understood and respected. Similarly, understanding team *roles and responsibilities* is critical. Patients and families deserve to understand who is contributing to their care and in what way. Additionally, team members should be clear with each other who is responsible for what aspects of care and capitalize on the wide scope of skills and competencies that are present in the team. The *communication* competency highlights the need to strive for clear, universal language and content, both inside of the team and when discussing plans with patients and families. Finally, *teams/teamwork* involves reviewing the team dynamics and outcomes to understand how the team effectiveness may be improved (IPEC, 2016).

Consider how these four competencies are fundamental to an effective warm handoff: a clear presentation of the potential problem (communication, values/ethics, and roles), a plan for who will follow up with further assessment and/or treatment (roles, communication, and teamwork), and how the plan is established and shared with the patient and family (values/ethics, roles, communication, and teamwork). Additionally, having a consistent message for the patients and families is also a very important factor. If a parent arrives to a pediatric clinic visit and then is offered an opportunity to speak to a mental health professional, the style, tone, and content of how that is communicated will likely determine the receptivity ("buy-in") of the families to this service. Financial issues may also present an obstacle to the delivery of mental health services. Health-care systems may charge separate fees on top of the cost of the visit per professional seen that day. If this is not communicated to the family, or the health-care system has not developed solutions to this potential barrier, families may be surprised to discover they have unexpected consultation bills added to their visit and decline further behavioral health services.

Integrated primary care models aim to identify, triage, and treat (when appropriate) behavioral health issues. There is no universal gold standard for effective integrated pediatric primary care. For example, coordinated care and colocated models may be preferred in settings where resources are limited, especially when considering space and time/clinical flow factors. Settings in which the organizational and/or clinic cultures promote and facilitate collaboration between medical and behavioral health practitioners [and trainees] are more likely to have success. Yet, other settings may have systemic and logistical barriers that require creativity in implementing an integrated care model. To address these issues, a number of important considerations should be considered. How easy it is for interprofessional team members to readily access one another? Do medical and behavioral health providers practice alongside each other to help facilitate impromptu conversation and "curbside" consultations? If not, what other modes of expeditious access are available: encrypted texting, telemedicine, email, and regularly scheduled interdisciplinary team meetings? Developing a business model for a sustainable integrated care program in the current health-care economic climate continues to be a challenge. However, the creation of new collaborative care codes for behavioral health integration has been developed that may support some of the currently unreimbursed time spent participating in non-face-to-face patient care, such as in treatment planning collaboration, psychiatric consultation, and care coordination (Centers for Medicare and Medicaid Services, 2018).

The "Who" in Integrated Primary Care

As highlighted above, integrated care models vary widely and are predictably impacted by economic, population, and health-care system variables. One important factor to consider is the type(s) of professional that will be providing the behavioral health arm of the team-based care. There is a movement in the medical culture for providers to practice at the "top" of their licenses, with extenders (e.g., advanced practice nurses and physician assistants) increasing patient access to standard care and allowing physicians to focus on more complex cases with higher reimbursement potential (Moawad, 2017). Similarly, in any given pediatric setting, there may be a variety of behavioral health professionals (e.g., masters-level counselors and social workers), child development specialists (e.g., child life), and health-care educators and providers (e.g., nurse clinicians, dieticians, health educators). However, the unique skill sets offered by these various disciplines are not always clear to our interprofessional colleagues and system administrators. Without a clear understanding of the benefits related to the areas of unique expertise of pediatric psychologists vs. nondoctoral providers—as well as workforce availability—practices may opt for less-expensive behavioral health providers. Indeed, most studies examining outcomes of collaborative care models have described practices that rely on care managers or other nondoctoral providers.

As a rapidly evolving subspecialty, pediatric psychologists bring unique skills of benefit to the primary care setting. In addition to providing evidence-based training in screening, assessment, and interventions, most pediatric psychologists have specialized training in the program development, evidence-based protocols, quality improvement, health promotion, and adherence. They often have training to provide supervision and mentorship to interprofessional trainees, including medical residents and other behavioral health trainees (Stancin & Perrin, 2014). Integrated primary care practices may utilize psychologists in leadership/supervision roles including the provision of support for more complex patient presentations. It is essential that psychologists convey the nature of our specialized training and skills so they are afforded the opportunity to practice at the highest levels of their licenses.

Clinical Practice Essentials

As we shift from theoretical models to actual patient presentations in pediatric integrated primary care, consider that pediatric and adult primary care practices have distinct foci. While adult integrated behavioral health care is responsive and reactive to morbidity, pediatric mental and medical health systems tend to focus somewhat more on early intervention and prevention of chronic health problems and disease (Stancin & Perrin, 2014). As a result, the types of problems encountered in pediatric primary care can range from normalizing milestones and basic behavior principles used to navigate typical child development (e.g., sleep and toilet training, managing tantrums) to addressing specific stressors (e.g., bullying, learning problems, phobias), to exploring emerging health issues with behavioral origins (e.g., obesity, medication adherence), to responding to acute risk and pathology (e.g., suicide assessments, emerging psychosis).

Psychologists can play a critical role in assessing and managing problems in pediatric primary care and in other more specialized pediatric clinics and emergency room settings. PPCPs in primary care serve, in part, as medical gatekeepers and decision-makers: they regularly screen and assess medical/developmental concerns, determine acuity, and facilitate admission to inpatient medical settings as needed. In an integrated primary and specialty care setting, psychologists can serve a similar role, by screening for and assessing general psychosocial and more urgent mental health concerns (e.g., suicidal ideation, homicidal ideation, and self-harm). Understandably, in order to function within time and space constraints, efficiency in identifying and triaging behavioral health needs in the clinical setting is crucial.

Mental health issues account for more than 20% of visits in primary care (Cherry & Schappert, 2014), and recent studies suggest that nearly half patients in pediatric specialty clinics screen positive for some mental health concern (Shemesh et al., 2016). Data from the MCPAP suggests that PPCPs generally accessed available behavioral health consultation for clarity on diagnoses, community resources, medication consultations, school issues, and mental health crises (Sarvet et al., 2010). These data also highlighted the range of behavioral health presentations, including ADHD, common internalizing and externalizing disorders, developmental disorders, trauma, eating disorders, substance use, and psychotic disorders (Sarvet et al., 2010). However, this list does not include other consultations common in our own pediatric clinic, including sleep issues, barriers to adherence, toilet training, and feeding problems, among others. Specialized training in applied child development, developmental psychopathology, and the interconnectedness of physical and mental health is essential for effective practice and endemic to the training of most pediatric psychologists.

One of the challenges of integrated care is that it does not fit traditional mental health models used in training programs, and the setting, time constraints, and logistical issues often require adaptations of evidence-based interventions. Several studies have demonstrated effectiveness of adapted interventions to address behavior problems, obesity, depression, and transdiagnostic presentations in pediatric primary care (Asarnow, Rozenman, Wiblin, & Zeltzer, 2015; Fleischman et al., 2016; Richardson et al., 2014; Weersing, Rozenman, Maher-Bridge, & Campo, 2012).

Suicide

One particularly urgent issue in pediatric primary care is suicidality. Suicide currently represents the second leading cause of death in 10- to 24-year-olds in the United States (WISQARS, 2017). In 2017, approximately 1 in 6 American high school students reported that they had seriously considered attempting suicide in the past year, and 1 in 13 students reported that they had attempted suicide in the past year (Kann et al., 2018). In a traditional, nonintegrated outpatient pediatric setting, patients who endorse suicidal ideation in the pediatric visit are generally sent urgently to an emergency room, where they can wait many hours for a mental health assessment, and many will be discharged home with a list of referrals for mental health services (Doshi, Boudreaux, Wang, Pelletier, & Camargo, 2005). This process is not only inefficient and costly for families and managed care providers, but it can also be a stressful (Allen, Carpenter, Sheets, Miccio, & Ross, 2003) and even traumatic experience for a young person to spend hours in a fast-paced emergency department setting, watching other psychiatric or critically ill or injured patients.

In a fully integrated care setting, PPCPs concerned about self-harm and suicidality can access a mental health professional for an immediate risk assessment and determination of acuity and need (e.g., engage in safety planning and discharge with appropriate supervision or facilitate admission to an inpatient psychiatric setting). One integrated care program (MetroHealth) demonstrated that 90% of suicide/risk assessments presenting in the primary care clinic resulted in successful de-escalation of the crisis and a safety plan outcome that did not require further emergency room visits or inpatient psychiatric hospitalizations (Pereira et al., 2016).

When an inpatient psychiatric hospitalization is deemed necessary, the outpatient primary care team often needs to communicate the results of the assessment to a psychiatric emergency room team, who then conduct their own assessment, and communicate results to an inpatient psychiatric team. Upon discharge, the inpatient team needs to communicate patient outcomes and coordinate psychological follow-up with the outpatient team. This last step is particularly important given that patients are at higher risk for suicide in the week immediately following discharge from an inpatient psychiatric hospitalization. Pediatric psychologists integrated in primary care clinics can help to coordinate the difficult transition from inpatient psychiatric hospitalization to outpatient treatment by working closely with the inpatient medical team.

Acute and Chronic Health Issues

Psychologists in integrated care settings also collaborate closely with *inpatient medical* teams to manage issues of adjustment and treatment adherence for children with chronic and acute medical conditions. Children with chronic medical conditions who face inpatient stays are discharged for regular outpatient follow-up with PPCPs and specialty care providers. Integrated care psychologists can help families translate the treatment recommendations of the inpatient medical team into practically implemented strategies, as well as to help the outpatient medical providers understand patient and family barriers and potential resistance to implementing medical advice and recommendations.

Young people managing chronic illness often struggle to accept and adjust to symptoms, like chronic pain, special diet, and restriction of daily activities. Many young people with chronic medical conditions report feeling hopeless and isolated from peers, while others suffer anxiety surrounding frequent medical procedures and surgeries. Mental health professionals in outpatient pediatric primary settings are in a unique position to work to promote positive social, emotional, and behavioral adjustment for patients with chronic medical conditions.

Workforce Development

While health systems increasingly move toward integrated models of care, mental health training still largely focuses on traditional models of care. In graduate school, psychology trainees typically learn to provide traditional outpatient therapy (i.e., weekly 50-min individual sessions with a therapist) in an outpatient training clinic. Trainees wishing to specialize in pediatric psychology may choose to seek hospital-based training opportunities to develop expertise in a medical subspecialty (e.g., oncology, neurology, endocrinology) or to gain experience working in other treatment settings (e.g., inpatient consultation-liaison, psychiatric inpatient units). To date, few programs offer such training opportunities in an integrated care, leaving the mental health workforce underprepared to meet the ever-growing demand for integration. In fact, until relatively recently, there were few generally agreed-upon training competencies around which to build a specialized training program. In 2012, the American Psychological Association (APA) initiated a call for the creation of an Interorganizational Work Group to identify competencies for psychology practice in primary care (McDaniel et al., 2014) which were then further defined and tailored for pediatric populations (Hoffses et al., 2016). These competencies are important not only to standardize training and best practices in primary care but also serve to clearly identify and differentiate the role of psychologists from that of other behavioral health professionals in primary care. Furthermore, they capture the multifaceted role of integrated primary care psychologists, including application and adaptation of evidence-based clinical interventions, consuming and producing research on integrated primary care, building and navigating interprofessional relationships, training the next generation of integrated primary care psychologists, and serving as leaders and advocates in the community.

Many pediatric primary care settings incorporate interprofessional learners and supervisors at varying levels. The inherent complexities in creating integrated care teams (complex and interwoven medical and behavioral health issues, variety of training and practice cultures, and economic and financial pressures of productivity and reimbursement) underscore that training across developmental levels of learners and practitioners is critical to maintaining and cultivating a responsive and effective, sustainable integrated primary care practice.

Special Considerations

Facilitating Psychiatry Access

The national shortage of child psychiatrists has created a high demand for pediatric psychopharmacological intervention. Marwaha et al. (2017)

piloted a model in which predoctoral psychology interns embedded in pediatric primary care clinics acted as access point to activate a formal psychopharmacological medication consultation with the collaborating pediatric psychiatrist. This model aided in (1) extending pediatric psychiatry service in the hospital, (2) preventing a bottleneck of referrals to outpatient psychiatry for simple medication requests, and (3) enhancing the psychopharmacological knowledge of psychology and pediatric residents (Marwaha et al., 2017).

Culturally Informed Care

Studies suggest that African American, Hispanic, Asian American, and Native American families are less likely than White counterparts to utilize traditional specialty mental health services, even after accounting for symptom severity and other socioeconomic factors related to service utilization (Alegría et al., 2002). However, integrating mental health services into primary care has been shown to eliminate gaps between Hispanic (Bridges et al., 2014), African American (Ayalon, Areán, Linkins, Lynch, & Estes, 2007), and White adults' access to and utilization of specialized mental health services. Spielvogle, McCarty, and Richardson (2017) demonstrated effectiveness in addressing anxiety and depression in pediatric primary care, with the highest gains among Hispanic populations. Furthermore, disparities known to exist in the diagnosis and treatment of developmental disabilities (e.g., autism spectrum disorders) among minority children (Zablotsky, Black, & Blumberg, 2017) may be addressed through culturally sensitive developmental screening facilitated by psychologists integrated into pediatric clinics.

Resources

Pediatric psychology integration services should be tailored to fit the features of the setting so services may be organized differently for urban and rural communities. In urban communities with many mental health agencies and services to choose from, an integrated care model may focus on briefly addressing immediate patient concerns and helping them to connect to long-term services in the community. However, rural communities may have fewer community-based mental health services, so options to refer to outside agencies may be limited. Mental health providers in the primary care setting may represent one of the only mental health resources in a given area, and patients often have to travel long distances for specialty mental health services. Thus, in rural communities, same-day consultation in the primary care context may be preferable and more accessible for families than traditional weekly outpatient therapy appointments. It may also be beneficial to consider ways of extending mental health resources in a given area by using alternate models of service provision, like telehealth psychology, or by using trainees as extenders to increase the number of available behavioral health providers in the area. Families in urban communities face their own barriers to care (e.g., reliance on public transport). Thus, in both settings, mental health providers may need to be flexible with attendance policies to allow patients to easily reconnect with services even after missed appointments.

Concluding Remarks

As we close, consider this account of a fictional pediatric psychologist embedded in an integrated primary care clinic and how it highlights the variety of consultative roles required in a single day:

Dr. Gomes starts her day by meeting with hospital administrators to discuss reimbursement rates and current billable services for psychologists integrated into primary care. Later that morning, the pediatric endocrine specialist requests a consultation for an 8-year-old boy with diabetes who was recently discharged to the outpatient endocrine team after a prolonged inpatient admission for diabetic ketoacidosis. Dr. Gomes helps the endocrine team to assess barriers to adherence and helps to increase the fami-

ly's motivation to engage in effective care for the boy's diabetes. Dr. Gomes then observes a predoctoral psychology resident responds to a consult request in primary care for a 6-year-old patient presenting with tantrums, language delays, and difficulty with sleep onset. After the visit, Dr. Gomes discusses the management of the case with the psychology and pediatric resident, including how the communication of the consult was handled with the family and if the team felt that they were effective in meeting the needs of this patient and family. During lunch, Dr. Gomes delivers the weekly Pediatric Department Grand Rounds about the management of adolescent depression in primary care. As she returns to lunch for the afternoon pediatric clinic, Dr. Gomes receives a request for a consult regarding a 17-year-old patient with chronic daily headaches. During the visit, the patient endorses symptoms of hopelessness and anhedonia and makes a "joke" to Dr. Gomes that she would be "better off dead." Upon further assessment, the patient admits to acute suicidal ideation, with a specific plan and access. Dr. Gomes works jointly with the PPCP and the emergency department team to facilitate admission to the inpatient psychiatric unit. To wrap up the day, Dr. Gomes meets with her hospital's PPCPs to discuss how to use available trauma screeners to screen and identify children at risk for trauma in the growing Puerto Rican community moving into the city after the devastation left by Hurricane Maria.

Compared to traditional inpatient-based models of pediatric psychology consultation, integrated primary care affords an opportunity to screen, assess, triage, and intervene across a wide range of physical, developmental, behavioral, academic, mental health and psychosocial issues. With access to children presenting along a continuum of health and functioning, integrated pediatric primary care psychologists are afforded the opportunity to consult within primary care teams, teach and train interprofessional learners, and apply [adapted] evidence-based interventions to prevent and address pathology. Research on "what" developmental, behavioral, and social screening methods, assessment strategies, and behavioral interventions can be best applied to address problems in primary care settings is needed but is emerging.

References

Alegría, M., Canino, G., Ríos, R., Vera, M., Calderón, J., Rusch, D., & Ortega, A. N. (2002). Mental health care for Latinos: Inequalities in use of specialty mental health services among Latinos, African Americans, and non-Latino Whites. *Psychiatric Services, 53*(12), 1547–1555. https://doi.org/10.1176/appi.ps.53.12.1547

Allen, M. H., Carpenter, D., Sheets, J. L., Miccio, S., & Ross, R. (2003). What do consumers say they want and need during a psychiatric emergency? *Journal of Psychiatric Practice, 9*(1), 39–58. https://doi.org/10.1097/00131746-200301000-00005

American Pediatric Association. (2017). Recommendations for preventive pediatric health care [PDF file]. Retrieved from https://www.aap.org/en-us/Documents/periodicity_schedule.pdf

Asarnow, J. R., Rozenman, M., Wiblin, J., & Zeltzer, L. (2015). Integrated medical-behavioral care compared with usual primary care for child and adolescent behavioral health a meta-analysis. *JAMA Pediatrics, 169*(10), 929–937. https://doi.org/10.1001/jamapediatrics.2015.1141

Ayalon, L., Areán, P. A., Linkins, K., Lynch, M., & Estes, C. L. (2007). Integration of mental health services into primary care overcomes ethnic disparities in access to mental health services between black and white elderly. *The American Journal of Geriatric Psychiatry, 15*(10), 906–912. https://doi.org/10.1097/JGP.0b013e318135113e

Blount, A. (2015, April 10). A brief history of the integration of behavioral health in primary care [Web blog post]. Retrieved October 1, 2018 from https://www.cfha.net/blogpost/689173/213334/a-brief-history-of-the-integration-of-behavioral-health-in-primary-care

Bridges, A. J., Andrews, A. R., III, Villalobos, B. T., Pastrana, F. A., Cavell, T. A., & Gomez, D. (2014). Does integrated behavioral health care reduce mental health disparities for Latinos? Initial findings. *Journal of Latina/o Psychology, 2*(1), 37. https://doi.org/10.1037/lat0000009

Centers for Medicare and Medicaid Services. (2018, April 17). Frequently asked questions about billing medicare for behavioral health integration (BHI) services. Retrieved from https://www.cms.gov/Medicare/Medicare-Fee-for-Service-Payment/PhysicianFeeSched/Downloads/Behavioral-Health-Integration-FAQs.pdf

Cherry, D. K., & Schappert, S. M. (2014). Percentage of mental health-related primary care office visits, by age group-national ambulatory medical care survey, United States, 2010.

Collins, C., Hewson, D. L., Munger, R., & Wade, T. (2010). *Evolving models of behavioral health integration in primary care* (p. 504). New York, NY: Milbank Memorial Fund. https://doi.org/10.1599/EvolvingCare2010

Doarn, C. R., Pruitt, S., Jacobs, J., Harris, Y., Bott, D. M., Riley, W., … Oliver, A. L. (2014). Federal efforts to define and advance telehealth—A work in progress. *Telemedicine and e-Health, 20*(5), 409–418. https://doi.org/10.1089/tmj.2013.0336

Doshi, A., Boudreaux, E. D., Wang, N., Pelletier, A. J., & Camargo, C. A., Jr. (2005). National study of US emergency department visits for attempted suicide and self-inflicted injury, 1997–2001. *Annals of Emergency Medicine, 46*(4), 369–375. https://doi.org/10.1016/j.annemergmed.2005.04.018

Fleischman, A., Hourigan, S. E., Lyon, H. N., Landry, M. G., Reynolds, J., Steltz, S. K., … Ludwig, D. S. (2016). Creating an integrated care model for childhood obesity: A randomized pilot study utilizing telehealth in a community primary care setting. *Clinical Obesity, 6*(6), 380–388. https://doi.org/10.1111/cob.12166

Hager, B., Hasselberg, M., Arzubi, E., Betlinski, J., Duncan, M., Richman, J., & Raney, L. E. (2018). Leveraging behavioral health expertise: Practices and potential of the project ECHO approach to virtually integrating care in underserved areas. *Psychiatric Services, 69*(4), 366–369. https://doi.org/10.1176/appi.ps.201700211

Hegel, M. T., Imming, J., Cyr-Provost, M., Noel, P. H., Arean, P. A., & Unutzer, J. (2002). Role of behavioral health professionals in a collaborative stepped care treatment model for depression in primary care: Project IMPACT. *Families, Systems & Health, 20*(3), 265. https://doi.org/10.1037/h0089475

Hoffses, K. W., Ramirez, L. Y., Berdan, L., Tunick, R., Honaker, S. M., Meadows, T. J., … Stancin, T. (2016). Topical review: Building competency: Professional skills for pediatric psychologists in integrated primary care settings. *Journal of Pediatric Psychology, 41*(10), 1144–1160. https://doi.org/10.1093/jpepsy/jsw066

Interprofessional Education Collaborative. (2016). *Core competencies for interprofessional collaborative practice: 2016 update*. Washington, DC: Interprofessional Education Collaborative.

Kann, L., McManus, T., Harris, W. A., Shanklin, S. L., Flint, K. H., Queen, B., … Lim, C. (2018). Youth risk behavior surveillance—United States, 2017. *MMWR Surveillance Summaries, 67*(8), 1. https://doi.org/10.15585/mmwr.ss6708a1

Kessler, R. C., Amminger, G. P., Aguilar-Gaxiola, S., Alonso, J., Lee, S., & Ustun, T. B. (2007). Age of onset of mental disorders: A review of recent literature. *Current Opinion in Psychiatry, 20*(4), 359. https://doi.org/10.1097/YCO.0b013e32816ebc8c

Kolko, D. J., Campo, J., Kilbourne, A. M., Hart, J., Sakolsky, D., & Wisniewski, S. (2014). Collaborative care outcomes for pediatric behavioral health problems: A cluster randomized trial. *Pediatrics, 133*, e981–e992. https://doi.org/10.1542/peds.2013-2516

Lardieri, M. R., Lasky, G. B., & Raney, L. (2014). *Essential elements of effective integrated primary care and behavioral health teams*. Washington, DC: SAMHSA-HRSA Center for Integrated Health Solutions.

Marwaha, R., Pajek, J. A., Newton, K., Machado, E., Rae, M. W., & Stancin, T. (2017). Psychopharmacology consultation facilitated by integrated psychology residents in a pediatric continuity care clinic: A feasibility study. *Journal of the American Academy of Child & Adolescent Psychiatry, 56*(10), S214–S215. https://doi.org/10.1016/j.jaac.2017.09.183

McDaniel, S. H., Grus, C. L., Cubic, B. A., Hunter, C. L., Kearney, L. K., Schuman, C. C., … Miller, B. F. (2014). Competencies for psychology practice in primary care. *American Psychologist, 69*(4), 409.

McMillan, J. A., Land, M. L., Rodday, A. M., Wills, K., Green, C. M., & Leslie, L. K. (2018). Report of a joint association of pediatric program directors–American board of pediatrics workshop: Preparing future pediatricians for the mental health crisis. *The Journal of Pediatrics, 201*, 285–291. https://doi.org/10.1016/j.jpeds.2018.06.044

Moawad, H. (2017, May 3). Practicing at the top of your license. *MDMag*. Retrieved from https://www.mdmag.com/physicians-money-digest/contributor/heidi-moawad-md/2017/05/practicing-at-the-top-of-your-license

Patient Protection and Affordable Care Act. (2010). Patient protection and affordable care act. *Public Law, 111*(48), 759–762.

Pereira, L., Wallace, J., Brown, W., & Stancin, T. (2016, September). *Behavioral health utilization in an integrated pediatric continuity care clinic*. Poster presented at the annual meeting of the Society for Developmental and Behavioral Pediatrics conference, Savannah, GA.

Richardson, L. P., Ludman, E., McCauley, E., Lindenbaum, J., Larison, C., Zhou, C., … Katon, W. (2014). Collaborative care for adolescents with depression in primary care: A randomized clinical trial. *JAMA, 312*(8), 809–816. https://doi.org/10.1001/jama.2014.9259

Sarvet, B., Gold, J., Bostic, J. Q., Masek, B. J., Prince, J. B., Jeffers-Terry, M., … Straus, J. H. (2010). Improving access to mental health care for children: The Massachusetts Child Psychiatry Access Project. *Pediatrics, 126*, 1191–1200. https://doi.org/10.1542/peds.2009-1340

Shemesh, E., Lewis, B. J., Rubes, M., Ambrose, M. A., Cahill, M. K., Knight, C., … Annunziato, R. A. (2016). Mental health screening outcomes in a pediatric specialty care setting. *The Journal of Pediatrics, 168*, 193–197. https://doi.org/10.1016/j.jpeds.2015.09.046

Spielvogle, H., McCarty, C. A., & Richardson, L. P. (2017). Brief therapy for anxiety and depression in the pediatric primary care setting: Implications and next steps. *JAMA Pediatrics, 171*(10), 1006–1007. https://doi.org/10.1001/jamapediatrics.2017.2854

Stancin, T. (2016). Commentary: Integrated pediatric primary care: Moving from why to how. *Journal of Pediatric Psychology, 41*(10), 1161–1164. https://doi.org/10.1093/jpepsy/jsw074

Stancin, T., & Perrin, E. C. (2014). Psychologists and pediatricians: Opportunities for collaboration in primary care. *American Psychologist, 69*(4), 332. https://doi.org/10.1037/a0036046

Stancin, T., Perrin, E. C., & Ramirez, L. (2009). Pediatric psychology and primary care. In M. C. Roberts & R. G. Steele (Eds.), *Handbook of pediatric psychology* (pp. 630–646). New York, NY: Guilford Press.

Tynan, W. D. (2016). Commentary: Integrated primary care psychology evolving with the affordable care act. *Journal of Pediatric Psychology, 41*(10), 1165–1167. https://doi.org/10.1093/jpepsy/jsw086

Unützer, J., Katon, W., Williams, J. W., Jr., Callahan, C. M., Harpole, L., Hunkeler, E. M., … Oishi, S. M. (2001). Improving primary care for depression in late life: The design of a multicenter randomized trial. *Medical Care, 39*(8), 785–799. https://doi.org/10.1097/00005650-200108000-00005

Wang, P. S., Berglund, P. A., Olfson, M., & Kessler, R. C. (2004). Delays in initial treatment contact after first onset of a mental disorder. *Health Services Research, 39*(2), 393–416. https://doi.org/10.1111/j.1475-6773.2004.00234.x

Weersing, V. R., Rozenman, M. S., Maher-Bridge, M., & Campo, J. V. (2012). Anxiety, depression, and somatic distress: Developing a transdiagnostic internalizing toolbox for pediatric practice. *Cognitive and Behavioral Practice, 19*(1), 68–82. https://doi.org/10.1016/j.cbpra.2011.06.002

WISQARS. (2017, February 19). WISQARS leading causes of death reports. Retrieved from https://webappa.cdc.gov/sasweb/ncipc/leadcause.html

Zablotsky, B., Black, L. I., & Blumberg, S. J. (2017). Estimated prevalence of children with diagnosed developmental disabilities in the United States, 2014–2016. *NCHS Data Brief*, (291), 1–8.

A Short Course in Medicine for the Consulting Pediatric Psychologist: Essential Knowledge for the Nonphysician Clinician

Brooke Threlkeld, Kristie V. Schultz, Michael K. Sowell, and Sara Multerer

An integrated healthcare system with collaborative behavioral and medical professionals leads to improved health outcomes including increased access to indicated mental health diagnoses and treatments, reduced medical care utilization, and increased patient satisfaction (Conroy & Logan, 2014). Pediatric psychologists, with clinical health and child psychology training, are useful partners or consultants across medical specialties (Drotar, 1977). While value derived from integrated care is well-documented, there are multiple challenges to integration. One such challenge for behavioral health providers is learning the language of physician/medical colleagues. Furthermore, competency standards for pediatric psychologists recommend knowledge of acute and chronic medical illness/injury and medical intervention "from the medical literature" (Palermo et al., 2014, p. 969).

The following chapter represents a multidisciplinary, collaborative effort to create a brief guide to practical medical information for the pediatric psychologist working in a medical setting. Information presented is non-exhaustive, introductory, and focused on topics the authors find to be most common and relevant. There is special attention to emotional/behavioral considerations of various medical procedures and interventions throughout. Topics covered include medical specialty areas of expertise, diagnostic imaging, laboratory testing, common procedures, medication management, acronyms/abbreviations in medical terminology, useful resources for further reference, ethical and cultural considerations, and medically controversial topics. The ultimate goal of this review of medical information and resources is to further promote the successful collaboration and communication across healthcare specialists who have much to offer children and families facing complex health-related challenges.

Medical Specialties

Pediatric psychologists work with many different professions and specialties, in both inpatient and outpatient medical settings. Psychologists may work with physicians (e.g., Doctor of Medicine [MD] or Doctor of Osteopathy [DO]), nurses (e.g., registered nurse [RN] or licensed practical nurse [LPN]), advanced practice providers (e.g., advanced practice registered nurse [APRN] or

B. Threlkeld (✉) · K. V. Schultz (✉) · S. Multerer
Department of Pediatrics, Norton Children's Hospital, University of Louisville School of Medicine, Louisville, KY, USA
e-mail: brooke.threlkeld@louisville.edu; kristie.schultz@louisville.edu

M. K. Sowell
Department of Neurology, Norton Children's Hospital, University of Louisville School of Medicine, Louisville, KY, USA

B. D. Carter, K. A. Kullgren (eds.), *Clinical Handbook of Psychological Consultation in Pediatric Medical Settings*, Issues in Clinical Child Psychology, https://doi.org/10.1007/978-3-030-35598-2_7

physician assistant [PA]), or other providers (e.g., registered dietician [RD], physical therapist [PT], occupational therapist [OT], or certified social worker [CSW]). The Accreditation Council for Graduate Medical Education (ACGME) (n.d.) lists medical specialties and, within pediatrics, further delineates pediatric subspecialties, some of which are included here. Pediatric psychologists should be familiar with pediatric subspecialties and the care that they provide. For example, Pediatric Hematology Oncology (Hem-Onc) is concerned with blood diseases (e.g., deep venous thrombosis [DVT] or sickle cell disease [SCD]), as well as cancer and tumors (e.g., leukemia). Pediatric Cardiology sees patients for concerns associated with the heart and circulatory system (e.g., cardiomyopathy), and Pediatric Pulmonology is concerned with the lungs and respiratory system (e.g., asthma). Pediatric Gastroenterology focuses on conditions of the stomach and digestive tract (e.g., Crohn's disease), while Pediatric Endocrinology sees patients for concerns related to the endocrine system (e.g., diabetes). Pediatric Infectious Diseases focuses on the treatment and control of infections (e.g., human immunodeficiency virus [HIV]), Pediatric Nephrology treats the kidneys (e.g., chronic kidney disease [CKD]), and Pediatric Rheumatology treats the joints, muscles, and bones (e.g., fibromyalgia) (American Board of Medical Specialties, n.d.). In addition, while listed with ACGME as part of neurology rather than pediatrics, Child Neurology is concerned with the treatment of the nervous system (e.g., migraine, epilepsy).

Diagnostic Tools

A physician may order various imaging studies or laboratory studies to aid in diagnosis and treatment planning for pediatric patients in an inpatient or outpatient setting. Knowledge of various diagnostic studies is valuable for psychologists to best inform caregivers of what to expect and how to prepare a child in a developmentally appropriate manner to be most cooperative and successful across interventions.

Imaging Studies

There are several imaging modalities that can be useful in the medical setting. Common imaging tools with their most common indications are outlined below.

Radiograph/X-Ray

X-rays use ionizing radiation to generate images. The usefulness of X-rays is dependent on the atomic number of the substance being viewed and is most useful for substances that are very dense (e.g., bone) or substances that are not dense at all (e.g., air). X-ray images most often evaluate for fractures. A chest X-ray evaluates the lungs and is often used to diagnose pneumonia. Abdominal X-rays can also provide information about whether or not a patient is constipated or has signs of bowel obstruction. X-rays are often a valuable initial screening test, but the level of detail will not be as great as other imaging modalities. The primary disadvantage of X-ray is exposure to radiation (Woo Goo, Drubach, & Lee, 2018).

Emotional and Behavioral Considerations of X-rays

X-rays require a child/teen to remain still briefly and cause no significant pain or discomfort. Parents may be allowed to remain present but be required to wear a protective, weighted vest.

Ultrasound (US)

US is becoming much more prevalent in pediatrics as a type of imaging due to its lack of radiation or invasiveness. Rather than using X-rays, ultrasound (as the name suggests) uses sound waves to generate images from within the human body. Unfortunately, the accuracy of an ultrasound image is very user-dependent, especially in children. Some common uses for ultrasound in pediatric patients include (a) evaluation for intraventricular hemorrhage or signs of bleeding in the brain in premature infants; (b) visualization of the genitourinary system, including the kidneys and bladder; (c) evaluation of the liver and gallbladder; (d) evaluation of the anatomy of the heart (called echocardiography); and (e) evaluation for appendicitis (Woo Goo et al., 2018). In many centers, US has replaced the CT scan as the screening image of choice for appendicitis, and the list of US uses continues to grow. As technology evolves and images become clearer, US may become the standard of care in evaluation of many more pediatric conditions. The primary disadvantage of US is that it is user- and technician-dependent and therefore best done in a pediatric specialty setting. Primary advantages are that US is noninvasive and portable.

Emotional and Behavioral Considerations of US

US requires a child to remain still briefly and does not cause pain or discomfort, and caregivers may remain present for the duration of the study.

Computed Tomography (CT)

CT uses ionizing radiation to generate cross-sectional images from absorption of X-rays of the tissue examined (e.g., brain or spine). CT of the head is most commonly used in the emergency setting when an acute surgical emergency (e.g., head trauma with intracranial hemorrhage) must be excluded. CT is superior for imaging bone (e.g., skull fracture) or acute blood (e.g., subdural hematoma) and has the advantage of being more readily accessible and quicker (e.g., in the medically unstable patient). Disadvantages of CT include exposure to ionizing radiation, poor visualization of certain structures of the brain, and imaging typically limited to one (axial) plane (Morales & Shah, 2010).

In addition to the brain, CT is commonly used in the evaluation of abdominal pain. It shows more detail than an X-ray and is very useful in evaluating for the following conditions: appendicitis, pancreatitis, abdominal tumors, kidney stones, and kidney infections. CT is additionally used to evaluate the lungs, particularly if there is concern for certain types of cancer, chronic lung diseases, or pockets of infection (also called an abscess).

Emotional and Behavioral Considerations of CT

The child is required to lie on a small table that moves into a donut/circle-shaped machine. Younger children will often need to be sedated, though the imaging itself is only 5–10 min duration.

Magnetic Resonance Imaging (MRI)

MRIs are generated using principles of magnetism, capturing signal from water and organic molecules that produce a magnetic field. MRI generates some of the most detailed images of all the different types of imaging but is often not necessary if adequate images can be obtained with X-ray or CT. The brain and spine are the most common reasons for ordering an MRI in a pediatric patient. Other scenarios when an MRI may be useful are for bone and joint infections or to evaluate the pelvic anatomy, such as the ovaries and uterus.

MRI of the brain, widely used clinically since the mid- to late 1980s, is often the preferred modality for neurodiagnostic imaging. MRI may be obtained of the brain or spine or less commonly of the peripheral nerve or muscle. MRI is most commonly obtained in three planes (i.e., axial, coronal, and sagittal), thus allowing a better neuroanatomic localization. Other advantages include better visualization of some brain lesions and noninvasive visualization of blood vessels (e.g., magnetic resonance angiography-arteriography or magnetic resonance angiography-venography). Disadvantages of MRI include greater expense, longer duration, and poor/non-visualization of bone or acute blood (Morales & Shah, 2010).

Emotional and Behavioral Considerations of MRI

MRI requires a child to lie still for 45–90 min on a small table that moves into a tunnel-like space. The study is loud (similar to a jackhammer) and the space feels confining. Additionally, a brain MRI requires a child to wear a head coil that is most closely similar to a hockey mask, further exacerbating the feeling of being confined. Some young children (or youth with tics/motor disorders) require sedation to have an MRI. MRI in a child-friendly facility may provide headphones to listen to music/movies and allow the child to talk with the MRI technician.

Laboratory Testing

The list of available laboratory testing is exhaustive and is growing every day. There are some common lab tests that can be done in both inpatient and outpatient settings and are typically ordered for patients as part of an initial basic evaluation.

Complete Blood Count (CBC)

A CBC is a very common test. While the CBC can give one a lot of information, it must be interpreted in the context of the patient's symptoms and physical exam. It consists of four main components: the white blood cell count (WBC), the hemoglobin (Hgb), the hematocrit (Hct), and the platelet count. An elevation in the total WBC number can indicate signs of infection or inflammation somewhere in the body; however, this number is very nonspecific. The WBC can also be very high or very low with certain types of blood cancers and malignancies such as leukemia (Bain, 2001). The hemoglobin and hematocrit are different measures of the blood's ability to carry oxygen to the body. Low values are a sign of anemia, which can be from blood loss or chronic disease (Perkins & Hussong, 2001). The final piece of information gained from the CBC is called the platelet count. Platelets are very important cells in the blood clotting process. They can be low in genetic conditions, if the body is overwhelmed by infection, in many types of cancer, or even an autoimmune process. When the bone marrow is activated, either from infection or inflammation, the platelet number can also be high (Moriarty, 2001).

C-Reactive Protein (CRP)

The CRP is another general indicator of either infection or inflammation. It rises more quickly than the WBC count and is thought by many to be more indicative of an acute (or more recent) process. A normal CRP has a very high negative predictive value for infection; meaning, if this number is normal, it is very unlikely that the patient has a serious infection (Davidson, 2001).

Erythrocyte Sedimentation Rate (ESR)

An ESR is another nonspecific marker of inflammation. It takes a longer period of time for this marker to rise and thus is typically used to screen for the presence of more chronic inflammatory conditions, such as juvenile idiopathic arthritis (JIA), inflammatory bowel disease (IBD), or systemic lupus erythematosus (SLE or lupus), to name a few (Davidson, 2001).

Electrolyte Panels

There are several types of electrolyte panels, though they may be named differently depending on the institution. The most common types will likely be named the basic metabolic panel (BMP), the renal function panel (RFP), or the comprehensive metabolic panel (CMP). The BMP provides the following values: sodium, potassium, chloride, bicarbonate, blood urea nitrogen (BUN), creatinine, calcium, and glucose. The RFP will provide these values plus phosphate and magnesium. These screening labs can give a general idea of how a body is balancing electrolytes and can be particularly useful in evaluating how the kidneys are functioning. The CMP is more comprehensive (as the name suggests) and provides the information of the BMP and RFP with additional values, including aspartate aminotransferase (AST), alanine aminotransferase (ALT), alkaline phosphatase, and total bilirubin – these primarily evaluate if there is inflammation or obstruction occurring within the liver. It is not possible to go through the number of conditions that can cause derangements in these lab values, but abnormalities in any of the above tests can provide clues as to what might be causing the patient's symptoms (Batiuk, 2001).

Genetic Testing

The section above lists some common labs that are ordered on patients as general screening tools. There is also an exhaustive list of genetic testing that can be done to test for significant genetic sequences and syndromes that might predispose patients to disease. This is a rapidly growing area of science.

Pharmacogenomics

The term pharmacogenomics refers to the effect of one's genes on the body's response to medicine. This type of testing may also be referred to as "personalized medicine" (Mayo Clinic, n.d.). Pharmacogenetic tests look at a person's specific genes and can help determine which medication might be most effective for that person. The most common reason pharmacogenetic testing is used in children is to guide cancer therapies. While pharmacogenetic testing has benefit, there are some limitations, and it has yet to reach widespread use due to a lack of clear evidence of utility (Moaddeb & Haga, 2013). Pharmacogenetic testing does not exist for all medications, and a patient taking multiple medications may need to have more than one tests. Further, insurance coverage for this testing is variable.

Additionally, there can be ethical considerations in this type of testing. For example, the process of pharmacogenomic testing may reveal other gene abnormalities that are associated with other diseases. As a result, patients need to decide in advance if they would like this additional information revealed. Of note, there are federal laws that prohibit insurance companies from altering healthcare coverage based on genetic testing results (Mayo Clinic, n.d.).

Emotional and Behavioral Considerations of Laboratory Testing

Laboratory/genetic testing requires youth to participate in a blood draw that is relatively brief and minimally or moderately uncomfortable, depending on the subjective experience of a child. It is very common for children and teens to be fearful of needles and/or blood. Calm preparation, pain-relief creams, and distraction may all help children successfully provide blood to obtain necessary laboratory testing.

Overnight Polysomnography (PSG)

An overnight sleep study is most frequently used to diagnose and plan treatment for sleep-disordered breathing (obstructive sleep apnea), excessive daytime sleepiness (narcolepsy), or distinguish parasomnias from nocturnal seizures. PSG involves recording sleep staging, respiratory rate/effort, airflow, hemoglobin oxygen saturation, heart rate, arousals, leg/body movements, and snoring. Equipment/sensors include electroencephalogram (EEG), electromyogram (EMG), electrooculogram (EOG), oral and nasal thermal sensory and/or air pressure transducers, pulse oximeter, video, and microphone. PSGs are most often conducted in a hospital or free-standing sleep laboratory that serves both adults and children (Mindell & Owens, 2010).

Emotional and Behavioral Considerations of PSG

An overnight PSG requires a child to sleep in an unfamiliar environment with multiple wires, devices, and equipment that may feel unusual or uncomfortable. Parents are required to be present and are generally provided with a foldout chair in the room on which to sleep near their child. A child with anxiety may benefit from a tour of the sleep lab and equipment prior to participating in a sleep study.

Procedures and Intervention

Pediatric patients with acute or chronic illness may undergo various procedures and interventions that result in significant emotional distress or behavioral change. Psychologists should be familiar with common inpatient and outpatient medical intervention to best prepare a child and family for what to expect and understand the impact of an intervention on development and functioning.

Electroencephalography (EEG)

EEG is ordered most commonly in patients when there is concern for seizures. Electrodes are applied to the scalp corresponding to certain underlying regions of the brain, and electrical activity is recorded. Activation procedures such as sleep deprivation (only sleeping 4 h the night prior to EEG), hyperventilation (asking a child to blow on a pinwheel), and photic stimulation (exposure to flashing lights) are typically employed in order to increase the likelihood of identifying a seizure. Epileptiform activity (i.e., spikes and sharp waves) suggests a tendency to seizures and may indicate sites of origin for them. In some cases, EEG may be combined with video recording to correlate sudden changes in behavior with electrical activity of the brain. This may be accomplished in an epilepsy monitoring unit (EMU). Video EEG may be ordered to localize a site of origin for epilepsy or to distinguish epileptic seizures (i.e., electrical activity from the brain resulting in abrupt change in behavior) versus non-epileptic events (Morales & Shah, 2010).

Emotional and Behavioral Considerations of EEG

A routine outpatient EEG takes 20–40 min and caregivers may remain present for the duration of the test. Inpatient, longer duration, and ambulatory EEGs are also an option as warranted. The placement of the electrodes and cleaning the area of the scalp after may be somewhat awkward for a child, but the test itself does not cause any pain/discomfort. The other behavioral consideration is intentional sleep deprivation that may briefly but negatively affect a child's energy level, mood, and sleep schedule.

Lumbar Puncture (LP)

LP is a procedure to collect cerebrospinal fluid (CSF) for diagnostic purposes. Neuroimaging with CT or MRI of the brain is generally completed first. An LP is placement of a needle under sterile technique into the lumbar CSF space (lower, middle back) after local anesthetic is applied. Opening pressure is obtained (especially useful to determine if pseudotumor cerebri or idiopathic intracranial hypertension is present), and CSF is collected in tubes and sent to the laboratory for evaluation. The most common complication of an LP is a "post-LP headache," which is a persistent CSF leak and a headache that occurs upon sitting up and is relieved by lying down. This generally resolves with conservative management in approximately 72 h (Soni, 2010).

Emotional and Behavioral Considerations of LP

This procedure takes approximately 10 min and caregivers may remain present. Though the area of needle placement is anesthetized, a deep pressure sensation is felt. Conscious sedation may be required in younger children.

Blood Products and Transfusions

A transfusion is giving of donated blood or any of its main components (plasma, platelets, red blood cells, or white blood cells) to a patient, usually through an intravenous line (IV). The primary reason a patient would need a transfusion would be if they are low on blood or a blood product. The reasons for having low levels of blood or its components will vary but are commonly seen in settings of trauma, cancer, or critical illness. Typically, whole blood is broken down into these main components for the purposes of transfusion: packed red blood cells (PRBC), platelets, and fresh frozen plasma (FFP). Intravenous immunoglobulin (IVIG) is an infusion of antibodies, a type of infection-fighting cell. IVIG will commonly be used in autoimmune conditions or immune deficiencies. Transfusions of blood or its products can be controversial, and the process of transfusion also carries some risk to the patient. With any type of transfusion, there is a risk of a transfusion reaction that typically includes fever, chills, or difficulty in breathing (Seeber & Shander, 2013).

Emotional and Behavioral Considerations of Blood Transfusions

Transfusions vary in invasiveness and duration. Caregivers may remain present throughout, and distraction from needle pokes in the form of social engagement or other (electronic) entertainment is generally available in a pediatric setting.

Gastrointestinal (GI) Tract Procedures

In addition to ultrasound, symptoms associated with digestion may be evaluated with endoscopy and biopsy (small tissue sample removed for further evaluation). An endoscope is a flexible, lighted tube with a camera (smaller than a pencil) that can be inserted into the body to observe and biopsy tissue at different points in the digestive tract.

Esophagogastroduodenoscopy (EGD or upper gastrointestinal endoscopy) provides information about the upper digestive tract, including the esophagus, stomach, and upper small intestine. The endoscope is inserted through the mouth into the stomach and small intestine to observe and take a biopsy. This procedure is generally done under full anesthesia. Also performed under full anesthesia, a colonoscopy evaluates the colon/large intestine and rectum through an endoscope inserted into the rectum. In preparation for a colonoscopy (or for problems with chronic constipation), a child or teen may be prescribed a bowel clean out procedure involving oral laxatives and/or enemas (Hoffenberg et al., 2018).

Emotional and Behavioral Considerations of GI Procedures

GI imaging and procedures can be invasive and uncomfortable and will require anesthesia/sedation. A child or teen will certainly benefit from preparation for such procedures. Additionally, a bowel clean out process takes at least 12 h and may be done as an inpatient in preparation for a colonoscopy the following day. An outpatient clean out involves drinking a significant amount of fluid and frequent bathroom breaks.

Medication Management

Medications used in an inpatient or outpatient pediatric setting can be broadly divided into categories. For purposes of this chapter, emphasis will be placed on medications used as an adjunct to behavioral treatment and/or medications with emotional/behavioral side effects.

Anticonvulsants

The Food and Drug Administration (FDA) issued an alert on January 31, 2008 to healthcare providers regarding the risk of suicidal thoughts and behavior with antiepileptic drugs (AEDs). AEDs are associated with a variety of cognitive and behavioral side effects. The American Epilepsy Society position is and remains that, in the vast majority of patients with epilepsy, the benefits of treatment outweigh the risks (American Epilepsy Society, 2008).

Primary effect: Anticonvulsants are prescribed to individuals with seizure disorders to reduce the risk of having further seizures. Examples include phenobarbital, carbamazepine, topiramate, and zonisamide. Side effects: Sedation, ataxia, agitation/aggression, depression, suicidal or homicidal ideation in children, nightmares, allergic skin reactions, and liver dysfunction (Guilfoyle et al., 2018; Halma et al., 2014).

Antidepressants

Primary effect: Antidepressants (e.g., SSRI, SSRI/SNRI, tricyclic antidepressants, others) are prescribed as an adjunct to psychotherapy in the treatment of depressive disorders and/or anxiety disorders. Examples include citalopram, escitalopram, sertraline, paroxetine, and bupropion. Side effects: Dry mouth, blurred vision, constipation, diarrhea, suicidal or homicidal ideation in children, nightmares, unusual thoughts, weight gain, agitation, irritability, and sexual problems.

Antihistamines

Primary effect: Antihistamines are most commonly prescribed to combat the symptoms of allergic rhinitis (congestion, itchy watery eyes, sneezing). Examples include diphenhydramine, hydroxyzine, loratadine, and cetirizine. Side effects: Dry mouth, drowsiness, dizziness, nausea and vomiting, restlessness or moodiness (in some children), blurred vision, and confusion. Note: Antihistamines are sometimes used to treat anxiousness and sleep disturbance (Milgrom & Bender, 1995).

Anxiolytics

Primary effect: Anxiolytic medications (such as benzodiazepines) are used for the treatment of anxiety disorders and their related psychological and physical symptoms. Examples include alprazolam, lorazepam, and clonazepam. Side effects: Drowsiness, sedation, confusion, dependence and withdrawal symptoms, and weight gain.

Opioids

Primary effect: Prescription opioids can be used to treat moderate-to-severe pain and are often prescribed for short-term use following surgery or injury or for terminal health conditions such as cancer. Examples include morphine (reference standard), codeine, and oxycodone. Side effects: Drowsiness, sedation, confusion, dependence and withdrawal symptoms, constipation, and weight gain (Centers for Disease Control and Prevention [CDC], 2017). Due to problematic side effect profile and abuse potential, opioids are not recommended for first-line treatment of chronic pain in pediatric patients (PAINS Project, 2017).

Atypical Antipsychotics

Primary effect: Atypical antipsychotic medications are used to treat depression, anxiety, and psychosis. They have been found to improve delusions and hallucinations in patients who fail to respond to other antipsychotic drugs and to reduce the risk of suicide. Examples include aripiprazole and risperidone. Side effects: Sedation, constipation, dizziness, weight gain, diabetes mellitus, hyperlipidemia, cardiac rhythm disturbances, sexual dysfunction, and extrapyramidal side effects (e.g., tremor, chorea, dystonia) (Meltzer, 2004; Üçok & Gaebel, 2008).

Stimulants

Primary effect: Stimulants are intended to reduce hyperactivity, fidgetiness, impulsivity, and inattentiveness, primarily associated with ADHD. Examples include methylphenidate, dextroamphetamine, and dexmethylphenidate hydrochloride. Side effects: Potential side effects include headache, gastrointestinal distress, elevated blood pressure, loss of appetite, weight loss, nervousness, and possibly exacerbation of tics. Note: Examples of non-stimulant medications also used to treat ADHD are atomoxetine and guanfacine.

Sympathomimetics

Primary effect: Most commonly used to facilitate bronchodilation and alleviate the symptoms of asthma. Side effects: Anxiousness, jitteriness, tremor, and nervousness.

Corticosteroids

Primary effect: Glucocorticoids (also referred to as simply steroids) are most commonly administered to reduce an inflammatory- or immune-mediated reaction. Examples include the acute treatment of asthma, migraine, or a variety of rheumatologic or digestive conditions. Side effects: Insomnia, agitation/aggression, emotional instability, and a host of side effects involving other organ systems; thus, most providers attempt to prescribe at the lowest dosage and duration (Drozdowicz & Bostwick, 2014).

Medication prescriptions often include abbreviations for dosage information and instruction; some of the common abbreviations are listed in Table 1.

Table 1 Prescription abbreviations

Abbreviation	Meaning	Abbreviation	Meaning
a.c.	Before meals	q( )h	Every ( ) hours
b.i.d.	Twice a day	q.h.s.	At every bedtime
p.c.	After meals	q.i.d.	Four times per day
p.r.n.	As needed	q.m.	Every morning
p.o.	By mouth, orally	q.n.	Every night
q.h.	Every hour	t.i.d.	Three times a day

Common Medical Acronyms/Abbreviations

Medical abbreviations and acronyms are frequently used in healthcare documentation and are used as a common language among medical professionals. Some of the common abbreviations and acronyms are included in Table 2, but many other abbreviations exist, such as those presented throughout this chapter that are not additionally identified in Table 2. All of the abbreviations and acronyms used in Table 2 are found in *Dorland's Dictionary of Medical Acronyms and Abbreviations* (2016). The Joint Commission on Accreditation of Hospitals (JCAH) also has a list of prohibited medical abbreviations, acronyms, and symbols (see https://www.jointcommission.org/facts_about_do_not_use_list/), and no item on that list should be used in medical documentation. Each medical system or institution may use its own abbreviations, and providers should therefore consult with their institution to obtain a list of approved or prohibited abbreviations and acronyms.

Additional Ethical and Cultural Considerations

Informed Consent

All caregivers and patients can expect to participate in an informed consent and assent process for any (clinical or research) procedure or intervention. In 2016, the American Academy of

Table 2 Common medical abbreviations and acronyms

Abbreviation or acronym	Meaning
AAP	American Academy of Pediatrics
ACE	Adverse childhood experience
AMA	American Medical Association; against medical advice
AMS	Altered mental status
BMT	Bone marrow transplant
BP	Blood pressure
CBC	Complete blood cell count
CC	Chief complaint
CKD	Chronic kidney disease
CF	Cystic fibrosis
C/O	Complaining of
CP	Cerebral palsy
CSF	Cerebrospinal fluid
CT	Computed tomography
DKA	Diabetic ketoacidosis
DM	Diabetes mellitus
DNR	Do not resuscitate
DVT	Deep venous thrombosis
Dx	Diagnosis
ECMO	Extracorporeal membrane oxygenation
ED	Emergency department
EEG	Electroencephalography
EGD	Esophagogastroduodenoscopy
EKG	Electrocardiogram
EMR	Electronic medical record
EMS	Emergency medical services
ETOH	Ethanol
GERD	Gastroesophageal reflux disease
GI	Gastrointestinal
GYN	Gynecology
GSR	Galvanic skin response
HA	Headache
HbA1c	Glycosylated hemoglobin
Hgb	Hemoglobin
H/O	History of
HTN	Hypertension
H&P	History and physical examination
HPI	History of present illness
HR	Heart rate
IBD	Inflammatory bowel disease
IM	Intramuscular
IV	Intravenous
IVIG	Intravenous immunoglobulin
JIA	Juvenile idiopathic arthritis
LLQ	Lower left quadrant
LP	Lumbar puncture

(continued)

Table 2 (continued)

Abbreviation or acronym	Meaning
LUQ	Left upper quadrant
M&M	Morbidity and mortality
MRI	Magnetic resonance imaging
MRSA	Methicillin-resistant *Staphylococcus aureus*
MUS	Medically unexplained symptoms
N&V	Nausea and vomiting
NPO	Nothing by mouth
NS	Normal saline
PCOS	Polycystic ovary syndrome
PCP	Primary care physician/provider
PICC	Peripherally inserted central catheter
PICU	Pediatric intensive care unit
PMD	Primary physician
PMH	Past medical history
POTS	Postural orthostatic tachycardia syndrome
Pt	Patient
RBC	Red blood cell
RLQ	Right lower quadrant
ROS	Review of systems
RUQ	Right upper quadrant
SLE	Systemic lupus erythematosus
SOB	Shortness of breath
S/P	Status post[operative]
SQ	Subcutaneous
Sx	Signs; symptoms
TB	Tuberculosis
UA	Urinalysis
UNOS	United Network for Organ Sharing
UOP	Urinary output
URI	Upper respiratory infection
WBC	White blood cell count
WNL	Within normal limits

Note: Many of the abbreviations and acronyms above may have other meanings as well

Pediatrics (AAP) published an updated position statement related to the process of informed consent. This document posits that informed consent should be seen as an essential and active part of healthcare with developmentally informed involvement of the child's or adolescent's opinion in medical decision-making. Informed consent incorporates three responsibilities: disclosure of information related to diagnosis/treatment (including potential risks, benefits, and uncertainties to patients and surrogates); assessment of patient and surrogate understanding of the information and capacity for medical decision-making; and obtaining voluntary informed consent before any intervention takes place. The collaborative consent and treatment process should maximize benefit and minimize harm. Should conflict arise, consultation with an ethics committee, psychologist, psychiatrist, chaplain, or palliative care team is recommended, while legal intervention is considered a last resort. The three broad categories when a minor can legally, independently make medical decisions are related to specific diagnostic/care categories (i.e., sexual/mental health), the "mature minor" exception (adolescent is deemed cognitively and psychosocially mature enough to make independent medical decisions), and legal emancipation. Finally, physicians must also be aware of all research-specific and local/state laws relevant to the consent and assent process (Katz & Webb, 2016).

Objections to Medical Care

Physicians have a right to express moral/conscientious objection to provision of a treatment or intervention, but ethical practice requires a physician to disclose this individual objection as a part of the informed consent process and provide appropriate referrals for ongoing care as needed (American Academy of Pediatrics, Committee on Bioethics, 2009).

There are also various cultural/religious groups that may object to all or certain medical intervention. Competent adults may refuse lifesaving care for themselves, but the US Supreme Court has ruled that parents may not deny their children necessary medical care. The AAP supports provision of lifesaving medical care for all seriously ill children despite parental religious beliefs that oppose such intervention (Jenny & The Committee on Child Abuse and Neglect, 2007).

Medical Neglect

Physicians are obligated to assess and respond to possible medical neglect or the failure of a caregiver to recognize or respond to a child's medical needs. A caregiver response is only considered neglect if harm is evident, appropriate healthcare is available, and the caregiver understands the medical situation and advice. The assessment process of potential medical neglect must be culturally sensitive, thorough, and collaborative. Again, legal intervention should be considered a last resort (Jenny & The Committee on Child Abuse and Neglect, 2007).

Medically Controversial Topics

Medically Difficult to Explain Diagnoses

Psychologists benefit from being aware of potentially controversial topics in medicine. The following conditions/diagnoses may be controversial due to the understanding of etiology, maintenance, and management of these conditions, which may be provider- or institution-specific and/or not well-defined in the pediatric medical/psychological literature: pediatric autoimmune neuropsychiatric disorders associated with streptococcal infections (PANDAS), Lyme disease, juvenile fibromyalgia, systemic exertion intolerance disease (SEID) or myalgic encephalomyelitis (ME; sometimes abbreviated as ME/CFS and previously known as chronic fatigue syndrome), headache/concussion, postural orthostatic tachycardia syndrome (POTS), chronic regional pain syndrome (CRPS), psychogenic/paroxysmal nonepileptic seizure/spells (PNES), or any condition that may be understood as somatic, psychogenic, nonorganic, functional, or medically difficult to explain. The term "functional" is currently preferred and refers to symptoms resulting in impairment of functioning that lack an identified structural etiology (e.g., functional abdominal pain is impairing level of belly pain in the presence of a thorough and normal abdominal/GI medical evaluation). Cautious evaluation of scientific evidence and a collaborative, interdisciplinary approach to diagnosis and management is warranted for any such condition. Validation of individual patient and family experience and focus on evidence-based interventions targeting functional restoration is generally most beneficial (Carter & Threlkeld, 2012; Williams & Zahka, 2017).

Cannabinoids/Medical Marijuana

Marijuana has two chemical substances—cannabidiol (CBD) and tetrahydrocannabinol (THC). CBD has less intoxicating effect, and CBD-derived products are becoming more widely available. There are a few (pill) forms of medical marijuana approved for use in adults receiving chemotherapy or experiencing AIDS-associated nausea/vomiting, and these are generally prescribed when other interventions have failed (American Academy of Neurology, 2014). In June of 2018, the FDA approved the first drug derived from CBD to treat refractory seizures associated with Dravet and Lennox-Gastaut syndromes (LGS) in youth (Epilepsy Foundation, 2018). There are ongoing trials of CBD-derived medications for various other medical conditions for adults and children. Many national organizations have position statements related to the use of cannabinoids or medical marijuana (i.e., the American Academy of Neurology, the Epilepsy Foundation, the American Psychiatric Association). The American Academy of Pediatrics and American Psychological Association also have several publications/statements related to the use of marijuana in pediatric populations. The acceptance and use of these products will vary across settings and provider and, of course, time, as research develops.

Recommended Resources

The field of pediatric medicine is complex and ever evolving. The authors recommend utilizing the following resources for further information/reference. Some resources may require purchased subscription, but most are generally accessible via a university/college library system (Table 3).

Table 3 Recommended resources for additional reference

Name	Website	Description
Medscape	www.medscape.com	Free-access website designed for clinicians to access healthcare/disease-specific information, continuing education
UpToDate	www.uptodate.com	Subscription-required, peer-reviewed website designed for healthcare providers to improve patient care
DynaMedPlus	www.dynamed.com	Subscription-required website with various clinical healthcare information designed for providers, affiliated with EBSCO
MedlinePlus	http://medlineplus.gov	Free-access health information from NIH/US National Library of Medicine
Epocrates	www.epocrates.com	Medical reference app with free and paid content
Lexicomp	www.online.lexi.com	Subscription-required website or app with clinical drug information designed for prescribing providers
New England Journal of Medicine on YouTube	www.youtube.com/user/NEJMvideo	Free-access video-based content of various medical information and brief video slideshow summaries of journal articles
Coping Club	www.copingclub.com	Free-access website of videos of children/teens for other children/teens related to coping with medical procedures/illness
HealthyChildren	www.healthychildren.org	Free-access information related to pediatric healthcare from the AAP, designed for caregivers (English and Spanish content)
KidsHealth	www.kidshealth.org	Free-access pediatric healthcare information with content for parents, teens, kids, and educators
Children's Hospitals websites	Find through any search engine	Many hospitals maintain websites with valuable videos and handouts designed for patients and families and/or healthcare providers

References

Accreditation Council for Graduate Medical Education. (n.d.). Retrieved from https://www.acgme.org/Specialties/Overview/pfcatid/16

American Academy of Neurology. (2014). Summary of systematic review for patients and their families: Medical marijuana in certain neurological disorders. Retrieved from https://www.aan.com/Guidelines/home/GetGuidelineContent/650

American Association of Pediatrics, Committee on Bioethics. (2009). Policy statement—Physician refusal to provide information or treatment on the basis of claims of conscience. *Pediatrics, 124*(6), 1689–1693. https://doi.org/10.1542/peds.2009-2222

American Board of Medical Specialties. (n.d.). Retrieved from https://www.abms.org/member-boards/contact-an-abms-member-board/american-board-of-pediatrics/

American Epilepsy Society. (2008). AES position on risk of suicidal thoughts and behavior with anti-epileptic medications. Retrieved from https://www.aesnet.org/about_aes/position_statements/aespositiononriskofsuicidalthoughtsbehaviorwithantiepilepticmedications

Bain, B. J. (2001). White blood cells. In S. L. Jones (Ed.), *Clinical laboratory pearls* (pp. 97–138). Philadelphia, PA: Lippincott Williams & Wilkins.

Batiuk, T. D. (2001). Electrolytes and fluid balance. In S. L. Jones (Ed.), *Clinical laboratory pearls* (pp. 310–318). Philadelphia, PA: Lippincott Williams & Wilkins.

Carter, B. D., & Threlkeld, B. M. (2012). Psychosocial perspectives in the treatment of pediatric chronic pain. *Pediatric Rheumatology, 10*, 15. https://doi.org/10.1186/1546-0096-10-15

Centers for Disease Control and Prevention. (2017). Prescription opioids. Retrieved from https://www.cdc.gov/drugoverdose/opioids/prescribed.html

Conroy, C., & Logan, D. E. (2014). Pediatric multidisciplinary and interdisciplinary teams and interventions. In M. C. Roberts, B. S. Aylward, & Y. P. Wu (Eds.), *Clinical practice of pediatric psychology* (pp. 93–108). New York, NY: The Guilford Press.

Davidson, D. D. (2001). Inflammation and repair. In S. L. Jones (Ed.), *Clinical laboratory pearls* (pp. 447–450). Philadelphia, PA: Lippincott Williams & Wilkins.

Dorland's dictionary of medical acronyms & abbreviations (7th ed.). (2016). Philadelphia, PA: Elsevier.

Drotar, D. (1977). Clinical psychological practice in a pediatric hospital. *Professional Psychology, 8*(1), 72–80. https://doi.org/10.1037/0735-7028.8.1.72

Drozdowicz, L. B., & Bostwick, J. M. (2014). Psychiatric adverse effects of pediatric corticosteroid use. *Mayo Clinic Proceedings, 89*(6), 817–834.

Epilepsy Foundation. (2018). Medical marijuana and epilepsy. Retrieved from https://www.epilepsy.com/learn/treating-seizures-and-epilepsy/other-treatment-approaches/medical-marijuana-and-epilepsy

Guilfoyle, S. M., Follansbee-Junger, K., Smith, A. W., Combs, A., Ollier, S., Hater, B., & Modi, A. C. (2018). Antiepileptic drug behavioral side effects and baseline hyperactivity in children and adolescents with new onset epilepsy. *Epilepsia, 59*(1), 146–154.

Halma, E., de Louw, A. J., Klinkenberg, S., Aldenkamp, A. P., Ijff, D. M., & Majoie, M. (2014). Behavioral side-effects of levetiracetam in children with epilepsy: A systematic review. *Seizure, 23*(9), 685–691. https://doi.org/10.1016/j.seizure.2014.06.004

Hoffenberg, E. J., Furuta, G. T., Kobak, G., Walker, T., Soden, J., Kramer, R. E., & Brumbaugh, D. (2018). Gastrointestinal tract. In W. W. Hay, R. R. Deterding, M. J. Levin, & M. J. Abzug (Eds.), *Current diagnosis and treatment: Pediatrics* (24th ed., pp. 626–668). New York, NY: McGraw Hill Education.

Jenny, C., & The Committee on Child Abuse and Neglect. (2007). Recognizing and responding to medical neglect. *Pediatrics, 120*(6), 1385–1389. https://doi.org/10.1542/peds.2007-2903

Katz, A., & Webb, S. (2016). Informed consent in decision-making in pediatric practice. *Pediatrics, 138*(2), 1–7.

Mayo Clinic. (n.d.). Center for individualized medicine: Drug-gene testing. Retrieved from http://mayoresearch.mayo.edu/center-for-individualized-medicine/drug-gene-testing.asp

Meltzer, H. Y. (2004). What's atypical about atypical antipsychotic drugs? *Current Opinion in Pharmacology, 4*(1), 53–57.

Milgrom, H., & Bender, B. (1995). Behavioral side effects of medications used to treat asthma and allergic rhinitis. *Pediatrics in Review, 16*(9), 333–335.

Mindell, J. A., & Owens, J. A. (2010). *A clinical guide to pediatric sleep: Diagnosis and management of sleep problems* (2nd ed.). Philadelphia, PA: Lippincott Williams & Wilkins.

Moaddeb, J., & Haga, S. B. (2013). Pharmacogenetic testing: Current evidence of clinical utility. *Therapeutic Advances in Drug Safety, 4*(4), 155 169.

Morales, R. E., & Shah, D. G. (2010). Fundamentals of neuroradiology. In W. J. Weiner, C. G. Goetz, R. K. Shin, & S. L. Lewis (Eds.), *Neurology for the non-neurologist* (pp. 43–62). Philadelphia, PA: Lippincott Williams & Wilkins.

Moriarty, A. T. (2001). Platelets, coagulation, fibrinolysis. In S. L. Jones (Ed.), *Clinical laboratory pearls* (pp. 139–161). Philadelphia, PA: Lippincott Williams & Wilkins.

PAINS Project. (2017). Pediatric chronic pain: Prevalence, economic impact, and its relevance to the current opioid epidemic. *Policy & Educational Brief, 10*, 2–7. Retrieved from http://painsproject.org/aipm/wpcontent/uploads/2017/09/PAINS_Policy_Brief_10_web.pdf

Palermo, T. M., Janicke, D. M., McQuaid, E. L., Mullins, L. L., Robins, P. M., & Wu, Y. P. (2014). Recommendations for training in pediatric psychology: Defining core competencies across training levels. *Journal of Pediatric Psychology, 39*, 965–984.

Perkins, S. L., & Hussong, J. W. (2001). Red blood cells. In S. L. Jones (Ed.), *Clinical laboratory pearls* (pp. 61–96). Philadelphia, PA: Lippincott Williams & Wilkins.

Seeber, P., & Shander, A. (2013). *Basics of blood management* (2nd ed.). Hoboken, NJ: Wiley-Blackwell.

Soni, M. (2010). Clinical use of neurologic diagnostic tests. In W. J. Weiner, C. G. Goetz, R. K. Shin, & S. L. Lewis (Eds.), *Neurology for the non-neurologist* (pp. 33–42). Philadelphia, PA: Lippincott Williams & Wilkins.

Üçok, A., & Gaebel, W. (2008). Side effects of atypical antipsychotics: A brief overview. *World Psychiatry, 7*(1), 58–62.

Williams, S. E., & Zahka, N. E. (2017). *Treating somatic symptoms in children and adolescents*. New York, NY: The Guilford Press.

Woo Goo, H., Drubach, L. A., & Lee, E. Y. (2018). Imaging techniques. In B. Cooley (Ed.), *Caffey's pediatric diagnostic imaging* (13th ed., pp. 457–467). Philadelphia, PA: Elsevier.

Collaborating with Psychosocial Colleagues in the Hospital Setting

Amanda L. Thompson and Megan Connolly

By nature of our specialty training and expertise, pediatric psychologists collaborate closely with a variety of medical providers—physicians (both specialist and primary care), advance practice providers, nurses, and more—in order to promote the health and development of children and adolescents in various pediatric health contexts. In most cases, pediatric psychologists are also working closely with a number of other psychosocial colleagues, including social workers, child life specialists, and chaplains, and based on availability of resources, additional support services such as art therapists, music therapists, educational supports (e.g., education specialists, school liaisons, or teachers), and patient navigators. These psychosocial providers each have unique training and areas of competency that together provide a model of interprofessional care that addresses many vital aspects of patient and family psychological, social, emotional, and spiritual well-being.

A. L. Thompson (✉) · M. Connolly
Department of Pediatrics, Children's National Hospital, George Washington University School of Medicine and Health Sciences, Washington, DC, USA

Department of Psychiatry and Behavioral Science, Children's National Hospital, George Washington University School of Medicine and Health Sciences, Washington, DC, USA
e-mail: Amanda.Thompson@inova.org

Guidelines within professional psychology support the role of psychologists in their efforts to collaborate with other psychosocial providers. Specifically, the American Psychological Association's Ethics Code (APA, 2002, 2010, 2016) and Guidelines for Psychological Practice in Health Care Delivery Systems (APA, 2013) emphasize that psychologists cooperate with other professionals in order to serve their patients effectively and appropriately. In addition, the core competencies for training in pediatric psychology highlight that trainees must be proficient in working "effectively with colleagues from other disciplines (e.g., nursing, pediatrics, social work) to maintain a climate of mutual respect and shared values" (Palermo et al., 2014, p. 972). Even more, some specific illness areas, like pediatric oncology, have integrated open and respectful collaboration among psychosocial providers into their standards of psychosocial care (Patenaude, Pelletier, & Bingen, 2015).

Despite these guidelines, there is little research specific to collaboration among psychosocial providers within the hospital setting. Instead, as this type of psychosocial collaboration within pediatric healthcare has become more the rule than the exception, pediatric psychologists must look to the broader literature on interprofessional collaboration, teamwork, and team-based healthcare for guidance on models of engagement between providers and determinants of successful

B. D. Carter, K. A. Kullgren (eds.), *Clinical Handbook of Psychological Consultation in Pediatric Medical Settings*, Issues in Clinical Child Psychology, https://doi.org/10.1007/978-3-030-35598-2_8

collaboration. In this chapter, we present these models, as well as many of the essential elements of successful psychosocial collaboration, strategies for promoting collaboration (while highlighting common barriers that may interfere with successful teamwork and patient care), and directions for future research.

Psychosocial Teams

For the purposes of this chapter, the term "team" will be used to describe two or more providers (in this case, psychosocial providers) who work collaboratively with patients and their caregivers to accomplish shared goals (Ervin, Kahn, Cohen, & Weingart, 2018; Mitchell et al., 2012). Psychosocial teams, it must be noted, may vary greatly between institutions and even between units, divisions, or departments within the same institutions. Depending on organizational factors like hospital/division size, staffing, resources, and leadership structure, teams can be large or small, with goals that are focused and time-limited or more general and sustained (Mitchell et al., 2012). Some psychosocial teams are well-defined and centralized with a single reporting structure (i.e., all report to the same manager) and providers that only offer care to one disease group, while others are less well-defined and more dispersed, with providers reporting to multiple managers and maintaining multiple care-team responsibilities. A pediatric psychologist, then, may be embedded within a specific hospital unit as part of a formal, well-established psychosocial team that provides care to patients with one specific clinical condition or set of conditions (e.g., all patients with diabetes). Alternatively, a generalist consultation-liaison (CL), pediatric psychologist may interact with a fluid and dynamic psychosocial team on multiple cases across multiple units throughout the day (e.g., a social worker in the NICU, a child life specialist in Gastroenterology).

Certainly, the appropriate team structure varies by situation, the needs of the patient population, availability of staff and other resources, and more (Mitchell et al., 2012). Despite these differences, however, it is generally assumed that the involvement of more than one discipline is valuable and has benefits to the patients, families, and medical teams seeking consultation and support. Within the increasingly complex setting of modern healthcare, an interdisciplinary team approach seems best suited to address the equally complex psychosocial needs of the patients and families in our care (Baggott & Kelly, 2002; Gibson, 2009).

Interprofessional Collaboration and Teamwork

Professional collaboration exists along a spectrum, and unique terms have been used to define different levels of engagement between disciplines. The common team descriptions "multidisciplinary" and "interdisciplinary" are often used interchangeably but, in fact, represent very distinct models of provider engagement and interaction. According to Choi and Pak (2006), in a *multidisciplinary* team, members function as independent specialists rather than interactive team members; they treat patients independently and share information with each other after the fact. For example, during a multidisciplinary long-term follow-up clinic for survivors of childhood cancer, a social worker, psychologist, and education specialist may each individually assess a patient, generally at the discretion of the team leader, usually a physician. Providers typically submit their individual recommendations via documentation in the electronic medical record (EMR). While these team members may consult about the case and discuss their impressions following their initial assessments, another team member's assessment generally does not factor into the psychologist's assessment or recommendations at the time of the assessment. An *interdisciplinary* team, on the other hand, seeks a more sophisticated level of collaboration, in which members of different disciplines and training backgrounds combine their knowledge and mutually develop an integrated plan of care (Choi & Pak, 2006). As an example, team members working together in an interdisciplinary long-term follow-up clinic for survivors of childhood cancer, then, may see the patient individually before discussing the patient and the plan of care. Importantly, in this model, members share their individual assessments based on their areas of expertise but then develop a joint treatment plan for the patient wherein one member's assessment informs another member's recommendation. Even more, team members using this model may meet together with the patient to provide their collective impressions and recommendations. Some interdisciplinary teams in the pediatric healthcare setting may even meet with the patient and family to conduct an assessment together, integrating care and expertise from the start. Multidisciplinarity, then, is an additive process, with providers working in parallel, while interdisciplinarity is a synthesis or integration, with providers working jointly, and where, in effect, the "whole is greater than the sum of its parts."

As these models apply to teams in all fields (e.g., healthcare, policy, research, industry), the healthcare domain, specifically, has proposed that interdisciplinarity be conceptualized as "interprofessionality" or "interprofessional collaboration" in order to emphasize the development of a cohesive practice between professionals of different disciplines (D'Amour & Oandasan, 2005). *Interprofessional* collaboration is framed as an integrated approach to the needs of patients and families that "involves continuous interaction and knowledge sharing between professionals..." "to solve or explore a variety of education and care issues all while seeking to optimize patient's participant" in their care (D'Amour & Oandasan, 2005, p. 9). In practice, then, it refers to cooperating, nonhierarchical independent equals who contribute to a shared vision of health; it is not to be confused with providers who work independently but happen to liaise with one another over a given period of time (Herbert, 2005; Scholes & Vaughan, 2002).

Although we lack any empirical evidence specific to psychosocial collaboration, research indicates that interprofessional healthcare collaboration benefits patients and families *and* providers and teams. When providers share their expertise and experience within the team environment, patients and families have access to the highest and most diverse level of knowledge and expertise and the fullest range of services available, and patient outcomes are positively impacted (Drotar, 2002; Gibson, 2009; Mitchell et al., 2012; Zwarenstein, Reeves, & Perrier, 2005). Collaboration has been linked to improved patient satisfaction, higher quality of care, and better ability to meet the needs of family, as well as improved team morale, greater job satisfaction, increased efficiency, and better team member mental health (Firth-Cozens, 2001; Majzun, 1998; West, Borrill, & Unsworth, 1998; Yeager, 2005). On the other hand, lack of interprofessional collaboration and communication can result in fragmentation of care, lower quality and satisfaction of care, and worse patient outcomes (Baggs et al., 1999; Joint Commission on Accreditation of Healthcare Organizations, 2005; Larson, 1999; Majzun, 1998).

Elements of Successful Psychosocial Collaboration

The significant heterogeneity in size, composition, patient population, and treatment settings is a challenge to defining optimal interprofessional psychosocial collaboration or to providing specific guidance on the best structure and function for teams. Nevertheless, there is a substantial body of literature—much of which is well beyond the scope of this chapter (Hackman, 2014; Mitchell et al., 2012; Salas, Shuffler, Thayer, Bedwell, & Lazzara, 2015)—that supports the notion that effective teams and successful collaborations in healthcare appear to be guided by the same basic unifying principles and strategies. Most relevant to collaboration and coordination among psychosocial providers in the medical setting are the principles of (1) shared goals, (2) role clarity, and (3) effective communication. Table 1 summarizes these elements, their key features, and strategies to enhance their effectiveness as described in the text that follows.

Table 1 Essential elements of an effective psychosocial team

Essential element	Key features	Strategies to enhance effectiveness
Shared goals	– Patient/family centered – Clearly articulated – Broad (mission/vision) and specific (per patient)	– Ensure meeting space and time for goal creation and for regular evaluation and refinement – Create written plans of care, accessible to all members, that explicitly include shared goals – Identification of shared goals
Role clarity	– Clear expectations for team member's role, function, and responsibilities – Can reduce confusion, frustration, conflict, and territorialism – Can optimize team efficiency and effectiveness and reduce professional burnout	– Develop clear understanding of one's own role, expertise, and boundaries and ability to communicate same (e.g., handout or elevator speech) – Educate oneself about the role of psychosocial colleagues (e.g., meeting with team members to learn about training, skillsets, interests; shadowing opportunities; reading documentation of patient/family interactions and session) – Maintain written, unambiguous job descriptions – Address role overlap directly and confront conflict in a timely manner – Ensure meeting space and time for open discussion about roles and skills of team members – Revisit issues as team composition changes
Effective communication	– Most important determining factor of an effective collaborative healthcare team – Impacts other aspects of collaboration, like mutual respect and trust	– Set high standard for consistent, clear, professional communication and hold members accountable – Ensure meeting space and time for discussion of communication processes, patterns, and protocols – Hold provider-to-provider or care coordination rounds (daily or weekly) with a clear purpose and organizational structure – Arrange for handoffs between providers – Organize family-centered rounds/multidisciplinary family meetings – Conduct psychosocial rounds for certain care teams – Document coordinated care plans – Document consistently and clearly in the medical record – Use informal communication methods frequently (e.g., phone, email, face to face) – Create and implement standardized protocols, policies, and procedures for documentation

Shared Goals

As described previously, the notion of a shared goal is integral to the definition of "team" (Mitchell et al., 2012; Salas et al., 2015), as team-based medicine involves the expertise and coordinated efforts of two or more clinicians working together on a shared task or goal (Ervin et al., 2018). For a psychosocial team to collaborate well together and provide the highest quality of care to patients and families, shared goals should be organized around the needs and perspective of patients and families and be clearly articulated, understood, and supported by all members (Mitchell et al., 2012). Discussion of shared goals is important for the team in the broader sense (e.g., preparation of a mission and/or vision statement) but also in each individual case where psychosocial collaboration is occurring. For example, team members may find it helpful to agree on clear, unifying goals of reducing distress associated with inpatient admissions, improving adherence to treatment recommendations, or supporting family decision-making, among others. Shared, patient-oriented goals should be regularly evaluated and refined as needed (in psychosocial rounds, patient/family meetings, etc.) so that team members remain cognizant of and focused on those goals when providing care for patients and families. Ongoing discussions about team and patient care goals allows for decisions to be made about expected and desired outcomes, clarification and prioritization of goals, and opportunities to clarify intent, prevent misunderstandings, and acknowledge and/or resolve any issues that may arise with regard to competing goals. Written plans of care that explicitly delineate shared psychosocial goals may be particularly helpful as a tool for ongoing care coordination.

Role Clarity

Coordination and collaboration among psychosocial providers is most effective when there are clear expectations about each team member's role, function, and responsibilities. Role clarity can optimize team efficiency and effectiveness (Mitchell et al., 2012), as it likely reduces duplication of effort (i.e., more than one provider offering the same service), and has been associated with improved clinician well-being and decreased professional burnout (Brunetto, Farr-Wharton, & Shacklock, 2011; Smith et al., 2018; So, West, & Dawson, 2011). On the other hand, role ambiguity has been found to impact communication between team members, reduce appreciation of one another's expertise, and reduce quality of patient care (Ervin et al., 2018; Lingard, Espin, Evans, & Hawryluck, 2004).

Compared to teams with more distinct areas of expertise, role clarity can present particular challenges on psychosocial teams, as skillsets among various helping professionals can have significant overlap. Multiple team members, for example, may have experience (to varying degrees) with providing supportive counseling, methods of distraction, and/or relaxation strategies to patients and families. Social workers, child life specialists, psychologists, and educational consultants/liaisons may all play a role in academic support and school reentry for children with chronic illness. Pediatric psychologists may share expertise in teaching children to swallow pills with the child life specialist and in teaching guided imagery with the music therapist. In some cases, these overlaps can increase the potential for confusion and frustration about roles/responsibilities and lead to misunderstandings and breakdowns in communication. Left unchecked, these confusions can also lead to significant conflict and territorialism among team members, which can ultimately erode team trust and impact patient care.

The structure and composition of psychosocial teams differ in each setting, and roles may look quite different depending on number of providers, expectations from leadership, provider training, experience, and time at institution, among other factors. It is not uncommon for psychosocial providers on small teams to take on multiple, or even unconventional, roles and responsibilities out of necessity—some of which may even fall outside of the traditional scope of practice. Because of these nuances, it is difficult to define the typical scope of practice for the various providers on the psychosocial team; instead, it is important to recognize the potential for overlap, seek out opportunities to learn about the roles and responsibilities of all team members, and share one's own competencies, expertise, and contributions to the multidisciplinary care of patients and families.

In fact, pediatric psychologists have obligations regarding role clarification, as outlined by the APA Ethics Code and the Guidelines for Psychological Practice in Health Care Delivery Systems (APA, 2002, 2010, 2013, 2016). Specifically, "psychologists are prepared to clarify their distinct roles and services and how these relate to those of other health care professionals" (APA, 2013; Guideline 3). When psychologists have a clear understanding of their role, they will be more equipped to clearly communicate their expertise and boundaries to others. It is their job, then, to foster others' understanding of their skills and potential contributions in their practice environment to providers of different non-psychologist disciplines. Pediatric psychologists must be prepared to articulate their individual contributions with confidence, describing how their knowledge, skills, training, education, and experience complement and enhance those of other professionals. For example, in developing psychology services as part of a new medical specialty, psychologists may find it helpful to have a brief and simple handout that outlines the services provided by pediatric psychology that are distinct from and complimentary to other psychosocial services within the hospital. Similarly, if a psychologist is consulting to a medical team that is less familiar with pediatric psychology services, having an "elevator speech" prepared regarding the role of pediatric psychology will be critical. Focusing on what psychology *can* provide to patients and families (i.e., rather than what other services are unable to provide) is an important and respectful approach to clarifying pediatric psychology's role with other team members. Example language for introducing psychology services and the consultative model is provided in Table 2.

In order to facilitate role clarity, not only do pediatric psychologists need a comprehensive understanding of their own profession, but they also must educate themselves about the roles of their psychosocial colleagues and engage in open discussion about the most effective provision of needed services (APA, 2013). Every psychosocial provider possesses a diverse and unique knowledge base acquired through different training pathways and therefore has an important contribution (Yeager, 2005) that only serves to enrich interprofessional treatment planning for patients and families. Online resources are available to better understand psychosocial health professionals like music therapy (American Music Therapy Association; www.musictherapy.org), art therapy (American Art Therapy Association; arttherapy.org), Child Life (www.childlife.org), education specialists (Hospital Educator and Academic Liaison Association; www.healassociation.org), and chaplains (Pediatric Chaplain Network; pediatricchaplains.org). Better still, meeting with psychosocial colleagues one-on-one and in person or shadowing a colleague's practice in vivo can helpful ways to learn about others' training, skillsets, and interests; these opportunities may be particularly helpful for new providers as part of a standardized orientation protocol. Through mutual understanding, team members can better recognize their distinct and overlapping roles, avoid making misinformed assumptions about one another, and resist the inclination toward exclusive professional turfs and the emergence of professional silos (D'Amour & Oandasan, 2005).

Team leaders play a critical role in facilitating role clarification on psychosocial teams. First and foremost, they must lead by example and be a model of professionalism and positive communication within the team. They can develop clear, unambiguous job descriptions, be transparent with all team members about expectations for providers in each role, hold team members accountable for those expectations, address role overlap directly, and confront any conflict that arises in a timely manner (Mitchell et al., 2012). Leaders will need to encourage and provide frequent opportunities for open and honest discussion about the skills, interests, and preferences of individual team members. In doing so, they can help to ensure that the discipline-specific expertise of providers are well-aligned with the team's shared goals. As new members join the team and others leave, leaders will have to revisit these issues in order to address shifting roles and responsibilities and help to maintain a healthy equilibrium within the team dynamic.

Effective Communication

To optimize patient care, APA not only values team-oriented collaborative care for psychologists practicing within a healthcare setting but specifically highlights the role of effective and timely communication with other healthcare professionals (APA, 2013, Guideline 7). This is not surprising, as communication is generally considered the most important determining factor of an effective collaborative healthcare team and one that strongly impacts other aspects of collaboration, like mutual respect and trust (San Martín-Rodríguez, Beaulieu, D'Amour, & Ferrada-Videla, 2005). As helping professionals, psychosocial providers typically have refined communication skills and, for those working in pediatrics, training that has focused specifically on communication within the medical setting. Pediatric psychologists, in particular, are well-trained in enhancing communication with patients, as they are often assessing and sharing

Table 2 Introducing Psychology Services and the Consultative Model (an example)

Key points	Example	Considerations
1. Describe the consultative model.	*"We are available for consultations both when patients are inpatient and when they are here for a medical outpatient appointment. We use a model where psychology is embedded in the medical team so that team members can consult us directly with a specific referral question in mind."* *OR* *"Because we serve patients throughout the entire hospital, we are available for consultations when patients are admitted to the unit and you have concerns about their psychological functioning. We try to work as closely as possible with you and their family during the patient's admission."*	• Does your team complete automatic consultations for all patients or a subset of patients? Or, are you referral only? • Does your team offer brief consultations, short-term therapy, and/or long-term therapy? • In what setting does your team see patients?
2. Provide examples of common referral questions.	*"Our most common referral questions or concerns include difficulty adjusting to a diagnosis, treatment, or the hospitalization, difficulties with pain management, concern for symptoms of depression or procedural anxiety, poor sleep hygiene, behavioral challenges, or difficulties with adherence."*	• Consider who your colleagues are and the most common concerns they are likely to see in your setting. • Consider adjusting your language accordingly (e.g., are you speaking to another psychosocial provider or medical colleague?).
3. Describe the process to enhance expectations.	*"When we are consulted, we typically gather some initial information from the referring provider so that we have an understanding of the team's concerns. We will then see the family for an initial assessment. After the initial assessment, we provide recommendations directly to the family and speak with the referring provider to discuss our assessment and observations. This way, we can continue to work together to support the family. We document our assessment and recommendations in the medical record."*	• Help the provider to understand (1) the process by which you complete a consultation, (2) how you typically convey information back to the family, and (3) how you typically convey information back to the provider (e.g., in person, by phone, using a paging system, referring to the medical chart).
4. Typical outcomes.	*"Our recommendations might include (1) brief evidence-based interventions that we provide directly to the patient/family, (2) ongoing collaboration with other services and providers, and/or (3) additional resources or referrals that we provide to the family."*	• Does your team offer direct intervention services to families? • What does ongoing collaboration look like in your setting? • Does your team provide referrals to families?

with the team the particular stressors, vulnerabilities, and strengths of the child and their family; facilitating appropriate communication around consent and treatment decisions; managing conflicts and negotiating differences of opinions among patients, families, and healthcare providers; and providing recommendations to caregivers and medical teams to support and enhance patient and family quality of life.

Despite limited research on the diverse communications of psychosocial providers within a medical team, there are many ways to facilitate interprofessional communication for the purposes of information sharing and joint decision-making. In general, a high-functioning team prioritizes and continuously evaluates its communication skills and has well-defined processes for efficient, bidirectional, and closed-loop communication. More specifically, team conferences, team-patient and family dialogue, patient care rounds, and documented coordinated care plans within the medical record are all effective communication strategies (Patenaude et al., 2015). Psychosocial leaders can facilitate effective communication by setting a high standard for consistent, clear, professional communication among team members, allowing ample time for team members to meet to discuss direct care and team processes, and recognizing signs of tension and conflict as triggers to reexamine team communication patterns and protocols (Mitchell et al., 2012).

Models of Rounds

Although there is limited literature on team meetings (i.e., "rounds") among psychosocial team members specifically, our medical colleagues have long utilized rounds to enhance team communication. Depending on the team's goals and responsibilities, prioritizing daily or weekly meetings with all team members can be a particularly helpful model for maintaining timely communication as it relates to patient care. Within the medical team context, rounds have been shown to be effective in improving patient outcomes (Kim, Barnato, Angus, Fleisher, & Kahn, 2010) and have been associated with improved staff and patient/family satisfaction (Rappaport, Ketterer, Nilforoshan, & Sharif, 2012), better understanding of information, increased confidence in the medical team, and reduced parental anxiety (Rea, Rao, Hill, Saylor, & Cousino, 2018). Furthermore, when family members join rounds, they report increased knowledge of the team members' roles (Rappaport et al., 2012), which may help to minimize confusion and discomfort when in an unfamiliar setting, such as an inpatient setting. However, simply holding multidisciplinary team meetings does not necessarily result in more effective decision-making (Raine et al., 2014). Perhaps not surprisingly, the success of rounds appears to be mediated by a team's ability to have a clear purpose (i.e., shared goals), agreed-upon processes, and a general team atmosphere that facilitates inclusion of team members and families (Raine et al., 2014). Despite the limited research on rounds within the psychosocial field, psychosocial teams can draw on the medical team models of collaborative communication.

Coordinated, family-centered care may involve various models of rounds, including (1) provider-to-provider or care coordination rounds (which consist solely of team members), (2) "weekly handoffs" between providers, and/or (3) family-centered rounds or multidisciplinary family meetings where families share in decision-making (Sisterhen, Blaszak, Woods, & Smith, 2007). Specific goals for care coordination rounds in an inpatient setting may include reviewing treatment decisions, discharge goals, and identifying discharge needs so that discharge is approached from a proactive, rather than reactive, perspective (White et al., 2017). Multidisciplinary weekly handoffs may be specifically useful when psychosocial teams provide coverage for patients and families on an alternating basis. Handoffs are an opportunity for teams to gather and discuss relevant information about presenting concerns, relevant past or current stressors, and longer-term treatment goals prior to a change in team (White et al., 2017). In this way, both inpatient and outpatient providers are encouraged to be involved, to the extent possible, for continuity of care related to short- and long-term treatment goals. Lastly, family meetings can serve as an opportunity for various psychosocial team members to meet jointly with families to discuss how the family and patient in particular have been coping with an admission or outpatient treatment. Families have the benefit from being able to present questions and concerns in a group setting where psychosocial team members can speak broadly to the family's questions and respond more specifically by discipline so that the family feels their needs are adequately met. Similar to family meetings for providing team recommendations, teams may also consider utilizing integrative clinics wherein team members may jointly meet with a patient and family or providers meet individually with patients and families and use a "handoff" approach so that team members are working closely with one another to complete an initial assessment and provide consolidated recommendations to patients and families. Regardless of the specific model of rounds used, interdisciplinary—or interprofessional—communication can remain a goal of the team's use of rounds, such that rounds serves as an opportunity for team members to share impressions and develop a joint plan of care.

Psychosocial Rounds

One model that is common in some settings is the implementation of weekly, care coordination *psychosocial* rounds. These team meetings may take on different formats but generally consist of the entire psychosocial team (e.g., psychologists, social workers, child life specialists, art therapists, music therapists, education specialists, liaisons, or teachers, patient navigators, chaplains, etc.) and, as appropriate and available, the inclusion of medical colleagues, such as attending physicians, medical fellows, nursing staff, and/or palliative care team members. Goals of psychosocial rounds may include review of newly diagnosed patients, discussion of challenging patient situations, and coordination of interprofessional care plans. Depending on the specific patient population, rounds may include both inpatient and outpatient providers and incorporate discussion of both types of cases, particularly in fields where patients regularly receive care across settings. Specific patient concerns that may be appropriate to discuss in the interprofessional psychosocial rounds setting may include: patient emotional/behavioral issues and/or family dynamics that may be interfering with treatment, challenges surrounding adherence to medications, difficult patient/family-team dynamics, barriers and potential solutions to supporting follow-up care, coordinated nonpharmacological pain management treatment plans, ethical considerations for patient care, and end-of-life and bereavement support. To maximize the use of time, it may be helpful to identify a weekly discussant or leader who prioritizes cases, paces the meeting, and facilitates flow of discussion.

Additional Means of Communication

In addition to rounds, both formal communication (e.g., documentation in the medical record) and informal communication (e.g., speaking in person or contacting team members by email or phone) may help to facilitate patient care across psychosocial providers. Specifically, the institution's digital capacity (e.g., the EMR, e-mail, portable phones, etc.) should be utilized to facilitate easy and continuous communication among team members. Formal documentation within the medical record can make clinical impressions and recommendations readily available to other team members. Thoughtful consideration, however, should be paid to the limits and implications of documentation given the potential ready access to providers in other departments and to patients and families. To that end, psychosocial providers should maintain comprehensive understanding of the system in which they practice to understand the implications of informed consent, documentation, and record keeping systems in accordance with ethical guidelines of their profession, the Health Insurance Portability and Accountability Act (HIPPA), and other state and federal laws (APA, 2013, Guideline 2; Patenaude et al., 2015). Additionally, there may be variability in the psychosocial subspecialties that have access to review or document within the medical record. Therefore, it is important to not only consider the potential benefits and consequences of access to the medical record within the institution but also other means of communication available to team members, such as telephone calls and email use, while adhering to institution-specific, state, or federal policies related to email use. Above all, it is imperative that documentation and interprofessional communication "reflect appropriate understanding of what information is essential for team members and/or family members to know, when specific permission is needed, and what different rules apply under extraordinary conditions of risk of harm" (Patenaude et al., 2015, p. S872). Policies, procedures, or protocols for interprofessional documentation may be helpful in standardizing communication among providers and maintaining clear expectations regarding timing, content, and access of included information.

Future Directions

While the medical field continues to move toward an increasingly integrated model, to date, there is minimal research on interprofessional collaboration and its outcomes within the pediatric hospital setting and even less specific to collaboration among psychosocial professionals. As such, we simply do not know how to tell, empirically, when collaboration is working well. How does a team know it is functioning effectively? How is "effective functioning" defined, and how does it relate to improvements in patient care and outcomes? In order to answer these questions, we must engage with our psychosocial colleagues in *interprofessional research* focused on the measurement of team processes, function, and outcomes. We can identify best practices for and essential elements of interprofessional psychosocial care and compare different team-based models in order to better articulate what works well, for whom, and when. Measurement of team processes and outcomes can help to identify key barriers to effective interprofessional collaboration and suggest strategies that may help to overcome them (Mitchell et al., 2012). Psychosocial teams should consider taking advantage of quality improvement (QI) methodologies (an inherently interdisciplinary endeavor) to improve processes and make systems changes that will result in improvements for team members, patients, and/or families. Examples of specific QI projects may include implementing standardized psychosocial assessment protocols or inpatient behavioral incentive programs, reducing overall time from an initial consultation by a provider to the psychosocial team contacting the patient, or increasing the frequency of family-centered rounds.

Conclusion

Pediatric psychologists within hospital settings are caring for complex patients within complex systems (e.g., family, community, healthcare system). Just as the medical needs of most of these patients are beyond the expertise of any single provider, so too may be their psychosocial needs. Therefore, providing true patient and family-centered care requires interprofessional collaboration and effective teamwork (Freeth, 2001). As a pediatric psychologist, psychosocial collaboration involves frequent interaction with providers in the fields of social work, child life, education, creative and therapeutic arts, and more and requires a mutual respect for each profession's contribution toward patient care. Even within the "helping professions," it is naïve to think that effective teamwork comes easily, develops spontaneously, or appears through good will alone (Gibson, 2009). Strategies aimed at developing shared goals, defining clear roles for providers, and communicating effectively are critical, along with psychosocial leaders who demonstrate respect for and knowledge of each profession's different skillsets. Further, leaders play a valuable role in teaching and modeling for others how to transcend professional turfs. Ultimately, however, willingness to collaborate with our psychosocial colleagues is a voluntary endeavor. We choose whether to contribute to and support a positive team culture, to work to build trust with colleagues, and to uphold the ethical principles of our profession. In doing so, we remain focused on the needs of the patients and families we serve and make the intentional commitment to providing the highest quality of care.

References

American Psychological Association. (2002). Ethical principles of psychologists and code of conduct. *American Psychologist, 57*(12), 1060–1073.

American Psychological Association. (2010). Ethical principals of psychologists and code of conduct including 2010 amendments. Retrieved from https://www.apa.org/ethics/code/

American Psychological Association. (2013). Guidelines for psychological practice in health care delivery systems. *American Psychologist, 68*(1), 1.

American Psychological Association. (2016). Ethical principals of psychologists and code of conduct including 2016 amendments. Retrieved from https://www.apa.org/ethics/code/

Baggott, C. R., & Kelly, K. P. (2002). Interdisciplinary collaboration. In G. Fochtman & G. V. Foley (Eds.), *Nursing care of children and adolescents with cancer* (3rd ed., pp. 626–639). Philadelphia, PA: W.B. Saunders.

Baggs, J. G., Schmitt, M. H., Mushlin, A. I., Mitchell, P. H., Eldredge, D. H., Oakes, D., & Hutson, A. D. (1999). Association between nurse-physician collaboration and patient outcomes in three intensive care units. *Critical Care Medicine, 27*(9), 1991–1998.

Brunetto, Y., Farr-Wharton, R., & Shacklock, K. (2011). Supervisor-nurse relationships, teamwork, role ambiguity and well-being: Public versus private sector nurses. *Asia Pacific Journal of Human Resources, 49*(2), 143–164.

Choi, B. C., & Pak, A. W. (2006). Multidisciplinarity, interdisciplinarity and transdisciplinarity in health research, services, education and policy: 1. Definitions, objectives, and evidence of effectiveness. *Clinical and Investigative Medicine, 29*(6), 351.

D'Amour, D., & Oandasan, I. (2005). Interprofessionality as the field of interprofessional practice and interprofessional education: An emerging concept. *Journal of Interprofessional Care, 19*(sup1), 8–20.

Drotar, D. (2002). Reflections on interdisciplinary collaboration in the new millennium: Perspectives and challenges. *Journal of Developmental & Behavioral Pediatrics, 23*(3), 175–180.

Ervin, J. N., Kahn, J. M., Cohen, T. R., & Weingart, L. R. (2018). Teamwork in the intensive care unit. *American Psychologist, 73*(4), 468.

Firth-Cozens, J. (2001). Cultures for improving patient safety through learning: The role of teamwork. *BMJ Quality & Safety, 10*(Suppl 2), ii26–ii31.

Freeth, D. (2001). Sustaining interprofessional collaboration. *Journal of Interprofessional Care, 15*(1), 37–46.

Gibson, F. (2009). Multiprofessional collaboration in children's cancer care: Believed to be a good thing but how do we know when it works well? *European Journal of Cancer Care, 18*(4), 327–329.

Hackman, R. (2014). *What makes for a great team?* Washington, DC: American Psychological Association.

Herbert, C. P. (2005). Changing the culture: Interprofessional education for collaborative patient centered practice in Canada. *Journal of Interprofessional Care, 19*(Suppl 1), 1–4.

Joint Commission on Accreditation of Healthcare Organizations. (2005). *The Joint Commission guide to improving staff communication*. Oakbrook Terrace, IL: Joint Commission Resources.

Kim, M. M., Barnato, A. E., Angus, D. C., Fleisher, L. F., & Kahn, J. M. (2010). The effect of multidisciplinary care teams on intensive care unit mortality. *Archives of Internal Medicine, 170*(4), 369–376.

Larson, E. (1999). The impact of the physician-nurse interaction on patient care. *Holistic Nursing Practice, 13*, 38–46.

Lingard, L., Espin, S., Evans, C., & Hawryluck, L. (2004). The rules of the game: Interprofessional collaboration on the intensive care unit team. *Critical Care, 8*(6), R403.

Majzun, R. (1998). The role of teamwork in improving patient satisfaction. *Group Practice Journal, 47*, 12–17.

Mitchell, P., Wynia, M., Golden, R., McNellis, B., Okun, S., Webb, C. E., … Von Kohorn, I. (2012). *Core principles and values of effective team-based health care*. Washington, DC: National Academy of Sciences.

Palermo, T. M., Janicke, D. M., McQuaid, E. L., Mullins, L. L., Robins, P. M., & Wu, Y. P. (2014). Recommendations for training in pediatric psychology: Defining core competencies across training levels. *Journal of Pediatric Psychology, 39*(9), 965–984.

Patenaude, A. F., Pelletier, W., & Bingen, K. (2015). Communication, documentation, and training standards in pediatric psychosocial oncology. *Pediatric Blood & Cancer, 62*(S5), S870–S895.

Raine, R., Wallace, I., Nic a'Bháird, C., Xanthopoulou, P., Lanceley, A., Clarke, A., … Ferlie, E. (2014). Improving the effectiveness of multidisciplinary team meetings for patients with chronic diseases: A prospective observational study. *Health Services and Delivery Research, 2*(37), 1–172.

Rappaport, D. I., Ketterer, T. A., Nilforoshan, V., & Sharif, I. (2012). Family-centered rounds: Views of families, nurses, trainees, and attending physicians. *Clinical Pediatrics, 51*(3), 260–266.

Rea, K. E., Rao, P., Hill, E., Saylor, K. M., & Cousino, M. K. (2018). Families' experiences with pediatric family-centered rounds: A systematic review. *Pediatrics, 141*(3), e20171883.

Salas, E., Shuffler, M. L., Thayer, A. L., Bedwell, W. L., & Lazzara, E. H. (2015). Understanding and improving teamwork in organizations: A scientifically based practical guide. *Human Resource Management, 54*(4), 599–622.

San Martín-Rodríguez, L., Beaulieu, M. D., D'Amour, D., & Ferrada-Videla, M. (2005). The determinants of successful collaboration: A review of theoretical and empirical studies. *Journal of Interprofessional Care, 19*(Suppl 1), 132–147.

Scholes, J., & Vaughan, B. (2002). Cross boundary working: Implications for the multiprofessional team. *Journal of Clinical Nursing, 11*(3), 399–408.

Sisterhen, L. L., Blaszak, R. T., Woods, M. B., & Smith, C. E. (2007). Defining family-centered rounds. *Teaching and Learning in Medicine, 19*(3), 319–322.

Smith, C. D., Balatbat, C., Corbridge, S., Dopp, A. L., Fried, J., Harter, R., … Sinsky, C. (2018). *Implementing optimal team based care to reduce clinician burnout. NAM perspectives*. Discussion Paper. Washington, DC: National Academy of Medicine. Retrieved from https://nam.edu/implementing-optimal-teambased-care-to-reduce-clinician-burnout/

So, T. T., West, M. A., & Dawson, J. F. (2011). Team-based working and employee well-being: A cross-cultural comparison of United Kingdom and Hong Kong health services. *European Journal of Work and Organizational Psychology, 20*(3), 305–325.

West, M., Borrill, C. A., & Unsworth, K. L. (1998). Team effectiveness in organizations. In C. L. Cooper & I. Robertson (Eds.), *International review of industrial and organizational psychology* (Vol. 13, pp. 1–48). Chichester, UK: Wiley.

White, C. M., Thomson, J. E., Statile, A. M., Auger, K. A., Unaka, N., Carroll, M., … Brady, P. W. (2017). Development of a new care model for hospitalized children with medical complexity. *Hospital Pediatrics, 7*, 410–414.

Yeager, S. (2005). Interdisciplinary collaboration: The heart and soul of health care. *Critical Care Nursing Clinics, 17*(2), 143–148.

Zwarenstein, M., Reeves, S., & Perrier, L. (2005). Effectiveness of pre-licensure interprofessional education and post-licensure collaborative interventions. *Journal of Interprofessional Care, 19*(Suppl 1), 148–165.

Collaborating with Child Psychiatry

Hillary S. Blake, Amy E. Williams, Julianne Giust, and Ann M. Lagges

Introduction

Pediatric consultation-liaison (CL) psychologists spend a great deal of time collaborating with pediatricians, nurses, and other care providers in a hospital setting. Given the nature of the CL psychologist's role, it is not uncommon to collaborate more frequently with consulting medical teams than with our mental health colleagues (e.g., psychiatrists). However, effectively collaborating with our child psychiatry colleagues is important to maximize the quality of care we provide for consult patients. Given variability in organizational structures for CL teams, the structure and methods to facilitate collaboration between CL psychologists and psychiatrists will also vary across hospital systems.

Unfortunately, there is a dearth of research on mental health outcomes when psychiatry and psychology CL services are combined. However, there is some evidence to suggest that outcomes are likely to be improved when psychiatrists and psychologists effectively collaborate to provide CL services. First, for several mental health conditions, including depression (March et al., 2004), evidence-based medicine indicates better outcomes with treatments that combine psychiatric expertise (medication management) and psychology expertise (therapy). Further, the integrated care literature supports more efficient care and better outcomes when psychiatry and psychology work collaboratively with primary care providers (Osofsky, Osofsky, Wells, & Weems, 2014). This chapter focuses on the benefits of collaboration with psychiatry during CL work, the pros and cons of different collaboration models, and strategies to facilitate effective collaborations.

Collaboration Between Psychiatry and Psychology in Non-CL Settings

While there is scant discussion on "collaborative care" between psychologists and psychiatrists, there is some review of "split treatment" in the psychiatry literature. "Split treatment" describes care in which the patient is receiving treatment from more than one caregiver, most commonly referring to a psychiatrist providing psychopharmacology and a psychotherapist providing therapy (Balon, 2001; Gitlin & Miklowitz, 2016). Research supports that many mental health disorders benefit from combined treatments of psychotherapy and psychopharmacology. However, psychopharmacologists are a very limited resource and may feel pressure to focus solely on psychopharmacology contributing to decreasing incidences of psychiatrists providing both services.

H. S. Blake (✉) · A. E. Williams
J. Giust · A. M. Lagges
Department of Psychiatry, Riley Hospital for Children, Indiana University School of Medicine, Indianapolis, IN, USA
e-mail: hcstanle@iupui.edu

B. D. Carter, K. A. Kullgren (eds.), *Clinical Handbook of Psychological Consultation in Pediatric Medical Settings*, Issues in Clinical Child Psychology, https://doi.org/10.1007/978-3-030-35598-2_9

The "split treatment" model has become common in mental health care (i.e., when a psychiatrist provides psychopharmacology services and collaborates with a therapist who provides psychotherapy) and review of it can be helpful in considering the positives and negatives of collaboration between psychologists and psychiatrists in CL roles.

There are many positive aspects noted for "split treatment" (which we will refer to from this point as collaboration between psychiatrists and psychologists). With more than one provider, the care will benefit from different specialized knowledge bases and skills, lending unique clinical lenses for gleaning of information, conceptualization of the patient, and developing treatment plans (Balon, 2001; Gitlin & Miklowitz, 2016; Woodward, 2002). Further, the patient potentially gains more treatment time, increased resources, and better coverage of care during provider vacation or leave. Working together, the two providers may also be able to use their different relationships with the patient to help resolve conflict with either patient-provider relationship or to enhance adherence to one another's treatment plan. In addition, the shared provider experience may provide reciprocal support with difficult cases.

There are also negative aspects of collaborative care in comparison to one provider doing both interventions. The patient may give discrepant information to each provider, leading one provider to act on information and possibly derail the other's care plan (Balon, 2001). Such experiences can lead to splitting of the team and possibly termination of one provider's care. If communication between the two providers lapses, the psychiatrist may inappropriately prescribe at times when an issue may be better worked through in therapy, or perhaps stop an antidepressant when the patient has recently reported suicidal ideation in therapy (Balon, 2001). Another concern is that having two providers can reinforce the mind-body split (Gabbard & Kay, 2001; Gitlin & Miklowitz, 2016; Woodward, 2002). This may be an even greater concern in consultation-liaison work where a psychiatrist and psychologist are seeing the patient independently. This is where close collaboration between the psychiatrist and psychologist can facilitate patient and family understanding of the important interplay of psychological and physical factors.

It is reasonable to think that many psychotherapists and psychopharmacologists agree that good communication is essential to collaborative care; however, a review of a survey completed by 61 psychiatrists in 2012 suggests that communication between collaborating mental health providers occurs infrequently (Kalman, Kalman, & Granet, 2012). For the 875 patients that were being seen by two providers for psychopharmacology and psychotherapy for greater than 6 months, respondents reported no communication with the other provider on 24% of the patients, and only 18% of the respondents reported quarterly communication with the psychotherapist (Kalman et al., 2012).

In summary, while there are many benefits to collaboration between psychiatrists and psychologists (or psychotherapists) in an outpatient setting, it can be logistically challenging to maintain the extent of communication necessary for collaboration, and even in the best of collaborations there are potential problem areas that may arise. Similar dynamics are likely to occur in collaborations between psychiatrists and psychologists in consultation-liaison settings, highlighting the need to make intentional efforts to establish and maintain regular effective collaborations with our psychiatry colleagues.

Collaboration Between Psychiatry and Psychology in Pediatric CL Settings

Pediatric psychology/psychiatry CL services vary considerably in structure across different organizations. Recent surveys of psychology (Kullgren et al., 2015) and psychiatry (Shaw, Pao, Holland, & DeMaso, 2016) CL services have been published and provide some insight into the structure of these programs and extent of collaboration between psychiatry and psychology providers. A survey of 118 pediatric CL psychologists found that just over half (56%) of their pediatric hospital settings had separate CL psychology and CL psychiatry services, and most reported not having a psychiatrist on their team (mode = 0) (Kullgren et al., 2015). This may be a reflection of departmental structure for the surveyed CL psychology services as only 26% of these services were housed in a department/division of psychiatry compared to 41% housed in a psychology department/division (Kullgren et al., 2015). A survey of pediatric CL *psychiatry* services, in primarily academically affiliated or children's hospital settings, found that just under half of these programs included a psychologist (Shaw et al., 2016). A similar survey of 48 pediatric CL *psychiatry* services found that only 11% had separate CL psychiatry and CL psychology services (Shaw, Wamboldt, Bursch, & Stuber, 2006).

The discrepancy between these surveys in percentage of hospitals with separate CL psychiatry and psychology services (56% vs. 11%) may reflect sampling biases in the two surveys due to sampling of psychologists (Kullgren et al., 2015) vs. psychiatrists (Shaw et al., 2006) as survey respondents. Interpretation of these results suggests that pediatric CL services that are labeled as psychiatry services, and/or directed by psychiatrists, may be more likely to include interdisciplinary (both psychiatry and psychology) teams, whereas services labeled as CL psychology services and/or directed by psychologists may be less likely to include psychiatrists in their CL team. However, further research is needed to verify this hypothesis. In two separate reports, the majority (65–70%) (Shaw et al., 2006, 2016) of surveyed CL *psychiatry* services were directed by a psychiatrist (27% with joint directorship with a psychologist), and 10% were directed by a psychologist (6% with a joint directorship with a psychiatrist) (Shaw et al., 2006).

Models for Collaboration

As demonstrated through the survey data above, collaboration between psychiatrists and psychologists to provide pediatric CL services can occur through various models of care, including with or without integrated CL teams. An integrated CL team would include both psychiatry and psychology attendings and often a variety of other team members, possibly including social workers, nurse practitioners, psychology postdoctoral fellows, psychology interns, psychology practicum students, child psychiatry fellows, psychiatry residents, pediatric residents, and medical students (Kullgren et al., 2015). Trainees from multiple disciplines have been demonstrated to provide a significant proportion of clinical care on CL teams (Kullgren et al., 2015; Shaw et al., 2006). Integrated teams often have regular, daily or weekly, team meetings to discuss patient care, which can allow for the integration of each provider's unique expertise into each patient's care.

Literature supports that better integration of CL services with both medical and psychiatry colleagues leads to improved training of a variety of disciplines and improved patient care. Kullgren et al. (2015) noted the infrequent integration of psychology and psychiatry/medical teams on pediatric CL teams, particularly the lack of inclusion of medical student and resident trainees, as a "missed opportunity for interprofessional collaboration." Similarly, Shaw et al. (2006) expressed a belief that pediatric CL services that include both psychiatrists and psychologists "have a particular advantage in their ability to integrate multiple treatment modalities that are generally required in the management of children with complex medical issues." Fortunately, the majority (69%) of pediatric CL psychologists report having good working relationships with psychiatry colleagues and only infrequently (7%) report a typically poor working relationship (Kullgren et al., 2015).

Although data is lacking regarding the specific efficacy of integrated vs. separate, CL services including psychiatry and psychology, there is significant evidence in primary care to suggest that teams including both psychiatry and psychology result in significant improvement in treatment of mental health concerns in a primary care setting (Bodenheimer, 2007; Raney, 2015). Research indicates that multidisciplinary clinical teams obtain better patient health outcomes than teams that are not integrated (Wagner, 2000), and within integrated teams those that have an organizational structure and cohesive function (Bodenheimer, 2007; Bodenheimer & Grumbach, 2006), better team cohesion (Campbell et al., 2001), and more collaborative clinical environment (Bodenheimer, 2007) are more effective and have better patient health and satisfaction outcomes. It is reasonable to hypothesize similar improved care outcomes exist with integration of psychiatry and psychology CL services.

In contrast, limited or inefficient collaboration between CL psychiatrists and CL psychologists can present challenges to patient care. For example, problems may arise in systems where roles and communication between psychology and psychiatry are not well defined, especially when separate teams are accessed through different consultation routes. One issue that may arise when psychology and psychiatry work as separate teams is the primary team may inappropriately consult the less suitable team based on their perception of the patient problem. For example, the primary team may believe a patient's anxiety could only be managed by a medication and therefore needs a psychiatrist, or perhaps the team has misdiagnosed the problem as a functional issue leading them to consult a psychologist. This potential issue was highlighted by Aljarad, Osaimi, and Huthail (2008) in a study in which they looked at the perceived mental health diagnosis by the referring medical specialty of 157 physically ill adults compared to the mental health diagnosis reported by the CL service after evaluation. About 53% of the initial impressions by the referring team were reviewed to be inaccurate diagnoses, and only 49% referred for a depressive disorder were actually found to have a depressive disorder on assessment (Aljarad et al., 2008). Regular collaboration between psychiatry and psychology CL providers can minimize the potential negative impact of misperceptions by the primary team of the nature of the mental health problems of their patients. Review of the medical record, discussion with the primary team to better understand the consultation question, and communication between the psychologist and psychiatrist assist in a more appropriate and accurate consultation outcome. Continued review of a case after initial evaluation may also lead the psychiatrist or psychologist to involve the other discipline for differing expertise and treatment approaches. For example, the CL psychologist was consulted for assistance with agitation. However, upon reviewing the patient's medical record the CL psychiatrist had concern for delirium. As such, it was decided that the CL psychiatrist would complete the consult. In other cases, it may be apparent that a patient would benefit from both services and providers may choose to collaborate on care at the outset. This illustrates the importance of close collaboration between psychiatrists and psychologists even before the consult has taken place.

Psychology and Psychiatry Training and Competencies

Psychiatrists and psychologists have different training and expertise that when combined, can improve our conceptualizations and treatment plans for patients. To better understand how our different expertise can work together it is helpful to consider the differences in training and competency backgrounds. Pediatric psychologists typically attend graduate school and obtain a doctoral degree in some variant of health service psychology. During their doctoral training the psychologist completes a 1-year internship to obtain greater depth and breadth in their training while being supervised by licensed psychologists. In order to successfully complete internship, an intern must demonstrate competency and knowledge of assessment; intervention; diversity; consultation and interprofessional/interdisciplinary skills; supervision; research; ethical and legal standards; professional values, attitudes, and behavior; and communication and interpersonal skills (American Psychological Association, 2015). After completing internship it has become increasingly common for the psychologist to complete a 1- or 2-year postdoctoral fellowship to further specialize and strengthen their skills and competencies in pediatric psychology. At the end of a pediatric psychologist's training, it is recommended/expected that they demonstrate competence in the following six areas: science, professionalism, interpersonal skills, application, education, and systems (Palermo et al., 2014).

Training to become a child and adolescent psychiatrist begins with 4 years of medical school, which typically includes about 2 years of didactic curriculum followed by 2 years of clinical rotations. After earning a medical degree, the most traditional path continues through a 3-or-4-year adult psychiatry residency specializing in adult/pediatric medicine, neurology, and adult psychiatry followed by a 2-year child fellowship focused on psychiatric work with children, adolescents, and their families. There are other pathways to becoming a child psychiatrist, including a 5-year triple board residency (combined training in Pediatrics, Adult Psychiatry, and Child Psychiatry) and the 6-year post pediatric portal program (AACAP, n.d.).

During a child psychiatrists' residency and fellowship they gain competency in professionalism, patient care and procedural skills, medical knowledge, practice-based learning and improvement, interpersonal and communication skills, scholarly activity, and system-based practice (ACGME, 2018). Board certified child psychiatrists are expected to have knowledge of child development, biological and clinical science (e.g., neuroscience, epidemiology, animal models of disease, genetics, statistics, and research design), psychopathology, treatment (e.g., psychopharmacology and psychotherapy), developmental assessment and diagnostics (e.g., mental status exam, diagnostic interviewing, differential diagnosis, rating scales, diagnostic imaging, medical/laboratory/genetic testing), issues in practice (e.g., legal issues, ethics, cultural issues, etc.), and consultation (ABPN, 2017).

Overall, psychologists and psychiatrists have many areas that overlap in their training. However, in contrast to a psychologist's training, a psychiatrist has greater knowledge of medical issues, biological and clinical science, and psychopharmacology. Although psychiatrists receive training in screeners and a basic overview of psychological testing, psychiatrists are not competent in psychological assessments. Psychologists generally receive more in-depth training in research and psychotherapy; however, many psychiatry residency programs provide extensive training leading to competency in these areas.

Benefits of Combined Expertise of Psychiatry and Psychology

From our experiences as pediatric psychologists (HSB, AEW, AML) working in pediatric CL in both a separate psychology service and an integrated psychology/psychiatry service, we believe there are several potential benefits that can arise from working in close collaboration with our psychiatry colleagues. An obvious addition to the CL team that can be provided by a psychiatrist is expertise in psychotropic medications. As psychologists, we may at times have a bias toward psychotherapy or behavioral interventions due to our training and expertise, leading us to possibly be slower to consider medication options or not recognize situations in which medication management might be a helpful addition to the treatment plan. Psychiatrists also bring more depth of expertise to the identification, assessment, and treatment of cases involving challenging clinical presentations such as catatonia, extreme changes in mental status, delirium, etc., allowing us to be more efficient in the differential diagnosis of these conditions in our CL referrals. Finally, by virtue of their medical training a psychiatrist also provides more knowledge about medicine/pediatrics that can be extremely beneficial for several reasons: (1) helping psychologists fully understand the often very complicated health conditions and treatments our patients are experiencing, (2) improving psychologists' command of medical terminology and therefore our ability to communicate more effectively with our pediatric colleagues, and (3) improved medical sophistication of our diagnostic justifications for, or against, conditions such as Conversion Disorder and other perplexing Somatic Symptom Disorders. This may be particularly helpful in cases where symptoms are inconsistent with a primary psychological etiology and advocacy is needed to encourage further medical workup.

Barriers to Collaboration

While the above data, and experiences, indicate that integrated teams may have the potential to obtain better patient outcomes by facilitating more efficient and effective collaboration, sometimes integrated teams are not possible. The general integrated care literature cites several barriers to successful integration including funding lines, organizational structures, poor collaboration among corresponding leadership, and "turf wars" (Ling, Brereton, Conklin, Newbould, & Roland, 2012); and these barriers are likely to sometimes pose a challenge in integration of psychiatry and psychology CL services as well. For example, it can be difficult to have fully integrated teams when psychology and psychiatry are housed in different departments, and thus have different funding mechanisms, within the hospital or academic institution. Although most pediatric CL psychologists report having good working relationships with psychiatry colleagues (Kullgren et al., 2015), historical "turf wars" between our professions (Schindler, Berren, & Beigel, 1981) have likely contributed to the organizational structure of psychiatry and psychology CL teams and may at times contribute to lingering tendencies to isolate our practices from each other. Nonetheless, psychologists who work on teams that are separate from psychiatry CL services can still establish effective collaborations, and even provide integrated care services, with psychiatry colleagues, particularly if they are intentional about ensuring regular and effective communication and collaboration with psychiatry colleagues.

Guidelines for Effective Collaboration

As with any collaborative effort, consultation teams benefit from taking the time to truly develop a plan for how the collaboration will work. Establishing pathways of communication and defining roles and responsibilities can greatly increase the chance that the care provided by psychiatry and psychology is truly integrated, rather than simply co-located, and will reduce the possibility of duplicative or perhaps even contradictory efforts.

To facilitate effective collaboration, Gutheil (1994) describes the "eight Cs" (clarity, contract, communication, consent, contact, comprehensive view, credentialing, consultation) of collaborative treatment that provide guidelines for successful collaboration in care and for avoiding potential problems. Collaborative care providers are suggested to establish a contractual arrangement with clarified roles and responsibilities, determine the frequency of regular communication and when more urgent/emergent contact should occur, and assure patient understanding of roles and patient consent to the level of communication and collaboration planned (Gutheil, 1994). Further, collaborators should have a mutual understanding of the others' credentialing and experience (Gitlin & Miklowitz, 2016; Gutheil, 1994).

There are many obstacles potentially impeding regular and timely communication including coordination of schedules, non-billable nature of time spent on communication, power differentials in the dyad that may imply who contacts whom, and possible lack of physical proximity between the two providers (Gitlin & Miklowitz, 2016). As such, one of the easiest ways to ensure good communication among team members is to schedule daily, or nearly daily, team meetings or rounds during which all active patients are discussed. Carving out time each day can seem daunting, but having all disciplines together to discuss conceptualization and treatment planning is key to truly providing collaborative care. Without this type of frequent interaction and discussion of all patients, care can quickly become fragmented and less than optimal. For example, if a patient is quickly classified as a "behavioral patient," managed solely by the psychology side of the team, and never again discussed by the whole team, a new symptom that might actually be a sign of a medical complication or adverse reaction to a medication might be missed. When defining roles and responsibilities, it is usually easiest if either the psychologist or psychiatrist is designated as the lead provider for each patient.

That person takes the responsibility for leading discussion regarding conceptualization and treatment planning and also serves as the primary contact point for the consulting service.

Collaboration in Training and Education

As mentioned above, integrated CL services often have a variety of professionals in training including psychology postdoctoral fellows, psychology interns, psychology practicum students, child psychiatry fellows, psychiatry residents, pediatric and peds/med residents, pediatric subspecialty fellows, and medical students (Kullgren et al., 2015). Not only do psychologists and psychiatrists benefit from working on an integrated CL service, but the various trainees' education and depth of experience is enhanced when different disciplines train together.

While there appears to be a dearth of literature on the collaboration between psychiatry and psychology trainees, there is literature indicating several benefits to having psychology interns and pediatric residents train together. When psychology and pediatric residents train and attend didactics together, it appears to increase the likelihood that they will collaborate and work together in the future (Pidano, Arora, Gipson, Hudson, & Schellinger, 2018). Integrated training assists in promoting common language, referrals, and increased collaboration when working with complex cases (Jee, Baldwin, Dadiz, Jones, & Alpert-Gillis, 2018). Pediatric residents also find it valuable to observe psychology trainees interact with patients and vice versa (Jee et al., 2018), as they report learning new strategies for conducting clinical interviews and asking questions (Pisani, leRoux, & Siegel, 2011).

From our experience, when psychiatry and psychology trainees work together on teams, it enhances their knowledge of the other profession's education, training, and unique expertise. It is imperative that each profession fully understand the skills and services offered by pediatric psychiatrists and psychologists to assist with formulating clear (and answerable) referral questions. Furthermore, it is valuable for psychology trainees to work beside their child psychiatry colleagues to further their competence by increasing their knowledge of medical conditions, their understanding of the bidirectional influence of medical conditions and mood/behavior, gaining a basic working knowledge of laboratory results, and their awareness of the efficacy and limitations of psychotropic medications. Similarly, psychiatry residents can learn from the psychology trainee's knowledge of assessments (e.g., cognitive and academic), research, and often more in-depth training in the various modalities of psychotherapy and specialty interventions such as clinical biofeedback. Combined training allows trainees to supervise and role-play with one another, which can further foster learning. Additionally, training together allows psychiatrists and psychologists the opportunity to collaborate on scholarly activities such as research and quality improvement projects.

Case Examples

The following two case examples demonstrate the usefulness of collaboration between CL psychiatrists and psychologists.

Case Example 1

Jen is a 14-year-old girl with Autism Spectrum Disorder, seizure disorder, and self-injurious behaviors (SIB) who was admitted for intravenous antibiotics for forearm skin infection secondary to self-inflicted bites. The primary team consulted the consultation-liaison psychiatrist for medication management of agitation and SIB. In talking further with the primary team, they express concern about difficulty with wound healing and potential future infections due to Jen's ongoing biting behaviors. They also reported concerns that Jen is persistently biting herself and hitting nurses and is easily agitated with care. Working together on an integrated CL service, the psychologist and psychiatrist discuss the case, potential medical workup, and behavioral and pharmacological interventions. They agree to evaluate the patient together. During the interview, mother reported that Jen will use one- to two-word phrases and has a moderate intellectual disability. She screams, bites, and hits during transitions or when she is unable to have access to a desired tangible item. When Jen has a tantrum, mother will either "give in" or give her gummy worms to stop the behavior. Mother reported that during the past month her behaviors have escalated and that she cannot identify any recent life changes. Mother noted that Jen has not had mental health services or medication in the past to help with her behavior problems. Mom does note that Jen has had diphenhydramine previously for hives and that she was very agitated on this medication. Jen has had prior issues with constipation and has not had a bowel movement in a week, according to her mother. Additionally, she was prescribed a new antiepileptic medication a month ago, which has seemed to make her more irritable. Mother also reported that with the medication change Jen has had more episodes than typical for her seizures. Furthermore, Jen often has an increase in her aggression when in pain.

After the evaluation, the CL psychologist and psychiatrist discuss the case and develop a conceptualization that contributions to her self-injurious behavior and agitation are multifactorial and include her baseline communication limitations, difficulty adjusting to the hospital setting, arm pain due to her wounds, constipation, possible side effect of her new antiepileptic medication, and possibly worsening seizure disorder. The psychiatrist recommends the primary team consult neurology for possible EEG and review of current medication choice given that the timeline for Jen's exacerbation of baseline symptoms aligns with her medication changes. It is recommended to evaluate and treat her constipation and review her current pain treatment regimen. In addition, olanzapine (atypical antipsychotic) is recommended "as needed" for moderate to severe agitation while in the hospital if de-escalation techniques cannot be successfully used. The psychologist recommends and creates visual boards representing important aspects of care with preferred rewards and models how to use this with the mother, patient, and nursing staff. In addition, the psychologist works with mother on blocking and planned ignoring of self-injurious and negative behaviors, as well as positive attention toward preferred behaviors.

As illustrated in this case, patient presentations that have both a strong behavioral component and medical component benefit nicely from having both a psychiatrist and a psychologist collaborating in provision of CL services. In Jen's case, the conceptualization of the patient was improved by having the psychologist and psychiatrist work collaboratively. The psychologist was able to assist with behavioral interventions and recognizing the impact of the pain, while the psychiatrist was effective in assisting with medication management and encouraging consultations from other medical subspecialties, i.e., neurology.

Case Example 2

John is a 12-year-old male who was admitted for burns. A psych consult was requested to "assist with coping." After discussing the case in consult team rounds, it was decided that the psychologist would complete the initial interview and take the lead on the case. During the interview, it was disclosed that John, his friend, and John's father were sitting by a firepit when John's father went inside to get some water. In his father's absence, John took kerosene from the family shed and as he was pouring kerosene on the fire, he accidentally spilled some on his clothing causing it to ignite. He has 52% total surface area burns, including burns to his trunk, the lower third of his face, and to his dominant hand requiring thumb and fore finger amputation. John had no baseline mental health problems (i.e., depression, anxiety, ADHD). Since admission to the hospital for his burn injury, the parents and medical staff reported that John was irritable and had a flat affect. He had expressed concern that he could no longer be able to play on his baseball team because of his hand injury. John exhibited several symptoms of Acute Stress Disorder (nightmares, intrusive thoughts of the accident and of dressing changes, feeling guilty, an increased startle response) and it was very difficult to get John to talk about the incident as he became very anxious when he was asked to do so. John's dressing changes took significantly longer than they should due to John's anxiety, panic attacks prior to dressing changes, and avoidant behavior. The primary team had given him lorazepam (an anxiolytic) at the start of the dressing change and found it mildly helpful in decreasing his anxiety. The psychologist provided psychoeducation on trauma symptoms to John's parents and taught the patient behavioral techniques such as visualization and distraction to manage anxiety and promote relaxation (he was unable to engage in progressive muscle relaxation and diaphragmatic breathing due to the nature of his burns). The psychologist also worked with the primary team to decrease the number of dressing changes and medical interventions occurring in the patient's room, moving him to the bathroom when possible to do these interventions, in an effort to create a "safe space" in his patient room. In addition, the psychologist worked with John to identify themes in his nightmares and help him rescript or create and visualize the content of his nightmares to be less threatening. Despite these behavioral interventions, John continued to have nightmares and panic attacks and his anxiety had only slightly improved. In addition, his sleep became more disturbed by the nightmares, causing him to get only 3 to 4 h of sleep a night and affecting his ability to cope during the day.

In consult team rounds, the psychologist discussed the case with the psychiatrist, and it was decided that the psychiatrist would evaluate John to see if medication would be appropriate for his nightmares and panic attacks. Since John's symptoms had only started a week prior and he did not have a history of anxiety or depression, the psychiatrist planned to continue to monitor the need for consideration of a more long-acting medication (e.g., a SSRI) while therapeutic interventions were implemented. Additionally, the psychiatrist recommended prazosin (an antihypertensive drug that appears to have some efficacy in decreasing anxiety via dampening the norepinephrine effects likely contributing to the nightmares) to help with his nightmares. It was also decided that the psychologist would accompany John to his next dressing change to assist with behavioral techniques, e.g., coaching John in imagery techniques, providing distractions, and modeling positive self-statements. With the titration of the medication and psychologist coaching during his dressing change, his anxiety decreased significantly. John did not have any additional panic attacks and the dressing change was not prolonged as it previously had been. John's sleep also improved, and he no longer experienced nightmares.

In this case, close collaboration between the psychologist and the psychiatrist was essential to achieving desired outcomes. Given the severity of John's anxiety and trauma symptoms at admission, the behavioral techniques the psychologist utilized were of minimal efficacy. The psychiatrist prescribed a medication beneficial in treating his nightmares and improved his sleep. The intervention allowed the psychologist's treatment strategies to become more effective and optimized John's treatment.

Conclusion

In conclusion, there is limited research on the collaboration of psychiatry and psychology, especially in CL settings, and future research is needed to better understand the benefits of collaboration. Despite the sparse literature, existing evidence suggests close collaboration between psychiatry and psychology in providing pediatric CL services is likely to result in more efficient care with better outcomes. When psychiatry and psychology providers collaborate effectively, they are able to capitalize on and integrate each of their unique strengths to create a more robust psychological conceptualization of the patient leading to an often more efficient and effective treatment plan. In addition to patients benefitting from collaboration between psychiatry and psychology for CL services, trainees can also benefit from training with both psychiatrists and psychologists and alongside other disciplines.

References

Accreditation Council for Graduate Medical Education (ACGME). (2018). ACGME common program requirements (fellowship). Retrieved from https://www.acgme.org/Portals/0/PFAssets/ProgramRequirements/CPRFellowship2019.pdf

Aljarad, A. M., Osaimi, F. D. A., & Huthail, Y. R. A. (2008). Accuracy of psychiatric diagnoses in consultation liaison psychiatry. *Journal of Taibah University Medical Sciences, 3*(2), 123–128.

American Academy of Child and Adolescent Psychiatry (AACAP). (n.d.). Child and adolescent psychiatry training. Retrieved from https://www.aacap.org/aacap/Medical_Students_and_Residents/Residents_and_Fellows/Child_and_Adolescent_Psychiatry_Training.aspx

American Board of Psychiatry and Neurology (ABPN). (2017). Certification examination in child and adolescent psychiatry. Retrieved from https://www.abpn.com/wp-content/uploads/2017/10/2018_Child_and_Adolescent_Psychiatry_CERT_Content_Specifications.pdf

American Psychological Association. (2015). Standard for accreditation for health service psychology. Washington, DC: American Psychological Association. Retrieved from https://www.apa.org/ed/accreditation/about/policies/standards-of-accreditation.pdf

Balon, R. (2001). Positive and negative aspects of split treatment. *Psychiatric Annals, 31*(10), 598–603.

Bodenheimer, T. (2007). Building teams in primary care: Lessons learned. Oakland, CA: California Healthcare Foundation. Retrieved from: https://www.chcf.org/wp-content/uploads/2017/12/PDF-BuildingTeamsInPrimaryCareLessons.pdf

Bodenheimer, T., & Grumbach, K. (2006). *Improving primary care: Strategies and tools for a better practice*. New York, NY: McGraw-Hill.

Campbell, S. M., Hann, M., Hacker, J., Burns, C., Oliver, D., Thapar, A., … Roland, M. O. (2001). Identifying predictors of high quality care in English general practice: Observational study. *British Medical Journal, 323*(7316), 784–787.

Gabbard, G. O., & Kay, J. (2001). The fate of integrated treatment: Whatever happened to the biopsychosocial psychiatrist? *American Journal of Psychiatry, 158*(12), 1956–1963. https://doi.org/10.1176/appi.ajp.158.12.1956

Gitlin, M. J., & Miklowitz, D. J. (2016). Split treatment: Recommendations for optimal use in the care of psychiatric patients. *Annals of Clinical Psychiatry, 28*(2), 132–137.

Gutheil, T. G. (1994). Risk management at the margins: Less-familiar topics in psychiatric malpractice. *Harvard Review of Psychiatry, 2*(4), 214–221.

Jee, S. H., Baldwin, C., Dadiz, R., Jones, M., & Alpert-Gillis, L. (2018). Integrated mental health training for pediatric and psychology trainees using standardized patient encounters. *Academic Pediatrics, 18*(1), 119–121. https://doi.org/10.1016/j.acap.2017.06.014

Kalman, T. P., Kalman, V. N., & Granet, R. (2012). Do psychopharmacologists speak to psychotherapists? A survey of practicing clinicians. *Psychodynamic Psychiatry, 40*(2), 275–285.

Kullgren, K. A., Tsang, K. K., Ernst, M. M., Carter, B. D., Scott, E. L., & Sullivan, S. K. (2015). Inpatient pediatric psychology consultation-liaison practice survey: Corrected version. *Clinical Practice in Pediatric Psychology, 3*(4), 340–351.

Ling, T., Brereton, L., Conklin, A., Newbould, J., & Roland, M. (2012). Barriers and facilitators to integrating care: Experiences from the English Integrated Care Pilots. *International Journal of Integrated Care, 12*(5), e129. https://doi.org/10.5334/ijic.982

March, J., Silva, S., Petrycki, S., Curry, J., Wells, K., & Fairbank, J. (2004). Fluoxetine, cognitive-behavioral therapy, and their combination for adolescents with depression: Treatment for Adolescents with Depression Study (TADS) randomized controlled trial. *JAMA, 292*(7), 807–820. https://doi.org/10.1001/jama.292.7.807

Osofsky, H. J., Osofsky, J. D., Wells, J. H., & Weems, C. (2014). Integrated care: Meeting mental health needs after the Gulf oil spill. *Psychiatric Services, 65*(3), 280–283. https://doi.org/10.1176/appi.ps.201300470

Palermo, T. M., Janicke, D. M., McQuaid, E. L., Mullins, L. L., Robins, P. M., & Wu, Y. P. (2014). Recommendations for training in pediatric psychology: Defining core competencies across training levels. *Journal of Pediatric Psychology, 39*(9), 965–984. https://doi.org/10.1093/jpepsy/jsu015

Pidano, A. E., Arora, P., Gipson, P. Y., Hudson, B. O., & Schellinger, K. B. (2018). Psychologists and pediatricians in the primary care sandbox: Communication is key to cooperative play. *Journal of Clinical Psychology in a Medical Settings, 25*(1), 32–42. https://doi.org/10.1007/s10880-017-9522-y

Pisani, A. R., leRoux, P., & Siegel, D. M. (2011). Educating residents in behavioral health care and collaboration: Integrated clinical training of pediatric residents and psychology fellows. *Academic Medicine, 86*(2), 166–173. https://doi.org/10.1097/ACM.0b013e318204fd94

Raney, L. E. (2015). Integrating primary care and behavioral health: The role of the psychiatrist in the collaborative care model. *American Journal of Psychiatry, 172*(8), 721–728. https://doi.org/10.1176/appi.ajp.2015.15010017

Schindler, F. E., Berren, M. R., & Beigel, A. (1981). A study of the causes of conflict between psychiatrists and psychologists. *Hospital & Community Psychiatry, 32*(4), 263–266.

Shaw, R. J., Pao, M., Holland, J. E., & DeMaso, D. R. (2016). Practice patterns revisited in pediatric psychosomatic medicine. *Psychosomatics, 57*(6), 576–585. https://doi.org/10.1016/j.psym.2016.05.006

Shaw, R. J., Wamboldt, M., Bursch, B., & Stuber, M. (2006). Practice patterns in pediatric consultation-liaison psychiatry: A national survey. *Psychosomatics, 47*(1), 43–49. https://doi.org/10.1176/appi.psy.47.1.43

Wagner, E. H. (2000). The role of patient care teams in chronic disease management. *British Medical Journal, 320*(7234), 569–572.

Woodward, B. (2002). Anticipating and avoiding pitfalls in split treatment. *Psychiatric Times, 19*, 22.

Consultation-Liaison Psychologists' Role in Medical Education

Crystal Cederna-Meko and Rebecca Ellens

Pediatric medical education is evolving considerably alongside shifts in the scope of practice, educational needs, and instructional methods (Simpson, Marcdante, Souza, Anderson, & Holmboe, 2018). Innovative and interprofessional approaches to medical education are increasingly relied upon to cover historically under-addressed content areas, yet training often remains inadequate. Pediatric consultation-liaison (CL) psychologists are well positioned to fill many of the gaps between expected and actual learner outcomes. In what follows, current learners, learning needs, approaches to education, and opportunities for psychologists within medical education are reviewed. Thereafter, adaptations to support individualized learning, and strategies to promote sustainable medical education involvement are highlighted. The chapter ends with a hypothetical case review outlining the roles of three CL psychologists within a pediatric residency program

C. Cederna-Meko (✉) · R. Ellens
Department of Pediatrics and Human Development, Michigan State University College of Human Medicine, Hurley Children's Hospital, Flint, MI, USA
e-mail: ccedern1@hurleymc.com

Pediatric Medical Residents Defined

During their 4 years of medical school, medical students complete coursework and clinical experiences essential to medical practice including clerkships (i.e., brief clinical experiences) in psychiatry and pediatrics. In the final year of medical school, individuals interested in providing care and advocacy for children apply to train in a pediatric residency program. During their first year, pediatric residents endorse completion of a variety of scholarly and clinically relevant activities (AAMC, 2018a). Early involvement in residency-relevant experiences is unsurprising given the popularity of pediatrics as a specialty and resulting competition for residency positions (AAMC, 2018b).

Educational Standards Informing Pediatric Medical Education

Pediatric residencies are 3-year training programs designed to impart extensive medical knowledge and skills specific to pediatrics. Graduates are prepared for general pediatrics practice or entry into a fellowship program for further specialization. To ensure graduation readiness, the Accreditation Council for Graduate Medical Education (ACGME) accredits residency programs (ACGME, 2018). ACGME

B. D. Carter, K. A. Kullgren (eds.), *Clinical Handbook of Psychological Consultation in Pediatric Medical Settings*, Issues in Clinical Child Psychology, https://doi.org/10.1007/978-3-030-35598-2_10

program requirements have undergone significant revision over time. Highlights pertinent to CL psychologists within pediatric medical education include the following: implementation of a 1-month developmental-behavioral pediatrics rotation within pediatric residencies (1997), the establishment of six domains of competence essential to physician practice (i.e., patient care, medical knowledge, professionalism, interpersonal and communication skills, systems-based practice, and practice-based learning; 2000–2002), and the transition from program requirements stipulating the educational process to requirements focused on educational outcomes (2013; Desy, Reed, & Wolanskyj, 2017).

The shift to outcome-based educational standards prompted the ACGME to develop physician competencies (i.e., milestones). Within pediatrics, the ACGME milestones consist of 21 sub-competencies or expected behaviors that fall within the aforementioned six domains of competence (ACGME & American Board of Pediatrics [ABP], 2017). Pediatric residencies have since had to identify multimodal, multimethod means of assessing resident competency in accordance with the milestones (ACGME, 2017). While milestones focus more granularly on individual behaviors, the ABP (n.d.) has also preliminarily identified pediatric-specific activities that residents should be competent to perform independently by residency completion (i.e., entrustable professional activities (EPAs)). Currently, programs are encouraged, but not required, to monitor residents' progress toward independent performance of the EPAs (Holmboe, ten Cate, Durning, & Hawkins, 2018). As data emerge in support of the EPAs, increasing emphasis on their adoption is likely.

The educational environment provided by sponsoring institutions is also monitored and thus informed, in part, by the ACGME. During periodic Clinical Learning Environment Review visits, site visitors assess an institution's effectiveness in supporting pre-specified focus areas. Thereafter, verbal and written feedback for improvement is provided to institutional leadership to guide future improvement efforts. Presently, the ACGME reviews six initiatives including patient safety, healthcare quality, supervision, care transitions, well-being, and professionalism (ACGME, CLER Evaluation Committee, 2017). Well-being was the most recent addition to the areas under review and emerged in response to the disproportionately high rates of depression, burnout, and suicide among physicians (Matta et al., 2015; Shanafelt et al., 2015). Moving forward, focus areas will continue to adapt to capture educational and patient care needs and consequently influence many aspects of medical education.

Additional Factors Shaping Pediatric Medical Education

An outcome closely monitored by the ACGME and a common prerequisite to practice, the ABP certification examination (i.e., board exam) is a 7-h, multiple choice test composed of 25 content domains deemed essential to pediatric practice (ABP, 2018). Board topics relevant to psychologists engaged in medical education include the following: common behavior problems, normal child development, psychosocial and developmental screening, neurodevelopmental and psychiatric conditions, substance use/abuse, adolescent behavioral health issues, societal issues such as immigration and violence, familial issues such as divorce and adoption, professionalism, cross-cultural issues, research methods, and quality improvement methodology. Given the stakes associated with board performance, residencies work hard to ensure program content prepares residents to succeed. Consequently, residency curriculum overlaps considerably with exam content.

The breadth of psychologist-relevant exam content reflects the increasing scope of mental and behavioral health practice within pediatrics. Both the American Academy of Pediatrics (AAP; AAP Committee on Psychosocial Aspects of Child and Family Health & Task Force on Mental Health, 2009) and the ABP (2013) published mental health, behavioral health, and specific developmental-behavioral health competencies. The AAP and Bright Futures (2017) also publish recommendations for when pediatricians should conduct developmental and behavioral health screenings to aid in early problem detection. And, in support of expediting access to treatment, the AAP endorses guidelines advising pediatricians to diagnose, initiate first-line treatment, and monitor treatment efficacy for attention-deficit/hyperactivity disorder (AAP Subcommittee on Attention-Deficit/Hyperactivity Disorder & Steering Committee on Quality Improvement and Management, 2011) and adolescent depression (Cheung et al., 2018; Zuckerbrot et al., 2018). As mental health provider shortages increase (Andrilla, Patterson, Garberson, Coulthard, & Larson, 2018), so too will the scope of pediatric practice residents must master during residency training.

Contemporary teaching practices that support improved learner competence have also influenced medical education. Such teaching practices encourage residents to self-reflect, develop learning goals, create action plans, and evaluate outcomes (Sandars, 2009; Sawatsky, Ratelle, Bonnes, Egginton, & Beckman, 2017). Meanwhile, faculty are encouraged to engage in more collaborative educational approaches (Taylor & Hamdy, 2013), while programs maintain safe learning environments (van den Eertwegh, van Dalen, van Dulmen, van der Vleuten, & Scherpbier, 2014) and appoint expert faculty to observe or be observed during patient care activities (Hampton, Richardson, Bostwick, Ward, & Green, 2015). Interprofessional education (Ward, Zagoloff, Rieck, & Robiner, 2018) and the use of multimodal, multimedia-infused, experiential, and interactive teaching methods (Papanagnou et al., 2016; Ramnanan & Pound, 2017) have also been promoted. The abundance of instructional advancements reflects the current medical education climate—rapidly evolving, innovation-encouraging, and embracing of change.

Inadequately Met Needs Within Pediatric Medical Education

Despite advances aimed at improving residents' readiness to address behavioral and mental health issues, further improvements are needed (McMillan, Land, & Leslie, 2017). Pediatricians and residents report low confidence in their ability to assess, identify, and manage behavioral and mental health issues and cite inadequate training as a key contributing factor (Horwitz et al., 2015). Hampton et al. (2015) conducted focus groups with pediatric residents to determine where current training falls short. Residents involved endorsed insufficient training in mental health, interpersonal and communication skills, and skills relevant to working in interprofessional teams. To improve training, residents in the study expressed interest in having more access to mental health specialists and related clinical services (Hampton et al., 2015), a recommendation supported by stakeholders (e.g., AAP Committee on Psychosocial Aspects of Child and Family Health & Task Force on Mental Health, 2009; Ward et al., 2018).

In another study, Shahidullah et al. (2018) examined the perceptions of 148 out of 214 pediatric residency program directors in the United States and similarly found behavioral health training to be insufficient. Identified barriers to better training included not enough faculty, inadequate administrative support to enhance behavioral health training and workforce, and insufficient funding. Hernandez, Hopkins, and Dudas (2018) also attributed unsatisfactory learning outcomes to inadequate time for educational activities. As this brief review suggests, multiple factors contribute to suboptimal physician comfort and competence in addressing behavioral and mental health issues.

Opportunities for Consultation-Liaison Psychologists Within Medical Education

Psychologists are well represented within pediatric residency programs (Shahidullah et al., 2018) and academic health centers (Robiner, Dixon, Miner, & Hong, 2014). However, additional deliberate medical education involvement is needed to improve resident outcomes. Clinically, most CL psychologists provide patient-centered care to a broad patient population (Carter et al., 2017), utilize a biopsychosocial framework, engage patients in health-promoting interventions (Kazak, Nash, Hiroto, & Kaslow, 2017), and rely on skilled interviewing techniques. In addition to their clinical expertise, psychologists' understanding of cognition and learning supports their involvement in developing scientifically driven, educationally rich experiences deemed by Simpson et al. (2018) as essential to meeting resident needs. Frequent involvement in psychology training programs (Mackner, Swift, Heidgerken, Stalets, & Linscheid, 2003) also affords them strong supervisory skills that apply to residents.

Pediatric Medical Education on the Medical Unit

CL psychologists can participate in resident education within the medical unit in a variety of ways (see Table 1). Patient rounds present a powerful opportunity for bedside education (Peters & ten Cate, 2014). Topics taught during rounds can be case specific, such as how to explain to a school-aged child the need for insulin injections and blood glucose checks. More generalizable topics, such as how to promote social/emotional health in toddlers during hospitalization, can also be presented. In addition to teaching, psychologists can model, conduct structured observations, and provide feedback (e.g., Rao et al., 2018) on a number of skills. Immediately after rounds, brief case-based discussions can aid residents in generalizing lessons learned beyond individual patient encounters.

Table 1 Pediatric medical education on the medical unit

Activity
• Curbside consultation • Direct observation • Formal consultation • Patient encounter • Patient rounds
Sample instructional/teaching methods
• Coaching • Direct learner observation, assessment, and/or evaluation • Facilitation of resident-constructed learning goals • Feedback • Guided resident self-reflection • Modeling • On-the-fly, case-based, and bedside education • Outcome evaluation

Patient-specific interactions can also be rich learning moments. In addition to imparting knowledge and skills, informal curbside consultations enable psychologists to share clinical reasoning processes, suggest areas for further evaluation, and encourage consideration of alternative explanations for observed behaviors (Vogel, Kirkpatrick, Collings, Cederna-Meko, & Grey, 2012). Even when curbside consultations are simply to clarify the need for formal consultation, the resulting dialogue improves knowledge of the indications for including various disciplines in future patient care.

Formal consultations also offer multiple learning opportunities. Residents may observe a consultation with a defined learning goal, such as identifying pre-specified interpersonal and communication skills in action. Under a psychologist's supervision, they may also complete portions of the evaluation relevant to their training. Similar to the brief educational opportunities after rounds, psychologists can provide feedback to promote growth and engage residents in a variety of clinical discussions after completing consultations.

Psychologists can also conduct direct observations of residents on the medical unit. Observations can include aspects of history taking such as agenda setting and sharing a diagnosis; they can also center around the interpersonal and communicative aspects of physical examinations (e.g., asking or telling before touching, providing feedback on exam findings) or the resident's approach to assessing and managing psychology-relevant topics. Outside the patient encounter, psychologists can observe patient sign-outs between residents, as well as resident interactions with peers, nurses, and consultants. Through direct observation, resident competence in various milestones and related professional activities can be monitored while providing feedback to residents to further their growth. In a competency-based educational era, such educational interactions amidst patient care are likely to promote competency gains that exceed the standard curriculum.

Pediatric Medical Education Beyond the Medical Unit

As Table 2 illustrates, educational opportunities extend beyond the medical unit. CL psychologists can present didactics for residents on a range of topics pertinent to pediatric practice and the board exam. Faculty trainings focused upon competency-based teaching and evaluative tools such as direct observation methods, delivering effective feedback, supporting individualized learning plans, curriculum development, and resident evaluation would also be of benefit. Common venues for presenting on the aforementioned topics include grand rounds, faculty development sessions, and program- or graduate medical education-wide didactics. Pediatric education committee meetings are another venue for delivering brief, albeit meaningful, faculty training experiences.

Within any given institution are multiple established activities in which psychologist presence and participation is meaningful. Psychologists can highlight the psychosocial aspects of care during inpatient case presentations and co-facilitate journal clubs. Strength in systems-based practice lends itself nicely to involvement in morbidity and mortality conferences. And advanced therapeutic skills enable psychologists to suggest scripts for responding to challenging patient scenarios as they arise during oncology or trauma conferences. Additional venues of relevance may include staff meetings focused upon patient care (e.g., morning report, case conference, safety huddles, quality meetings) and committees concerned with initiatives such as ethical/legal issues, multicultural inclusion, and well-being. Consulting with departmental and hospital leadership to identify opportunities outside the medical unit is encouraged.

Psychologists can also apply expertise in assessment and research to support nonclinical programmatic aims. They may assist residencies in meeting scholarly activity requirements by collaborating, teaching and training, mentoring, and/or serving as a liaison between residents and faculty (Abramson et al., 2018). Proficiency in assessment and program development enables completion of needs assessments and curricular design to address identified program deficiencies (Kazak et al., 2017). Assessment and psychometric knowledge can also inform the development of standardized, systematic interviewing methods and approaches to resident evaluation (e.g., Hanna-Attisha et al., 2016). Residencies value the aforementioned contributions, along with others that facilitate a psychologically safe and effective learning environment, enhance resident evaluation, and ultimately improve resident competence.

Essential Resources and Support

For psychologists not yet involved in medical education or seeking to strengthen their role(s), a few key considerations are advised. The following highlights strategies to support effective and ongoing medical education involvement.

Job Description and Productivity Expectations

While highly beneficial to their learning, resident involvement in CL psychologist's clinical activity will reduce service efficiency, as will the insertion of instructional activities between clinical tasks. Considerable resources are also required to construct and deliver high-quality didactics, observe and provide feedback to residents, and fulfill other medical education roles. To ensure sufficient support, involvement in medical education should be detailed within one's job duties and responsibilities, with adequate time and compensation allotted (Hernandez et al., 2018). Within productivity-driven settings where education aligns with the institutional mission, tying medical education roles to educational value units (EVUs) may offset reductions in

Table 2 Examples of psychologist contributions to medical education beyond the medical unit

Curriculum development and evaluation	• Problem identification/formal needs assessment • Curriculum development, implementation, and evaluation – *Target populations*: Community-based and core faculty, graduate medical education at-large, institution at-large, pediatric residents, program administration – *Example Topics*: Subsets of content specifications for the ABP certification examination, evidence-based medicine, interpersonal and communication skills, interprofessional education and practice, professionalism, well-being	Resident evaluation	• Problem identification/formal needs assessment • Identification, development, and implementation of multi-method, multisource data to inform semiannual resident evaluation • Incorporation of the pediatric-specific entrustable professional activities into the program's competency-based evaluation system • Selection and/or development of assessment tools • Faculty development specific to resident and competency-based evaluation • Participation in the clinical competency committee
Didactic delivery, attendance, and participation	• Problem identification/formal needs assessment • Resident didactic development, delivery, and participation • Faculty development sessions – *Example resident didactic venues*: Case presentations; grand rounds; institution-specific meetings, committees, and councils; morbidity and mortality conferences; resident seminars – *Example faculty development venues*: Committee meetings, local and regional conferences, on-site workshops and seminars, resident didactics	Resident performance problem support	• Behaviorally based problem identification • Development of behaviorally based expectations for improvement and measurable outcomes • Development of strategies to support improvement • Participation in remediation • Monitoring of remediation plan outcomes
Resident interviewing and recruitment	• Identification of program-valued, measurable characteristics • Development of behaviorally anchored rating scales for characteristics of interest • Development of standardized interview content by characteristic • Faculty development (interviewer specific and overall) • Participation in resident interviews and resident selection	Scholarly activity contributions, monitoring, and implementation	• Scholarly activity completion in collaboration with program faculty and residents • Program-specific scholarly activity requirement development, implementation, and/or monitoring • Evidence-based medicine curriculum delivery or participation • Journal club facilitation • Mentoring specific to resident research • Service as a research liaison between faculty and residents

clinically derived productivity (D'Angelo & Gallagher, 2016). In July 2019, the ACGME will also enhance support for psychologists within medical education by expanding core faculty eligibility within residency programs to nonphysicians (ACGME, 2018). The shift to competency-based education, identification of unmet needs within pediatrics, emergence of mission-based productivity standards specific to educational activity, and upcoming recognition of psychologists by the ACGME place CL psychologists in a strong position to negotiate for education-related protected time and funding.

Innovative Leaders and Environments

Psychologists can thrive when immersed in a proactive environment with leaders who see change as opportunity and strive for continuous quality improvement. In such environments, psychologists are viewed as equals to physician colleagues (Kazak et al., 2017), with distinct areas of expertise that are valued and respected. From this position, medical education contributions can follow in a variety of ways that align with psychologists' broad skill set. These are also settings that support interprofessional training and recognize the value-added benefits of multidisciplinary involvement despite potential reductions in clinical productivity (Ward et al., 2018). Within such settings, it is not unusual for psychologists to share the same staff privileges, office space, departmental affiliations, and benefits as physicians. In this manner, innovative leaders and educational environments support patient, learner, and programmatic contributions that promote successful outcomes, regardless of the source or precedent.

Networking, Collaboration, and Program Participation

Identifying areas of demand in the residency program that align with personal areas of expertise is strongly encouraged. Depending on the faculty composition, CL psychologists may find overlap between their areas of expertise and those of others within the residency program. Role delineation is supported by gaining familiarity with the program, learning about the roles/interests of existing faculty, and establishing meaningful relationships with program staff and residents. Strategies to enhance familiarity include collaborations in patient care, attending program-coordinated events and didactics, participating in committees, and adding to discussions during departmental meetings. Translating one's expertise into meaningful contributions also requires awareness of one's strengths and unique point of view within a predominantly physician team (Ward et al., 2018). For example, one could apply expertise in treatment planning during a clinical competency committee meeting to assist in developing a plan for strengthening a resident's communication skills. Finally, seeking and maintaining strong mentorship will support the process of networking and increasing program integration considerably (Hong & Robiner, 2016).

CL Psychologists and Medical Education in Action

The following hypothetical case illustrates several valuable roles of psychologists within medical education. CL psychologists 1, 2, and 3 are embedded within a large public hospital in the United States. Each is considered non-core faculty of the hospital-affiliated, ACGME-accredited pediatric residency program and a member of the department of pediatrics. Although each psychologist has a predominantly clinical role, 1 day per week is allotted for clearly defined medical education activities.

Throughout the academic year, the psychologists provide large group didactics as part of the residency's weekly seminar series. The requested topics are broad, spanning traditional pediatric psychology content and other topics such as toxic stress, social determinants of health, and culturally sensitive communication. Two of the psychologists also present small group didactics within the residents' 1-month rotation in developmental-behavioral pediatrics. The small group presentation topics correspond to the rotation's weekly curriculum and include motivational interviewing (week 1), normal development and developmental variations (week 2), neurodevelopmental and psychiatric conditions (week 3), and common subclinical behavior problems of childhood (week 4).

Within didactics, the psychologists provide evidence-based information tailored to the needs of practicing pediatricians, incorporate interaction and skill-based practice with feedback, review video clips to illustrate phenomena in action, and include case-based learning opportunities. On a rotating basis, the psychologists also attend case presentations, morbidity and mortality conferences, and large group didactics presented by pediatric residency faculty. When in attendance, they contribute relevant psychosocial perspectives and aspects of systems-based care, interpersonal and communication skills, and professionalism.

As part of her contribution to the developmental-behavioral pediatrics rotation, CL psychologist 1 has residents assigned to shadow her inpatient consultations on the general pediatrics units 2 days each week. During one such rotation she has two first-year residents, learner A and learner B, assigned to work with her. In order to efficiently cultivate a safe learning environment, CL psychologist 1 engages the two residents in a brief discussion that includes an introduction to the role of pediatric psychology in relation to patient care and this learning experience. She then elicits a brief history and review of self-identified goals from learner A and learner B.

Learner A is an international medical graduate who completed a pediatric residency training program in Nepal, where she stayed and practiced pediatrics for 1 year prior to entering the current residency program. Learner B is an American medical graduate who was accepted into the residency program immediately following medical school. Both residents express interest in general pediatrics after residency. As such, CL psychologist 1 discusses their need for broad developmental and behavioral exposure, including strategies for differentiating normal from abnormal, as well as appropriate management and referral practices for common behavioral and mental health problems. With this guidance, learner A defines a goal of developing comfort in screening for depression and risk for self-harm, activities described as outside the scope of her previous practice and thus of little familiarity. After describing minimal clinical exposure to toddlers during her pediatric clerkship, learner B expresses a desire to master toddler development and learn how to establish rapport with young patients.

In support of learner A and learner B's learning objectives, CL psychologist 1 selects three consultations for the residents to shadow. She encourages learner A to attend to differences in the evaluation of depressive symptoms for a 16-year-old male presenting with chronic abdominal pain compared to a 4-year-old with new onset acute lymphocytic leukemia. The psychologist encourages learner B to pay attention to the methods of establishing and maintaining a therapeutic alliance with the 4-year-old patient and to the approach to surveying development in a 3-year-old patient presenting with fecal impaction and chronic constipation. After the consultations, CL psychologist 1 elicits from each resident what was learned, answers resident-driven questions for 2–3 min, then provides a 5-min didactic highlighting a few key points illustrated during the patient encounters.

CL psychologist 2 allots a portion of his medical education time to routinely participating in morning rounds on the intensive care units along with participation in curbside consultations, resident observation with feedback, and brief education. He meets learner A and learner B while they are on a pediatric intensive care rotation. During rounds, the psychologist discusses the developmental and psychosocial aspects of patient presentations and treatment plans, demonstrates professionalism, and exhibits patient-centered communication skills. After rounds and while still in the intensive care unit, CL psychologist 2 participates in curbside consultations as prompted by learners, attending physicians, and the psychologist himself. On one such occasion, learner A inquires into the appropriateness of a formal psychology consultation after observing an adolescent patient's pervasively flat affect and minimal engagement since hospital admission. From this interaction, learner A acquires the indications for a formal consultation and places the order. The patient is then seen by CL psychologist 2, after which learner A's concerns are substantiated and brief education regarding the presenting problem and management are provided.

CL psychologist 3 dedicates a portion of her medical education time to advancing the interpersonal and communication skills of senior pediatric residents. After conducting a needs assessment, comfort and skills in motivational interviewing are identified as significant opportunities for improvement. Consequently, CL psychologist 3 develops and implements a curriculum that includes monthly didactics, low-stakes role-playing with immediate feedback, and live observation of residents' medical encounters within the continuity clinic. Upon identifying learner A and learner B's plans for general pediatric practice, CL psychologist 3 observes and provides feedback specific to motivational interviewing within primary care. She highlights strengths then missed opportunities. Specifically, they review the promotion of safe sleep practices during a 3-month well-child visit and role-play how the skills might look in action. CL psychologist 3 then assists learner A and learner B in generating action plans for improvement. At the end of four observations and following improvement plan implementation, learner A and B report enhanced comfort and motivational interviewing skills in the primary care setting.

In addition to the aforementioned roles, each psychologist participates in residency program-supporting activities. CL psychologists 1 and 2 update the developmental-behavioral pediatrics curriculum using the six-step approach outlined by Thomas, Kern, Hughes, and Chen (2016). The two continue to monitor meaningful outcomes of the rotation in the spirit of the program's continuous quality improvement philosophy. CL psychologist 3 provides faculty development sessions and one-on-one training in support of the competency-based resident evaluation process. She also supports the residency program in identifying reliable and valid assessment strategies to inform semiannual resident evaluations.

During their annual faculty evaluations with the pediatric residency program director, CL psychologists 1, 2, and 3 were recognized for their valuable educational roles. Specific examples of how each promoted resident growth in domains of competence and professional activities were given. Performance on in-training exams in the content areas taught by the psychologists was also reviewed, with novel ideas for enhancing resident knowledge of content specifications subsequently generated. Each psychologist was asked to continue their existing efforts within the residency program, and one was asked to seek administrative support for additional protected education time. Specifically, owing to her skill in engaging residents and creating a safe space to discuss challenging issues, CL psychologist 3 was asked to lead the program's implementation of institutionally driven resident well-being initiatives. At graduation, learners A and B eagerly informed CL psychologists 1 and 2 of their successful attainment of general pediatrics positions and of their readiness for practice in part on account of several memorable beside teaching moments with the psychologists.

Concluding Remarks

This chapter focused on the roles and accompanying benefits of CL psychologists within medical education. Pediatrics as a field and medical education at-large are continuously advancing. The need for content experts to aid residency programs in teaching, monitoring, and evaluating resident progression toward competence for independent practice is great. To this end, psychologists can lend highly applicable knowledge, skills, and attributes. Through their efforts, psychologists will find themselves increasingly at home participating and/or leading a variety of educational activities among an interdisciplinary team of colleagues. In turn, the astute psychologist will note a deepening appreciation for the inextricable link between psychology and medicine and for the many unexpected yet welcomed ways psychology and medicine shape one another. While needs within medical education will evolve, the indispensable role for psychologists in addressing them will endure.

References

Abramson, E. L., Naifeh, M. M., Stevenson, M. D., Mauer, E., Hammad, H. T., Gerber, L. M., & Li, S.-T. T. (2018). Scholarly activity training during residency: Are we hitting the mark? A national assessment of pediatric residents. *Academic Pediatrics, 18*(5), 542–549. https://doi.org/10.1016/j.acap.2018.02.002

Accreditation Council for Graduate Medical Education. (2017). ACGME common program requirements. Retrieved from https://www.acgme.org/Portals/0/PFAssets/ProgramRequirements/CPRs_2017-07-01.pdf

Accreditation Council for Graduate Medical Education. (2018). ACGME common program requirements (residency). Retrieved from https://www.acgme.org/Portals/0/PFAssets/Program Requirements/CPRResidency2019.pdf

Accreditation Council for Graduate Medical Education & American Board of Pediatrics. (2017). The pediatrics milestone project. Retrieved from https://acgme.org/Portals/0/PDFs/Milestones/PediatricsMilestones.pdf

Accreditation Council for Graduate Medical Education, CLER Evaluation Committee. (2017). CLER pathways to excellence: Expectations for an optimal clinical learning environment to achieve safe and high quality patient care, Version 1.1. Retrieved from https://www.acgme.org/Portals/0/PDFs/CLER/CLER_Pathways_V1.1_Digital_Final.pdf

American Academy of Pediatrics, Committee on Psychosocial Aspects of Child and Family Health & Task Force on Mental Health. (2009). The future of pediatrics: Mental health competencies for pediatric primary care. *Pediatrics, 124*(1), 410–421. https://doi.org/10.1542/peds.2009-1061

American Academy of Pediatrics, Subcommittee on Attention-Deficit/Hyperactivity Disorder & Steering Committee on Quality Improvement and Management. (2011). ADHD: Clinical practice guideline for the diagnosis, evaluation, and treatment of attention-deficit/hyperactivity disorder in children and adolescents. *Pediatrics, 128*(5), 1007–1022. https://doi.org/10.1542/peds.2011-2654

American Board of Pediatrics. (2013). Curricular components for general pediatrics EPA 9. Retrieved from https://www.abp.org/sites/abp/files/pdf/gen_peds_epa_9.pdf

American Board of Pediatrics. (2018). Booklet of information: A guide to board certification in pediatrics. Retrieved from https://www.abp.org/sites/abp/files/pdf/certboi.pdf

American Board of Pediatrics. (n.d.). Entrustable professional activities for general pediatrics. Retrieved from https://www.abp.org/entrustable-professional-activities-epas

Andrilla, C. H. A., Patterson, D. G., Garberson, L. A., Coulthard, C., & Larson, E. H. (2018). Geographic variation in the supply of selected behavioral health providers. *American Journal of Preventive Medicine, 54*(6S3), S199–S207. https://doi.org/10.1016/j.amepre.2018.01.004

Association of American Medical Colleges. (2018a). Table B1. Test scores and experiences of first-year residents, by specialty: 2017–2018 first-year residents. Retrieved from https://www.aamc.org/data/493918/report-on-residents-2018-b1table.html

Association of American Medical Colleges. (2018b). Table B3. Number of active residents, by type of medical school, GME specialty, and sex: 2017–2018 active residents. Retrieved from https://www.aamc.org/data/493922/report-on-residents-2018-b3table.html

Bright Futures & American Academy of Pediatrics. (2017). Recommendations for preventive pediatric health care. Retrieved from https://www.aap.org/enus/Documents/periodicity_schedule.pdf

Carter, B. D., Kronenberger, W. G., Scott, E. L., Kullgren, K. A., Piazza-Waggoner, C., & Brady, C. E. (2017). Inpatient pediatric consultation-liaison. In R. G. Steele & M. Roberts (Eds.), *Handbook of pediatric psychology* (5th ed., pp. 105–118). New York, NY: Guilford Press.

Cheung, A. H., Zuckerbrot, R. A., Jensen, P. S., Laraque, D., Stein, R. E. K., & GLAD-PC Steering Group. (2018). Guidelines for adolescent depression in primary care (GLAD-PC): Part II. Treatment and ongoing management. *Pediatrics, 141*(18), e20174082. https://doi.org/10.1542/peds.2017-4082

D'Angelo, E. J., & Gallagher, K. (2016). Capturing psychologists' work in academic health settings: The role of the educational value unit (EVU). *Journal of Clinical Psychology in Medical Settings, 23*, 21–32. https://doi.org/10.1007/s10880-016-9453-z

Desy, J. R., Reed, D. A., & Wolanskyj, A. P. (2017). Milestones and millennials: A perfect pairing—Competency-based medical education and the learning preferences of Generation Y. *Mayo Clinic Proceedings, 92*(2), 243–250. https://doi.org/10.1016/j.mayocp.2016.10.026

Hampton, E., Richardson, J. E., Bostwick, S., Ward, M. J., & Green, C. (2015). The current and ideal state of mental health training: Pediatric resident perspectives. *Teaching and Learning in Medicine, 27*(2), 147–154. https://doi.org/10.1080/10401334.2015.1011653

Hanna-Attisha, M., Cederna-Meko, C. L., Casey, S., Trimm, F., Goslings, S., & Harper, R. (2016, February). Beyond "tell me about yourself?": Using multiple mini interview to overcome interview and selection challenges. Workshop presented at the 2016 ACGME annual educational conference, Harbor Spring, MA.

Hernandez, R. G., Hopkins, A., & Dudas, R. A. (2018). The evolution of graduate medical education over the past decade: Building a new pediatric residency program in an era of innovation. *Medical Teacher, 40*(6), 615–621. https://doi.org/10.1080/0142159X.2018.1455969

Holmboe, E. S., ten Cate, O., Durning, S. J., & Hawkins, R. E. (2018). Assessment challenges in the era of ouctomes-based education. In E. S. Holmboe, S. J. Durning, & R. E. Hawkins (Eds.), *Practical guide to the evaluation of clinical competence* (pp. 1–21). Philadelphia, PA: Elsevier.

Hong, B. A., & Robiner, W. N. (2016). Psychologists in academic health centers and medical centers: Being visible, relevant and integral. *Journal of Clinical Psychology in Medical Settings, 23*(1), 11–20. https://doi.org/10.1007/s10880-016-9450-2

Horwitz, S. M., Storfer-Isser, A., Kerker, B. D., Szilagyi, M., Garner, A., O'Connor, K. G., … Stein, R. E. (2015). Barriers to the identification and management of psychosocial problems: Changes from 2004 to 2013. *Academic Pediatrics, 15*(6), 613–620. https://doi.org/10.1016/j.acap.2015.08.006

Kazak, A. E., Nash, J. M., Hiroto, K., & Kaslow, N. J. (2017). Psychologists in patient-centered medical homes (PCMHs): Roles, evidence, opportunities, and challenges. *American Psychologist, 72*(1), 1–12. https://doi.org/10.1037/a0040382

Mackner, L. M., Swift, E. E., Heidgerken, A. D., Stalets, M. M., & Linscheid, T. M. (2003). Training in pediatric psychology: A survey of predoctoral internship programs. *Journal of Pediatric Psychology, 28*(6), 433–441. https://doi.org/10.1093/jpepsy/jsg033

Matta, D. A., Ramos, M. A., Bansal, N., Khan, R., Guille, C., Di Angelantonio, E., & Sen, S. (2015). Prevalence of depression and depressive symptoms among resident physicians: A systematic review and meta-analysis. *JAMA, 314*(22), 2373–2383. https://doi.org/10.1001/jama.2015.15845

McMillan, J. A., Land, M., Jr., & Leslie, L. K. (2017). Pediatric residency education and the behavioral and mental health crisis: A call to action. *Pediatrics, 139*(1), e20162141. https://doi.org/10.1542/peds.2016-2141

Papanagnou, D., Serrano, A., Barkley, K., Chandra, S., Governatori, N., Piela, N., … Shin, R. (2016). Does tailoring instructional style to a medical student's self-perceived learning style improve performance when teaching intravenous catheter placement? A randomized controlled study. *BMC Medical Education, 16*(1), 205. https://doi.org/10.1186/s12909-016-0720-3

Peters, M., & ten Cate, O. (2014). Bedside teaching in medical education: A literature review. *Perspectives on Medical Education, 3*(2), 76–88. https://doi.org/10.1007/s40037-013-0083-y

Ramnanan, C. J., & Pound, L. D. (2017). Advances in medical education and practice: Student perceptions of the flipped classroom. *Advances in Medical Education and Practice, 2017*(8), 63–73. https://doi.org/10.2147/AMEP.S109037

Rao, P., Hill, E., Palka, C., Rea, K., Jones, K., Balzer, K., … Cousino, M. (2018). Improving pediatric resident communication during family-centered rounds using a novel simulation-based curriculum. *MedEdPORTAL, 14*, 10733. https://doi.org/10.15766/mep_2374-8265.10733

Robiner, W. N., Dixon, K. E., Miner, J. L., & Hong, B. A. (2014). Psychologists in medical schools and academic medical centers: Over 100 years of growth, influence, and partnership. *American Psychologist, 69*(3), 230–248. https://doi.org/10.1037/a0035472

Sandars, J. (2009). The use of reflection in medical education: AMEE Guide No. 44. *Medical Teacher, 31*(8), 685–695. https://doi.org/10.1080/01421590903050374

Sawatsky, A. P., Ratelle, J. T., Bonnes, S. L., Egginton, J. S., & Beckman, T. J. (2017). A model of self-directed learning in internal medicine residency: A qualitative study using grounded theory. *BMC Medical Education, 17*(1), 31. https://doi.org/10.1186/s12909-017-0869-4

Shahidullah, J. D., Kettlewell, P. W., Palejwala, M. H., Forman, S. G., Billups, A., Anismatta, S. L., & Madsen, B. (2018). Behavioral health training in pediatric residency programs. *Journal of Developmental and Behavioral Pediatrics, 39*(4), 292–302. https://doi.org/10.1097/DBP.0000000000000548

Shanafelt, T. D., Hasan, O., Dyrbye, L., Sinsky, C., Satele, D., Sloan, J., & West, C. P. (2015). Changes in burnout and satisfaction with work-life balance in physicians and the general US working population between 2011 and 2014. *Mayo Clinic Proceedings, 90*(12), 1600–1613. https://doi.org/10.1016/j.mayocp.2015.08.023

Simpson, D., Marcdante, K., Souza, K. H., Anderson, A., & Holmboe, E. (2018). Job roles of the 2025 medical educator. *Journal of Graduate Medical Education, 10*(3), 243–246.

Taylor, D. C. M., & Hamdy, H. (2013). Adult learning theories: Implications for learning and teaching in medical education: AMEE Guide No. 83. *Medical Teacher, 35*(11), e1561–e1572. https://doi.org/10.3109/0142159X.2013.828153

Thomas, P. A., Kern, D. E., Hughes, M. T., & Chen, B. Y. (Eds.). (2016). *Curriculum development for medical education: A six step approach* (3rd ed.). Baltimore, MD: Johns Hopkins University Press.

van den Eertwegh, V., van Dalen, J., van Dulmen, S., van der Vleuten, C., & Scherpbier, A. (2014). Residents' perceived barriers to communication skills learning: Comparing two medical working contexts in postgraduate training. *Patient Education and Counseling, 95*(1), 91–97. https://doi.org/10.1016/j.pec.2014.01.002

Vogel, M. E., Kirkpatrick, H. A., Collings, A. S., Cederna-Meko, C. L., & Grey, M. J. (2012). Integrated care: Maturing the relationship between psychology and primary care. *Professional Psychology: Research and*

Practice, 43(4), 271–280. https://doi.org/10.1037/a0029204

Ward, W., Zagoloff, A., Rieck, C., & Robiner, W. (2018). Interprofessional education: Opportunities and challenges for psychology. *Journal of Clinical Psychology in Medical Settings, 25*(3), 250–266. https://doi.org/10.1007/s10880-017-9538-3

Zuckerbrot, R. A., Cheung, A., Jensen, P. S., Stein, R. E. K., Laraque, D., & GLAD-PC Steering Group. (2018). Guidelines for adolescent depression in primary care (GLAD-PC): Part I. Practice preparation, identification, assessment, and initial management. *Pediatrics, 141*(3), e20174081. https://doi.org/10.1542/peds.2017-4081

Assessment in Pediatric Psychology Consultation-Liaison

Dana Albright, Teryn Bruni, and William Kronenberger

As a key pillar of psychological practice, assessment in the context of consultation and liaison (CL) psychology must be conducted in a manner that is pragmatic, flexible, and adaptable to meet the unique needs of the healthcare setting. Practices remain grounded in strong assessment principles with the aim of the providing sound clinical services and informed treatment approaches. The purpose of assessment in CL is to characterize behaviors and symptoms, to assist in differentiation of the referral problem definition, to guide intervention, and to facilitate appropriate case disposition, as opposed to providing a more comprehensive evaluation. Most often the primary modality of evaluation consists of a clinical interview focused on the referral concern along with a brief survey of relevant background information. When the decision is made to employ more formal assessment tools, instrument selection is typically targeted to a specific clinical population or presenting clinical concern, e.g., adherence, in order to aid in the differential diagnosis/functional analysis of the presenting problems and the formulation of corresponding targeted recommendations. Acknowledging the more targeted nature of assessment in pediatric CL work, we will review the primary assessment approaches used by the pediatric CL psychologist and explore important considerations in the selection and use of screening and assessment tools, before concluding with an illustrative CL-specific case presentation.

D. Albright (✉) · T. Bruni
Department of Pediatrics, C.S. Mott Children's Hospital, University of Michigan School of Medicine, Ann Arbor, MI, USA
e-mail: maydk@med.umich.edu

W. Kronenberger
Department of Psychiatry, Riley Hospital for Children, Indiana University School of Medicine, Indianapolis, IN, USA

Assessment Modalities in the CL Setting

Clinical Interview

A strong clinical interview is the backbone of consultation assessment practices and should inform the process of instrument selection for a more targeted assessment. The CL clinical interview typically mirrors the format employed in a general child psychology setting including the following: a review of the presenting problem(s) and key symptoms, family functioning, academic functioning, social functioning, mental and physical health history of the patient and family, current mental health status, developmental history, and behavioral functioning. Additionally, CL clinical interviews are often tailored to address health-specific information. Common areas covered include patient and parent/guardian

B. D. Carter, K. A. Kullgren (eds.), *Clinical Handbook of Psychological Consultation in Pediatric Medical Settings*, Issues in Clinical Child Psychology, https://doi.org/10.1007/978-3-030-35598-2_11

knowledge of the child's medical condition, coping/adjustment to new diagnosis, adherence to medical regimen, family involvement in medical care, coping and adherence with procedures/appointments/hospitalizations, and illness impact on school, social, and other activities. Unstructured clinical interviews allow for the highest level of individualization with limited time resources, but semi-structured interview components (e.g., from the KSADS-PL for DSM-5; https://www.pediatricbipolar.pitt.edu/resources/instruments) may also be used to provide consistency.

Screening Measures

Screening instruments (Table 1) are often used to assess populations of patients (e.g., all diabetes patients referred for psychological consultation) for the possible presence or absence of psychological concerns that may impact coping, adjustment, adherence, etc. Universal mental health screening as part of regular standard of care involves surveying the mental health status of all patients seen in a particular setting, e.g., pediatric heart failure clinic (American Academy of Pediatrics, 2009). This type of screening allows for early detection of concerns and has been shown to facilitate more open discussion between patients and their physicians regarding behavioral health concerns (Wissow et al., 2013). Regularly administered screening measures can also be used to distribute psychological resources (e.g., prevention and early intervention efforts) or for identifying patients in need of more intensive services (Kazak, Schneider, Didonato, & Pai, 2015). Alternatively, screening instruments may be used to gain a better understanding of the psychosocial needs of a specific patient and help in the selection of additional, more targeted instruments. Screening measures, due to their brevity and ease of scoring, are particularly suited for most busy medical settings. On the downside, it can be challenging to provide timely follow-up and identify easily accessible resources for those patients identified by screening assessment as having serious and/or emergent mental health concerns (e.g., suicidality, psychosis). Close coordination with other medical team members, e.g., social work, case management,

Table 1 Universal screeners

Name of assessment	Brief description	Age range	Respondent	Administration method
Ages and Stages Questionnaire (ASQ-3; ASQ:SE-2) (Squires, Bricker, & Twombly, 2015; Squires, Twombly, Bricker, & Potter, 2009)	Assesses development in young children	1 month to 5 years	Parent	Rating scale
Parent Evaluation of Developmental Status (PEDS) (Glascoe, 1997)	Developmental-behavioral screening measure for young children that screens for behavioral, social, emotional, mental health, and autism	Birth to age 8	Parent	Rating scale
Patient Health Questionnaire Modified for Teens (PHQ-9) (Kroenke, Spitzer, & Williams, 2001)	Brief assessment of presence and severity of depression symptoms over a 2-week period	11–17	Self	Rating scale
Pediatric Symptom Checklist (PSC) (Gardner et al., 1999)	Psychosocial screener that aims to identify children at risk for emotional, behavioral, and cognitive problems	6–16	Parent Self	Rating scale
Strengths and Difficulties Questionnaire (Goodman, 1997)	Behavioral screening questionnaire measuring positive and negative behavioral attributes	3–16	Parent Teacher	Rating scale

nursing staff, etc., is important to make sure that problems identified through screening initiatives are adequately addressed.

Broadband Behavior Checklists

Broadband behavior checklist measures can be used as screening tools but are also useful for gathering information about a wide range of presenting problem areas. Broadband measures typically assess internalizing and externalizing symptoms, school problems, social behavior, and adaptive functioning using parent, teacher, and/or child report and are particularly useful for cases when multiple adjustment problems are present or when there is uncertainty about the nature of the adjustment problem. Widely used broadband behavior checklists include the Achenbach System of Empirically Based Assessment (ASEBA) measures (including the Child Behavior Checklist (CBCL)) and Behavior Assessment System for Children (BASC) (Table 2). In addition to broadband behavior checklists designed to assess behavior in the home or school environment, the Pediatric Inpatient Behavior Scale (PIBS) is a broadband parent- or nurse-completed behavior checklist measuring child behavior in the pediatric hospital, which can be especially helpful in a CL evaluation (Kronenberger et al., 1997).

Narrowband Behavior Checklists

Narrowband measures focus on a specific domain of behavior or functioning such as aggression, attention, or anxiety, typically identified by using a behavior checklist format. Children referred for CL services often vary widely in their behavioral response to such experiences as physical symptoms, hospitalization, treatments, and their side effects, presenting with behavioral symptoms ranging from angry outbursts to anxiety and withdrawal. Narrowband behavior checklists can be used to identify the nature and severity of specific domains of behavioral symptoms in order to assist in case formulations, suggest additional assessment, guide treatment, and monitor outcomes. They are particularly helpful when the domain of concern is known or suspected (e.g., depression, social adjustment), and additional information is needed about severity or subtypes of symptoms within the domain. There are a plethora of narrowband measures (Table 3), reflecting the large number of symptom domains.

Table 2 Broadband measures

Name of assessment	Brief description	Age range	Respondent	Administration method
Behavior Assessment System for Children (BASC-3) (Reynolds & Kamphaus, 2009)	Assesses a broad range of behavioral and self-perceptions. Includes several subscales and diagnostic scales	2–25	Parent Teacher Self	Rating scale
Child Behavior Checklist (CBCL) (Achenbach, 2009)	Assesses a broad range of behavioral and emotional concerns	1½–18	Parent Teacher Self	Rating scale
Conners Comprehensive Behavior Rating Scales (Conner's CBRS) (Conners, 2008)	Assesses emotional, social, behavior and academic problems across settings	6–18	Parent Teacher Self	Rating scale
Eyberg Child Behavior Inventory (Eyberg & Pincus, 1999)	Assesses frequency of child behavior problems and degree to which behavior is perceived as a problem	2–16	Parent	Rating scale
Pediatric Inpatient Behavioral Scale (PIBS) (Kronenberger, Carter, & Thomas, 1997)	Assesses behavior during hospitalization	6–17	Parent Nurse	Rating scale
Psychological Assessment Tool (PAT) (Kazak et al., 2011)	Assesses the level of psychosocial risk in pediatric health	2½–18	Parent	Rating scale

Table 3 Narrowband and neurocognitive/developmental measures

Name of assessment	Type/domain	Brief description	Age range	Respondent	Administration method
BDEFS (Barkley Deficits in Executive Functioning Scale) (Barkley, 2012)	Executive functioning	Questionnaire measure of executive functioning	6–81	Parent Teacher Self	Rating scale
BRIEF-2 (Behavior Rating Inventory of Executive Function) (Gioia, Isquith, Guy, & Kenworthy, 2015)	Executive functioning	Questionnaire measure of executive functioning	2–90	Parent Teacher Self	Rating scale
CAMPIS (Child-Adult Medical Procedure Interaction Scale) (Blount, Sturges, & Powers, 1990)	Pain	Observer rating scale of pain behaviors and distress during a procedure	Child	Observer	Rating scale
Child Depression Inventory (CDI-2), second edition (Kovacs, 2010)	Psychological adjustment, depression	Assesses the presence of depressive symptoms in children	7–17	Parent Teacher Self Self (short)	Rating scale
Child Observed Coping Scale (COCS) (Kronenberger et al., 1996)	Coping	Parent, teacher, or nurse report of child coping	6–17	Parent teacher nurse	Rating scale
DP-3 (Developmental Profile) (Alpern, 2007)	Development	Questionnaire/interview of development	0–12	Parent	Rating scale or interview
Generalized Anxiety Disorder 2-Item (GAD-2) (Spitzer, Kroenke, Williams, & Löwe, 2006)	Screener, anxiety	A two-item screener to identify risk for anxiety	Lifespan (late childhood—Adolescent recommended)	Self	Rating scale
Gilliam autism rating scale (GARS-3), third edition (Gilliam, 2014)	Autism	Parent perception of the presence of symptoms consistent with a diagnosis of ASD (assesses symptom frequency and severity)	3–22	Parent	Rating scale
K-BIT-2 (Kaufman Brief Intelligence Test) (Kaufman & Kaufman, 2004)	Cognition, IQ	Brief test of verbal and nonverbal cognitive abilities	4–90	Self	Individually administered test
Kidcope (Spirito, Stark, & Williams, 1988)	Coping	Self-report measure of coping	6–17	Self	Rating scale
LEAF (Learning, Executive, and Attention Functioning Scale) (Castellanos, Kronenberger, & Pisoni, 2018)	Executive functioning, learning	Questionnaire measure of executive functioning, learning, and related cognitive skills	3–90	Parent Teacher Self	Rating scale

Modified Checklist for Autism in Toddlers (M-CHAT) (Robins, Fein, & Barton, 1999)	Screener, autism	Brief screening measures to assess risk for autism spectrum disorder among young children	16–30 months	Parent	Rating scale
Multidimensional Anxiety Scale for Children (MASC) (March, 1997)	Psychological adjustment, anxiety	Assesses the presence of symptoms related to variety of anxiety disorders that occur in children	8–19	Parent Teacher Self	Rating scale
OSBD (Observational Scale of Behavioral Distress) (Jay, Ozolins, Elliott, & Caldwell, 1983)	Pain, distress	Observer rating scale of pain behaviors and distress during a procedure	Child	Observer	Rating scale
PPQ (Pediatric Pain Questionnaire) (Varni, Thompson, & Hanson, 1987)	Pain	Parent, child, and clinician questionnaire measure of several dimensions of pain	Child	Self, parent, clinician	Rating scale
Reynolds Adolescent Depression Scale (RADS-2), second edition (Reynolds, 2004)	Psychological adjustment, depression	Assesses the presence and severity of depressive symptoms in children	11–20	Self	Rating scale
Screen of Child Anxiety Related Emotional Disorders (SCARED) (Birmaher et al., 1999)	Psychological adjustment, anxiety	Measures the presence of several anxiety disorder symptoms in children	8–18	Parent Self	Rating scale
Vanderbilt ADHD Diagnostic Scales (Wolraich et al., 2003)	Screener, ADHD	Assesses core symptoms of ADHD including those consistent with inattention and hyperactivity/impulsivity	6–12	Parent Teacher	Rating scale
WASI-II (Wechsler Abbreviated Scale of Intelligence) (Wechsler, 2011)	Cognition, IQ	Brief test of verbal and nonverbal cognitive abilities	6–90	Self	Individually administered test

Functional Behavioral Assessment

Behavioral assessment can also be conducted to identify environmental influences on patient behavior. Functional behavior assessment (FBA) provides a structured method for identifying antecedents and consequences surrounding a specific behavior (Cipani, 2018). FBA can be indirect, where controlling contingencies are identified through semi-structured interviews or questionnaires designed to identify behavior function. Examples of semi-structured interviews have been outlined by Cipani (2018). An example of a structured functional assessment measure is the Questions About Behavior Function questionnaire (QABF; Paclawskyj, Matson, Rush, Smalls, & Vollmer, 2000). The QABF includes 25 items which are each weighted to one of five function categories (i.e., attention, escape, nonsocial, physical, and tangible) to determine the likely function of a specific behavior.

FBA also involves recording antecedents and consequences of a particular behavior in real time as the behavior is occurring. This may be particularly helpful for inpatient settings. Common functions of behavior include access to attention, escape from non-preferred tasks, and access to tangible items. Accurate identification of behavior function should guide intervention approaches. For more information on specific FBA strategies and approaches, readers are encouraged to review Cipani's (2018) guide on conducting functional assessment in educational and mental health settings.

Neurocognitive Measures

Neurocognitive testing refers to assessment of the information processing abilities of the brain, including evaluation of verbal knowledge, fluid reasoning, memory, attention, executive functioning, visual-spatial, and global cognitive abilities (Kronenberger & Pisoni, 2018). Although comprehensive neurocognitive testing is rarely a primary reason for pediatric psychology consultation, brief neurocognitive testing or screening may be important in specific cases. CL-based neurocognitive assessment is most often performed to assess neurocognitive functions relevant to addressing the goals of the consultation or to screen neurocognitive functions in order to identify or understand areas of concern. Neurocognitive assessment by the CL team typically involves the use of questionnaires or brief individually administered tests (Table 3).

Individually administered brief tests of verbal abilities, nonverbal abilities, and academic achievement may also be helpful for describing a child's comprehension or learning abilities, which may affect understanding of their medical condition, communication with healthcare professionals, and/or academic success. Questionnaire measures of neurocognitive functioning are brief, easy to administer, and correspond to real-world behaviors as observed by caregivers. However, questionnaire results overlap only modestly with those from individually administered tests, with correlations typically in the 0.3–0.4 range (Barkley, 2012). When only a brief screening battery is used, interpretation should be limited to the validity and scope of the tests. Referral for more comprehensive follow-up is essential if significant concerns are present or if results will be used to guide long-term interventions or education.

Pain Measures

Assessment of pain symptoms and their effects on functioning are common reasons for consultation in pediatric medical settings, as are questions regarding treatment. Pain increases distress and anxiety and can lead to avoidance and nonadherence. Several types of pain assessment tools exist, as well as tools that provide information about how the child is coping with pain (see Table 3 for specific measures): **Intensity measures** ask the child to rate the level of pain on a numeric or visual scale, such as a 1–10 scale, a location on a line, a color, or pictures of faces. Intensity measures are brief, commonly used, easy to obtain, simple to administer, and well-validated, but are affected by insight, understanding, and motivation of the child. In contrast to self-report intensity measures, **observer report behavior rating scales** measure pain based on behavior characteristic of pain experiences or pain-related distress. Observer report behavior rating scales correspond to actual behavior, provide detailed assessment of behavior, require little child engagement in the assessment process, and have been validated, but they can be complex, time-consuming, and affected by the quality of the rater and familiarity of the rater with child behavior. **Diary measures** are used to record pain experiences over time during multiple pain episodes. Finally, **self-report questionnaires** assess different dimensions of pain including location, intensity, duration, and sensory, emotional, and/or environmental/cultural experience of the pain (Cohen et al., 2008; Turk & Melzack, 2011).

CL psychologists should consider the complex, multidimensional, biopsychosocial nature of pain when developing strategies for assessment. Obtaining both self-report and observer report data can provide a more comprehensive and accurate characterization of pain. Furthermore, assessing not only intensity but also other qualities of pain, as well as the impact of pain on distress, beliefs, behaviors, and social outcomes, will provide formulations to guide specific pain management approaches.

Functional Impairment Measures

Functional impairment, or the extent to which the patient's problem interferes with his or her ability to engage in daily physical, social, occupational, and interpersonal activities (Stein & Jessop, 1990), is an important aspect of a CL assessment. Functional impairment can be summarized with informal clinical assessment or formal measures. As a part of a clinical interview, questions about the child's functioning in areas such as self-care, community skills, health and safety skills, social skills, academic skills, self-direction, and independent living skills can provide valuable information. Structured measures such as the Child Activity Limitations Interview (CALI) (Palermo, Lewandowski, Long, & Burant, 2008), Functional Disabilities Inventory (FDI) (Claar & Walker, 2006), and Functional Status II (R) (Stein & Jessop, 1990) provide information about functional impairment related to having a physical condition. For more comprehensive measurement of adaptive functioning, the Vineland Adaptive Behavior Scales (Sparrow, Cicchetti, & Balla, 2005) has both questionnaire and interview formats.

Progress Monitoring

CL psychologists can play an important role in monitoring patient progress and change over time. While any assessment instrument can be used at 2 points in time to monitor progress or change in a target area, some specific instruments are designed specifically for progress monitoring. These include the BASC-3 Flex Monitor (Reynolds & Kamphaus, 2009), behaviorally anchored rating scales such as the Clinical Global Impressions Scale (CGI; Busner & Targum, 2007; Guy, 1976), or proxy measures, such as the number of school absences per month. Progress monitoring tools should be short and easy to administer and should be sensitive enough to detect small changes over time.

Considerations for Assessment in CL

Time Considerations

Traditional psychological assessments often occur over the course of several hours or even across a few days; however, this is impractical in a CL setting. Brief screening should take no longer than 15 min and be directly relevant to treatment planning and outcome assessment (Groth-Marnat, 2009). When administering one or more psychological tests, the **length of the assessment battery** is a primary consideration. Limiting the assessment to the fewest number of measures and items to answer the specific targeted questions serves not only the psychologist by reducing the associated time demand but also assists other providers consuming the patient data. Patient questionnaire "fatigue" can also occur. Choosing an efficient **administration method** is also an important consideration to manage the time and effort required for assessments. For example, paper-and-pencil or electronic questionnaires completed by caregivers place little burden on the child. Structured interviews with caregivers are more time-consuming and require more clinician involvement but may be helpful. Individually administered performance tests such as ability tests are more demanding on the child (whose performance may be adversely affected by setting factors such as anxiety and distractions of the hospital setting) and are usually used sparingly. Electronically administered (by computer or tablet) tests can be fast and demand relatively little clinician time, but may be more expensive (in terms of equipment, license, and per-use costs) than paper-and-pencil tests that have a one-time cost or that are free to use.

Scoring and interpretation present additional effort and burden. Methods to reduce scoring and interpretation burden are using measures that can be quickly and easily hand-scored and interpreted (Castellanos et al., 2018) and using electronic scoring, particularly if an electronic process was used to acquire the data from the respondent. All rating scales in Tables 1–3 are very easy and brief to administer because of their questionnaire format, and most of them can be quickly scored, reducing burden on the CL team.

Billing

Billing for assessment services is the primary way to obtain resources and time to integrate testing into the CL process, and understanding the options for additional current procedural terminology (CPT codes) is essential to appropriately bill (www.aapc.com). CPT coding differentiates between types of testing (i.e., psychological testing services, neuropsychological testing services, single test result, and automated testing and result) and the specific activities required by a psychologist through the course of an assessment (i.e., administration vs. interpretation). The standard psychological diagnostic interview code (90791) is typically used for the clinical interview portion of the consultation, which is not a time-based code and can be used in isolation or as part of a more comprehensive assessment that also includes testing. CPT codes for testing were revised in January 2019 to more accurately capture activities involved in testing by psychologists (APA Practice Organization, 2018). CL psychologists can also bill for computer scored/automated psychological testing.

As with all consultation services, obtaining payment for psychological testing in the CL context can be challenging. Strategies to maximize payment include preauthorizing with insurance, documenting extensively, and adjusting the use of testing so that it falls within a time/cost range that might be covered by insurance. Nevertheless, external funding is frequently necessary to support the assessment services of a CL team. The American Psychological Association Practice Organization is a helpful tool for updated billing information for psychological assessment.

Follow-Up and Communication with Medical Team

It is important for psychologists to communicate assessment results clearly and efficiently to other psychologists, medical team members, patients, and families. Clinicians embedded in a medical service may be in a position to communicate assessment findings directly to the team and the patient/family within the context of the medical appointment, initiating follow-up recommendations as needed. Some embedded psychologists have the capacity to schedule return visits with patients to follow-up on recommendations, to engage in ongoing progress monitoring, or to conduct further assessment. If follow-up visits are not feasible and results cannot be provided in the context of the medical visit itself, follow-up with patients regarding assessment results can also be done via phone communication, letters, or patient access to select electronic health records. Communication with the medical team regarding assessment results can be accomplished within a variety of modalities including multidisciplinary team meetings, informal ("curbside") consultation in the context of daily work, written letters, and the electronic health record (EHR). Finally, telemedicine or telehealth is a growing service in many medical settings and presents the opportunity for the psychologist to present results to families or medical team members in real time over video, allowing for interactive feedback.

Referrals for Further Evaluations

Referrals for follow-up after consultation services are common for both assessment and treatment. In the realm of assessment, follow-up testing is commonly indicated for children who screen positive for problem/concern areas during the consultation or for children who need more extensive neurocognitive or psychoeducational testing. In the current climate of limited mental health resources in the United States, appropriately screening patients who would benefit from further evaluations is also important to maximize efficient use of resources and avoid unnecessary additional or extensive evaluations. The role of the CL psychologist can be to provide a clear referral question for the evaluation, summarize important background information, and provide results of tests completed during the consultation.

Assessment in Outpatient Contexts

In addition to inpatient CL work, pediatric psychologists perform CL services in different capacities across a wide array of multidisciplinary outpatient clinics. These include integrated primary care settings as well as programs addressing specific chronic illness management (e.g., pain, transplant, etc.). Specific clinics present with unique assessment needs, and the time and scope of assessment will depend on the nature of the psychologist's role in a particular clinic. Considerations for psychological testing are similar in outpatient CL settings to those in inpatient CL settings, as described earlier in the chapter.

Similar to multidisciplinary settings, assessment practices in primary care are shaped by the needs of the setting, which demand brief, problem-focused assessment that can be easily communicated to physicians and patients (Cummings, O'Donohue, & Cummings, 2009). The goal of assessment in primary care is to identify specific presenting concerns and provide evidence-based treatment options, ideally using screening tools and brief measures. Thus, the specific measures used in primary care are similar to those used by psychologists who work within outpatient multidisciplinary teams. Psychologists in primary care may also participate in more universal screening initiatives, such as prevention, early detection, and early intervention, as well as functional assessment methods to directly inform behavioral recommendations.

Case Illustration of CL Assessment

Tom was a 15-year-old with spina bifida referred to the inpatient CL service during a hospitalization for treatment of multiple severe pressure ulcers, requiring surgical debridement, wound care, and antibiotic treatment (specific characteristics of the case have been altered for confidentiality and privacy). He was referred to the pediatric psychology CL service because of concerns that poor hygiene, negative attitude, and insufficient adherence to mobility/activity recommendations had contributed to the development of the pressure ulcers. Medical history included myelomeningocele (L4 level) repaired and shunted at birth, with no significant complications, bleeds, or infections. Tom used a wheelchair to ambulate and had no sensation or movement in the lower extremities. He was followed as an outpatient in the spina bifida clinic, where healthcare personnel had been working with him on reducing weight and increasing activity. He was educated at home in an online program and was socially isolated with the exception of contact over social media and online video games. He described his typical activities and interests as consisting of using the computer and playing video games, with no regular exercise. He lived with his mother and had no siblings. Mother worked full time on weekdays and part time on evenings and weekends, and financial resources were very limited. Prior to the consultation, Tom had no prior contact with mental health professionals other than sporadic meetings with medical social workers through the spina bifida clinic and some assessment and informal meetings with a school psychologist.

Both nursing and the attending team expressed concerns that Tom seemed detached, unmotivated, and possibly depressed. Tom's physician and nurses in the spina bifida clinic also noted that he seemed to have difficulty focusing and understanding educational materials and interactions about the importance of activity and hygiene for good health. Questions were raised about his intelligence, attention, and ability to understand how inactivity and poor hygiene could contribute to pressure ulcers. There was also speculation about whether his disengagement and avoidance of school were reflective of fundamental neurocognitive or learning delays.

As a part of the CL evaluation, Tom was administered assessment instruments to better understand his behavioral, emotional, and neurocognitive functioning. On the PIBS completed separately by two nurses, Tom received raw scores of 1.50 and 1.67 on the withdrawal scale (negative mood and social withdrawal), exceeding 1 SD above the mean of a hospitalized pediatric sample; no other PIBS subscale was elevated, but the positive sociability score of 0.25 by both nurses was well below average. A BASC-2 (Reynolds & Kamphaus, 2004) completed by mother produced T-score elevations >65 for depression, somatization, and withdrawal and T-scores of <35 for social skills and leadership. On the self-report BASC-2, Tom elevated the somatization and depression subscales. On the K-BIT-2, Tom's verbal score of 102 was significantly greater than his nonverbal score of 79. Tom's mother completed a LEAF scale, producing clinical elevations of the following subscales: comprehension and conceptual learning, processing speed, visual-spatial organization, sustained sequential processing, working memory, novel problem-solving, mathematics skills, and written expression skills.

In the context of information obtained from interview, background information, and behavior observations, results of the PIBS and BASC-2 were consistent with the presence of moderate to severe depressive symptoms and social skills delays with significant social isolation. Results of neurocognitive screening tests showed average verbal knowledge and fund of information but significantly delayed nonverbal reasoning. Mother's LEAF was consistent with K-BIT-2 nonverbal testing results indicating delayed concept formation, visual-spatial, and novel problem-solving skills. LEAF results also suggested delays in the executive functioning domains of working memory, planning, and sustained mental effort. Further evaluation of math and written expression was suggested by LEAF results. These neurocognitive screening results overlap with deficits in assembled cognitive processes (organizing and integrating details of information to construct meaningful wholes), which have been identified as neurocognitive risks for some children with spina bifida (Fletcher & Dennis, 2010).

Based on evaluation findings, the CL team identified depressive symptoms (particularly mood, activity level, and social withdrawal), nonverbal concept formation and organization, and delays in some domains of executive functioning (particularly working memory) as key psychological problems and targets for further assessment and intervention. Brief cognitive-behavioral therapy, an activity schedule, use of accommodations and assistive devices to address concept formation and executive functioning delays (repetition learning, use of mnemonic strategies to enhance memory, conceptual explanations at a level consistent with ability, use of prominent pictures and schedules as reminders), and a behavior plan were put in place during hospitalization to address depressive symptoms, reduce withdrawal, and improve adherence. Social-environmental stresses and challenges, including family and school issues, were also evaluated and addressed. Tom's progress during hospitalization was measured with completion of the PIBS scale by a nurse and mother every 2–3 days, showing consistent improvement in withdrawal and positive sociability scores, although his oppositional-noncompliant score increased during the first 2–3 days of the intervention. At discharge, referrals were made to the child neuropsychology service for more extensive evaluation and follow-up with the school system and to a pediatric psychologist for outpatient treatment.

References

Achenbach, T. M. (2009). *The Achenbach system of empirically based assessment (ASEBA): Development, findings, theory, and applications*. Burlington, VT: University of Vermont Research Center for Children, Youth, & Families.

Alpern, G. D. (2007). *Developmental profile-3*. Torrance, CA: Western Publishing Services.

American Academy of Pediatrics Task Force on Mental Health. (2009). Policy statement, the future of pediatrics: Mental health competencies for the care of children and adolescents in primary care settings. *Pediatrics, 124*, 410–421.

APA Practice Organization. (2018). https://www.apapracticecentral.org/reimbursement

Barkley, R. A. (2012). *Barkley deficits in executive functioning scale—Children and adolescents (BDEFS-CA)*. New York, NY: Guilford Press.

Birmaher, B., Brent, D. A., Chiappetta, L., Bridge, J., Monga, S., & Baugher, M. (1999). Psychometric properties of the screen for child anxiety related emotional disorders (SCARED): A replication study. *Journal of the American Academy of Child and Adolescent Psychiatry, 38*, 1230–1236.

Blount, R. L., Sturges, J. W., & Powers, S. W. (1990). Analysis of child and adult behavioral variations by phase of medical procedure. *Behavior Therapy, 21*(1), 33–48.

Briggs-Gowan, M. J., & Carter, A. S. (2002). *Brief-infant toddler social and emotional assessment (BITSEA): Manual. Version 2.0*. New Haven, CT: Yale University.

Busner, J., & Targum, S. D. (2007). The clinical global impressions scale: Applying a research tool in clinical practice. *Psychiatry, 4*(7), 28–37.

Castellanos, I., Kronenberger, W. G., & Pisoni, D. B. (2018). Questionnaire-based assessment of executive functioning: Psychometrics. *Applied Neuropsychology: Child, 7*(2), 93–109. https://doi.org/10.1080/21622965.2016.1248557

Cipani, E. (2018). *Functional behavioral assessment, diagnosis, and treatment: A complete system for education and mental health settings* (3rd ed.). New York, NY: Springer Publishing Company.

Claar, R. L., & Walker, L. S. (2006). Functional assessment of pediatric pain patients: Psychometric properties of the functional disability inventory. *Pain, 121*(1–2), 77–84.

Cohen, L. L., Lemanek, K., Blount, R. L., Dahlquist, L. M., Lim, C. S., Palermo, T. M., … Weiss, K. E. (2008). Evidence-based assessment of pediatric pain. *Journal of Pediatric Psychology, 33*(9), 939–955.

Conners, C. K. (2008). *Conners comprehensive behavior rating scales (Conners CBRS)*. North Tonawanda, NY: Multi-Health Systems (MHS).

Cummings, N. A., O'Donohue, W. T., & Cummings, J. L. (2009). The financial dimension of integrated behavioral/primary care. *Journal of Clinical Psychology in Medical Settings, 16*(1), 31–39.

Eyberg, S., & Pincus, D. (1999). *Eyberg Child Behavior Inventory & Sutter-Eyberg Student Behavior Inventory-Revised: Professional manual*. Odessa, FL: Psychological Assessment Resources.

Fletcher, J. M., & Dennis, M. (2010). Spina bifida and hydrocephalus. Pediatric neuropsychology: Research, theory, and practice, 2, 3–25.

Gardner, W., Murphy, M., Childs, G., Kelleher, K., Pagano, M., Jellinek, M., … Chiappetta, L. (1999). The PSC-17: A brief pediatric symptom checklist with psychosocial problem subscales. A report from PROS and ASPN. *Ambulatory Child Health, 5*(3), 225–236.

Gilliam, J. E. (2014). *Gilliam autism rating scale: GARS 2*. Austin, TX: Pro-ed.

Gioia, G. A., Isquith, P. K., Guy, S. C., & Kenworthy, L. (2015). *Behavior rating inventory of executive function-2 manual*. Lutz, FL: Psychological Assessment Resources.

Glascoe, F. P. (1997). *Parents' evaluation of developmental status (PEDS)*. Nashville, TN: Ellsworth & Vandermeer Press, Ltd..

Goodman, R. (1997). The strengths and difficulties questionnaire: A research note. *Journal of Child Psychology and Psychiatry, 38*, 581–586.

Groth-Marnat, G. (2009). *Handbook of psychological assessment*. Hoboken, NJ: Wiley.

Guy, W. (1976). *ECDEU assessment manual for psychopharmacology* (pp. 534–537). Rockville, MD: US Department of Health, and Welfare.

Jay, S. M., Ozolins, M., Elliott, C. H., & Caldwell, S. (1983). Assessment of children's distress during painful medical procedures. *Health Psychology, 2*(2), 133–147. https://doi.org/10.1037/0278-6133.2.2.133

Kaufman, A. S., & Kaufman, N. L. (2004). *Kaufman brief intelligence test* (2nd ed.). Minneapolis, MN: NCS Pearson.

Kazak, A. E., Barakat, L. P., Ditaranto, S., Biros, D., Hwang, W. T., Beele, D., … Reilly, A. (2011). Screening for psychosocial risk at cancer diagnosis: The psychosocial assessment Tool (PAT). *Journal of the Pediatric Hematology Oncology, 33*, 289–294.

Kazak, A. E., Schneider, S., Didonato, S., & Pai, A. L. (2015). Family psychosocial risk screening guided by the pediatric psychosocial preventative health model (PPPHM) using the psychosocial assessment tool (PAT). *Acta Oncologica, 54*(5), 574–580.

Kovacs, M. (2010). *Children's depression inventory 2 (CDI 2)*. North Tonawanda, NY: Multi-Health Systems (MHS).

Kroenke, K., Spitzer, R. L., & Williams, J. B. (2001). The PHQ-9: Validity of a brief depression severity measure. *Journal of General Internal Medicine, 16*(9), 606–613.

Kronenberger, W. G., Carter, B. D., Stewart, J., Morrow, C., Martin, K., Gowan, D., & Sender, L. (1996). Psychological adjustment of children in the pretransplant phase of bone marrow transplantation: Relationships with parent distress, parent stress, and child coping. *Journal of Clinical Psychology in Medical Settings, 3*(4), 319–335. https://doi.org/10.1007/BF01994017

Kronenberger, W. G., Carter, B. D., & Thomas, D. (1997). Assessment of behavior problems in pediatric inpatient settings: Development of the pediatric inpatient behavior scale. *Children's Health Care, 26*(4), 211–232. https://doi.org/10.1207/s15326888chc2604_1

Kronenberger, W. G., & Pisoni, D. B. (2018). Neurocognitive functioning in deaf children with cochlear implants. In H. Knoors & M. Marschark (Eds.), *Evidence-based practices in deaf education*. London, UK: Oxford University Press.

March, J. S. (1997). *Manual for the multidimensional anxiety scale for children (MASC)*. Toronto, ON: Multi-Health Systems.

Paclawskyj, T. R., Matson, J. L., Rush, K. S., Smalls, Y., & Vollmer, T. R. (2000). Questions about behavioral function (QABF): A behavioral checklist for functional assessment of aberrant behavior. *Research in Developmental Disabilities, 21*(3), 223–229.

Palermo, T. M., Lewandowski, A. S., Long, A. C., & Burant, C. J. (2008). Validation of a self-report questionnaire version of the child activity limitations interview (CALI): The CALI-21. *Pain, 139*(3), 644–652.

Reynolds, C. R., & Kamphaus, R. W. (2009). *Behavior assessment system for children (BASC-2): Progress monitor (PM)* (2nd ed.). Bloomington, MN: Pearson.

Reynolds, W. M. (2004). The Reynolds Adolescent Depression Scale-Second Edition (RADS-2). In M. J. Hilsenroth & D. L. Segal (Eds.), Comprehensive handbook of psychological assessment, Vol. 2. Personality assessment (p. 224–236). John Wiley & Sons Inc.

Roberts, M. C., Mitchell, M. C., & McNeal, R. (2003). The Evolving Field of Pediatric Psychology: Critical Issues and Future Challenges. In M. C. Roberts (Ed.), Handbook of pediatric psychology (p. 3–18). The Guilford Press.

Robins, D. L., Fein, D., & Barton, M. (1999). *The modified checklist for autism in toddlers (M-CHAT)*. Self-published.

Sparrow, S. S., Cicchetti, D. V., & Balla, D. A. (2005). *Vineland adaptive behavior scales: Survey forms manual* (2nd ed.). Circle Pines, MN: AGS Publishing.

Spirito, A., Stark, L. J., & Williams, C. (1988). Development of a brief coping checklist for use with pediatric populations. *Journal of Pediatric Psychology, 13*(4), 555–574. https://doi.org/10.1093/jpepsy/13.4.555

Spitzer, R. L., Kroenke, K., Williams, J. B., & Löwe, B. (2006). A brief measure for assessing generalized anxiety disorder: The GAD-7. *Archives of Internal Medicine, 166*(10), 1092–1097.

Squires, J., Bricker, D., & Twombly, E. (2015). *Ages and stages questionnaires: Social-emotional (ASQ:SE-2): A parent-completed child monitoring system for social-emotional behaviors*. Baltimore, MD: Paul H. Brookes Publishing.

Squires, J., Twombly, E., Bricker, D., & Potter, L. (2009). *Ages and stages questionnaires, User's guide* (3rd ed.). Baltimore, MD: Paul H. Brookes Publishing.

Stein, R. E., & Jessop, D. J. (1990). Functional status II (R): A measure of child health status. *Medical Care, 28*, 1041–1055.

Turk, D. C., & Melzack, R. (2011). *Handbook of pain assessment* (3rd ed.). New York, NY: Guilford Press.

Varni, J. W., Thompson, K. L., & Hanson, V. (1987). The Varni/Thompson pediatric pain questionnaire: I. Chronic musculoskeletal pain in juvenile rheumatoid arthritis. *Pain, 28*(1), 27–38. https://doi.org/10.1016/0304-3959(87)91056-6

Wechsler, D. (2011). *Wechsler abbreviated scale of intelligence (WASI-II)* (2nd ed.). San Antonio, TX: Pearson.

Wissow, L. S., Brown, J., Fothergill, K. E., Gadomski, A., Hacker, K., Salmon, P., & Zelkowitz, R. (2013). Universal mental health screening in pediatric primary care: A systematic review. *Journal of the American Academy of Child & Adolescent Psychiatry, 52*(11), 1134–1147.

Wolraich, M. L., Lambert, W., Doffing, M. A., Bickman, L., Simmons, T., & Worley, K. (2003). Psychometric properties of the Vanderbilt ADHD diagnostic parent rating scale in a referred population. *Journal of Pediatric Psychology, 28*(8), 559–568.

Part II

Clinical Conditions and Interventions

The Problem of Pain: Acute Pain and Procedures

Nicole E. MacKenzie, Perri R. Tutelman, and Christine T. Chambers

Introduction

Case Study—Charlotte

Charlotte is an 8-year-old girl diagnosed with sickle cell disease, a blood disorder where hemoglobin cells become impaired in their ability to transport oxygen throughout the body. Determining this diagnosis involved many blood tests which Charlotte met with intense fear, often crying and having tantrums, resulting in many hospital staff being present in order for the blood work to be completed. With her treatment plan of monthly blood transfusions set to begin, which involves the insertion of intravenous (IV) catheters, Charlotte's family and healthcare team are extremely concerned about how she will handle these procedures and are unsure of how they will manage her strong reactions. Her parents have not yet told her about her treatments for fear that she will become very distressed.

Acute pain is a common childhood experience. From routine procedures (e.g., venipuncture) to specialized medical treatments (e.g., lumbar punctures, surgery), acute pain in children represents a prevalent health issue. Research has shown that in a typical pediatric hospital setting, more than 75% of pediatric inpatients undergo at least one painful procedure (an average number of 6.3 painful procedures a day; Stevens et al., 2011), and only one-third to half of these children receive any form of pain management (Friedrichsdorf et al., 2015).

Proper management of children's acute pain is critical to consider from a biopsychosocial perspective, as children's pain experiences can be influenced by biological, psychological, and social factors. First, repeated exposure to acute pain can impact children's thoughts, feelings, and reactivity to pain in the short and long term. For example, painful procedures are not only remembered negatively in the future, but are also related to higher levels of distress during future procedures which can lead to a learned fear toward medical procedures (Noel, Pavlova, McCallum, & Vinall, 2017). Second, there are physiological implications, including increased inflammation in the brain and disrupted somato-

N. E. MacKenzie · P. R. Tutelman
Department of Psychology and Neuroscience, Dalhousie University, Halifax, NS, Canada

Centre for Pediatric Pain Research, IWK Health Centre, Halifax, NS, Canada

C. T. Chambers (✉)
Department of Psychology and Neuroscience, Dalhousie University, Halifax, NS, Canada

Centre for Pediatric Pain Research, IWK Health Centre, Halifax, NS, Canada

Department of Pediatrics, Dalhousie University, Halifax, NS, Canada
e-mail: Christine.Chambers@Dal.Ca

B. D. Carter, K. A. Kullgren (eds.), *Clinical Handbook of Psychological Consultation in Pediatric Medical Settings*, Issues in Clinical Child Psychology, https://doi.org/10.1007/978-3-030-35598-2_12

sensory cortex functioning (Fitzgerald & Walker, 2009). Third, parents and children's pain catastrophizing can also influence the distress and pain a child may experience during their painful procedure (Birnie, Chambers, Chorney, Fernandez, & McGrath, 2016).

Overall, there are several facets to consider when working to manage acute pain during medical procedures, as well as several methods for managing it. The objective of this chapter is to summarize best practices in pediatric psychology consultations for acute pain management including evidence-based approaches to effective pain assessment and management. Further, this chapter outlines how to make assessment and treatment decisions in tandem with child and treatment factors throughout the course of painful medical treatment and procedures.

Navigating Referrals for Acute Pain Management

Referrals to psychology for children's pain management have become an increasingly common. Top reasons for a referral to psychology in hospitals include anxiety related to procedural pain (Piazza-Waggoner, Roddenberry, Yeomans-Maldonado, Noll, & Ernst, 2013) which can include factors related to preparation for medical procedures like venipuncture, intravenous line start, lumbar puncture, port access, and surgical procedures. Another common reason for referral is to improve both child and parent coping and communication skills during painful procedures and to provide education around pain management strategies. Through the use of these strategies, developed in tandem with the psychologist and family, the ultimate goal is to reduce child and family stress and ultimately improve post-procedure outcomes.

Key Aspects of the Referral

There are several key biopsychosocial factors which must be carefully considered when reviewing the referral to psychology for pediatric procedural pain management. The type of information which is presented and required may differ across clinical settings. These common referral components are described in further detail:

Child factors. Consideration of the child's age is critical in guiding the selection of appropriate pain assessment tools and pain interventions (see sections below for more detailed information), as interventions can have varying impact levels on different age groups (Birnie et al., 2014). As well, children's past medical experiences can influence the way in which the child copes with the procedure depending on the memory of the experience (Noel, Pavlova, et al., 2017). Understanding of these past experiences could be obtained through consulting with the child, family, or relevant healthcare providers.

Family factors. The family members present during the child's medical procedure, as well as their own past experiences with needles, can impact the child's experience. This includes whether both parents or a single parent will be present or if any siblings will attend. It could be helpful to encourage parents to consider their potential reactions to their child's painful medical procedure, such as parent catastrophizing about their child's pain which can influence the distress and pain a child may experience (Birnie et al., 2016). Cultural factors around communication or customs may also need to be considered, as these factors can influence how children express their pain, both verbally and nonverbally, as well as the caregiver's recognition and response to their child's pain (Kristjansdottir et al., 2018).

Primary and comorbid medical conditions. It is important to be aware of the primary medical condition being treated, as well as comorbid conditions, including other chronic or acute illnesses, developmental or intellectual disorders, and other relevant psychological concerns including trauma, abuse, depression, anxiety, disordered eating, and psychotic disorders. For example, a child with a visual-motor impairment would likely not benefit from a virtual reality intervention.

Additionally, knowledge of other diagnoses may call for further investigation in symptoms or treatments which could potentially impact their pain sensitivity.

Pain history. Consider whether this child has an extensive or relatively unremarkable history of pain, remembering to ask about both chronic and procedural pain. If there is a history of pain, it would be of value to know what level of pain tolerance the child has, as well as whether there are pain management strategies which have been effective or ineffective in the past. Past experiences with pain may not only influence the child's sensitivity to pain but also impact the efficacy of pain treatment methods and strategies (Taddio et al., 2009). For example, as children are repeatedly exposed to painful medical procedures with inadequate pain management, their experience of pain becomes more intense with time and interventions become less effective over time.

Treatment plan/planned procedures. When creating a pain management plan, it is important to know what the medical treatment plan is and what types of painful procedures it will include. As well, it could be helpful to know how painful the procedures themselves are, how much pain should be expected post-procedure, and what the expected side effects of the treatment are. It is important to remember that the conceptualization of a medical procedure as major or minor is subjective and therefore the amount of pain may not necessarily reflect the size of the procedure. Additionally, it is important to know what medications the child is taking and how might this affect the child's mental state. These factors are important to be aware of as pharmacological treatment could impact the efficacy of pain management strategies.

Organizational context. The setting in which the psychologist is seeing the child has the potential to impact the type of pain management plan which can be implemented. Settings in which psychologists may be seeing patients include inpatient units (for short- or long-term stays), consultation-liaison settings, private practice, or primary care clinics (among others). The length of time a psychologist is able to see a client for can range from a single consult to a longer-term follow-up period, and the amount of time available to work with clients can be directly impacted by this time frame. Thus, the type of assessment method selection as well as the intervention method should be selected in consideration of the amount of time available to work with the child. Further, the resources available to the family to engage psychological services may also need to be taken into account and therefore may dictate the assessment and intervention selected.

Evaluation and Assessment for Procedural Pain Management

A comprehensive assessment of the child from a biopsychosocial perspective is necessary in order to develop a tailored pain management plan. Key aspects of this assessment include consideration of the following factors (adapted from Guite, Logan, Simons, Blood, & Kerns, 2011):

Expectations of the child, family, and medical team

- What do the child, family, and medical team aim to achieve?
- Are these goals realistic?
- What goals are common and which conflict?

Child anticipatory anxiety toward painful procedures

- Assess trait and state anxiety level.
- Assess the child's level of fear and distress related to their medical procedures.
- If there are needles involved in the procedures, identify if the child experiences needle phobia and fear of needle pain through self-report and observation.
- Assess the child's attitudes and concerns related to the upcoming procedure(s).

Parent understanding of their child's pain experience

- Assess how each parent typically reacts before, during, and after their child's medical procedures (consider previous vaccination experiences where there is no medical history).
- Assess each parent's attitudes and concerns related to the upcoming procedure(s).
- Identify parent strengths in assisting with pain management and coaching of their child.

Gauging parent willingness to be involved in pain management

Potential questions to gauge the extent to which parents may want to be involved include:

- How comfortable are parents in helping to manage their child's pain during procedures?
- What kind of a role do parents see for themselves in their child's pain management?
- What are some ways parents have helped their child cope with painful procedures?
- Are parents interested in learning strategies they can use to manage their child's pain?

Validated tools could also be considered, where appropriate, to assess constructs like parent catastrophizing, including the Pain Catastrophizing Scale for Parents [PCS-P] (Goubert, Eccleston, Vervoort, Jordan, & Crombez, 2006). Brief tools like this could be administered as part of the intake and consultation process.

Assessing Acute Pain in Children

The psychologist wanted to know more about Charlotte's experiences with painful procedures in order to properly prepare her for IV catheter insertion. Prior to her most recent blood work, the psychologist had Charlotte complete the State-Trait Anxiety Inventory for Children (State form) to assess for anxiety-related symptoms and her state anxiety levels. Post blood work, Charlotte completed Faces Pain Scale—Revised to assess the amount of pain she experienced. The psychologist also had Charlotte's parents describe a typical blood work procedure, explaining what happens before, during, and after the procedure to understand the full scope of how Charlotte typically reacts to needles and how she might react during an IV insertion. With both sources of information, the psychologist was able to begin to form a comprehensive assessment of sources of distress and reactions during future IV insertion procedures.

Proper pain assessment is the first step to proper pain management. There are a number of validated methods to assess acute pain in infants, children, and adolescents (see Table 1). The setting may dictate the type of assessment the psychologist is able to conduct given time and resource availability and therefore the number of items included in each measure is outlined within this table to facilitate the decision-making process for psychologists regarding selection of an assessment method. As well, some forms have been developed for research purposes and are therefore lengthy. When selecting assessment tools, it is important to account for time resources available to carry out the desired assessment.

Pain is inherently a subjective phenomenon, and thus, child self-reported pain should be obtained whenever possible. A recent study systematically reviewed the literature on self-reported pain intensity measures for children (Birnie, Hundert, Lalloo, Nguyen, & Stinson, 2019) and found over 60 published measures. Based on the current research base, three measures were strongly recommended for the self-report of children's acute pain intensity: the Numerical Rating Scale (NRS), Faces Pain Scale—Revised (FPS-R), and Color Analogue Scale (CAS).

One of the most common ways to assess pain in children is through an 11-point Numerical Rating Scale (NRS), which asks children to rate their pain on a scale of 0–10, either verbally or visually. Research on children's descriptors of pain supports the use of the phrase "no hurt" for the lower anchor and "the worst hurt you could ever imagine" as the top anchor for school-aged children (Young et al., 2017). The NRS is considered a "well-established measure"

Table 1 Assessment tools

Developmental category	Administration style	Assessment tools
Infancy (less than 1 year)	Observation	Premature Infant Pain Profile [PIPP] (Stevens, Johnston, Petryshen, & Taddio, 1996) 7 items *∗For preterm and term infants <2 months of age*
	Observation	The Revised Face, Legs, Activity, Crying, and Consolability [r-FLACC] Scale (Malviya, Voepel-Lewis, Burke, Merkel, & Tait, 2006) *∗For infants <2 months of age* 30 items
	Observation	Non-communicating Child's Pain Checklist—Revised [NCCPC-R] (Breau Lynn, Finley, McGrath, & Camfield, 2002) 30 items
	Proxy report	Parent report
Early childhood (1–6 years)	Self report	The Faces Pain Scale—Revised [FPS-R] (Hicks, von Baeyer, Spafford, van Korlaar, & Goodenough, 2001) Single rating
	Self report	The Pieces of Hurt Tool (Hester, 1979) Single rating
	Observation	Non-communicating Child's Pain Checklist—Revised [NCCPC-R] (Breau Lynn et al., 2002) 30 items
	Observation	Child Facial Coding System [CFCS] (Gilbert et al., 1999) 11 items
	Observation	Observational Scale of Behavioral Distress—Revised [OSBD-R] (Elliott, Jay, & Woody, 1987) 11 items
	Observation	The Revised Face, Legs, Activity, Crying, and Consolability [r-FLACC] Scale (Malviya et al., 2006) 30 items
	Proxy report	Parent report
School-aged to adolescence (7–18 years)	Self report	Verbal Numeric Rating Scale [VNRS] (Young, Carter, & von Baeyer, 2017) Single rating
	Self report	The Faces Pain Scale—Revised [FPS-R] (Hicks et al., 2001) Single rating
	Self report	Colored Analogue Scale [CAS] (McGrath et al., 1996) Single rating
	Self report	Visual Analogue Scale Single rating
	Self report	Fear of Pain Questionnaire—Short Form [FPQ-SF] (Asmundson, Bovell, Carleton, & McWilliams, 2008) 30 items
	Observation	Observational Scale of Behavioral Distress—Revised [OSBD-R] (Elliott et al., 1987) 11 items
	Observation	Procedure Behavior Checklist [PBCL] (LeBaron & Zeltzer, 1984) 8 items
	Observation	Child-Adult Medical Procedure Interaction Scale—Revised [CAMPIS-R] (Blount et al., 1997) 6 items
	Observation	Parents' Postoperative Pain Measure [PPPM] (Chambers, Reid, McGrath, & Finley, 1996) 15 items
	Proxy report	Parent report

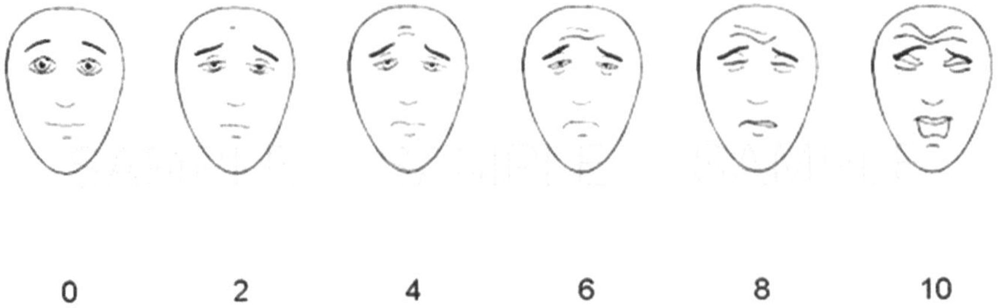

Fig. 1 The FPS-R allows children to identify their pain level using faces, reducing cognitive demand

for self-reported pain intensity in children as young as 6 years of age (Birnie, Noel, Chambers, Uman, & Parker, 2018).

The FPS-R is a faces scale that asks children to match their level of hurt to one of the six faces presented that range from "no pain" to "very much pain" (see Fig. 1). The FPS-R is a desirable self-report pain tool for use with children given that it reduces the cognitive demands of numerical and spatial competency, as seen in the NRS. The FPS-R is validated for use in children as young as 7 years of age and has instructions available in over 50 different languages. The FPS-R can be freely downloaded for clinical use at www.iasp-pain.org/fpsr. This tool is very brief, simple to administer, and appropriate for children and adolescents, making it appropriate for use in most settings psychologists may be working in.

The CAS (McGrath et al., 1996) resembles a thermometer with gradations in color, area, and length. Children are asked to slide a marker along the scale to the position that indicates the intensity of their pain. The CAS is recommended to assess self-reported acute pain in children ages 8 years and older.

While self-report is the gold standard for assessment, it may not always be possible due to the child's age, developmental level, or state of consciousness. When a child's self-report is not available, it can be estimated by proxy report (e.g., parent report) or through validated observational measures. A summary of recommended tools for the assessment of acute pain in children can be found in the table below.

When using these measures during a first appointment with a family, it can also be helpful to interview the patient and their parents to ask about past procedural pain experiences. When meeting with families for an initial appointment, there are several topics which could be covered during discussion (see Table 2 for example topics). Not only is the interview an opportunity to begin establishing rapport with families, but these topics also allow the psychologist to keep the interview focused while also ensuring sufficient breadth of information is obtained. The information obtained through the interview can then be bolstered by the information collected through other measures which can provide quantitative data which can be tracked and assessed over time to look for evidence of change.

Table 2 Semi-structured interview topics

Initial meeting with parents and patient
• Explain the role of the psychologist • Current coping strategies • Previous interventions and outcomes, including medical, psychological, behavioral
Semi-structured interview with patients
• Level of distress during procedures • Perception of control • Goals for treatment and support
Semi-structured interview with parents
• Patient's medical and developmental history • Family functioning (e.g., constellation, functioning, impact of child's pain) • Emotional concerns
Behavioral observations
• Parent responses to pain behaviors during procedures • Parent and patient response to prior interventions • General observations of parent and patient interactions during the interview

Note. Adapted from Cunningham and Banez (2006)

Strategies for Acute Procedural Pain Management

As with the selection of assessment tools, it is essential to select the intervention carefully while considering the following key points:

Environmental factors
- Consider features of the clinic or hospital environment, including:
  The number of people in the room during the procedure
  Whether the space is noisy or quiet
- Where choices are possible, ask patients what their preferences are for the environment.

Parent and family factors
- Parent nervousness and catastrophizing—coach parents in working through their nerves so they do not project onto their child (Birnie et al., 2016).
- Discourage parents' use of problem-focused language including the following:
  "I'm sorry you have to do this," "It'll be over soon," or "It'll be quick."
- Encourage positive and specific phrases like "you did a great job taking deep breaths."
- Sibling influences—interactions with siblings which are pain focused may actually result in more painful experiences for the child undergoing the procedure (Schinkel, Chambers, Corkum, & Jacques, 2018).

Strategies for Managing Acute Pain

Table 3 presents evidence-based strategies for the management of a range of painful procedures from a biopsychosocial perspective. These strategies are based on a recent Cochrane review which identified the most effective pain management strategies for reducing needle pain and distress in children (Birnie et al., 2018) and a clinical practice guideline for healthcare providers (Taddio et al., 2015). It is strongly encouraged that these strategies be used in tandem where possible as physical (e.g., positioning) and pharmacological (e.g., analgesic creams) strategies can complement psychological interventions (Birnie et al., 2018). Therefore, when administering any of these strategies, collaboration with nurses and other healthcare providers (e.g., nurses, physicians, pharmacists, child life specialists) is important in ensuring these strategies can be applied effectively and support can be provided with nonpsychological strategies, in terms of resources (e.g., directing parents to where they can purchase analgesic cream).

When selecting an appropriate pain management strategy, there are some key considerations to keep in mind.

Child Factors
- Preferences for activities during procedures (consider what resources are available in your specific setting).
- Provide choice of strategies to maintain engagement and support.

Procedure-Related Factors
- Can the strategies offered be accommodated given the procedure and environment?
- Is there enough room to accommodate the child, staff, psychologist, and parents?
- Are there any restrictions regarding the type of equipment that can enter the procedure room?

Organizational Considerations
- When selecting an appropriate intervention strategy, the resources available should be taken into account. Interventions which require more planning and longer time commitments may not be appropriate when the psychologist is providing a single consultation or working with the family during a single procedure. More brief interventions would be more appropriate in these settings, such as distraction or physical interventions. Alternatively, in private practice or inpatient settings where psychologists are able to follow patients for longer periods of time, more intensive and complex psychological interventions would be more appropriate. Table 3 highlights these interventions and considerations.

In collaboration with Charlotte's parents, the psychologist developed a pain management plan in order to help Charlotte cope with her upcom-

Table 3 Interventions

Type of intervention	Examples	Considerations
Distraction	*Active distraction* • Parent distraction • Playing with a toy • Reading a story • Distraction cards • Interactive handheld games *Passive distraction* • Watching a movie or video • Listening to music • Listening to a story	For patients who are easily overstimulated, consider selecting a more passive (or less stimulating) distraction technique. Note that some children may prefer to watch the injection/procedure and may not want to be distracted. These strategies are appropriate in most medical settings
Combined CBT	Combinations of two or more cognitive and behavioral strategies: • Distraction • Modeling and rehearsal • Breathing • Suggested relaxation • Guided imagery (see Appendix for script) • Positive coping statements • Cognitive restructuring	Consider the ability of the patient to engage in abstract thought when selecting CBT strategies. Strategies such as suggested relaxation, guided imagery, and cognitive restructuring may be best used in settings where the client has time to meet with a psychologist prior to a procedure in order to be prepared to engage with these strategies
Hypnosis	• Direct hypnosis (e.g., analgesic) • Indirect, therapist, or self-led hypnosis (e.g., Magic Glove)	These can be effective even in early childhood. See Birnie et al. (2014) for a comprehensive review of hypnosis for pain management. Note that training on pediatric hypnosis is needed prior to use. These strategies may also be best used in a setting where the psychologist is able to meet with the child with enough time to discuss and practice the strategy
Preparation and information provision	• Picture book detailing procedure • Tour of procedure room • Verbal explanation • Include sensory and procedural information (Jaaniste, Hayes, & Von Baeyer, 2007)	Consider how far in advance preparation information should be provided based on developmental stage. It is recommended that children younger than 6 receive less than 5 days' notice, whereas children older than 6 receive at least 5 days' notice. In inpatient situations, consider showing the child the procedure space if appropriate
Breathing	• Blowing bubbles, party blower, pinwheel • Inflating a balloon during venipuncture • Deep breathing during procedure	Ensure the patient does not have any respiratory conditions before suggesting any breathing interventions. These strategies are appropriate in most settings
Positioning	• Infants should be held be a parent • Young children also be held or sit in their parent's lap • Older children may prefer to sit up on their own	Children should be given the opportunity to choose the positioning style which they prefer. In inpatient settings, consult with medical staff on any restrictions regarding positions prior to adjusting the child
Technological interventions	• Virtual reality (distraction) • Subcutaneous port (e.g., Port-a-Cath®) • Humanoid robots (e.g., MEDi; see Fig. 3)	Should be considered on a patient by patient basis
Infant interventions	• Breastfeeding • Sucrose	Sucrose on the pacifier or put directly in the infant's mouth is a simple breastfeeding alternative for infants who are not breastfed or fathers accompanying their infants
Pharmacological interventions	• Analgesic creams, gels, and lotions (e.g., EMLA, lidocaine-based creams, etc.)	Be aware of how long these products take to have an effect and how long the effect lasts; advise parents to apply accordingly

Note. Adapted from Birnie et al. (2018)

ing blood transfusion. This included telling Charlotte about her upcoming procedure one week in advance and reviewing what she could expect during the procedure. The family also collaboratively reviewed intervention options and agreed that an analgesic cream would be applied in advance of the IV catheter insertion. Charlotte also decided that she would like to play an electronic game to help keep her distracted during the IV catheter insertion.

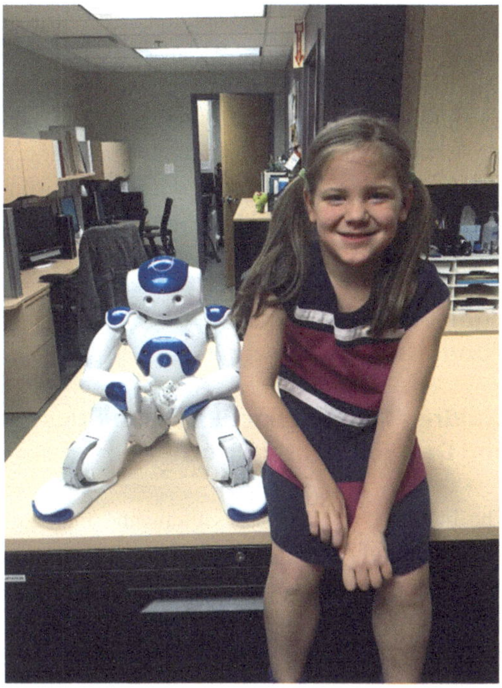

Fig. 3 Humanoid robots like MEDi can help distract children during procedures like venipuncture and vaccinations

Engaging Parents in Acute Pain Management Strategies

Parents should also be provided with education on these pain management strategies, so they may also utilize them with their children. Initiatives like *It Doesn't Have to Hurt* provide parents with evidence-based strategies for pain management in plain language. Parents can be directed to the *It Doesn't Have to Hurt* YouTube video or parent resource sheet (Chambers et al., 2013; see Fig. 2) which outlines pain manage-

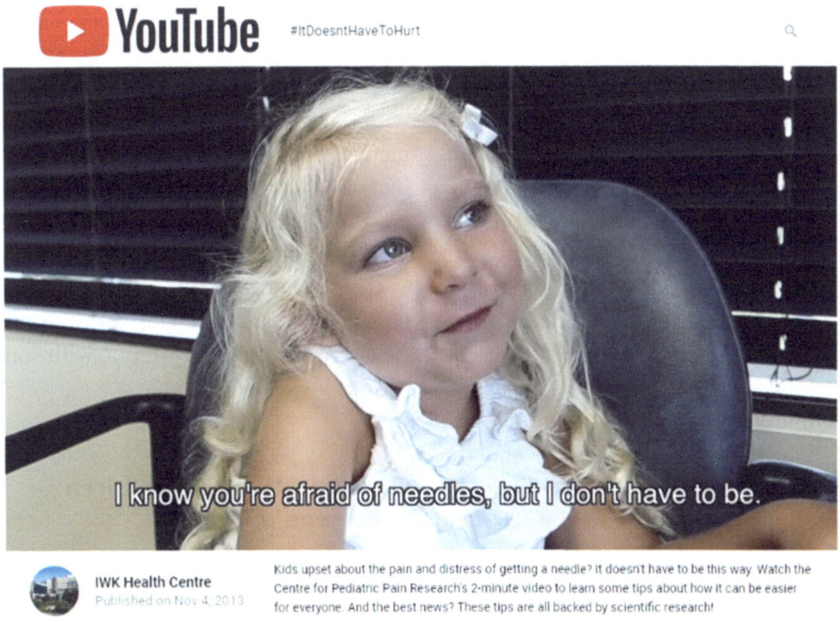

Fig. 2 A screenshot of the *It Doesn't Have to Hurt* parent video, demonstrating how strategies for needle pain management can be used

ment strategies which parents can easily utilize during needle procedures. Parent resources specific to infant procedural pain management are also available through online fact sheets and YouTube videos, including evidence-based resources such as *Be Sweet to Babies* (Harrison, Larocque, Reszel, Harrold, & Aubertin, 2017).

Considerations for Special Populations

Children with Intellectual Disabilities and Developmental Disorders

The literature on pain assessment and management in children with intellectual or developmental disabilities (I/DD) is scant but rapidly growing. Many children with I/DD have associated disabilities or health conditions that often require painful procedures and therapies (Belew et al., 2013). Acute pain assessment and management in this population can be complex and requires careful consideration of potential biopsychosocial factors which may be present, including cognitive, verbal, and/or motor impairments. While modifications and adjustments may be necessary, many of the same principles apply.

While self-report is the gold standard for pain assessment in typically developing school-aged children and adolescents, the reliability of this method for children with I/DD is uncertain. Higher functioning children and adolescents with I/DD may be able to complete self-reports. However, these should be supplemented with additional pain measures. Currently, the use of observational measures is considered best practice for pain assessment in children with I/DD. Commonly used observational tools to assess pain in children with I/DD include the NCCPC-R (Breau Lynn et al., 2002) and the r-FLAAC (Malviya et al., 2006; see Table 1). Indeed, these tools are limited by the fact that some children with I/DD display atypical pain expression. Pain assessment results in children with I/DD should be interpreted with the individual child in mind.

The assessment of pain in this population is of particular importance, given some demonstrated variability in their reactivity to pain. For example, children with some I/DD have been shown to demonstrate less intense or even a complete absence of a reaction to pain compared to their typically developing counterparts, as well as little to no crying following a painful occurrence (Gilbert-MacLeod, Craig, Rocha, & Mathias, 2000). The case of autism spectrum disorder (ASD) is quite complex, and research has shown children with ASD to be less behaviorally reactive to pain induced by venipuncture, however, were also shown to have increased heart rates during venipuncture compared to matched typically developing peers (Tordjman et al., 2009). These less intense reactions, however, should not be mistaken to mean that children in these populations are not experiencing pain.

It has also been shown that children with ASD demonstrate intense facial reactions to pain during venipuncture (Nader, Oberlander, Chambers, & Craig, 2004). Assessing pain in this population has an added level of complexity as parent reports of their child with ASD's pain are often discordant with rater observations of pain during procedures, whereas there was generally better concordance between raters and parents of typically developing children (Nader et al., 2004). Effective assessment of pain in children with developmental disorders therefore needs to include a multimodal model of pain assessment, including parent report, child self-report, and both observational and physiological assessments (Knoll, McMurtry, & Chambers, 2013).

The management of procedural and acute pain children with I/DD is very similar to that of typically developing children, with some modifications presented in Table 4.

Considerations for Children with Needle Phobia

It is normative for children to demonstrate some fear about needle procedures, and the aforementioned strategies are appropriate for most children.

Table 4 Pain management strategies for children with I/DD

Strategy	What's involved
Social stories	• Breaking down the procedure for a child in easily understood language through the perspective of a fictitious child • Provides children with cues on how a procedure will progress, what they can expect, and how they are expected to participate • Provides coping options for children when they face difficulties during their procedures
Visual cues	• Images to cue children with what will happen before (i.e., any prep), during (i.e., coping techniques), and after (i.e., reward) • Image cards which can be attached using hook-and-loop fasteners or a small magnetic board are helpful to prepare with the patient
Other interventions	• Analgesic creams, gels, and lotions (e.g., EMLA, lidocaine-based creams, etc.)

However, there is a subgroup of children who can be classified as having a needle phobia (or *trypanophobia*) and may require additional targeted treatments beyond the strategies presented this far. Exposure-based therapy involves slowly showing the child stimuli related to needles and the needle-based procedure has been shown to be effective in managing needle fear in young children (McMurtry et al., 2016). This type of intervention may be best suited to children who have time before their procedure is scheduled to happen and may not always be possible in inpatient settings, for example. In children who are known to faint during needle procedures, applied muscle tension has been shown to be effective in keeping children's blood pressure elevated during needle procedures (McMurtry et al., 2016). This intervention involves tensing the muscles with brief releases in between (i.e., approximately 5 s). Resources which discuss interventions for addressing needle phobia in childhood are also available to consult for more in-depth information on this topic (for reference, see McMurtry, Noel, et al., 2015; McMurtry, Pillai Riddell, et al., 2015).

Post-Procedure Pain Management

Continuing to manage pain after the procedure is complete is critical to maintaining the comfort of the pediatric patient. The following are strategies and scripts which can be used to coach parents on effective language post-procedure and provide reinforcement to children.

Reinforcement for Use of Pain Management Strategies

Positive reinforcement:

- Language to reinforce aspects of the procedure and engagement with strategies that went well ("You did a great job holding your arm still that whole time")

Rewards for completing the procedure:

- Time with a game or other desirable activity
- Stickers or prize if extrinsic motivation would be helpful

Memory reframing (adapted from Noel, McMurtry, Pavlova, & Taddio, 2017):

- An emerging and novel area of research where memories about a painful experience are restructured to create a sense of positivity and confidence for future procedures
- Strong and frequent emphasis on successful use and efficacy of pain management strategies ("Remember how you took those deep breaths and you said it helped you not feel scared?")
- Reframing negative memories or exaggerations of pain and fear ("I remember you said it didn't hurt as much as you thought it would")

Coaching Parents for Constructive Language

Encourage behavior-oriented, specific, and constructive feedback:

- Focus on a positive aspect of the procedure as well as how a certain strategy was used well to encourage successful use of it in the future. Ensure feedback is specific and meaningful.

- "You did a great job taking deep breaths" rather than "You did a great job."
- "You were brave when you held still the whole time" rather than "You were brave."
- "It must have been helpful for you to watch that video because you did a great job of staying calm" rather than "That video must have been helpful."

Discharge Planning

Engage in reflection personally and with the child and family to identify strengths and areas which need development for future procedures:

- Psychologist: Were all pertinent factors accounted for in this case? Were they attended to suitably when developing and executing the plan? What could be improved upon?
- Patient: Was the patient able to successfully engage in the plan and strategies? Were the patient's goals met? What did they feel went well? Where do they feel they could learn more?
- Parents: Were they confident in their ability to engage in the pain management plan? Were they satisfied with how their child's pain was managed? Upon reflecting on the perceived strengths of the pain management plan and identification of areas for development, begin to strategize about how these new goals can be integrated into future procedural pain management plans, for the present families and others in the future.

Charlotte's first blood transfusion went well overall. Though she did become nervous at the time of the IV catheter insertion, she stated feeling better having the numbing cream applied and it was evident that she made a good effort to remain engaged with her game. Upon completion of the IV insertion, Charlotte was praised by her parents and the psychologist, reinforcing her effort to remain calm and focused.

Conclusion

Acute pain is a common and important issue for children. It is critical for the pediatric psychologist to approach their assessments and treatment plans from a biopsychosocial context, considering not only the patient's presenting problem and characteristics but also considering the young patient's family, cultural context, and collective goals. This will ensure the treatment plan is collaborative in how it is developed so all parties can remain engaged in the pain management plan. By setting common goals with patients and families early on, it allows for strong rapport which will ultimately facilitate the successful use of any of the pain management strategies presented here. Finally, by engaging in reflection and future planning with families following a procedure, the psychologist is able to reinforce their support of the family as they continue to use pain management strategies throughout their child's medical treatment.

Appendix: Guided Imagery Script

You are lying down on your back. ... Start to take slow, deep breaths into your belly. Make your belly bigger as you breathe in, and let it flatten down as you breathe out. [Perhaps the child wants to place a small stuffed animal on his or her belly.] Don't worry about your breathing. Just let it happen. You can feel your whole body begin to relax with each breath ... breathing out stress and worry ... breathing in relaxation and calm. Centering yourself ... inwardly smile. Deep breathing, relaxing ... now imagine a warm ball of light in your belly. Every time you take a breath in, the warm ball of light climbs up the front of your body, becoming bigger, expanding. It is now in your chest, making it feel warm and light ... with another inhalation, it travels up into your throat and neck ... each time you breathe in, the warm ball of light grows bigger ... it is filling you. ... Your face is now filled with this warm light and your jaw loosens ... let your mouth open slightly.... The ball of light reaches the top of your head ... relaxing your scalp ... it travels with each inward breath down the back of your head to your spine ... warming and relaxing your entire back ... softening each bone in your back. The ball of light rolls slowly down both arms ... then to your hands ... making them heavy and warm. ... This warm flow slowly moves into each of your legs ... travelling to your knees ... ankles ... softly on to your feet ... warming you ... each toe and bone in your foot is relaxed ... softened. This is everywhere. Keep breathing and let all your tension and worry be gone ... quiet ... melted away. Go back to any area that has any tightness and bring the warm ball of healing light back to it. Take your time. You are warm, relaxed, happy, and safe. Your body is heavy and comfortable ... filled with relaxation.

References

Asmundson, G. J. G., Bovell, C. V., Carleton, R. N., & McWilliams, L. A. (2008). The Fear of Pain Questionnaire-Short Form (FPQ-SF): Factorial validity and psychometric properties. *Pain, 134*(1–2), 51–58. https://doi.org/10.1016/j.pain.2007.03.033

Belew, J. L., Barney, C. C., Schwantes, S. A., Tibboel, D., Valkenburg, A. J., & Symons, F. J. (2013). Pain in children with intellectual or developmental disabilities. In P. J. McGrath, B. J. Stevens, S. M. Walker, & W. T. Zempsky (Eds.), *Oxford textbook of paediatric pain* (Vol. 1). Oxford, UK: Oxford University Press. https://doi.org/10.1093/med/9780199642656.003.0016

Birnie, K. A., Chambers, C. T., Chorney, J., Fernandez, C. V., & McGrath, P. J. (2016). Dyadic analysis of child and parent trait and state pain catastrophizing in the process of children's pain communication. *Pain, 157*(4), 938–948. https://doi.org/10.1097/j.pain.0000000000000461

Birnie, K. A., Hundert, A. S., Lalloo, C., Nguyen, C., & Stinson, J. N. (2019). Recommendations for selection of self-report pain intensity measures in children and adolescents: a systematic review and quality assessment of measurement properties. *Pain, 160*, 5–18. https://doi.org/10.1097/j.pain.0000000000001377

Birnie, K. A., Noel, M., Chambers, C. T., Uman, L. S., & Parker, J. A. (2018). Psychological interventions for needle-related procedural pain and distress in children and adolescents. *Cochrane Database of Systematic Reviews*, John Wiley and Sons Ltd. https://doi.org/10.1002/14651858.CD005179.pub4

Birnie, K. A., Noel, M., Parker, J. A., Chambers, C. T., Uman, L. S., Kisely, S. R., & McGrath, P. J. (2014). Systematic review and meta-analysis of distraction and hypnosis for needle-related pain and distress in children and adolescents. *Journal of Pediatric Psychology, 39*(8), 783–808. https://doi.org/10.1093/jpepsy/jsu029

Blount, R. L., Cohen, L. L., Frank, N. C., Bachanas, P. J., Smith, A. J., Manimala, M. R., & Pate, J. T. (1997). The child-adult medical procedure interaction scale-revised: An assessment of validity. *Journal of Pediatric Psychology, 22*(1), 73–88. https://doi.org/10.1093/jpepsy/22.1.73

Breau Lynn, M., Finley, G. A., McGrath, P. J., & Camfield, C. S. (2002). Validation of the non-communicating children's pain checklist—Postoperative version. *Anesthesiology, 96*(3), 528–535. Retrieved from https://anesthesiology.pubs.asahq.org/journal.aspx

Chambers, C. T., Reid, G. J., McGrath, P. J., & Finley, G. A. (1996). Development and preliminary validation of a postoperative pain measure for parents. *Pain, 68*(2–3), 307–313. Retrieved from http://www.ncbi.nlm.nih.gov/pubmed/9121819

Chambers, C. T., Taddio, A., Stinson, J. N., Campbell-Yeo, M., Halperin, S., & Parker, J. A. (2013). It doesn't have to hurt: Strategies for helping children with shots and needles (A YouTube video for parents). Retrieved from https://www.youtube.com/watch?v=vIJnNF1U2ZI

Cunningham, C. L., & Banez, G. (Eds.) (2006). Recurrent abdominal pain. In *Pediatric gastrointestinal disorders: Biopsychosocial assessment and treatment* (pp. 93–116). New York, NY: Springer. https://doi.org/10.1007/b135749

Elliott, C. H., Jay, S. M., & Woody, P. (1987). An observation scale for measuring children's distress during medical procedures. *Journal of Pediatric Psychology, 12*(4), 543–551. https://doi.org/10.1093/jpepsy/12.4.543

Fitzgerald, M., & Walker, S. M. (2009). Infant pain management: A developmental neurobiological approach. *Nature Clinical Practice Neurology, 5*(1), 35–50. https://doi.org/10.1038/ncpneuro0984

Friedrichsdorf, S. J., Postier, A., Eull, D., Weidner, C., Foster, L., Gilbert, M., & Campbell, F. (2015). Pain outcomes in a US children's hospital: A prospective cross-sectional survey. *Hospital Pediatrics, 5*(1), 18–26. https://doi.org/10.1542/hpeds.2014-0084

Gilbert-MacLeod, C. A., Craig, K. D., Rocha, E. M., & Mathias, M. D. (2000). Everyday pain responses in children with and without developmental delays. *Journal of Pediatric Psychology, 25*(5), 301–308. https://doi.org/10.1093/jpepsy/25.5.301

Gilbert, C. A., Lilley, C. M., Craig, K. D., McGrath, P. J., Court, C. A., Bennett, S. M., & Montgomery, C. J. (1999). Postoperative pain expression in preschool children: Validation of the child facial coding system. *The Clinical Journal of Pain, 15*(3), 192–200. https://doi.org/10.1097/00002508-199909000-00006

Goubert, L., Eccleston, C., Vervoort, T., Jordan, A., & Crombez, G. (2006). Parental catastrophizing about their child's pain. The parent version of the Pain Catastrophizing Scale (PCS-P): A preliminary validation. *Pain, 123*(3), 254–263. https://doi.org/10.1016/j.pain.2006.02.035

Guite, J. W., Logan, D. E., Simons, L. E., Blood, E. A., & Kerns, R. D. (2011). Readiness to change in pediatric chronic pain: Initial validation of adolescent and parent versions of the pain stages of change questionnaire. *Pain, 152*(10), 2301–2311. https://doi.org/10.1016/j.pain.2011.06.019

Harrison, D., Larocque, C., Reszel, J., Harrold, J., & Aubertin, C. (2017). Be sweet to babies during painful procedures: A pilot evaluation of a parent-targeted video. *Advances in Neonatal Care, 17*(5), 372–380. https://doi.org/10.1097/ANC.0000000000000425

Hester, N. K. (1979). The preoperational child's reaction to immunization. *Nursing Research, 28*(4), 250–255. Retrieved from http://www.ncbi.nlm.nih.gov/pubmed/255924

Hicks, C. L., von Baeyer, C. L., Spafford, P. A., van Korlaar, I., & Goodenough, B. (2001). The Faces Pain Scale-Revised: Toward a common metric in pediatric pain measurement. *Pain, 93*(2), 173–183. https://doi.org/10.1016/S0304-3959(01)00314-1

Jaaniste, T., Hayes, B., & Von Baeyer, C. L. (2007). Providing children with information about forthcoming medical procedures: A review and synthesis. *Clinical Psychology: Science and Practice, 14*(2), 124–143. https://doi.org/10.1111/j.1468-2850.2007.00072.x

Knoll, A. K., McMurtry, C. M., & Chambers, C. T. (2013). Pain in children with Autism Spectrum Disorder: Experience, expression, and assessment. *Pediatric Pain Letter, 15*(2), 23–28.

Kristjansdottir, O., McGrath, P. J., Finley, G. A., Kristjansdottir, G., Siripul, P., Mackinnon, S. P., & Yoshida, Y. (2018). Cultural influences on parental responses to children's pain. *Pain, 159*(10), 2035–2049. Retrieved from https://journals.lww.com/pain/Fulltext/2018/10000/Cultural_influences_on_parental_responses_to.15.aspx

LeBaron, S., & Zeltzer, L. (1984). Assessment of acute pain and anxiety in children and adolescents by self-reports, observer reports, and a behavior checklist. *Journal of Consulting and Clinical Psychology, 52*(5), 729–738. https://doi.org/10.1037/0022-006X.52.5.729

Malviya, S., Voepel-Lewis, T., Burke, C., Merkel, S., & Tait, A. R. (2006). The revised FLACC observational pain tool: Improved reliability and validity for pain assessment in children with cognitive impairment. *Pediatric Anesthesia, 16*(3), 258–265. https://doi.org/10.1111/j.1460-9592.2005.01773.x

McGrath, P. A., Seifert, C. E., Speechley, K. N., Booth, J. C., Stitt, L., & Gibson, M. C. (1996). A new analogue scale for assessing children's pain: An initial validation study. *Pain, 64*(3), 435–443. Retrieved from http://www.ncbi.nlm.nih.gov/pubmed/8783307

McMurtry, C. M., Noel, M., Taddio, A., Antony, M. M., Asmundson, G. J. G., Riddell, R. P., … Shah, V. (2015). Interventions for individuals with high levels of needle fear: Systematic review of randomized controlled trials and quasi-randomized controlled trials. *The Clinical Journal of Pain, 31*(10 Suppl), S109–S123. https://doi.org/10.1097/AJP.0000000000000273

McMurtry, C. M., Pillai Riddell, R., Taddio, A., Racine, N., Asmundson, G. J. G., Noel, M., … Shah, V. (2015). Far from "Just a Poke": Common painful needle procedures and the development of needle fear. *The Clinical Journal of Pain, 31*(10 Suppl), S3–S11. https://doi.org/10.1097/AJP.0000000000000272

McMurtry, C. M., Taddio, A., Noel, M., Antony, M. M., Chambers, C. T., Asmundson, G. J. G., … Scott, J. (2016). Exposure-based Interventions for the management of individuals with high levels of needle fear across the lifespan: A clinical practice guideline and call for further research. *Cognitive Behaviour Therapy, 45*(3), 217–235. https://doi.org/10.1080/16506073.2016.1157204

Nader, R., Oberlander, T. F., Chambers, C. T., & Craig, K. D. (2004). Expression of pain in children with autism. *The Clinical Journal of Pain, 20*(2), 88–97. https://doi.org/10.1097/00002508-200403000-00005

Noel, M., McMurtry, C. M., Pavlova, M., & Taddio, A. (2017). Brief clinical report: A systematic review and meta-analysis of pain memory-reframing interventions for children's needle procedures. *Pain Practice, 18*(1), 123–129. https://doi.org/10.1111/papr.12572

Noel, M., Pavlova, M., McCallum, L., & Vinall, J. (2017). Remembering the hurt of childhood: A psychological review and call for future research. *Canadian Psychology/Psychologie Canadienne, 58*(1), 58–68. https://doi.org/10.1037/cap0000098

Piazza-Waggoner, C., Roddenberry, A., Yeomans-Maldonado, G., Noll, J., & M. Ernst, M. (2013). Inpatient pediatric psychology consultation-liaison program development: 5-year practice patterns and implications for trends in health care. *Clinical Practice in Pediatric Psychology, 1*(1), 28–41. https://doi.org/10.1037/cpp0000008

Schinkel, M. G., Chambers, C. T., Corkum, P., & Jacques, S. (2018). Dyadic analysis of siblings' relationship quality, behavioural responses, and pain experiences during experimental pain. *Pain, 159*(8), 1569–1579. https://doi.org/10.1097/j.pain.0000000000001244

Stevens, B. J., Abbott, L. K., Yamada, J., Harrison, D., Stinson, J., Taddio, A., … Finley, G. A. (2011). Epidemiology and management of painful procedures in children in Canadian hospitals. *Canadian Medical Association Journal = Journal de l'Association Medicale Canadienne, 183*(7), E403–E410. https://doi.org/10.1503/cmaj.101341

Stevens, B., Johnston, C., Petryshen, P., & Taddio, A. (1996). Premature infant pain profile: Development and initial validation. *The Clinical Journal of Pain, 12*(1), 13–22. https://doi.org/10.1097/00002508-199603000-00004

Taddio, A., Chambers, C. T., Halperin, S. A., Ipp, M., Lockett, D., Rieder, M. J., & Shah, V. (2009). Inadequate pain management during routine childhood immunizations: The nerve of it. *Clinical Therapeutics, 31*(Suppl 2), S152–S167. https://doi.org/10.1016/j.clinthera.2009.07.022

Taddio, A., McMurtry, C. M., Shah, V., Riddell, R. P., Chambers, C. T., Noel, M., … Bleeker, E. V. (2015). Reducing pain during vaccine injections: Clinical practice guideline. *Canadian Medical Association Journal, 187*(13), 975–982. https://doi.org/10.1503/cmaj.150391

Tordjman, S., Anderson, G. M., Botbol, M., Brailly-Tabard, S., Perez-Diaz, F., Graignic, R., … Bronsard, G. (2009). Pain reactivity and plasma beta-endorphin in children and adolescents with autistic disorder. *PLoS One, 4*(8), e5289. https://doi.org/10.1371/journal.pone.0005289

Young, M. A., Carter, B., & von Baeyer, C. L. (2017). Optimizing numeric pain rating scale administration for children: The effects of verbal anchor phrases. *Canadian Journal of Pain, 1*(1), 191–198. https://doi.org/10.1080/24740527.2017.1398587

The Problem of Pain: Chronic Pain

Emily Foxen-Craft, Amy E. Williams, and Eric L. Scott

Children and adolescents with chronic pain are often encountered in a consultation-liaison (CL) setting during an acute on chronic exacerbation of pain. Families are often experiencing significant emotional distress and may be resistant to discharging without improvement in pain or at least a plan for improving pain. Physicians may feel significant frustration as there is often not an inpatient (or quick) solution for the child's chronic pain and they may struggle with what interventions to provide and when to discharge a child with a chronic pain condition who continues to report significant pain. The CL psychologist can play an important role in the care of these patients with goals to improve patient/family coping strategies and minimize distress, develop plans to limit unnecessary medical admissions and treatments, and facilitate transition to more comprehensive outpatient treatment programs. This chapter provides information germane to CL psychologists encountering inpatients and outpatients with ongoing pain that need initial evaluation and recommendations for further treatment.

Electronic supplementary material: The online version of this chapter (https://doi.org/10.1007/978-3-030-35598-2_13) contains supplementary material, which is available to authorized users.

E. Foxen-Craft
Department of Pediatrics, C.S. Mott Children's Hospital, University of Michigan Medical School, Ann Arbor, MI, USA

A. E. Williams
Department of Psychiatry, Riley Hospital for Children, Indiana University School of Medicine, Indianapolis, IN, USA

E. L. Scott (✉)
Department of Pediatrics, C.S. Mott Children's Hospital, University of Michigan Medical School, Ann Arbor, MI, USA

Department of Anesthesiology, C.S. Mott Children's Hospital, University of Michigan School of Medicine, Ann Arbor, MI, USA
e-mail: erlscott@med.umich.edu

Diagnosis

Chronic pain, i.e., in pediatric patients of greater than 3 months duration, is prevalent in children and adolescents with studies indicating 11–38% experience chronic pain (King et al., 2011). Pediatric chronic pain is associated with functional impairment, decreased quality of life (Huguet & Miro, 2008), and psychological comorbidities (Noel, Groenewald, Beals-Erickson, Gebert, & Palermo, 2016; Vinall, Pavlova, Asmundson, Rasic, & Noel, 2016). Estimates indicate about one-third of children and adolescents with chronic pain continue to have pain into adulthood (Brattberg, 2004; Gieteling, Bierma-Zeinstra, Passchier, & Berger, 2008). Inpatient census reports of patients experiencing pain prior to their hospitalization indicate

B. D. Carter, K. A. Kullgren (eds.), *Clinical Handbook of Psychological Consultation in Pediatric Medical Settings*, Issues in Clinical Child Psychology, https://doi.org/10.1007/978-3-030-35598-2_13

up to 20–30% of patients come to the hospital with existing pain (Postier et al., 2018; Walther-Larsen et al., 2017). In addition to substantial individual and family impacts of chronic pediatric pain, the societal impact is significant with an estimated societal cost in the USA of $19.5 billion annually (Groenewald, Essner, Wright, Fesinmeyer, & Palermo, 2014). Epidemiological studies indicate headaches, abdominal pain, and musculoskeletal pain are common chronic pain diagnoses in pediatric patients (King et al., 2011). Children and adolescents may also present with chronic pain associated with an underlying medical diagnosis (e.g., sickle cell disease or juvenile rheumatoid arthritis) or with neuropathic pain (e.g., complex regional pain syndrome (CRPS)). Regardless of the pain etiology, a CL psychologist can be of benefit in helping the patient decrease pain and associated functional limitations, improve pain coping, improve adherence to treatments that reduce pain/improve health, and treat psychological comorbidities.

From a psychological perspective, several diagnoses may be considered when working with patients with chronic pain. Many children and adolescents with chronic pain, particularly those for whom a psychology consult is requested, will meet criteria for a *somatic symptom disorder with predominant pain* (American Psychiatric Association, 2013). It is important to note this diagnosis is equally applicable to a patient whose pain is thought to be predominantly functional in origin as it is to a patient whose pain has a clear medical/organic etiology (see chapter "Somatic Symptom and Related Disorders"). Rather than being reflective of the cause of the pain, this diagnosis indicates a problematic reaction to the pain, including functional impairments, distress, or excessive time focused on symptoms. Given the influential role of psychological factors in pain modulation (see section "Medical Basics" below), it is clear that pain will nearly always be influenced by psychological variables in a patient's life. Thus, the diagnosis of *psychological factors affecting other medical condition* (American Psychiatric Association, 2013) can be indicated in situations where psychosocial factors (e.g., comorbid depression, anxiety, or behavior disorder) are having a significant impact on pain or pain coping, but symptoms associated directly with pain do not meet criteria for a somatic symptom disorder. We have observed clinically that many patients with *conversion disorder* (American Psychiatric Association, 2013) have a pain component to their symptom presentation; however, this would not be a likely diagnosis if pain is the only/primary symptom.

As noted above, many children and adolescents with chronic pain will have comorbid psychiatric diagnoses (Noel et al., 2016; Vinall et al., 2016), such as anxiety and depression, which should also be considered in the psychiatric differential for pediatric patients with chronic pain. It is also possible that the pediatric patient with chronic pain may not have a relevant psychiatric diagnosis, but can still benefit significantly from psychological interventions. In the absence of a clinically significant mental health diagnosis, the primary medical diagnosis may be used with a Health and Behavior code (H&B code) for billing to allow the patient to receive appropriate health psychology services.

Medical Basics: Basic Neurophysiology of Pain Perception and Modulation

In working with chronic pain populations it is essential to understand basic physiological mechanisms involved and to communicate this to the patient and family. Pain sensation originates in peripheral sensory nerves called nociceptors which, when activated by noxious stimulation, send signals to afferent neurons in the dorsal horn of the spinal cord (Price & Bushnell, 2004). Primary afferent neurons transmit signals to a distributed brain network including somatosensory cortices, limbic structures (amygdala), the anterior cingulate cortex, and hypothalamus. Pain sensations trigger brief emotional responses, cognitive appraisals regarding threat, and physiological reactions to the pain.

Psychological processes can act upon this afferent pain pathway to modulate nociceptive transmission and either facilitate or inhibit pain (Price & Bushnell, 2004). Psychological factors known to modulate pain include attention, cognitive variables (e.g., cognitive appraisals, catastrophizing, coping strategies), operant conditioning, psychological conditions (e.g., anxiety, depression), and emotional states (Price & Bushnell, 2004). Impairments in normal endogenous pain modulation (i.e., decreased inhibition or increased facilitation) may create a "pro-nociceptive" state that predisposes development of chronic pain (Yarnitsky, 2010). Central sensitization reflects alterations in central nervous system nociceptive pathways resulting in hyperexcitability of nociceptors, and increased pain, and is frequently observed in persons with chronic pain (Woolf, 2011).

Melzack and Wall's (1965) gate control theory is often utilized to explain pain modulation to patients. This theory proposes a theoretical "gate" at the level of the spinal cord through which pain signals must pass. The gate control theory proposes that various behavioral, psychological, and physiological factors can change how open or closed the gate is, thereby increasing or decreasing the number of pain signals transmitted to the brain. This provides a framework for conceptualizing how psychological interventions can impact pain sensation by maximizing behavioral, cognitive, and environmental factors that inhibit pain (i.e., close the pain gate) and eliminating/minimizing factors that facilitate pain (i.e., open the pain gate).

Psychological Formulation of Pediatric Chronic Pain

A biopsychosocial approach to conceptualization of pediatric chronic pain is typically utilized to account for the impacts of psychological and social variables. Palermo (2012) has proposed a model for conceptualizing pediatric chronic pain that accounts for the biological considerations in pain (e.g., sex, age, physical health), within the context of the individual's psychological factors (e.g., coping, mood, anxiety, beliefs/appraisals), nested within the social environment (e.g., parenting and family factors, peer influences, socioeconomic status, culture), and also considers the role of individual health behaviors (e.g., sleep, physical activity).

In a medical inpatient CL setting, time constraints often require abbreviated evaluations compared to outpatient settings, and thus it is recommended to focus interviews on information necessary to develop a treatment plan for the inpatient setting and for referral for appropriate outpatient treatment. Time permitting, it is helpful to gain an understanding of the history of the chronic pain condition in full (including frequency of emergency room visits or hospitalizations for pain) and factors associated with what is often an acute on chronic exacerbation of pain resulting in the current hospitalization. More complete explanations of biopsychosocial contributions to pediatric chronic pain can be found elsewhere (Law, Noel, Nagel, & Dahlquist, 2017; Palermo, 2012); in this chapter we focus on biopsychosocial variables that are most important for CL psychologists to guide evidence-based interventions in the inpatient setting.

Biological Variables

The CL psychologist should develop a clear understanding of the patient's physical health and pain history, which can be gathered through discussion with consulting physicians, chart review, and interview with the patient and caregivers. Important factors to consider include the pain etiology (e.g., is pain suspected to be primarily functional or organic), how long the pain has been present, the typical course for pain symptoms (e.g., waxing and waning, progressive worsening), triggers for increased or decreased pain, and what kind of medical treatments the patient utilizes and finds helpful. Although not modifiable through therapy interventions, it is important to note some additional biological characteristics that are associated with increased pain including increasing age and pubertal status, female sex, and genetics (Palermo, 2012).

It is also helpful to consider how physiological processes such as central sensitization (Woolf,

2011) and/or a pro-nociceptive (Yarnitsky, 2010) pattern of pain modulation (as discussed in section "Medical Basics" above) might be contributing to the patient's chronic pain. This information facilitates understanding of how psychological interventions can be helpful and often plays a significant role in engaging the patient and family in psychological interventions. Currently, it is not standard of care to complete physiological assessments of pain processing or modulation; however, patient history and/or knowledge about pain processing and modulation in general can inform conceptualization of these processes in an individual patient.

Psychological Variables

Psychological comorbidities such as depression, anxiety, and behavior disorders are common among children and adolescents with chronic pain (occurring in as many as 25%), sometimes beginning prior to the onset of pain (Tegethoff, Belardi, Stalujanis, & Meinlschmidt, 2015). Further, children and adolescents with chronic pain are at greater risk for lifetime occurrence of depression and anxiety when assessed in adulthood (Noel et al., 2016). Depression is associated with greater functional disability in pediatric patients with chronic pain (Kashikar-Zuck, Goldschneider, Powers, Vaught, & Hershey, 2001). These data imply a bidirectional relationship with mental illness having the potential to contribute to development or exacerbation of pain and pain having the potential to contribute to development or exacerbation of mental illness (Palermo, 2012). In healthy individuals, research indicates negative emotions (of low to moderate intensity) facilitate pain (i.e., open the pain gate) and positive emotions inhibit pain (i.e., close the pain gate) (Rhudy, Williams, McCabe, Nguyen, & Rambo, 2005; Williams & Rhudy, 2009). This pattern of modulation may be disrupted in persons with chronic pain, providing further justification for psychological interventions targeting emotional factors.

Thinking styles and cognitive attributions (such as pain catastrophizing, pain-related injustice perceptions, fear of pain, and pain self-efficacy) also impact pain outcomes in children and adolescents with chronic pain. Pain catastrophizing has been demonstrated to have strong associations with quality of life, anxiety, and depression and moderate associations with pain intensity and physical disability (Miller, Meints, & Hirsh, 2018). Children's perceptions of pain-related injustice (i.e., unfairness and blame associated with their pain) are associated with increased pain and poorer functioning (Miller et al., 2018; Miller, Scott, Trost, & Hirsh, 2016). Fear of pain, or the perception of potential pain triggers as threatening, is associated with higher pain intensity and pain-related disability (Fisher, Heathcote, Eccleston, Simons, & Palermo, 2018; Simons, Sieberg, Carpino, Logan, & Berde, 2011). Pain self-efficacy is the belief that one is able to cope with and function effectively despite pain and is associated with lower levels of pain-related disability (Kalapurakkel, Carpino, Lebel, & Simons, 2015). These associations illustrate the importance of assessing how the child/adolescent and their family think about their pain, its impact on their life, and their ability to effectively cope with pain.

Health Habits

Important health habits to consider include sleep and physical activity (Palermo, 2012). Evidence indicates children and adolescents with chronic pain have poor sleep compared to healthy peers, and lower sleep efficiency is predictive of more functional limitations (Valrie, Bromberg, Palermo, & Schanberg, 2013). There is a bidirectional relationship between sleep and pain such that poor sleep is often associated with increased pain the following day, and increased pain is associated with disrupted sleep the following night (Valrie et al., 2013). In addition to baseline sleep disruption, it is important to assess changes in sleep during inpatient hospitalization since children and adolescents often have increased sleep difficulty in the hospital and are at risk for sleep-phase shifting during hospital stays. If sleep is an area of concern, brief interventions can be implemented in the CL setting including sleep hygiene and stimulus control (Palermo, 2012), and referral to sleep medicine specialists and/or for more extensive cognitive behavioral interventions targeting sleep may be indicated.

Physical activity is also important to consider, with high levels of sedentary activity associated with risk for chronic pain in children and adolescents (Auvinen, Tammelin, Taimela, Zitting, & Karppinen, 2008; Paananen et al., 2010) and, in contrast, very high levels of physical activity associated with risk for pain associated with traumatic injuries (Auvinen et al., 2008; El-Metwally, Salminen, Auvinen, Macfarlane, & Mikkelsson, 2007). Further, children and adolescents with chronic pain often have a decline in physical activity during the course of their pain condition, as evidenced by research showing functional impairments in children/adolescents with chronic pain (Huguet & Miro, 2008; Kashikar-Zuck et al., 2001). Obesity is also associated with chronic pain in children and adolescents (Wilson, Samuelson, & Palermo, 2010).

Social Variables

Operant conditioning, particularly negative reinforcement, has been shown to play a significant role in pain behaviors (Sanders, 2002); as such, it is important to assess how family members, peers, and others respond to pain behaviors. Responses to pain that result in a temporary reduction of pain (resting, parental comfort) or avoidance/escape of an unpleasant experience (avoidance of non-preferred activity such as chores or school) may negatively reinforce, and thus maintain or exacerbate, pain behaviors (Sanders, 2002). Solicitous responding to pain (e.g., attending to pain, allowing activity limitations) by parents is associated with increased pain and pain behaviors (Claar, Simons, & Logan, 2008). High levels of pain catastrophizing among mothers of children/adolescents with pain are associated with greater pain reports. Poorer family functioning (e.g., frequent arguments, poor communication) is associated with increased pain-related disability (Lewandowski, Palermo, Stinson, Handley, & Chambers, 2010). Further, children who have a parent with chronic pain have an increased risk for chronic pain themselves (Hoftun, Romundstad, & Rygg, 2013), which can be hypothesized to be due to both genetics and modeling or other social contributions to pain (Palermo, 2012). To assess these potential impacts on pain it can be helpful to ask about daily routines, functional limitations, how the family decides to limit functioning, impacts on peer relationships, and barriers to managing pain in the home and at school. Recommended self-report assessment measures are presented in Table 1.

Table 1 Suggested self-report assessments for pediatric chronic pain

Domain	Suggested Measures
Pain intensity[a]	Brief Pain Inventory Visual Analog Scale[a] Numeric Rating Scales[a]
Pain location/ widespreadness	SUPERKIDZ Body Map
Physical functioning[a]	PedsQL[a] Oswestry Disability Index Functional Disability Inventory[a] PROMIS Mobility
Emotional functioning[a]	PROMIS Depressive Symptoms PROMIS Anxiety PROMIS Psychological Stress Pain Catastrophizing Scale Children's Depression Inventory[a] Revised Child Anxiety and Depression Scale[a] PedsQL
Role functioning[a]	School attendance PedMIDAS (headache) PedsQL
Symptoms and adverse events[a]	Symptom Severity Index
Global judgment of satisfaction with treatment[a]	Global question with specifiers
Sleep[a]	PROMIS Sleep PROMIS Fatigue Pittsburgh Sleep Questionnaire Sleep Habits Questionnaire
Motivation	Pain Stages of Change

Notes: Clinicians should consider age normative data, as well as how aspects of reliability and validity may be relevant to the clinical context. For some of these measures, child and parent-proxy versions are available. Most of these questionnaires are available in the public domain

[a]Core outcome domain recommended by PedIMMPACT (Pediatric Initiative on Methods, Measurement, and Pain Assessment in Clinical Trials), a professional consensus meeting that identified core outcome domains and measurements that should be considered in clinical trials of treatments for acute and chronic pain in children and adolescents

Engagement in Psychological Treatment

Consistent with CL services more generally, children and adolescents hospitalized with chronic pain typically do not present to the hospital setting in search of psychological care and have varying levels of receptivity to CL psychology services. Therefore, it is important that efforts are made to educate the patient/family to establish "buy-in" for the relevance and benefits of psychological interventions. To do this, psychoeducation about psychological influences on pain is crucial, often involving education about the gate control theory (Melzack & Wall, 1965). Additionally, the use of clinical analogies to describe pain, pain modulation, and treatment can be helpful for increasing patient's understanding and buy-in. Coakley and Schechter (Coakley & Schechter, 2013) provide several examples of useful clinical analogies when working with children with pain. Additionally, it can be helpful to highlight or elaborate on examples the child/teen mentions regarding their own experiences that illustrates the interaction between pain and psychological or behavioral factors.

A developmental approach to the child's pain provides a framework for helping move resistant or hesitant families toward increasing buy-in for psychological interventions. It can be beneficial to first assess the child and family's conceptualization of pain and introduce new concepts or examples to move them toward a more biopsychosocial approach. For example, in some cases a patient/family is resistant to a suspected functional etiology for the patient's pain. While the eventual goal may be to help the family better understand and accept a functional etiology, this may be difficult to achieve during the brief encounter of an inpatient consult, particularly during an acute pain exacerbation. Rather, the goal of an inpatient consult can be to help the patient/family understand that *regardless of the etiology for pain,* psychological factors play a role and psychological interventions can be of help for coping with pain.

Intervention

Substantial evidence to date supports the effectiveness of the use of psychological therapies in treating pediatric chronic pain (Eccleston et al., 2012). The inpatient admission represents a unique opportunity to provide evidence-based intervention to a captive audience in acute pain and distress; however, due to the nature of inpatient CL, time is often limited and effort may be focused on facilitating discharge. Therefore, the clinician should focus on case formulation and specific goals that will facilitate a discharge to successful outpatient intervention. Motivational interviewing techniques may be particularly useful in obtaining engagement in treatment and patients' and parents' willingness to try new behaviors or coping skills (Simons & Basch, 2016). For example, open-ended questions, affirmations, reflections, and summarizing can be used to facilitate an environment in which the patient and family feel comfortable discussing their ambivalence about pain self-management and/or psychological treatment for pain (Rosengren, 2018). Through this discussion patient's personal goals/values and motivations (e.g., desire for less pain, goal to return to social or athletic activities) for pain self-management can be identified, focused on, and facilitated to strengthen motivation to participate in treatment. Parent education regarding differential attention to non-pain behaviors can reduce pain behaviors in the inpatient setting and at home through the transition to outpatient therapy. Similarly, the patient and/or family can be engaged in short-term goal setting to increase functioning to facilitate discharge, such as goals for movement or walking (Palermo, Wilson, Peters, Lewandowski, & Somhegyi, 2009). For some patients, the focus of motivational interviewing can be to develop the willingness to engage in self-management of pain during the next stage of treatment which may include return to school (see below) (Logan, Conroy, Sieberg, & Simons, 2012). Additional pain-coping techniques may be adapted for implementation in an inpatient setting. For instance, creative thinking regarding opportunities for distraction can be useful. Similarly, though extensive biofeedback training may not be feasible, brief training in biofeedback-facilitated relaxation may ameliorate some distress, provide a concrete illustration of the mind-body connection, and provide a positive coping technique to a child in pain and distress (see chapter "Technological Innovations in Pediatric Psychological Consultation") (Table 2).

Pain-focused CBT has ample evidence to support treatment of pediatric chronic pain (Eccleston et al., 2012), but a full course of pain-focused CBT may not be feasible during a brief inpatient stay. Instead, the inpatient CL clinician can provide training on core skills that may be relevant and helpful to an engaged patient, such as identifying and challenging a few key cognitive distortions. Finally, the clinician can help the patient and family problem-solve barriers that would impede adherence to discharge recommendations and transition to outpatient treatment, as well as proactively problem-solve concerns to prevent readmission. Many times this will include re-integration into school after the hospitalization, especially if there was considerable number of days missed prior to the admission, and addressing affective distress over poor attendance and decreased performance in school and when depressive symptoms are present (Logan & Simons, 2010). Educating parents regarding the use of either an Individual Education Plan or 504 Plan to include academic accommodations can help remove some barriers to re-introduction into school. Stressing to parents the need to request an evaluation for either of these educational tools in writing is important. Common requests can include use of a rolling backpack to carry books, extra sets of books for classroom and home use, access to snacks and hydration, extra time for passing periods, use of computer or tablet for note taking, and access to notes from the teacher or trusted peer can all be rather readily included in such plans.

Table 2 Common interventions for children and youth

Education for parents and children
• *Managing Your Child's Chronic Pain*[a,b,c], Tonya Palermo
• *When Your Child Hurts*[a,b], Rachel Coakley
• *Pain Bytes*[a,b,c,d]
• Magination Press book titles regarding pain[a,b,d]
• Coping Club website[a,b,c,d]
Interventions
• Relaxation-based biofeedback[d]
• Cognitive-behavioral therapy[b,c]
• Hynosis[a,b,c]
• Mindfulness Based/Acceptance and Commitment Therapy[b,c]
• WebMap Mobile Application[b,c]
• Children's Health and Illness Recovery Program (CHIRP)[b,c]
• Fibroguide[b,c,d]

[a]Elementary school (6–10 years old)
[b]Middle school (11–14 years old)
[c]High school/early adult (15–20 years old)
[d]For additional information see online resource guide associated with this chapter

CL psychologists in the inpatient hospital setting should anticipate several common barriers to implementation of courses of evidence-based therapies commonly employed in pediatric pain clinics: (1) shortened length of stay (LOS) may prevent complete psychological interventions and treatment, (2) skepticism from patients and families about the necessity of conceptualization of their pain as chronic, and the psychologist's role in that care. The following section will describe relevant strategies to be most efficient and productive when encountering patients with pain on a hospital unit.

While LOS is short, hospital settings often provide access to numerous family and medical caregivers who can provide a wealth of information about the child's pain, which is not always readily available within an ambulatory setting. Participating in inpatient medical rounds; speaking with the patient's nurses, physicians, and ancillary care providers; observing the patient and family while hospitalized; and gathering information directly from the patient and family can provide an efficient multimodal evaluation (PROMIS measures).

Another set of barriers commonly encountered is surprise on the part of the patient that a psychologist is involved in their care. Patients may fear that a psychologist's involvement indicates the treatment team thinks their pain is made up, exaggerated, or, worse yet, "all in their head." This is a considerable barrier that pediatric psychologists on interdisciplinary teams frequently encounter. With practice, one can learn to respond to this with patience, reassurance, empathy, and sometimes well-placed humor. Additionally, when other professionals normalize the inclusion of mental health professionals, with phrasing like "this is how we treat pain here" or "pain is very complex and it requires professionals with many different skills to treat effectively," "the pain psychologist is a specialist who can help your child and our team provide the best possible care," or "dealing with pain can be very challenging and we want to ensure that your child's emotional health is considered when treating their illness," patients and families are more welcoming to the CL psychologist. CL psychologists need to ensure they provide the team with value-added content, e.g., targeted training by psychologists regarding topics like how to use motivational interviewing, how to use screening for depression, and how to talk to families about difficult topics like somatic symptoms or trauma. Additionally, CL psychologists can talk with the patient and family about how the emotional experience of pain is shaped by thoughts and emotions, not caused by them, to help allay fears that their pain is going to be minimized or dismissed by the team as simply fabricated. Finally, educating patients as to the scope and limits of the interventions, which is focused on pain and working toward discharge, can be helpful in reducing defensiveness. For example, topics like parental complex trauma, parental pain, and problematic peer relationships the patient has at school, while important to note, will be unlikely to be resolved while in the hospital, but should be noted in documentation and longer-term treatment plans. Deep and extended inquiries into these issues with the patient and family may overwhelm the patient and diminish rapport while serving no clear immediate purpose. As a consultant, your role is to build rapport with the family, assess their psychological needs, and provide initial interventions flexibly. The goal is generally to increase the likelihood that patients will follow up with psychological care after discharge. This is especially important for highly complex care that will require intense follow-up such as within a pediatric pain clinic or pediatric pain rehabilitation center.

Transition to Outpatient Care

Interdisciplinary collaboration is crucial to the successful outcome of an inpatient admission for pediatric chronic pain. The roles of the inpatient providers may vary based on the goals of the admission; however, they will likely include diagnosis and conceptualization of the presenting concern and developing a comprehensive plan for treatment. Typically, once competing diagnoses are eliminated, the CL psychologist can be instrumental in shifting the conversation with the patient and his or her family in the direction of rehabilitation. The clinician should help the family and the medical team validate the patient's pain while emphasizing the importance of developing a plan for restoring functioning. Specifically, after the evaluation is complete, the CL psychologist can begin preliminary intervention steps to set up the patient for continuing to progress in the outpatient setting. This likely includes educating the medical team and the family about chronic pain, including the biopsychosocial model, and the rationale and expectations for treatment. For instance, we have found inpatient-referred patients who are the most successful in our outpatient treatment programs have a strong foundation in understanding the nature of chronic pain, how function may improve before pain reduction occurs, and that any improvement will be the result of hard work and persistence to accomplish improved functioning. Effective communication, through visual depictions and metaphors, is especially important at this stage. A secondary focus of this preliminary intervention can be a brief introduction to coping techniques, such as developing a plan for a daily schedule at home after discharge, simple relaxation or distraction techniques, and parent management training. Finally, an important role for the CL psychologist will be the referral to an appropriate outpatient treatment program. Pediatric pain-focused treatment programs are constantly emerging and can vary considerably in which services are offered. An annually updated list of recognized programs for the United States and Canada can be found on the IASP Special Interest Group on Pain In Childhood's website.

Presence of clinician expertise and assurance of key environmental factors can facilitate optimal intervention for chronic pain in the inpatient consultation-liaison role. The clinician should be knowledgeable on the biopsychosocial model of pain and developmental factors related to pain presentations (Palermo, Valrie, & Karlson, 2014). Though comfort in flexibly applying psychosocial treatments for pain based on developmental appropriateness is paramount (Palermo, Eccleston, Lewandowski, Williams, & Morley, 2010), some foundational knowledge on medical aspects of painful conditions as well as medical treatments for pain can increase the clinician's conceptualization and communication regarding the intervention (see section entitled "Medical Basics" for details). To facilitate the intervention, ensuring the patient's room is quiet and has restrictions on interruptions by staff and other visitors is crucial to the sensitive discussion regarding concerns of chronic pain and especially essential for particular interventions such as relaxation training and biofeedback. The clinician should ensure parental or caregiver presence as developmentally appropriate, but clearly understand the role of systems theory here, that there may be powerful forces at play to keep the system in its current state, e.g., child and parent's separation anxiety could work to reduce parental insistence of school return. For instance, interventions for younger patients will likely focus on parent education and training, whereas interventions for adolescents may include relaxation and cognitive coping skills that can be taught individually to the patient and then reviewed with the parent for support. Supplementing and reinforcing concepts and skills with handouts and technological equipment (e.g., portable HRV or GSR devices) can be of assistance, particularly when concepts and skills are new to the patient and family, to facilitate engagement with treatment approach and practice of skills in the clinician's absence. For instance, depictions of the biopsychosocial model of pain, notes on relaxation instructions, worksheets on challenging cognitive distortions or meeting goals, or web applications for relaxation can be useful. Finally, informing the medical team of concepts and interventions taught can be helpful so that the medical team can continue to review and reinforce these throughout the patient's inpatient stay.

Outpatient Consultation

This section will address consultation in outpatient specialty and primary care clinics and coordination with outpatient mental health resources. In the case of patients seen initially for consultation in the hospital, this section will address next steps after discharge, e.g., short-term follow-up by the CL team.

Most cases of inpatient medical admission regarding chronic pain among children will require long-term follow-up for generalization and advancement of pain coping skills. Steps after discharge will be based on the particular needs of the patient and should be determined by the CL clinician in collaboration with other treatment providers, such as physicians and physical therapists. If the patient presents significant safety risks, such as suicidal ideation, a general psychiatry admission is likely indicated to stabilize these factors prior to any pain-focused treatment. Alternatively, if there is significant psychiatric comorbidity alongside pain concerns, a medical-psychiatric unit may be advisable. When primary concerns are related to pain, the CL clinician should match the level of services to the child's needs. In cases where disability levels are high, inpatient rehabilitation care may be indicated, available at a growing number of sites in the country. Increasing evidence supports the interdisciplinary intensive rehabilitation occurring within these programs that are designed to improve functioning, increase activity, and foster coping with pain (Hechler et al., 2015; Simons, Sieberg,

Pielech, Conroy, & Logan, 2012). Several considerations should be made when considering an inpatient rehabilitation admission versus a less intensive partial or day hospital stay: first, ensuring the family and patient are willing to support this level of care, and, second, consideration of extent of disability, e.g., ambulatory status, missed days of school, and ability to attend to activities of daily living. Lack of adequate progress in less intensive services often helps build the case for more intense care. For moderate levels of disability, the CL clinician may be able to refer to an intensive outpatient program where available. Such programs typically last 2–4 weeks, include interdisciplinary treatment in a day program setting, but require family involvement ensuring adherence to program recommendations outside of treatment hours and have demonstrated effectiveness (Simons et al., 2012). Finally, if disability levels are milder, individual outpatient treatment may be appropriate, in which case the CL psychologist can refer to an outpatient psychologist trained in treating pediatric chronic pain, sometimes available through the tertiary care setting or based in the community. *Any* to *many* of these programs typically involve long waitlists. Therefore, in addition to providing a referral, the CL psychologist can provide short-term follow-up care to facilitate the transition of care, as well as providing consultation and collaboration with the next provider.

Case Example

Sickle cell disease is the most common genetic blood disease among individuals in North America. Though acute, vaso-occlusive pain episodes are one of the sentinel symptoms of sickle cell disease, individuals commonly experience acute on chronic pain, often complicating treatment for this disease (Dampier et al., 2017).

Lu is a 17-year-old male with a diagnosis of sickle cell disease Hgb SS who experienced early complications of painful dactylitis, fevers, and chest pain requiring hospitalizations as a toddler. Currently, he is maintained on hydroxyurea, glutamine, methadone, and morphine, but due to frequent hospitalizations (6–8/year) lasting several days up to 2 weeks' duration, his team has growing concerns about his adherence and treatment efficacy (e.g., escalation of ED visits and hospitalizations, early requests for medication refills of his opioid medications, frequent inconsistencies in his report of medication use, stories of losing his medications, and negative urine screens for medications he was prescribed).

Psychosocial complications navigated by his team included his immigrant parents' status from a predominantly Muslim country of origin, his adherence to fasts during Ramadan which make taking maintenance doses of hydroxyurea difficult, and the death of his father during Lu's early years of life, living with his sister, her husband, and several children, while being away from his mother and brother who live in a large urban area on the west coast of the USA. The distance from his mother and difficult dynamics between him and his sister at times cause a good deal of distress for Lu; e.g., when his sister perceives that Lu is non-adherent to his medications, she calls Lu's mother. Lu then worries that his mother's level of distress will be detrimental to her health and lead to her untimely death, like he experienced with his father.

Results of neuropsychological testing revealed an individual with overall IQ estimated in the mid to upper 70s on brief IQ measures (Kaufman Brief Intelligence Test). Naturally, the treatment team was concerned that he may not understand complex treatment regimens or complex verbal instructions that require extensive conditional problem-solving.

In this particular situation, a psychologist embedded within the Comprehensive Hemoglobinopathies clinic and the consultation-liaison psychologist within the Children's Hospital were a part of a larger team including a hematologist, clinic nurse, Acute Pain Service, Palliative Care staff, Child Life, and a complex care team care coordinator. Both psychologists taught and reinforced skills Lu learned in the Sickle Cell clinic visits and frequent hospitalizations. Relaxation training (diaphragmatic breathing, progressive muscle relaxation), thermal biofeedback-assisted relaxation therapy, Beverly Thorn's Literacy Modified Cognitive Behavioral Therapy manual, the Children's Health and Illness Recovery Program Patient and Family Workbook (CHIRP; Carter, Kronenberger, Scott, & Brady, 2020), and behavioral strategies for medication adherence, e.g., use of pill boxes, schedules, and cell phone alarms placed on his calendar, were all elements of his successful treatment.

Ultimately, Lu was referred to an intensive outpatient pediatric pain clinic where physical therapy, occupational therapy, psychotherapy, art therapy, and recreational therapy were able to work with him over a 3-week session. Upon discharge from the pain clinic, he resumed regular school attendance, was more physically active, and was experiencing less pain. The set-up for the transition from the hospital to the outpatient setting was crucial, and without it, the move to the intensive outpatient clinic would not have been as successful.

References

American Psychiatric Association. (2013). *Diagnositic and statistical manual of mental health disorders: DSM-5* (5th ed.). Washington, DC: American Psychiatric Publishing.

Auvinen, J., Tammelin, T., Taimela, S., Zitting, P., & Karppinen, J. (2008). Associations of physical activity and inactivity with low back pain in adolescents. *Scandinavian Journal of Medicine & Science in Sports, 18*(2), 188–194.

Brattberg, G. (2004). Do pain problems in young school children persist into early adulthood? A 13-year follow-up. *European Journal of Pain, 8*(3), 187–199.

Carter, B. D., Kronenberger, W. G., Scott, E. L., & Brady, C. (2020). *CHIRP: Children's health and illness recovery program: Patient and family workbook*. New York, NY: Oxford University Press.

Claar, R. L., Simons, L. E., & Logan, D. E. (2008). Parental response to children's pain: The moderating impact of children's emotional distress on symptoms and disability. *Pain, 138*(1), 172–179.

Coakley, R., & Schechter, N. (2013). Chronic pain is like... The clinical use of analogy and metaphor in the treatment of chronic pain in children. *Pediatric Pain Letter: Commentaries on Pain in Infants, Children, and Adolescents, 15*(1), 1–8.

Dampier, C., Palermo, T. M., Darbari, D. S., Hassell, K., Smith, W., & Zempsky, W. (2017). AAPT diagnostic criteria for chronic sickle cell disease pain. *The Journal of Pain, 18*(5), 490–498.

Eccleston, C., Palermo, T. M., de Williams, A. C., Lewandowski, A., Morley, S., Fisher, E., & Law, E. (2012). Psychological therapies for the management of chronic and recurrent pain in children and adolescents. *Cochrane Database of Systematic Reviews*, (12), CD003968.

El-Metwally, A., Salminen, J. J., Auvinen, A., Macfarlane, G., & Mikkelsson, M. (2007). Risk factors for development of non-specific musculoskeletal pain in preteens and early adolescents: A prospective 1-year follow-up study. *BMC Musculoskeletal Disorders, 8*, 46.

Fisher, E., Heathcote, L. C., Eccleston, C., Simons, L. E., & Palermo, T. M. (2018). Assessment of pain anxiety, pain catastrophizing, and fear of pain in children and adolescents with chronic pain: A systematic review and meta-analysis. *Journal of Pediatric Psychology, 43*(3), 314–325.

Gieteling, M. J., Bierma-Zeinstra, S. M., Passchier, J., & Berger, M. Y. (2008). Prognosis of chronic or recurrent abdominal pain in children. *Journal of Pediatric Gastroenterology and Nutrition, 47*(3), 316–326.

Groenewald, C. B., Essner, B. S., Wright, D., Fesinmeyer, M. D., & Palermo, T. M. (2014). The economic costs of chronic pain among a cohort of treatment-seeking adolescents in the United States. *The Journal of Pain, 15*(9), 925–933.

Hechler, T., Kanstrup, M., Holley, A. L., Simons, L. E., Wicksell, R., Hirschfeld, G., & Zernikow, B. (2015). Systematic review on intensive interdisciplinary pain treatment of children with chronic pain. *Pediatrics, 136*, 115–127.

Hoftun, G. B., Romundstad, P. R., & Rygg, M. (2013). Association of parental chronic pain with chronic pain in the adolescent and young adult: Family linkage data from the HUNT study. *JAMA Pediatrics, 167*(1), 61–69.

Huguet, A., & Miro, J. (2008). The severity of chronic pediatric pain: An epidemiological study. *The Journal of Pain, 9*(3), 226–236.

Kalapurakkel, S., Carpino, E. A., Lebel, A., & Simons, L. E. (2015). "Pain Can't Stop Me": Examining pain self-efficacy and acceptance as resilience processes among youth with chronic headache. *Journal of Pediatric Psychology, 40*(9), 926–933.

Kashikar-Zuck, S., Goldschneider, K. R., Powers, S. W., Vaught, M. H., & Hershey, A. D. (2001). Depression and functional disability in chronic pediatric pain. *The Clinical Journal of Pain, 17*(4), 341–349.

King, S., Chambers, C. T., Huguet, A., MacNevin, R. C., McGrath, P. J., Parker, L., & MacDonald, A. J. (2011). The epidemiology of chronic pain in children and adolescents revisited: A systematic review. *Pain, 152*(12), 2729–2738.

Law, E. F., Noel, M., Nagel, M. S., & Dahlquist, L. M. (2017). Chronic and recurrent pain. In M. C. Roberts & R. G. Steele (Eds.), *Handbook of pediatric psychology* (5th ed., pp. 134–145). New York, NY: The Guilford Press.

Lewandowski, A. S., Palermo, T. M., Stinson, J., Handley, S., & Chambers, C. T. (2010). Systematic review of family functioning in families of children and adolescents with chronic pain. *The Journal of Pain, 11*(11), 1027–1038.

Logan, D. E., Conroy, C., Sieberg, C. B., & Simons, L. E. (2012). Changes in willingness to self-manage pain among children and adolescents and their parents enrolled in an intensive interdisciplinary pediatric pain treatment program. *Pain, 153*(9), 1863–1870.

Logan, D. E., & Simons, L. E. (2010). Development of a group intervention to improve school functioning in adolescents with chronic pain and depressive symptoms: A study of feasibility and preliminary efficacy. *Journal of Pediatric Psychology, 35*(8), 823–836.

Melzack, R., & Wall, P. D. (1965). Pain mechanisms: A new theory. *Science, 150*(3699), 971–979.

Miller, M. M., Meints, S. M., & Hirsh, A. T. (2018). Catastrophizing, pain, and functional outcomes for children with chronic pain: A meta-analytic review. *Pain, 159*, 2442.

Miller, M. M., Scott, E. L., Trost, Z., & Hirsh, A. T. (2016). Perceived injustice is associated with pain and functional outcomes in children and adolescents with chronic pain: A preliminary examination. *The Journal of Pain, 17*(11), 1217–1226.

Miller, M. M., Wuest, D., Williams, A. E., Scott, E. L., Trost, Z., & Hirsh, A. T. (2018). Injustice perceptions about pain: Parent-child discordance is associated with worse functional outcomes. *Pain, 159*(6), 1083–1089.

Noel, M., Groenewald, C. B., Beals-Erickson, S. E., Gebert, J. T., & Palermo, T. M. (2016). Chronic pain in adolescence and internalizing mental health disorders: A nationally representative study. *Pain, 157*(6), 1333–1338.

Paananen, M. V., Taimela, S. P., Auvinen, J. P., Tammelin, T. H., Kantomaa, M. T., Ebeling, H. E.,... Karppinen, J. I. (2010). Risk factors for persistence of multiple musculoskeletal pains in adolescence: A 2-year follow-up study. *European Journal of Pain, 14*(10), 1026–1032.

Palermo, T. M. (2012). *Cognitive-behavioral therapy for chronic pain in children and adolescents*. New York, NY: Oxford University Press.

Palermo, T. M., Eccleston, C., Lewandowski, A. S., Williams, A. C., & Morley, S. (2010). Randomized controlled trials of psychological therapies for management of chronic pain in children and adolescents: An updated meta-analytic review. *Pain, 148*(3), 387–397.

Palermo, T. M., Valrie, C. R., & Karlson, C. W. (2014). Family and parent influences on pediatric chronic pain: A developmental perspective. *The American Psychologist, 69*(2), 142–152.

Palermo, T. M., Wilson, A. C., Peters, M., Lewandowski, A., & Somhegyi, H. (2009). Randomized controlled trial of an internet-delivered family cognitive-behavioral therapy intervention for children and adolescents with chronic pain. *Pain, 146*(1–2), 205–213.

Postier, A. C., Eull, D., Schulz, C., Fitzgerald, M., Symalla, B., Watson, D.,... Friedrichsdorf, S. J. (2018). Pain experience in a US children's hospital: A point prevalence survey undertaken after the implementation of a system-wide protocol to eliminate or decrease pain caused by needles. *Hospital Pediatrics, 8*, 515–523.

Price, D. D., & Bushnell, M. C. (2004). Overview of pain dimensions and thier psychological modulation. In D. D. Price & M. C. Bushnell (Eds.), Psychological methods of pain control: Basic science and clinical perspectives (Vol. Progress in Pain research and Management, Vol. 29). Seattle: IASP Press.

Rhudy, J. L., Williams, A. E., McCabe, K. M., Nguyen, M. A., & Rambo, P. (2005). Affective modulation of nociception at spinal and supraspinal levels. *Psychophysiology, 42*(5), 579–587.

Rosengren, D. B. (2018). *Building motivational interviewing skills: A practitioner workbook* (2nd ed.). New York, NY: The Guilford Press.

Sanders, S. H. (2002). Operant conditioning with chronic pain: Back to basics. In D. C. Turk & R. J. Gatchel (Eds.), *Psychological approaches to pain management: A practitioner's handbook* (2nd ed., pp. 128–137). New York, NY: The Guilford Press.

Simons, L. E., & Basch, M. C. (2016). State of the art in biobehavioral approaches to the management of chronic pain in childhood. *Pain Management, 6*(1), 49–61.

Simons, L. E., Sieberg, C. B., Carpino, E., Logan, D., & Berde, C. (2011). The fear of pain questionnaire (FOPQ): Assessment of pain-related fear among children and adolescents with chronic pain. *The Journal of Pain, 12*(6), 677–686.

Simons, L. E., Sieberg, C. B., Pielech, M., Conroy, C., & Logan, D. E. (2012). What does it take? Comparing intensive rehabilitation to outpatient treatment for children with significant pain-related disability. *Journal of Pediatric Psychology, 38*(2), 213–223.

Tegethoff, M., Belardi, A., Stalujanis, E., & Meinlschmidt, G. (2015). Comorbidity of mental disorders and chronic pain: Chronology of onset in adolescents of a National Representative Cohort. *The Journal of Pain, 16*(10), 1054–1064.

Valrie, C. R., Bromberg, M. H., Palermo, T., & Schanberg, L. E. (2013). A systematic review of sleep in pediatric pain populations. *Journal of Developmental and Behavioral Pediatrics, 34*(2), 120–128.

Vinall, J., Pavlova, M., Asmundson, G. J., Rasic, N., & Noel, M. (2016). Mental health comorbidities in pediatric chronic pain: A narrative review of epidemiology, models, neurobiological mechanisms and treatment. *Children (Basel), 3*(4), E40.

Walther-Larsen, S., Pedersen, M. T., Friis, S. M., Aagaard, G. B., Romsing, J., Jeppesen, E. M., & Friedrichsdorf, S. J. (2017). Pain prevalence in hospitalized children: A prospective cross-sectional survey in four Danish university hospitals. *Acta Anaesthesiologica Scandinavica, 61*, 328–337.

Williams, A. E., & Rhudy, J. L. (2009). Supraspinal modulation of trigeminal nociception and pain. *Headache, 49*(5), 704–720.

Wilson, A. C., Samuelson, B., & Palermo, T. M. (2010). Obesity in children and adolescents with chronic pain: Associations with pain and activity limitations. *The Clinical Journal of Pain, 26*(8), 705–711.

Woolf, C. J. (2011). Central sensitization: Implications for the diagnosis and treatment of pain. *Pain, 152*(3 Suppl), S2–S15.

Yarnitsky, D. (2010). Conditioned pain modulation (the diffuse noxious inhibitory control-like effect): Its relevance for acute and chronic pain states. *Current Opinion in Anaesthesiology, 23*(5), 611–615.

Somatic Symptom and Related Disorders

Sara E. Williams, Nicole E. Zahka, and Kristin A. Kullgren

Diagnosis

Somatic symptom and related disorders (SSRD) represent a problem that is truly at the intersection of medicine and psychology. Somatic symptoms are defined broadly as physical symptoms in the absence of identifiable disease (Sharpe & Carson, 2001); they rise to the level of a disorder when a patient's concern about symptoms causes psychological distress and associated impairment. A hallmark feature of SSRD is that they seem related to an underlying medical condition, yet no disease is identified, or if there is a comorbid medical condition, the patient is more distressed and impaired than what would be expected based on the medical diagnosis alone (Silber, 2011). As such, children and adolescents with SSRD have a unique presentation that involves psychological *and* physical components, yet most are likely to present in a medical (rather than psychological) setting. As somatic symptoms are common among children and adolescents, a consultation-liaison (CL) psychologist is likely to come across patients with this presentation in practice. A collaborative, integrated medical psychological approach is needed for successful diagnosis and treatment of SSRD.

Children and adolescents with somatic symptoms represent a heterogeneous population in presentation, course, and outcome. Adolescents more commonly present with SSRD than young children, more females than males, and more from Caucasian, non-Hispanic backgrounds than other racial and ethnic groups (Campo & Fritsch, 1994). Among pediatric patients seeking medical consultation, up to 50% are estimated to have "medically unexplained" symptoms, and a subset have associated functional and emotional impairments (Andresen et al., 2011). A majority of youth with SSRD have comorbid organic medical diagnoses, history of psychiatric treatment, and primary symptoms of pain or neurologic symptoms (Bujoreanu, Randall, Thomson, & Ibeziako, 2014).

The fifth edition of the *Diagnostic and Statistical Manual of Mental Disorders* (DSM-5) devotes a diagnostic category to somatic symptom and related disorders (SSRD) to classify patients with prominent somatic symptoms and related

S. E. Williams (✉)
Department of Pediatrics, University of Cincinnati College of Medicine, Cincinnati, OH, USA

Division of Behavioral Medicine and Clinical Psychology, Cincinnati Children's Hospital Medical Center, Cincinnati, OH, USA
e-mail: Sara.Williams@cchmc.org

N. E. Zahka
Division of Behavioral Medicine and Clinical Psychology, Cincinnati Children's Hospital Medical Center, Cincinnati, OH, USA

K. A. Kullgren
Department of Pediatrics, C.S. Mott Children's Hospital, Michigan Medicine, Ann Arbor, MI, USA

B. D. Carter, K. A. Kullgren (eds.), *Clinical Handbook of Psychological Consultation in Pediatric Medical Settings*, Issues in Clinical Child Psychology, https://doi.org/10.1007/978-3-030-35598-2_14

distress/impairment (American Psychiatric Association, 2013). The category includes seven diagnoses: somatic symptom disorder, illness anxiety disorder, conversion disorder (functional neurological symptom disorder), psychological factors affecting other medical conditions, factitious disorder, other specified somatic symptom and related disorder, and unspecified somatic symptom and related disorder. The conceptualization of SSRD diagnoses represents a significant revision compared to previous versions of the DSM in that it moves away from "medically unexplained" symptoms, a defining feature of former diagnoses of somatoform disorder or hypochondriasis (Rief & Martin, 2014). The new DSM classification, in contrast, makes clear that symptoms do *not* have to be medically unexplained for a patient to qualify for most SSRD diagnoses (except for conversion disorder and pseudocyesis, in the other specified SSRD category).

SSRD diagnoses require presence of abnormal distress and impairment related to the experience of somatic symptoms, lasting between 3 to 6 months. As such, it is possible for patients to have organic medical diagnoses *and* SSRD diagnoses if associated distress and impairment is excessive to that expected from disease progression. If normative concern is present and impairment is not excessive, the patient would *not* qualify for SSRD diagnoses. In a population based study, while 22.7% of adolescents reported somatic symptoms, fewer than half met criteria for SSRD (van Geelen, Rydelius, & Hagquist, 2015).

While the focus of this chapter is on the primary diagnosis in this category, somatic symptom disorder, there are several important notes regarding the other diagnoses. Brief somatic symptom disorders (fewer than 6 months) are captured in the other specific SSRD category. Illness anxiety was designed for individuals who have anxiety around health in general, beyond a specific symptom. The presence of psychological or behavioral factors negatively affecting physical health counts for psychological factors affecting other medical conditions. Finally, physical symptoms associated with SSRD are considered real and involuntary, such that patients are actually experiencing them, across all diagnostic categories *except* for factitious disorder. Overall, SSRD diagnoses in the DSM-5 more effectively account for the biological, psychological, and social factors that impact the symptom experience compared to similar diagnostic categories in prior iterations of the DSM, hopefully leading to more effective understanding and treatment of symptoms (Rief & Martin, 2014).

Medical Basics

Studies on the etiology of somatic symptoms point to contributions of biological, psychological, and social factors. Genetically, traits associated with alexithymia and anxiety are related to SSRD; there are also high rates of identical twin concordance (Ellenstein, Kranick, & Hallett, 2011; Silber, 2011). Neurologically, differences in white matter integrity in brain regions associated with body perception (e.g., somatosensory cortex), brain chemistry, and motor response are more pronounced in patients with SSRD compared to healthy controls (Aybek et al., 2015; Zhang et al., 2015). This "somatosensory amplification" in the brain may result from stress, early life trauma, and/or inflammation (Perez, Barsky, Vago, Baslet, & Silbersweig, 2015). Psychologically, although often causally implicated for somatic symptoms, rates of trauma are not significantly different between adolescents with SSRD and national norms (Thomson, Randall, Ibeziako, & Bujoreanu, 2014). Youth with SSRD demonstrate fewer adaptive coping strategies and more intense emotional responses to stress compared to healthy peers (Walker, Garber, & Greene, 1993). In addition, low self-worth, poor social competence, early onset mood disorder, as well as anxiety and depression are associated with SSRD; however, not all children with SSRD have mood disorders (Beck, 2007). Finally, social factors are associated with intergenerational transmission of illness; patients with SSRD are more likely to come from home environments where illness behavior is modeled and more healthcare utilization occurs (Van Tilburg et al., 2015).

Medicine has historically used nonspecific, symptom-based terminologies for symptoms in the absence of disease, which has resulted in variability and poorly described or validated diagnoses (Aaron & Buchwald, 2001). Recently, there has been a movement to create unified and descriptive diagnoses to improve identification and treatment of somatic symptoms. A largely agreed upon term is "functional disorder" to indicate that symptoms are the result of body system dysfunction rather than organic disease, which is better accepted by patients than previous terms that further propagated mind-body dualism, such as "all in the head," hysterical, psychosomatic, psychogenic, somatoform, medically unexplained, and depression or stress related (Stone et al., 2002). There are functional disorders in nearly every medical specialty, such as functional gait disorder and non-epileptic episodes in Neurology, irritable bowel syndrome and functional abdominal pain in Gastroenterology, and syncope and non-cardiac chest pain in Cardiology.

Medically, it is important to apply the same scientific rigor and clinical decision-making for diagnosing functional disorders as organic disease; it is not just a diagnosis of exclusion. Functional disorders are identified from a combination of positive signs (e.g., inconsistencies in presentation, presence of nonorganic symptoms) *and* the absence of disease markers (Stone, Carson, & Sharpe, 2005a). Less than 5% of patients with functional disorders later receive an organic diagnosis (Crimlisk et al., 1998). To ensure patients have an adequate understanding of their functional disorder, psychologists should be familiar with medical terminologies and teach patients about the diagnosis in collaboration with the medical team. For patients with comorbid organic disease, the medical provider should give patients a clear framework for when symptoms represent disease exacerbation versus functional disorders, as treatment response typically differs based on the cause of symptoms.

Engagement

The first step to engaging patients and families in biopsychosocial treatment for SSRD is establishing the diagnosis. The reassurance of the medical provider about the real but nonthreatening nature of symptoms is necessary for patients and families to buy into SSRD diagnoses and psychology treatment recommendations. Because most patients with SSRD present to a medical setting, medical questions must first be answered before psychological diagnoses and treatment are pursued. Ideally, a suspected SSRD diagnosis is communicated by the physician as being on the differential early in the medical workup. For a psychologist in a CL setting, collaborative communication with the medical team is essential to present a coordinated message to families to reduce confusion and increase adherence to treatment recommendations.

When explaining functional disorders and SSRD from a medical perspective, several factors lead to acceptance and successful engagement in treatment by patients and families. Physicians providing good explanations for symptoms and diagnoses, clearly stating there is no organic disease, and empathizing with suffering are beneficial to patients (Ring, Dowrick, Humphris, Davies, & Salmon, 2005). Providing a positive diagnosis (e.g., "you have a functional disorder") and explanation of symptoms is associated with better patient outcomes compared to absence of a diagnosis (e.g., "we don't know what's wrong with you") (Stone et al., 2005a). Patients with SSRD show higher satisfaction, improved well-being, and reduced healthcare utilization when a positive diagnosis is received from a provider who helped them feel empowered, compared to providers who rejected the reality of symptoms or supported a dualistic mind versus body viewpoint (Salmon, Peters, & Stanley, 1999).

There are five basic tenets for medical providers and psychologists to follow when making a functional disorder or SSRD diagnosis: (1) explain what patients DO have based on symptom presentation (i.e., make a positive diagnosis versus stating the absence of a diagnosis); (2) tell them what they DON'T have based on diagnoses of exclusion (e.g., "the good news is that it's not epilepsy or cancer"); (3) show BELIEF in symptoms and disability, both in terms of showing empathy and explaining diagnoses (i.e., use metaphors like "it's a software problem, not a hardware problem" or "the fire is out but the alarm is still ringing"); (4) explain how COMMON functional symptoms are so patients know they are not alone; and (5) talk about treatments that DO work such as cognitive behavioral therapy (CBT), physical therapy (PT), and medical management (Stone, Carson, & Sharpe, 2005b). Overall, when everyone talks about symptoms and diagnoses in the same positive way, patients' outcomes improve (Sharpe & Carson, 2001).

Formulation

Once the diagnosis has been established and patients have been given a biopsychosocial understanding of symptoms from a medical standpoint, the psychologist can begin to conduct a psychological assessment. For many patients with somatic symptoms, the first time they encounter a psychologist is during a medical encounter. This puts the psychologist in a powerful position to provide patients and family with further education about the medical diagnosis in the context of the biopsychosocial model, conduct a medically sensitive psychological assessment, and set the stage for the importance of a functional approach to symptoms through CBT.

Building on the medical explanation for symptom onset, persistence, and impairment for patients with somatic symptoms, the psychologist's initial assessment and formulation should similarly focus on the patient's experience of, rather than causes for, symptoms. Depending on patients' status at the time of assessment, they may have been asked many times about what stressors caused their symptoms. Unfortunately, this common question emphasizes mind-body dualism and does not consider biological or social factors in the symptom experience. As these patients present with physical symptoms (not psychological complaints or social difficulties), it is important to tailor the assessment to the presenting problem—physical symptoms—first and then assess for other potentially contributing psychological and social factors. This validates the patients' concerns, reduces defensiveness about psychological factors that may be present, and increases the likelihood of formulating an accurate and effective case conceptualization and treatment plan. Biologically, focus questions on symptom pattern, frequency, duration, any alleviating/exacerbating factors, impact on sleep, and level of impairment. Psychologically, assess thoughts and feelings about symptoms (e.g., associated worries or sadness, changes in mood), in addition to historical symptoms of anxiety, depression, or other emotional/behavioral concerns. Although it is important to assess for trauma, as it is with any patient, it is also important to dispel the myth that SSRD are always, or even often, associated with trauma. Socially, assess functioning among family, peers, and school, and gain history into any preexisting learning or social challenges. Formal assessment measures may also be used to further investigate symptoms, disability, psychological comorbidities, and coping (Malas, Ortiz-Aguayo, Giles, & Ibeziako, 2017; Williams & Zahka, 2017).

Upon completion of the assessment, the psychologist, alone or in tandem with the medical team, can share the findings, including delivering a SSRD diagnosis to patients and families in a way that furthers buy-in to the diagnosis through use of the biopsychosocial model. Specific points that may aid in this explanation include stating belief in the reality of the symptoms, validating the impairment and distress associated with symptoms that have been confusing and hard to understand, and summarizing this presentation as captured by the SSRD diagnosis. Defensiveness about the diagnosis may be encountered based on several factors (e.g., previous medical experiences, unclear provider communication, dismissed symptoms, length of time to diagnosis). Candid conversations about family concerns and confusion or misinformation about the diagnosis are powerful to help patients and families accept the diagnosis, engage in CBT, and ultimately focus on returning patients to function. Even saying "I wonder if you're worried about talking to a psychologist because that means you might be crazy" can have a positive effect; if the clinician is able to say out loud what everyone may be thinking, it diffuses tension and allows for open communication, which can move treatment forward productively. Children may qualify for other psychological disorders (e.g., generalized anxiety disorder) in addition to SSRD, in which case it is important to make those diagnoses and treatment recommendations too, as unidentified and untreated comorbid psychological conditions negatively affect SSRD.

To better understand SSRD and their treatment, patients and families benefit from learning about the cognitive model (i.e., relation between thoughts, feelings, body responses, and actions) with a specific focus on body responses and the biology of the autonomic nervous system, as it provides a relatable explanation for *how* the mind-body connection results in intensification and maintenance of somatic symptoms. A useful analogy for describing the autonomic nervous system (ANS) is a comparison to the engine in a car, controlling the body's speed. The ANS is the body's engine and communication system between the brain and body; it controls involuntary body responses like breathing, heart rate, muscle tension, and digestion. The ANS has two branches, the sympathetic nervous system, or the body's gas pedal, and the parasympathetic nervous system, or the body's brake pedal. In response to a stressor (physical or emotional), the brain sends a message via the sympathetic nervous system to "hit the gas," activating the fight-or-flight response which leads to physical changes like increased heart and breathing rates, blood vessel constriction, muscle tension, inhibited digestion, and sweat production, and emotional changes like anxiety or fear, all designed to get the person away from or deal with the stressor. When the "danger" has passed, the brain "hits the brakes," by activating the rest-and-digest response via the parasympathetic nervous system, leading to decreased heart and breathing rates, blood vessel dilation, relaxed muscles, promotion of digestion, reduced sweat production, and lower anxiety. Without voluntary direction, the brain and the body effectively work together in a coordinated set of responses to respond to stressors and keep a person safe. However, when a patient has somatic symptoms, the ANS is dysregulated, the sympathetic nervous system is overactive, and the brain and the body are not working together efficiently. In fact, among patients with SSRD, the ANS has been found to react more intensely to perceived threat and does not habituate over time to stressors (Chrousos, 2009). In other words, in the presence or *even just in anticipation* of a stressor, the patient's ANS puts the gas pedal to the floor and goes careening down the highway, missing all signals that the danger has passed or was never even there, and forgets all about the brakes. As a result, symptoms are intense and unpleasant, and it gets harder for the system to regulate itself, leading to chronic sympathetic nervous system activation, persistent symptoms, and increased impairment.

Even for patients without comorbid anxiety, it is natural for worries to crop up related to ever-present symptoms as part of the sympathetic activation process. The irony is that worry only further activates the sympathetic nervous system, and as a result, the same symptoms patients worry about are more likely to happen. An analogy for the role of anticipatory anxiety is the experience of food poisoning; almost everyone has eaten something that did not agree with them, and now the mere thought of eating that food again results in a queasy feeling. Similarly, just paying attention to an itch intensifies the physical discomfort associated with that signal. Over time, the more patients pay attention to and anticipate symptoms, the more intense the symptoms and the more function is impacted. For these reasons, education about the ANS and corresponding analogies to illustrate the mind-body connection help patients and families understand why symptoms are happening, how they are maintained in a negative feedback loop, and, most importantly, set the stage for how they can be treated.

Intervention

With medical and psychological conceptualizations in place, a description of CBT can follow naturally as a way to understand how maladaptive thoughts, feelings, and actions influence symptoms and biological processes and how changing those patterns can regulate the ANS, improve function, and reduce impairment. Another way of positively presenting CBT is: "Essentially…an extension of the [biopsychosocial] explanation, a way of helping the patient to become aware of, examine, and if appropriate revise the way they think, respond emotionally and behave in response to symptoms. The aim is to maximize function and reduce symptoms—but not necessarily to abolish them. In formal CBT the patient meets a therapist every 1 or 2 weeks and practices new ways of thinking about and responding to their symptoms between these sessions" (Stone et al., 2016, p. i15). In this way, patients and families understand *how* CBT works, to address the mind-body connection in an active way to improve function and manage symptoms.

Clinically, there are a variety of ways in which CBT applies to patients with SSRD. A patient who presents with a functional abdominal pain and SSRD would likely work on thoughts and feelings related to and associated with pain episodes, with a focus on reduction of worry and anticipatory anxiety from the cognitive standpoint and learning relaxation strategies and distraction from a behavioral standpoint, while reinforcing functional participation in daily life. A patient who presents with a functional gait disorder and SSRD would likely work on thoughts and feelings related to disability, underlying stressors, and breaking the cycle of reinforcement of disability that has developed between the brain and the body by using reinforcement for behaviors that are desired (e.g., walking).

There is a strong evidence base for CBT in adults with SSRD and growing evidence in pediatric populations. A review of randomized control trials found CBT as the only and most effective treatment for adults with SSRD (Kroenke, 2007). Patients introduced to CBT through inpatient CL services are more motivated and likely to follow up with outpatient therapy after discharge from acute care (Schweickhardt, Larisch, Wirsching, & Fritzsche, 2007). Among children and adolescents with SSRD, PT alone was not successful in restoring functioning and reducing symptoms (FitzGerald, Southby, Haines, Hough, & Skinner, 2015). Several CBT protocols addressing unhelpful appraisals and distorted beliefs about symptoms were found to be feasible and efficacious among youth with SSRD (Carter, Kronenberger, Threlkeld, Townsend, & Pruitt, 2013; Whalley & Cane, 2017). Several mechanisms by which CBT works have been identified, including psychological changes (cognitive modification and improvements in perceptions of illness) and biological changes (improvements in gray matter and functional connectivity in somatically focused brain regions) (Christensen, Frostholm, Ørnbøl, & Schröder, 2015; Erpelding et al., 2016).

Adaptation

Evidence-based CBT for SSRD can and should be modified to fit the treatment setting, from a clinician having one point of contact during a medical clinic visit, to multiple visits during a hospitalization, to seeing patients on an ongoing outpatient basis. The core features of CBT for SSRD are psychoeducation, establishing a functional routine, behavioral strategies, and cognitive strategies. Psychoeducation is often provided during the diagnostic and assessment process for patients while in the hospital, during a clinic visit, or at the first outpatient session, as previously described in the formulation section. Functional, behavioral, and cognitive strategies should be taught to patients and families only *after* education is provided to ensure understanding and buy-in to the intervention. Strategies can be tailored to greatest area of need and delivered as time and treatment setting allows. This results in a flexible treatment approach that can be delivered in a sequence that makes the most sense for each patient. CBT techniques are used to improve function and build more adaptive coping with symptoms.

The first phase of CBT for SSRD is establishing a functional routine, including restoration of healthy habits. Information can be delivered in a one-time consult or it can be part of a multi-session intervention in an inpatient or outpatient setting. Symptoms and impairment that accompany SSRD often lead to significant disruption in patients' daily activities. They may have difficulty sleeping due to pain and difficulty walking due to a functional gait disorder or experience non-epileptic episodes that impact their ability to stay at school for a full day. Patients should adhere to a good sleep hygiene routine that allows for an adequate and consistent amount of sleep (about 8–10 h), as well as to be awake and out of bed during the day. They should eat on a regular schedule and remain well-hydrated (64–100 ounces of non-caffeinated beverages per day). Generally, an hour of physical activity is recommended, which can be a challenge for mobility-impaired patients to achieve. Psychologists should collaborate with other providers (e.g., physician, physical therapist) to achieve movement goals safely and realistically.

In addition, patients should keep a consistent daily schedule as an aid to functional restoration. This can be introduced in a clinic consultation or outpatient care for a family to follow at home or set up for patients during an inpatient admission. Once anchor points are established (e.g., sleep, school, meals), the rest of the schedule should be filled in with necessary activities (e.g., chores, exercise, homework) as well as pleasant or distracting activities that can also serve as rewards for positive function. A schedule provides a concrete structure for patients to begin the "how" of reducing their impairment by learning to say "it's time to..." rather than "do I feel like..." to shift attention away from symptoms and toward function.

Behavioral and cognitive strategies are best suited for patients who are seen more than just in consultation, either through short-term inpatient or longer-term outpatient intervention. Behavioral strategies for patients with SSRD act as coping tools to manage stressors, either external or internal (e.g., symptoms). It is important to note that for patients with SSRD, the word "stress" gets thrown around casually and often sends the wrong message, as "stress" is most commonly thought of as an emotional construct. Many patients with SSRD say they are not stressed due to the assumption of emotional stress, poor recognition of physical and emotional cues, or misattribution of cues (e.g., a queasy stomach before a big test represents food poisoning rather than anxiety). Because of variability in patients' understanding of "stress," it is necessary to both define and discuss it. Most patients admit to being overtired, overworked, and underhydrated which provides an opening to discuss the impact of different types of stressors on the brain, body, and ANS.

Behavioral strategies include distracting activities (i.e., directing attention away from symptoms through pleasant activities) and relaxation (e.g., diaphragmatic breathing, guided imagery, progressive muscle relaxation). Mindfulness and sensory grounding techniques share the goal of focusing attention purposefully *and* aiding in relaxation or "hitting the brakes." Biofeedback aids in delivery of behavioral strategies, as it empowers patients to see that they can change their body responses and visualize improved regulation of the ANS.

Finally, cognitive strategies are delivered and include emotion identification, reframing, attention bias, problem-solving, and goal setting. While a functional approach should drive intervention for SSRD, many a seasoned clinician has been sidelined by not paying enough attention to the emotional aspects of a patient's presentation. Sometimes in the effort to reassure patients that symptoms are not all in their heads, emotions may not get as much attention as they should. Functioning helps day-to-day management of symptoms and is an important first step; however, for all patients, especially those with more treatment-resistant presentations or strong emotions that may be contributing to or driving symptoms, emotions must also be addressed. Patients with SSRD sometimes have a hard time identifying even basic emotions and benefit from direct instruction about emotional constructs, including associated physical effects. Symptoms may be symbolic of psychological distress (e.g., a teenager who does not want to run track presents with leg paralysis). Asking patients "If you didn't have your symptoms, what would be the next biggest problem?" can help identify emotional challenges.

Whether or not patients have comorbid mood disorders, a natural increase in negative thinking and emotions occurs (and is necessary) in the experience of somatic symptoms. Or, negative thinking may not be related to symptoms but to something else entirely (e.g., falling behind in school), which still leads to increased symptoms and negative emotions. Cognitive reframing applies in both cases; teach patients to catch automatic negative thoughts and challenge them by generating more realistic or positive thoughts to improve emotions and symptom experiences. Standard cognitive reframing materials or worksheets can be modified to integrate body responses into the cognitive triad to show how thoughts, feelings, actions, and symptoms influence one another. Negative attention bias is a powerful concept to share with patients; when they anticipate a negative outcome related to symptoms, they are more likely to notice bodily cues and perceive threats as dangerous, rather than think adaptively about those cues, or notice positive/neutral cues. Finally, patients can be taught to problem-solve as a way of integrating their treatment knowledge to choose among the best functional, behavioral, and/or cognitive strategies when faced with stressors. It is useful to pull from the assessment to set goals for patients to work toward, such as returning to school, sports, or social activities.

Resources/Support

Guidelines for adults and schools supporting children with SSRD are helpful resources to provide during treatment. The desired support from adults is a *decreased* focus on symptoms and an *increased* focus on function so as not to further medicalize the condition and promote the child's functional return to all realms of life. For most adults, school personnel, and community members, this feels counterintuitive, as a typical response to children struggling with symptoms is to inquire about health, allow rest, and excuse from activities. Because of this, it is critical for clinicians working with patients with SSRD to provide education and support to families, school, and community so that the interventions children receive in treatment are supported in and outside of the home to reach true overall success.

Parents are typically the most accessible group to include in intervention, as they often accompany children to treatment. In a consult setting, it is important to provide at least basic reassurance for parents to allow children to function normally; in inpatient and outpatient intervention, consider devoting a full session to parent intervention. Children with SSRD are likely to have parents with histories of anxiety and somatic symptoms, which may make parents more sensitive and reactive to children's symptoms (Garber, Zeman, & Walker, 1990). Caregivers benefit from concrete tips on how to interact with children around symptoms, including five general concepts: (1) encourage normal activity with no special treatment if activity reduction is needed; (2) tolerate distress, both the child's and adult's; (3) do not ask about symptoms, and instead encourage use of coping skills when the child is struggling; (4) praise effort rather than outcome for functioning, and focus on what children *can* do; and (5) respond flexibly, because there is no one best solution to any problem (Williams & Zahka, 2017). In addition to a parent-focused session, when possible, include parents at the end of child-focused sessions to discuss how the family will support the child in practicing coping skills, such as asking "what will make it hard to do?" and "what might make it easier?"

School attendance is often challenging for children with SSRD, which makes it necessary to create a plan for school reentry as well as communicate with school personal to address any apprehension or uncertainty about supporting students in the school setting. Without the right information and plan, schools may unintentionally undo progress made in treatment by responding to symptoms as if they are a dangerous, acute medical event (e.g., call parents, call 911, not allow the child back), thereby reinforcing the cycle of symptoms and disability. It can be helpful for the clinician to create a template that describes SSRD generally (with space for specific information about a patient's specific presentation) and outlines that school attendance is expected as part of functional restoration, along with a list of suggested accommodations (Williams & Zahka, 2017). Common accommodations include: being allowed to carry a water bottle, have access to snacks, elevator pass if not able to use the stairs safely, self-modified activity in gym class, unlimited access to the bathroom, quiet place to engage in relaxation, extended time on tests, modified assignments, and extra time to make up missed work. It is important to communicate with the school that the child may show some variability in symptoms; they may be better able to distract themselves from their symptoms during less stressful times, such as during a favorite class, and may focus more on their symptoms and experience greater impairment during stressful times, such as during a test; however, this does not mean that the symptoms are voluntary or that the child is making them up. When possible, the clinician may attend a school planning meeting in person or by phone to address any concerns of the staff. Parents can request a 504 Plan or Individualized Education Program (IEP) to address accommodations more formally as necessary.

The Inpatient Setting

In the inpatient CL setting, there is a delicate balance between conducting a thorough biopsychosocial evaluation while taking care not to inadvertently reinforce an organic illness conceptualization via a lengthy medical admission with potentially low-yield medical interventions. As such, time is of the essence and the sooner that all relevant consultants (e.g., psychology, psychiatry, physical therapist, occupational therapist, subspecialists) can evaluate the patient, the better. Generally, psychology and/or psychiatry be consulted as soon as SSRD is on the differential, rather than waiting until the medical evaluation is complete. Ultimately, the best course to recovery takes place as an outpatient where return to typical function is the primary treatment goal, which cannot be met fully in the hospital. For patients where a safe return home is of concern (e.g., unable to ambulate) a targeted inpatient admission may be warranted (see case example). Otherwise, the goals of the inpatient admission are as follows: (1) complete a thorough biopsychosocial workup; (2) inform the family of the diagnosis, conceptualization, and treatment plan; (3) offer one or two brief intervention sessions for symptom management as a bridge to outpatient care (e.g., diaphragmatic breathing, return to school plan, daily schedule); and (4) facilitate outpatient care. As illustrated in the case example presented below, the CL psychologist plays a powerful role in setting the foundation for successful and collaborative treatment of SSRD.

When providing biopsychosocial assessment in the inpatient setting, communication about the diagnosis should follow the process as discussed earlier, but with the additional consideration for consistency in messaging across providers, such as holding a care conference with the family, collaborating medical providers, and the community pediatrician. A care conference is often a primary intervention for an inpatient admission, as it sets the foundation for interventions and focuses on a return to function. In many inpatient settings, the CL psychologist may not be able to conduct the course of outpatient care due to patient distance from the hospital, different area of expertise, or lack of outpatient clinic availability. Finding appropriate outpatient providers can be challenging, as many outpatient therapists lack confidence or experience in SSRD. Finding a local therapist who is able to perform CBT and willing to learn about SSRD treatment can be sufficient if the CL psychologist can provide consultation and treatment manual recommendations (Williams & Zahka, 2017).

The Outpatient Setting

The outpatient consultation setting has its own unique set of challenges. Psychologists consulting in multidisciplinary or primary care clinics may or may not have access to the same resources available to inpatient psychologists, such as access to and collaboration with other care providers (e.g., physical therapist, psychiatry) or access to the results of a medical workup. Regardless, collaboration with medical providers whether in person or through other communication is crucial to provide the family with an accurate diagnosis and treatment plan. If the patient will only have a one-time clinic visit, this could mirror the inpatient CL workup as discussed above. Depending on time constraints, the psychologist's only interventions may be the presentation of the diagnosis and resources. In this case, providing the family with supplementary reading materials or directing them to information regarding general coping strategies can be useful (see handouts). When the psychologist may have multiple contacts with the patient through subsequent multidisciplinary clinic visits or brief treatment, the interventions might be broken down by session as described above. The outpatient CL psychologist may consider transfer of care to a psychologist with a more flexible outpatient schedule to provide longer-term intervention, maintain gains, and/or address comorbid mental health concerns that may affect the SSRD presentation. Collaboration with the medical team and any other treating providers is key throughout to ensure consistent messaging across providers.

Case Example

An 11-year-old female presented to an outpatient neurology medical clinic for sudden onset leg weakness and difficulty walking. Previous history was significant for functional abdominal pain at age 9 and a recent bout of viral meningitis; otherwise she was healthy and typically developing. At the Neurology visit, the patient reported feeling like she was going to fall and had leg pain that worsened with walking. She also reported headache, fatigue, poor concentration, muscle soreness, weakness, poor appetite, and stomach pain. The exam was inconsistent, with findings of decreased temperature and sensation to mid shins, decreased vibratory sense of big toes, exaggerated reflexes of the right leg, and unusual gait (wide stance, unsteady). Diagnostic differential was postinfectious sensory neuropathy or central process of spinal cord. She was admitted to the inpatient Neurology service for further assessment.

During the inpatient stay, other inconsistencies were found, including intact reflexes, and sensation to touch and vibration, but not to temperature or pinprick from knee down. A normal MRI was reviewed. The physical therapist noted that the patient could walk appropriately when distracted. The patient was diagnosed with conversion disorder and discharged with outpatient Psychology and PT referrals. However, she returned to the pediatrician and hospital with worsening symptoms. Further testing ruled out other organic medical disorders. When she presented to the emergency room with a complete inability to walk, she was admitted to the hospital a third time.

At this point, a comprehensive, interdisciplinary approach was adopted, including CL Psychology and PT. In the psychological assessment, the patient did not identify a stressor associated with symptoms, though she maintained a high level of activity in athletic, social, and academic realms. She denied worry about symptoms and had difficulty identifying emotions in general. She disclosed a history of bullying and sibling conflict. The psychologist agreed with the conversion disorder diagnosis and provided further education to the patient and family.

The psychologist began intervention with a focus on functional restoration. First, a goal sheet was developed for the patient to earn rewards by following a daily schedule, reinforced by staff. Behavioral and cognitive interventions were taught, including diaphragmatic breathing, distraction, and cognitive restructuring to regulate emotions and symptoms. She and the family learned to identify stressors, including how her family needed to change to support her at home. Parent training was conducted to reinforce age-appropriate activities and effectively set limits.

Through this coordinated inpatient intervention, the patient made significant progress over the course of a week to ambulate appropriately and displayed greater awareness of how thoughts, feelings, actions, and family dynamics affected symptoms. The team communicated with the outpatient psychologist and physical therapist prior to discharge to ensure that the progress was maintained with unified treatment goals. During subsequent outpatient treatment, the patient and family remarked on how helpful the inpatient intervention was in terms of understanding patient's diagnosis, treatment goals, and recovery. The patient's gait continued to improve and she was eventually able to walk completely normally; although she experienced symptom flares from time to time, they typically resolved within a few days. The patient became aware of longstanding perfectionism, anxiety, and attention difficulty. She was referred to a psychiatrist for management of mood, which further aided her functional improvement.

Overall, this case example is a good representation of successful, coordinated care of a patient with functional somatic symptoms. There were multiple factors that contributed to her eventual success, including appropriate diagnostic workup, consistent and clear messages from the treatment team regarding the functional nature of her symptoms, involvement of CL Psychology and PT, family engagement, and coordination of care with outpatient providers. While common for multiple medical evaluations/hospitalizations to occur before adoption of an interdisciplinary approach, the patient and family would likely have benefitted from CL Psychology and PT involvement during the first hospitalization.

Appendix

Handout 1: Coping Skills Resource List

Start by taking good care of your body and keeping a daily routine every day of the week.

Hydration—*64–100 oz. fluids per day* Plant Nanny Waterlogged Daily Water Tracker Reminder	**Activity Pacing**—*daily schedule with time for activities and breaks* Schedule template: https://templates.office.com/en-au/Student-schedule-TM00000023 Google Calendar 24Me
Exercise—*1 h per day* My Fitness Pal Pocket Yoga Johnson & Johnson Official 7 min Workout Runkeeper Super Stretch Yoga	**Nutrition**—*well-balanced, consistent meals* Choose My Plate: https://www.choosemyplate.gov/ **Sleep**—*8–10 h per night, same bedtime and wake time with about an hour flex* White Noise Lite CBT-I Coach Relax Melodies: Sleep Sounds

Prevent, reduce, or manage impairment related to your symptoms by using your coping skills. You can change what you're doing, how you're thinking, or both. Try doing a favorite activity, taking some time to relax, or thinking in a neutral and realistic way

Diaphragmatic Breathing Learn the diaphragmatic breathing technique: https://www.youtube.com/watch?v=kgTL5G1ibIo Breathe2Relax Breathing Zone Breathe + Simple Breath Trainer (iTunes)	**Relaxation** GoNoodle—movement and mindfulness: https://www.gonoodle.com/ Stop Breathe & Think Stop Breathe & Think Kids Calm Headspace: Guided Meditation and Mindfulness Insight Timer-Meditation App
Biofeedback Heart Math Inner Balance: https://store.heartmath.com/innerbalance Belly Bio Interactive Breathing (iTunes) BreathMix (Google Play)	**Distracting Activities** Play a game, watch a show, do a craft, take a walk, text a friend, make a list, plan a party, look through photos, watch a funny video, listen to music, play iSpy
Thinking Strategies If you notice you're stuck in a negative thinking trap, ask yourself: "How likely is that to happen?" "Am I thinking too far ahead?" "What can I do to change that?" What's Up	**Coping Skills** Pacifica Virtual Hope Box Booster Buddy Mindshift Clear Fear WebMAP Mobile

All apps available on Google Play and iTunes unless otherwise noted

Handout 2: Somatic Symptom and Related Disorders Fact Sheet

Somatic symptom and related disorders (SSRD) are a set of diagnoses that are defined by the presence of physical symptoms, like muscle tremors, nausea, pain, or dizziness, often in the absence of an identifiable disease or injury. Patients receive one of these diagnoses when their concern about symptoms causes a lot of distress and keeps them from participating in their normal activities. Sometimes patients might also have a medical or mental health diagnosis at the same time, but the symptoms and distress are more impairing than expected.

Somatic symptoms are the result of how the brain processes different types of stressors—physical and emotional—and communicates this information to the body. Somatic symptoms are real, but they are not dangerous in terms of being related to a disease. Even still, they can be distressing for children and adolescents to experience, as well as for the adults who care for them. Because patients with SSRD have physical symptoms as their primary problem, they are usually first seen by a medical provider and expect to receive a medical cure, like a pill or a procedure. However, since somatic symptoms are due to how the brain processes stressors, the treatment is a primarily psychological treatment, or cognitive behavioral therapy (CBT), to learn how the brain and body are connected and how to manage symptoms more effectively.

CBT is an evidence-based treatment that teaches children coping skills to improve function in everyday activities and manage symptoms. CBT helps children understand the connections between their thoughts, feelings, actions, and body responses. Children learn how to manage and cope with their symptoms by changing what they are doing and how they are thinking about their symptoms, by learning skills like keeping their bodies healthy, relaxation, and thinking in a realistic way.

Parents, caregivers, and teachers have an important role in helping children by encouraging them to use coping skills and reducing attention to symptoms or impairment. Adults can also help children manage their symptoms by staying calm when symptoms occur, reducing check-ins, giving positive feedback for use of coping skills, and focusing on what the child can do instead of what they cannot. Depending on the child's level of impairment, parents may want to work with the school to develop a Section 504 plan for their child to provide accommodations as they work toward improving function.

Informational Resources

- Somatic Symptoms in Children: The 5 Ws Explained: https://blog.cincinnatichildrens.org/healthy-living/child-development-and-behavior/the-5ws-of-somatic-symptoms-in-children/
- Somatic Symptom and Related Disorders in Children: https://www.merckmanuals.com/home/children-s-health-issues/mental-health-disorders-in-children-and-adolescents/somatic-symptom-and-related-disorders-in-children
- American Academy of Child and Adolescent Psychiatry Facts for Families: https://www.aacap.org/aacap/families_and_youth/facts_for_families/fff-guide/Physical_Symptoms_of_Emotional_Distress-Somatic_Symptoms_and_Related_Disorders.aspx
- Kelty Mental Health Somatization: https://keltymentalhealth.ca/somatization
- Conversion Disorder: https://www.chop.edu/conditions-diseases/conversion-disorder
- 7 Steps to Getting a 504 Plan for Your Child: https://www.understood.org/en/school-learning/special-services/504-plan/7-steps-to-getting-a-504-plan-for-your-child

References

Aaron, L. A., & Buchwald, D. (2001). A review of the evidence for overlap among unexplained clinical conditions. *Annals of Internal Medicine, 134*(9 Part 2), 868–881.

American Psychiatric Association. (2013). *Diagnostic and statistical manual of mental disorders* (5th ed.). Arlington, VA: American Psychiatric Publishing.

Andresen, J. M., Woolfolk, R. L., Allen, L. A., Fragoso, M. A., Youngerman, N. L., Patrick-Miller, T. J., & Gara, M. A. (2011). Physical symptoms and psychosocial correlates of somatization in pediatric primary care. *Clinical Pediatrics, 50*(10), 904–909.

Aybek, S., Nicholson, T. R., O'Daly, O., Zelaya, F., Kanaan, R. A., & David, A. S. (2015). Emotion-motion interactions in conversion disorder: An FMRI study. *PLoS One, 10*(4), e0123273.

Beck, J. E. (2007). A developmental perspective on functional somatic symptoms. *Journal of Pediatric Psychology, 33*(5), 547–562.

Bujoreanu, S., Randall, E., Thomson, K., & Ibeziako, P. (2014). Characteristics of medically hospitalized pediatric patients with somatoform diagnoses. *Hospital Pediatrics, 4*(5), 283–290.

Campo, J. V., & Fritsch, S. L. (1994). Somatization in children and adolescents. *Journal of the American Academy of Child & Adolescent Psychiatry, 33*(9), 1223–1235.

Carter, B. D., Kronenberger, W. G., Threlkeld, B., Townsend, A., & Pruitt, A. (2013). The Children's Health & Illness Recovery Program (CHIRP): Feasibility and preliminary efficacy in a clinical sample of adolescents with chronic pain and fatigue. *Clinical Practice in Pediatric Psychology, 1*(2), 184.

Christensen, S. S., Frostholm, L., Ørnbøl, E., & Schröder, A. (2015). Changes in illness perceptions mediated the effect of cognitive behavioural therapy in severe functional somatic syndromes. *Journal of Psychosomatic Research, 78*(4), 363–370.

Chrousos, G. P. (2009). Stress and disorders of the stress system. *Nature Reviews Endocrinology, 5*(7), 374.

Crimlisk, H. L., Bhatia, K., Cope, H., David, A., Marsden, C. D., & Ron, M. A. (1998). Slater revisited: 6 year follow up study of patients with medically unexplained motor symptoms. *BMJ, 316*(7131), 582–586.

Ellenstein, A., Kranick, S. M., & Hallett, M. (2011). An update on psychogenic movement disorders. *Current Neurology and Neuroscience Reports, 11*(4), 396–403.

Erpelding, N., Simons, L., Lebel, A., Serrano, P., Pielech, M., Prabhu, S., … Borsook, D. (2016). Rapid treatment-induced brain changes in pediatric CRPS. *Brain Structure and Function, 221*(2), 1095–1111.

FitzGerald, T. L., Southby, A. K., Haines, T. P., Hough, J. P., & Skinner, E. H. (2015). Is physiotherapy effective in the management of child and adolescent conversion disorder? A systematic review. *Journal of Paediatrics and Child Health, 51*(2), 159–167.

Garber, J., Zeman, J., & Walker, L. S. (1990). Recurrent abdominal pain in children: Psychiatric diagnoses and parental psychopathology. *Journal of the American Academy of Child & Adolescent Psychiatry, 29*(4), 648–656.

Kroenke, K. (2007). Efficacy of treatment for somatoform disorders: A review of randomized controlled trials. *Psychosomatic Medicine, 69*(9), 881–888.

Malas, N., Ortiz-Aguayo, R., Giles, L., & Ibeziako, P. (2017). Pediatric somatic symptom disorders. *Current Psychiatry Reports, 19*(2), 11.

Perez, D. L., Barsky, A. J., Vago, D. R., Baslet, G., & Silbersweig, D. A. (2015). A neural circuit framework for somatosensory amplification in somatoform disorders. *The Journal of Neuropsychiatry and Clinical Neurosciences, 27*(1), e40–e50.

Rief, W., & Martin, A. (2014). How to use the new DSM-5 somatic symptom disorder diagnosis in research and practice: A critical evaluation and a proposal for modifications. *Annual Review of Clinical Psychology, 10*, 339.

Ring, A., Dowrick, C. F., Humphris, G. M., Davies, J., & Salmon, P. (2005). The somatising effect of clinical consultation: What patients and doctors say and do not say when patients present medically unexplained physical symptoms. *Social Science & Medicine, 61*(7), 1505–1515.

Salmon, P., Peters, S., & Stanley, I. (1999). Patients' perceptions of medical explanations for somatisation disorders: Qualitative analysis. *BMJ, 318*(7180), 372–376.

Schweickhardt, A., Larisch, A., Wirsching, M., & Fritzsche, K. (2007). Short-term psychotherapeutic interventions for somatizing patients in the general hospital: A randomized controlled study. *Psychotherapy and Psychosomatics, 76*(6), 339–346.

Sharpe, M., & Carson, A. (2001). "Unexplained" somatic symptoms, functional syndromes, and somatization: Do we need a paradigm shift? *Annals of Internal Medicine, 134*(9 Part 2), 926–930.

Silber, T. J. (2011). Somatization disorders: diagnosis, treatment, and prognosis. *Pediatrics in Review, 32*(2), 56–64.

Stone, J., Carson, A., & Sharpe, M. (2005a). Functional symptoms and signs in neurology: Assessment and diagnosis. *Journal of Neurology, Neurosurgery & Psychiatry, 76*(Suppl 1), i2–i12.

Stone, J., Carson, A., & Sharpe, M. (2005b). Functional symptoms in neurology: Management. *Journal of Neurology, Neurosurgery & Psychiatry, 76*(Suppl 1), i13–i21.

Stone, J., Hoeritzauer, I., Gelauff, J., Lehn, A., Gardiner, P., van Gils, A., & Carson, A. (2016). Functional disorders in neurology: Case studies. *Neurologic Clinics, 34*(3), 667–681.

Stone, J., Wojcik, W., Durrance, D., Carson, A., Lewis, S., MacKenzie, L., … Sharpe, M. (2002). What should we say to patients with symptoms unexplained by disease? The "number needed to offend". *BMJ, 325*(7378), 1449–1450.

Thomson, K., Randall, E., Ibeziako, P., & Bujoreanu, I. S. (2014). Somatoform disorders and trauma in medically-admitted children, adolescents, and young adults: Prevalence rates and psychosocial characteristics. *Psychosomatics, 55*(6), 630–639.

van Geelen, S. M., Rydelius, P.-A., & Hagquist, C. (2015). Somatic symptoms and psychological concerns in a general adolescent population: Exploring the relevance of DSM-5 somatic symptom disorder. *Journal of Psychosomatic Research, 79*(4), 251–258.

Van Tilburg, M. A., Levy, R. L., Walker, L. S., Von Korff, M., Feld, L. D., Garner, M., … Whitehead, W. E. (2015). Psychosocial mechanisms for the transmission of somatic symptoms from parents to children. *World Journal of Gastroenterology: WJG, 21*(18), 5532.

Walker, L. S., Garber, J., & Greene, J. W. (1993). Psychosocial correlates of recurrent childhood pain: A comparison of pediatric patients with recurrent abdominal pain, organic illness, and psychiatric disorders. *Journal of Abnormal Psychology, 102*(2), 248.

Whalley, M. G., & Cane, D. A. (2017). A cognitive-behavioral model of persistent postural-perceptual dizziness. *Cognitive and Behavioral Practice, 24*(1), 72–89.

Williams, S. E., & Zahka, N. E. (2017). *Treating somatic symptoms in children and adolescents*. New York, NY: Guilford Publications.

Zhang, J., Jiang, M., Yao, D., Dai, Y., Long, L., Yu, M., … Guo, W. (2015). Alterations in white matter integrity in first-episode, treatment-naive patients with somatization disorder. *Neuroscience Letters, 599*, 102–108.

Rumination Syndrome

Anthony Alioto and Kira S. Branch

Introduction

Rumination syndrome is a disorder in which the individual regurgitates recently ingested food from the stomach to the mouth, where it is either reswallowed or expelled. The disorder has been identified in infants, children, adolescents, and adults with a wide range of developmental abilities. Historically, rumination syndrome has been noted to have a low prevalence and to be more common in females (Khan, Hyman, Cocjin, & Di Lorenzo, 2000).

The precise etiology of rumination syndrome remains unknown at this time. Even so, many patients' histories are suggestive of a trigger at the onset of symptoms, such as an infectious or inflammatory gastrointestinal disease or stressors involving emotional arousal. After the initial stressor has resolved, the vomiting behavior and some sensory abnormalities appear to remain in place, with the behavior presenting somewhat like a habit disorder (Alioto & Di Lorenzo, 2017).

A. Alioto (✉) · K. S. Branch
Department of Pediatrics, Nemours/AIDHC, Wilmington, DE, USA

Thomas Jefferson University, Sidney Kimmel College of Medicine, Philadelphia, PA, USA
e-mail: Anthony.Alioto@nemours.org

While the disorder itself is not life-threatening, it typically has a significant medical and psychosocial impact on the patient and family (Monagas et al., 2017). As there are substantial differences in etiologic factors, phenotypic presentation, and treatment strategies between infantile and adolescent forms, coverage of all types of rumination is outside of the scope of the current chapter. Thus, the current chapter will focus solely on rumination syndrome in neurotypical older children and adolescents.

Epidemiology

Challenges in the recognition and diagnosis of rumination have made it difficult to fully determine its prevalence in children and adolescents. Further complicating this matter, the symptoms of rumination syndrome overlap with other functional gastrointestinal disorders, motility disorders, and eating disorders (Chial, Camilleri, Williams, Litzinger, & Perrault, 2003; Chitkara, Bredenoord, Talley, & Whitehead, 2006; Eckern, Stevens, & Mitchell, 1999; Graff, Surprise, Sarosiek, Twillman, & McCallum, 2002; O'Brien, Bruce, & Camilleri, 1995). Two studies of youth self-report of gastrointestinal symptoms found rumination symptoms present in anywhere from <1% in India (Bhatia et al., 2016) to 5% in Sri Lanka (Rajindrajith, Devanarayana, & Crispus Perera, 2012).

B. D. Carter, K. A. Kullgren (eds.), *Clinical Handbook of Psychological Consultation in Pediatric Medical Settings*, Issues in Clinical Child Psychology, https://doi.org/10.1007/978-3-030-35598-2_15

Diagnosis and Pathophysiology

The diagnosis of rumination syndrome should be a relatively straightforward endeavor, as rumination syndrome is a clinical diagnosis and is symptom based (O'Brien et al., 1995). No further investigation should be needed for patients who satisfy the Rome IV criteria for the condition (Table 1).

Even so, there are several factors that likely interfere with clinicians' ability to make a definitive diagnosis. First, there are a handful of other conditions that have overlapping symptoms and, per the Rome IV criteria, clinicians should be sure to rule out any organic conditions or an eating disorder diagnosis. While there are very few other gastrointestinal disorders associated with vomiting within seconds or minutes from food ingestion, clinicians should be sure to differentiate the symptom presentation from other disorders. Table 2 provides a listing of features differentiating rumination from other disorders (Alioto & Di Lorenzo, 2017).

Second, physicians and other clinicians seem to be less comfortable providing diagnoses that have a behavioral component and are functional in nature. Rumination syndrome is similar to other functional GI disorders where physicians may be more comfortable with an organic diagnosis rather than engaging in an intricate (and often uncomfortable) discussion with the patient and family about functional GI disorders.

Third, as rumination syndrome is a symptom-based functional GI disorder, there is no diagnostic test to conclusively diagnose the disorder. Because there is not a diagnostic test demonstrating a specific abnormality, clinicians often experience discomfort providing the diagnosis, and patients and families may not accept the diagnosis. As such, patients with rumination syndrome often are evaluated by multiple providers over many years before receiving the actual diagnosis (Alioto, Yacob, Yardley, & Di Lorenzo, 2015; Chial et al., 2003). While waiting for a diagnosis, patients often undergo many diagnostic and medical evaluations, which are costly and stressful and frequently uncover incidental findings that then further complicate the final diagnosis of rumination syndrome (Alioto, Di Lorenzo, Montgomery, & Yacob, 2017).

In order to understand the role that diagnostic testing may play in the evaluation of rumination syndrome, an appreciation of the pathophysiology is beneficial. The ingestion of food (or in some cases even the anticipation of ingesting food) initiates a cascade of behaviors, including contraction of the abdominal wall, opening of the lower and upper esophageal sphincter, and subsequent expulsion of food (Chitkara, Van Tilburg, Whitehead, & Talley, 2006). Literature from adult populations has indicated three different mechanisms of rumination: (1) the abdominal pressure increase that occurs before the retrograde flow (primary rumination), (2) an increase in abdominal pressure following the onset of a reflux event (secondary rumination), and (3) a supragastric belch, often associated with air swallowing, immediately followed by a

Table 1 Rome IV criteria for adolescent rumination syndrome

Diagnostic criteria[a] *must include* ***all*** *of the following*:

1. Repeated regurgitation and rechewing or expulsion of food that:
   (a) Begins soon after ingestion of a meal
   (b) Does not occur during sleep
2. Not preceded by retching.
3. After appropriate evaluation, the symptoms cannot be fully explained by another medical condition. An eating disorder must be ruled out.

[a]Criteria fulfilled for at least 2 months prior to diagnosis

Table 2 Differential diagnosis of rumination syndrome from other conditions presenting with emesis in adolescents

Diagnosis	Vomiting	Esophagitis	Prokinetics	Fundoplication
Rumination	During or minutes after meal	No	Not beneficial	Not beneficial
Achalasia	Hours after meal	Often (from stasis)	Not beneficial	Contraindicated
GERD	After large meals or when lying down	Often	Beneficial	Beneficial
Gastroparesis	Hours after meal	No	Beneficial	Not beneficial
Cyclic vomiting	Intermittent, unrelated to meal	During episodes	Not beneficial	Not beneficial

rumination event (supragastric belch-associated rumination; Kessing, Bredenoord, & Smout, 2014). Whether these different mechanisms are associated with different treatment strategies or prognosis is unclear.

While there is no test to diagnose this condition, manometry evaluations frequently are used to rule out other conditions (e.g., a bona fide motility disorder) while also providing visual "evidence" of the act of rumination occurring. For example, while antroduodenal manometry is not necessary to make the diagnosis, the characteristic synchronous increases in pressure (referred to as "r" waves) generated by the contraction of the skeletal abdominal muscles are seen across gastric and duodenal recording sites when rumination occurs. More recently, the use of esophageal manometry, a less invasive and time-consuming diagnostic test, has been demonstrated to provide similar objective evidence of rumination (Righini Grunder, Aspirot, & Faure, 2017).

Other frequently used diagnostic tests in rumination syndrome evaluations include impedance-manometry and gastric emptying. Impedance-manometry monitoring may help the clinician distinguish between rumination from GERD and from supragastric belching. The impedance study also will rule out nighttime reflux events in patients with rumination syndrome. Gastric emptying can help elucidate the role of impaired postprandial gastric accommodation in rumination (Thumshirn et al., 1998). It has been shown that approximately 40% of adolescents with rumination demonstrate a mild degree of gastroparesis (Chial et al., 2003). However, as patients often continuously regurgitate during the gastric emptying test, the results can be difficult to interpret.

In sum, the diagnosis of rumination syndrome is a symptom-based diagnosis that can be relatively easily distinguished from other gastrointestinal disorders. While there is no specific test for rumination syndrome, some diagnostic tests do allow for evaluation of comorbid conditions that may be contributory and allow for objective "evidence" of rumination that frequently feels reassuring for clinicians, patients, and families.

Patient and Family Engagement

Education and Reassurance

It is well-documented that accurate diagnosis and reassurance often provide considerable relief to families and patients (Banez & Gallagher, 2006; Kessing et al., 2014; Khan et al., 2000). Education and accurate description about rumination syndrome may allow for a reduction in anxiety, as well as patients being more active in their own treatment. The discussion of rumination syndrome from a biopsychosocial model allows families to understand the relationship between biological processes and emotional, behavioral, and social factors (Dalton & Czyzewski, 2009). Education should include how rumination syndrome is a symptom-based diagnosis, why further testing is not needed, and that treatment incorporates behavioral interventions.

Families benefit from a description of the pathophysiology of rumination, focusing on the contraction of the intercostal muscles and abdominal wall as the force behind the regurgitation of stomach contents (Barba et al., 2015). Food or fluid intake, the rise of dyspeptic symptoms, and the anticipation of eating or drinking are identified as potential triggers. Finally, it is important to discuss with the family the role of autonomic nervous system arousal (i.e., anxiety or worry) in rumination.

Language and Communication about Rumination Syndrome

Clinicians should closely attend to their word choices as they discuss and explain rumination syndrome. While many clinicians utilize the word "behavioral" in their descriptions with families to highlight the functional nature of the symptoms, most families interpret this word as meaning "on purpose." Families frequently misinterpret the referral to a behavioral health clinician as suggesting the symptoms are "in my head." Providing the interpretation of test results as "normal" also can reinforce the message that the symptoms are not real and are psychological in nature.

Families seem to respond well to an explanation of rumination syndrome that highlights several points. We discuss how, oftentimes, rumination begins with an illness that involves vomiting (e.g., influenza). At the time of illness, vomiting may have made sense and been an important part of recovery. However, after the illness passed, the gastric sensitivity remains as a learned response to having anything go into the stomach. The rumination is explained as a "leftover" behavior that has been learned, continues to serve the purpose of allowing the stomach to feel better, and can be unlearned.

Assessment and Formulation

Interview

Having the patient and parent provide a history can provide rich insights into the perception of the problem, what families have been told in the past by other clinicians, beliefs about the rumination, and the impact on quality of life. For the interview, we differentiate between vomiting (food being expelled) and rumination (food coming up the esophagus, perhaps into the mouth, being reswallowed). Standard inquiries include the following:

1. When did the problems with rumination begin? (inquire about any other concurrent stressors such as a viral illness, surgeries, emotional stressors, traumatic experiences).
2. When does rumination begin? Immediately after taking one sip or bite? During the meal? After completion of a meal?
3. What is the smallest amount of intake that can trigger rumination?
4. What are the associated postprandial sensory experiences (e.g., pain, nausea, burning)?
5. Is there burping or belching associated with eating?
6. Are there foods or drinks that do not result in rumination? Any that tend to make it worse?
7. Once rumination begins, is the patient able to reswallow regurgitant?
8. Is rumination worse with fluid, food, or a combination of both?
9. Have there been times in the past when rumination commenced and then terminated for a period of time?

Mealtime Behavioral Observation

The importance of observing the patient eat or drink and then ruminate cannot be overemphasized. Patients with a diagnosis of rumination syndrome often differ in regard to the antecedent sensory experience, the types or amounts of food or fluid that trigger rumination, or the manner in which they manage the rumination (e.g., reswallow, expel). The purpose of the observation of rumination is twofold: (1) it allows for further evaluation, and (2) it increases the patient's awareness of the behavior.

We conduct two mealtime observations while the patient is in the inpatient setting. For the first meal, patients are asked to eat a meal (of their choosing) at their natural pace and to ruminate and vomit as they normally would. Pertinent information includes the types and quantities of food they select, how often the patient ruminates during this meal (or if rumination starts after the meal ends), the rate of the patient's eating, the patient's posture, how they attempt to manage rumination, and observable symptoms (i.e., belching, retching). The observing clinician should inquire if the series of events observed are typical for meals at home or if the presentation is unusual in any way.

The second mealtime observation allows the clinician to better control several variables such as the type, amount, and pacing of intake, as well as encouraging the patient to attend to internal sensations and abdominal contractions. During the meal, the clinician directs the patient as to how much to eat or drink at 5-min intervals (Fig. 1). The clinician continuously records data such as the amount of food or fluid intake, the number of times the patient ruminates or vomits, and the patient's common dyspeptic symptoms every 5 min. The data often elucidates a gradual

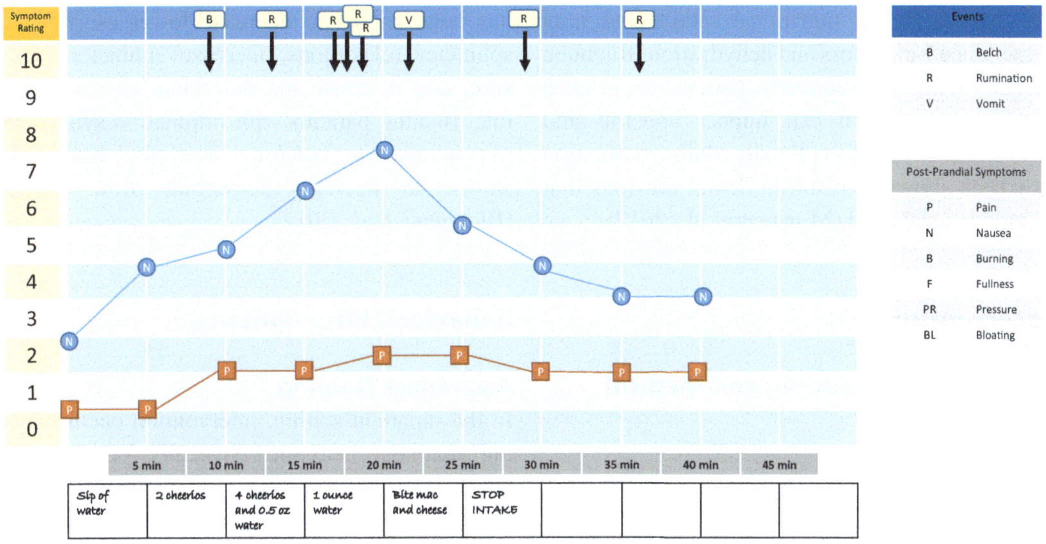

Fig. 1 Mealtime Observation Data Sheet

increase in dyspeptic symptoms, a gradual increase in rumination frequency and intensity, and a resolution of symptoms with emesis. The clinician shares this information with the patient to highlight the relationship between dyspeptic symptoms and rumination behavior. The observation mealtimes also allow the clinician to obtain a baseline for treatment, identifying the amount of food and/or fluid that can trigger rumination, as well as at the point in the meal rumination usually begins.

Environmental and Internal Factors

Environmental factors often influence the patient's rumination behavior. For example, some patients start to ruminate when food is present or when food first touches the tongue. Clinicians also should be aware of the presence of the patient's emesis container (e.g., the container into which patient vomits throughout the day). When this container is removed, patients often become more aware of rumination and show greater motivation to control vomiting.

Many patients have the expectation that everything they eat or drink will be ruminated and/or vomited, which often leads to self-talk or automatic thoughts (e.g., "This is going to hurt, I can't keep anything down"). These cognitions often serve to reduce motivation and potentially heighten autonomic arousal during mealtimes. Similar thoughts frequently are seen in patients with comorbid anxiety or depressive symptoms.

Mental Health Considerations

Similar to patients with other functional GI disorders, patients with rumination syndrome present with a range of psychiatric difficulties, with depression and anxiety the mostly commonly seen (Chial et al., 2003). With more severe presentations of rumination (as seen in an inpatient treatment setting), the presence of depression and anxiety is notably more common (27% and 40%, respectively; Alioto et al., 2015). Eating disorders also have been identified in a smaller portion of patients with rumination syndrome (Alioto et al., 2015; Chial et al., 2003). These comorbid difficulties should be thoroughly evaluated, as they often impact patients' ability to make progress.

Medical Considerations

Ruminating and vomiting on a daily basis typically has a deleterious impact on physical functioning. Patients typically have an alteration in their eating behaviors and nutritional intake and may experience weight loss and dehydration (Rachuba & Alioto, 2015). Frequently, patients experience constipation, which can impact appetite and abdominal discomfort. Finally, daily rumination has been shown to result in dental erosions that should be evaluated (Monagas et al., 2017).

Intervention

Supplemental Feeding and Medical Treatment

Behavioral treatment approaches typically take time and improvements with overall intake can be painfully gradual. As such, the patient's current nutritional status should be evaluated, and planning should be made with the expectation that improvements will not be immediate. Those with more severe rumination typically demonstrate significant weight loss and can require hospitalizations due to malnutrition and dehydration (Rachuba & Alioto, 2015). Thus, stabilization of nutrition and weight is strongly encouraged before beginning formal treatment for rumination. Stabilization can be achieved with naso-jejunal (NJ) or gastrojejunal (GJ) feeding catheters and should always be attempted prior to parenteral nutrition. In consideration of the supplemental feeding route, it should be noted that many patients with rumination cannot tolerate naso-gastric (NG) feeds, as they experience discomfort similarly to PO intake, easily ruminate the contents, and in turn dislodge or vomit their tube.

If constipation is determined to be an issue, it is recommended that this be treated aggressively (Boccia et al., 2008). Medications should also be considered to address other comorbid difficulties such as sleep and sensory difficulties such as nausea and early satiety (Rosen, Alioto, & Saps, 2016).

To date, pharmacological treatment of rumination in pediatric populations has not been demonstrated to be particularly effective. Baclofen, an agonist of the γ-aminobutyric acid B receptor, has been shown to decrease lower esophageal sphincter relaxations, increase sphincter pressure, and decrease the individual's swallowing rate. In adult patients with rumination syndrome or supragastric belching, baclofen has been shown to decrease retrograde flow events (Blondeau et al., 2012).

Behavioral Interventions

Awareness Training

In the inpatient setting, intervention occurs during treatment mealtimes (typically 3 times each day, lasting around 20–30 min). With the data from the observation meals as a baseline, the clinician designs mealtimes with the patient tracking rumination frequency, the intensity of dyspeptic symptoms, and vomiting at 5-min intervals (Fig. 2). It is relatively uncommon for the rumination behavior or dyspeptic symptoms to change during the first few days of intervention; however, these initial meals provide additional baseline information and increase the awareness of the patient and parent of the interplay between discomfort and rumination symptoms (Schroedl, Alioto, & Di Lorenzo, 2013).

The literature has suggested that biofeedback is a beneficial intervention in patients with rumination syndrome (Chial et al., 2003; Green, Alioto, Mousa, & Di Lorenzo, 2011; Olden, 2001; Shay et al., 1986), sometimes with little information about the rationale or method. Biofeedback can be utilized to further increase awareness of the physical response to rumination. For example, patients often benefit from the use of surface electromyography (sEMG), which monitors abdominal muscle contractions that occur during episodes of rumination (Alioto, Di Lorenzo, & Parzanese, 2014; Barba et al., 2015; Cunningham & Banez, 2006).

Gradual Refeeding

Previous research indicates the importance of having patients slowly reintroduce food and fluid intake (Chial & Camilleri, 2006). A gradual approach allows patients to practice and utilize

Daily Tracking Sheet

Day/Date: Monday, January 3

Session	Time	Food/Liquid/Amount	Rumination Waves	Nausea at end (0-10)	Stayed down or came out?
B	Whole Meal = 5 cheerios, 2 ounces water				
	Start	1 cheerio	II	2	**Down** Out
	5 min later	1 cheerio + 1 ounce	IIII	3	**Down** Out
	5 min later	1 cheerio	卌 I	5	**Down** Out
	5 min later	1 cheerio + 1 ounce	卌 III	7	Down **Out**
	5 min later	Meal ended due to vomiting			Down Out

Session	Time	Food/Liquid/Amount	Rumination Waves	Nausea at end (0-10)	Stayed down or came out?
L	Whole Meal = 6 cheerios, 2 ounces water				
	Start	1 cheerio	II	2	**Down** Out
	5 min later	1 cheerio	II	3	**Down** Out
	5 min later	2 cheerios	卌	3	**Down** Out
	5 min later	1 cheerio + 1 ounce	卌 III	4	**Down** Out
	5 min later	1 cheerio + 1 ounce	卌 III	4	**Down** Out

Session	Time	Food/Liquid/Amount	Rumination Waves	Nausea at end (0-10)	Stayed down or came out?
D	Whole Meal =				
	Start				Down Out
	5 min later				Down Out
	5 min later				Down Out
	5 min later				Down Out
	5 min later				Down Out

Fig. 2 Patient Mealtime Self-Report Tracking Sheet

their self-management skills while tolerating the discomfort that arises with gastric distension with increasing quantities of food. Beginning with easily digestible foods (e.g., simple carbohydrates such as pieces of cereal, animal crackers) can allow for initial successes, with food complexity increasing over time (Rachuba & Alioto, 2015). Frequent, small feeding trials also allow for constant re-exposure to a stressful stimulus (i.e., actual eating/drinking and/or anticipatory anxiety about eating/drinking). Supplemental feedings can be reduced proportionally as the patient is able to keep more food down (Rachuba & Alioto, 2015).

In our practice, we emphasize the importance of reswallowing any regurgitants that are returned to the mouth during a rumination event. Prior to treatment, patients may experience relief from their dyspeptic symptoms after vomiting (thereby negatively reinforcing the rumination/vomiting behaviors). Reswallowing allows the patient to maintain the discomfort while using self-regulation to improve the sensory experience while food remains in the stomach.

The Sensory Component

The patient's sensory experience after ingestion of food or drink is another internal cue for rumination. As discussed earlier, patients with rumination frequently describe a sense of nausea, pain, burning, pressure, bloating, or early satiety that intensifies with time and increased intake (Alioto et al., 2015; Barba et al., 2015; Tucker, Knowles, Wright, & Fox, 2013). These dyspeptic symptoms may function as a premonitory urge for abdominal wall contraction (i.e., the motor behavior) to occur, similar to what is seen in traditional motor tic or habit disorders (Alioto & Di Lorenzo, 2017).

Many approaches have been helpful for alleviating the sensory experience which may, in turn, reduce rumination. As mentioned earlier, pharmacological approaches (e.g., cyproheptadine, dicyclomine, omeprazole) may allow for a reduction of dyspeptic symptoms associated with eating. Shifting attention away from the discomfort (i.e., by engaging in an activity such as reading aloud) has also been beneficial for many patients (Barba et al., 2015; Chitkara, Van Tilburg, et al., 2006; Hejazi & McCallum, 2014). Reading aloud encourages patients to take diaphragmatic breaths with slow exhalation.

Biofeedback may provide further benefit to patients focused on reducing their overall arousal and triggering symptoms. Heart rate variability (HRV) biofeedback provides the patient with continuous feedback about their stress response/relaxation response. Also, autonomic nervous system dysregulation has been found to play a role in functional gastrointestinal disorders (Chelimsky, Boyle, Tusing, & Chelimsky, 2001; Cunningham & Banez, 2006). Biofeedback approaches (i.e., instruction on autonomic nervous system regulation) have been shown to be beneficial in patients with functional abdominal pain (Sowder, Gervitz, Shapiro, & Ebert, 2010). It is likely that similar mechanisms contribute to the challenges demonstrated by patients with rumination syndrome and biofeedback may also be beneficial in this population.

The Competing Response

A mainstay in the treatment of rumination syndrome is diaphragmatic breathing (Chitkara, Van Tilburg, et al., 2006; Halland, Pandolfino, & Barba, 2018; Kessing et al., 2014). Literature suggests that diaphragmatic breathing serves as a competing response to rumination (Hejazi & McCallum, 2014; Tucker et al., 2013; Wagaman, Williams, & Camilleri, 1998). As described earlier, the pathophysiology of rumination involves a simultaneous contraction of the intercostal and upper abdominal muscles and relaxation of the lower esophageal sphincter (Barba et al., 2015; Malcolm, Thumshirn, Camilleri, & Williams, 1997). This places significant pressure on the abdominal cavity, which results in intragastric pressure forcing gastric contents upward. Thus, the focus of behavioral therapy has been on the patient utilizing strategies (e.g., diaphragmatic breathing) to alleviate the impact of these contractions.

Barba et al. (2015) utilized an EMG biofeedback-focused approach to increase patient awareness of the use of abdominal muscles and thereby correct and reduce the contractions. The authors found that patients (adolescents and adults) were able to modify the behavior, decrease the number of rumination events during a meal, and maintain the gains up to 6 months later.

Treatment Adaptation

As discussed earlier, patients with rumination syndrome tend to be a heterogeneous group in terms of their rumination triggers, severity of rumination, and comorbid challenges and diagnoses. Thus, a one-size-fits-all approach to treatment is not suggested. Patients with less severe rumination may benefit from minimal intervention (e.g., one or several sessions of diaphragmatic breathing), while more complicated patients may require a multidisciplinary or interdisciplinary approach.

Programmatic approaches to the treatment of rumination syndrome have been discussed in the literature (Alioto et al., 2014; Alioto & Di Lorenzo, 2017; Chial et al., 2003; Green et al., 2011). Multidisciplinary/interdisciplinary approaches allow providers to address the patient's concerns in a complementary manner, as well as provide a more controlled environment for treatment. Treatment in an inpatient medical setting allows for close monitoring of associated medical difficulties. Such an interdisciplinary, intensive approach to treatment has been shown to provide short term (Alioto et al., 2015) and long-term improvements in rumination (Alioto & Di Lorenzo, 2018).

Most clinicians who see patients presenting with rumination syndrome will not have access to multiple clinicians in other disciplines familiar with treatment for rumination. In fact, for milder presentations where vomiting does not occur, outpatient approaches may be the best fit for treatment. Mealtime observations can easily occur in the office or clinic and modified as needed.

Challenges with office-based treatment typically arise with regard to the patient working on skills at home in the natural environment. While treatment involves working with smaller amounts of food, patients frequently return to their prior eating habits at home (including ruminating and vomiting). The clinician may consider having set "practice times" for the patient at home, understanding that there will be a return to regular eating habits in between practice times. Patients on supplemental feeds may be more likely to avoid returning to their prior eating habits, as their caloric and fluid needs are being met enterally.

Although biofeedback is not readily available for home use, clinicians may consider providing the patient with a recommendation for a respiration metronome phone app. These apps are often free and provide support for utilization of skills taught during sessions. If the clinician desires a relatively inexpensive biofeedback device, The Pip (www.thepip.com) may be considered. The Pip is a handheld skin conductance biofeedback device that utilizes a video game format and interacts with an app on smartphones and tablet devices.

Treatment Goals

It is highly recommended that clinicians set goals for treatment from the start of therapy. Many patients and families see complete resolution of rumination as the only desired outcome and therefore fail to appreciate the gradual gains. Short-term goals may include a reduction in the frequency, duration, or intensity of rumination, the ability to keep down more calories or fluid, reduction in enteral feedings, better ability to control the rumination contractions, and improvement in sensory experiences such as nausea or pain. Even in an intensive inpatient program, the majority of patients continue to ruminate by discharge, and full termination of rumination may not occur for several months (Alioto & Di Lorenzo, 2018). Outpatient follow-up will need to be arranged from both a medical and mental health/behavioral perspective.

Case Example

Tad was a 15-year-old male who experienced vomiting along with an episode of influenza. After recovery from the influenza symptoms, Tad vomited only after large meals. This ultimately progressed to not being able to retain any food or fluid intake. Regurgitation and vomiting would occur immediately after ingestion, and Tad carried a cup with him to vomit into. As a result,

Tad's weight dropped significantly, he was admitted to the hospital for malnutrition and dehydration, and naso-jejunal (NJ) feedings were initiated. Psychology was consulted during the admission, as prior testing was not suggestive of any organic difficulties, and rumination syndrome was the suspected diagnosis.

During the initial consultation, the psychologist explored the history of the vomiting and regurgitation. The diagnosis of rumination syndrome had been mentioned in the past; however, the family read on the Internet that the disorder only occurs in children with developmental disabilities or trauma and therefore did not feel that the diagnosis fit their child's presentation. An overview of rumination as well as review of past test results was provided to the family and an observation mealtime was conducted.

During the initial meal, Tad was asked to eat foods of his choosing at his own rate. Tad noticeably ate at a very rapid rate, with food being regurgitated almost immediately. During the second meal, the amount and timing of intake was regulated by the psychologist. It was observed that an item even as small as one Cheerio or one sip of water was vomited within 1 s of swallowing. No sensory aspect (e.g., pain, nausea) was noted by Tad during or after the mealtime. Abdominal contractions were clearly visible to the psychologist and were recognized by Tad once highlighted.

Impressions were discussed with the family that Tad's presentation was indicative of rumination syndrome and that it had progressed to the point where the rumination behavior had become a learned response to any amount of food or fluid being swallowed.

For treatment, the psychologist provided instruction on diaphragmatic breathing (respiration rate of 7 breaths/min). Biofeedback was utilized to support this intervention and to allow Tad to achieve self-regulation skills during mealtimes, and all emesis containers were removed from the room. Initially, the psychologist sought to find a quantity of food intake that would allow Tad to have success in reswallowing and keeping the food down while using self-regulation skills until rumination terminated. However, Tad was unable to keep down even a crumb of a Cheerio without regurgitation after swallowing. Therefore, initial sessions were conducted more like exposure sessions, with a crumb of a Cheerio held on the tongue in Tad's mouth while he used self-regulation skills. As Tad felt more comfortable with this, he was able to progress to swallowing the crumb, to keeping down one eighth of a Cheerio (with regurgitation and reswallowing) and ultimately a whole Cheerio.

While inpatient, mealtimes were scheduled for three times each day, with no food or fluid intake between mealtime sessions. Initially, sessions involved very small amounts such as one sip of water or one cheerio, with five 5-min trials, and use of biofeedback-assisted relaxation training. It was common for Tad to have up to 35 rumination contractions every 5 min. Tad was requested to continue to reswallow until rumination terminated on its own, typically around 1 h after the meal ended. Given the very gradual nature of progress, Tad was discharged with the NJ tube in place and outpatient sessions with the psychologist scheduled weekly.

During outpatient sessions, practice with mealtimes continued and specific mealtime practice sessions were designed to take place at home. After 1 week, Tad noted that he was able to keep down as many Cheerios as he wanted with little difficulty, but rumination would occur with any amount of any other food. By the second outpatient session 2 weeks later, Tad noted improvement with an increase in fluids and he had expanded to Goldfish crackers. Two weeks later (session 3), Tad presented to clinic with no NJ tube present, noting that rumination had stopped, that he was back to eating full meals with no rumination, and that he had removed the tube on his own.

Tad continued with no problems with rumination for around 6 weeks. He received a letter in the mail from his estranged father who was currently incarcerated, stating that he would be released soon. Within a day, rumination returned suddenly to its baseline level, the NJ tube was replaced 2 days later, and Tad began work with exposure to a crumb of Cheerio on his tongue, making gradual progress as he had done in the past.

Discussion

The case example above was selected in order to demonstrate several aspects of rumination syndrome and treatment. First, rumination may present in various forms, necessitating accommodation of the treatment approach. Second, the diagnosis of rumination may have been discussed with the family in the past, but due to misinterpretation of information, families may be reluctant to accept the diagnosis and treatment approach. Third, treatment progress may wax and wane within the same individual. Finally, a reappearance of symptoms can occur in response to an illness or stressor, and as such the clinician should engage in discussions of relapse prevention and how to re-engage in treatment should symptoms return.

References

Alioto, A., & Di Lorenzo, C. (2017). Rumination syndrome. In C. Faure, N. Thapar, & C. Di Lorenzo (Eds.), *Pediatric neurogastroenterology: Gastrointestinal motility and functional disorders in children* (2nd ed., pp. 437–444). Cham, Switzerland: Springer International Publishing.

Alioto, A., & Di Lorenzo, C. (2018). Long-term follow-up of adolescents treated for rumination syndrome in an inpatient setting. *Journal of Pediatric Gastroenterology and Nutrition, 66*(1), 21–25.

Alioto, A., Di Lorenzo, C., Montgomery, M. L., & Yacob, D. (2017). High cost and low yield: The diagnostic evaluation of rumination syndrome in pediatrics. *The Journal of Pediatrics, 185*, 155–159.

Alioto, A., Di Lorenzo, C., & Parzanese, M. (2014). Interdisciplinary intervention in adolescents with rumination syndrome. In C. Martin & T. Dovey (Eds.), *Pediatric gastrointestinal disorders: A psychosocial perspective* (pp. 151–169). London, UK: Radcliffe Publishing.

Alioto, A., Yacob, D., Yardley, H. L., & Di Lorenzo, C. (2015). Inpatient treatment of rumination syndrome: Outcomes and lessons learned. *Clinical Practice in Pediatric Psychology, 3*(4), 304–313.

Banez, G. A., & Gallagher, H. M. (2006). Recurrent abdominal pain. *Behavior Modification, 30*, 50–71.

Barba, E., Burri, E., Accarino, A., Malagelada, C., Rodriguez-Urrutia, A., Soldevilla, A., … Azpiroz, F. (2015). Biofeedback-guided control of abdominothoracic muscular activity reduces regurgitation episodes in patients with rumination. *Clinical Gastroenterology and Hepatology, 13*(1), 100–106.

Bhatia, V., Deswal, S., Seth, S., Kapoor, A., Sibal, A., & Gopalan, S. (2016). Prevalence of functional gastrointestinal disorders among adolescents in Delhi based on Rome III criteria: A school-based survey. *Indian Journal of Gastroenterology, 35*(4), 294–298.

Blondeau, K., Boecxstaens, V., Rommel, N., Farre, R., Depyper, S., Holvoet, L., … Tack, J. F. (2012). Baclofen improves symptoms and reduces postprandial flow events in patients with rumination and supragastric belching. *Clinical Gastroenterology and Hepatology, 10*(4), 379–384.

Boccia, G., Buonavolonta, R., Coccorullo, P., Manguso, F., Fuiano, L., & Staiano, A. (2008). Dyspeptic symptoms in children: The result of a constipation-induced cologastric brake? *Clinical Gastroenterology and Hepatology, 6*(5), 556–560.

Chelimsky, G., Boyle, J. T., Tusing, L., & Chelimsky, T. C. (2001). Autonomic abnormalities in children with functional abdominal pain: Coincidence or etiology? *Journal of Pediatric Gastroenterology and Nutrition, 33*(1), 47–53.

Chial, H. J., & Camilleri, M. (2006). A twenty-one-year-old college student with postprandial regurgitation and weight loss. *Clinical Gastroenterology and Hepatology, 4*, 1314–1317.

Chial, H. J., Camilleri, M., Williams, D. E., Litzinger, K., & Perrault, J. (2003). Rumination syndrome in children and adolescents: Diagnosis, treatment, and prognosis. *Pediatrics, 11*(1), 158–162.

Chitkara, D. K., Bredenoord, A. J., Talley, N. J., & Whitehead, W. E. (2006). Aerophagia and rumination: Recognition and therapy. *Current Treatment Options in Gastroenterology, 9*(4), 305–313.

Chitkara, D. K., Van Tilburg, M., Whitehead, W. E., & Talley, N. J. (2006). Teaching diaphragmatic breathing for rumination syndrome. *The American Journal of Gastroenterology, 101*(11), 2449–2452.

Cunningham, C. L., & Banez, G. A. (2006). Theoretical and historical basis for a biopsychosocial approach to pediatric gastrointestinal disorders. In C. L. Cunningham & G. A. Banez (Eds.), *Pediatric gastrointestinal disorders* (pp. 13–30). New York, NY: Springer.

Dalton, W. T., 3rd, & Czyzewski, D. I. (2009). Behavioral treatment of habitual rumination: Case reports. *Digestive Diseases and Sciences, 54*(8), 1804–1807.

Eckern, M., Stevens, W., & Mitchell, J. (1999). The relationship between rumination and eating disorders. *International Journal of Eating Disorders, 26*, 414–419.

Graff, J., Surprise, J., Sarosiek, I., Twillman, R., & McCallum, R. W. (2002). Rumination syndrome: Challenges with diagnosis and treatment. *The American Journal of Gastroenterology, 97*(Suppl), S48.

Green, A. D., Alioto, A., Mousa, H., & Di Lorenzo, C. (2011). Severe pediatric rumination syndrome: Successful interdisciplinary inpatient management. *Journal of Pediatric Gastroenterology and Nutrition, 52*(4), 414–418.

Halland, M., Pandolfino, J., & Barba, E. (2018). Diagnosis and treatment of rumination syndrome.

Clinical Gastroenterology and Hepatology, 16(10), 1549–1555.

Hejazi, R. A., & McCallum, R. W. (2014). Rumination syndrome: A review of current concepts and treatments. *The American Journal of Medical Sciences, 348*(4), 324–329.

Kessing, B. F., Bredenoord, A. J., & Smout, A. J. (2014). Objective manometric criteria for the rumination syndrome. *The American Journal of Gastroenterology, 109*(1), 52–59.

Khan, S., Hyman, P. E., Cocjin, J., & Di Lorenzo, C. (2000). Rumination syndrome in adolescents. *The Journal of Pediatrics, 136*(4), 528–531.

Malcolm, A., Thumshirn, M., Camilleri, M., & Williams, D. E. (1997). Rumination syndrome. *Mayo Clinic Proceedings, 72*, 646–652.

Monagas, J., Ritwick, P., Kolomensky, A., Acosta, J., Kay, D., Clendaniel, L., & Hyman, P. E. (2017). Rumination syndrome and dental erosions in children. *Journal of Pediatric Gastroenterology and Nutrition, 64*(6), 930–932.

O'Brien, M. D., Bruce, B. K., & Camilleri, M. (1995). The rumination syndrome: Clinical features rather than manometric diagnosis. *Gastroenterology, 108*(4), 1024–1029.

Olden, K. W. (2001). Rumination. *Current Treatment Options in Gastroenterology, 4*(4), 351–358.

Rachuba, K., & Alioto, A. (2015). Treatment of adolescent rumination syndrome: The role of the pediatric dietician. *PNPG Building Block for Life, 38*(4), 10–13.

Rajindrajith, S., Devanarayana, N. M., & Crispus Perera, B. J. (2012). Rumination syndrome in children and adolescents: A school survey assessing prevalence and symptomatology. *BMC Gastroenterology, 12*, 163.

Righini Grunder, F., Aspirot, A., & Faure, C. (2017). High-resolution esophageal manometry patterns in children and adolescents with rumination syndrome. *Journal of Pediatric Gastroenterology and Nutrition, 65*(6), 627–632.

Rosen, J. M., Alioto, A., & Saps, M. (2016). Advances in pain-predominant functional gastrointestinal disorders in the adolescent. *Adolescent Medicine: Stet of the Art Reviews, 27*(1), 34–56.

Schroedl, R. L., Alioto, A., & Di Lorenzo, C. (2013). Behavioral treatment for adolescent rumination syndrome: A case report. *Clinical Practice in Pediatric Psychology, 1*(1), 5.

Shay, S. S., Johnson, L. F., Wong, R. K., Curtis, D. J., Rosenthal, R., Lamott, J. R., & Owensby, L. C. (1986). Rumination, heartburn, and daytime gastroesophageal reflux. A case study with mechanisms defined and successfully treated with biofeedback therapy. *Journal of Clinical Gastroenterology, 8*(2), 115–126.

Sowder, E., Gervitz, R., Shapiro, W., & Ebert, C. (2010). Restoration of vagal tone: A possible mechanism for functional abdominal pain. *Applied Psychophysiology and Biofeedback, 35*, 199–206.

Thumshirn, M., Camilleri, M., Hanson, R. B., Williams, D. E., Schei, A. J., & Kammer, P. P. (1998). Gastric mechanosensory and lower esophageal sphincter function in rumination syndrome. *American Journal of Physiology, 275*(2 Pt 1), G314–G321.

Tucker, E., Knowles, K., Wright, J., & Fox, M. R. (2013). Rumination variations: Aetiology and classification of abnormal behavioural responses to digestive symptoms based on high-resolution manometry studies. *Alimentary Pharmacology & Therapeutics, 37*(2), 263–274.

Wagaman, J. R., Williams, D. E., & Camilleri. (1998). Behavioral intervention for the treatment of rumination. *Journal of Pediatric Gastroenterology and Nutrition, 27*(5), 596–598.

Organic Gastrointestinal Disorders

Michele H. Maddux, Amanda D. Deacy, and Jennifer M. Colombo

Diagnosis

Gastrointestinal (GI) symptoms in children are very common and frequently nonspecific, thus making the diagnosis of a GI disorder or disease challenging. Children presenting with GI symptoms may have an acute self-limited illness, a functional GI disorder, or an organic GI disease which may be temporary or lifelong. When approaching a child with a GI complaint, it is critical to obtain an accurate history. Asking specific questions about the symptom onset, frequency and severity of symptoms, and any aggravating or relieving factors can be especially helpful. The specific details of the GI complaint gathered during history taking are used to generate a differential diagnosis. The differential diagnosis is based primarily on the clinician's experience, pattern of disease recognition, constellation of symptoms, and probability of the disease which may depend on several factors such as age and gender of child, time course of the symptoms, time of year, family history, etc. (Aronoff & Del Vecchio, 2016). The clinician may use physical exam findings, medication trials, laboratory testing, radiologic studies, and/or other testing such as upper and lower endoscopy with biopsies to help narrow the list and rule out diagnoses that do not appropriately explain the child's symptoms.

M. H. Maddux (✉) · A. D. Deacy · J. M. Colombo
Department of Pediatrics, Children's Mercy-Kansas City, University of Missouri-Kansas City, MO, USA
e-mail: mhmaddux@cmh.edu

Medical Basics

Summarizing all organic GI disorders in children is beyond the scope of this chapter; therefore, only the most common organic GI diseases encountered in consultation settings will be reviewed and presented here.

Gastroesophageal Reflux Disease (GERD)

Gastroesophageal reflux is a normal process that refers, simply, to the backward flow of gastric contents into the esophagus. When the presence of gastric contents in the esophagus leads to bothersome symptoms, this normal process becomes a disease. GERD can present as back arching, regurgitation or vomiting, feeding refusal, and poor weight gain in infants and as epigastric pain, heartburn, and regurgitation in older children. For most children with uncomplicated symptoms of GERD, empiric acid suppression treatment with an H2 receptor antagonist or a proton pump inhibitor can help treat the symptoms without the need for further testing (Rosen et al., 2018).

B. D. Carter, K. A. Kullgren (eds.), *Clinical Handbook of Psychological Consultation in Pediatric Medical Settings*, Issues in Clinical Child Psychology, https://doi.org/10.1007/978-3-030-35598-2_16

Eosinophilic Esophagitis (EoE)

Eosinophilic esophagitis is an allergic inflammatory disease characterized by eosinophil cells infiltrating the lining of the esophagus, confirmed by upper endoscopy and biopsy of the esophagus (Markowitz & Liacouras, 2016). The symptoms of EoE include vomiting, regurgitation, upper abdominal pain, difficulty swallowing, feeding refusal, and food impaction. This is a chronic condition with lifelong implications as most children with EoE are treated with dietary elimination with or without swallowed corticosteroids. Dietary elimination ranges in complexity from removal of specific identified food allergens to total elimination diets using amino acid-based formula only (Markowitz & Liacouras, 2016).

Celiac Disease

Celiac disease is an autoimmune disorder triggered by a sensitivity to gluten (i.e., a protein found in wheat, barley, and rye) and occurs only in children and adults who possess the necessary genetic makeup for the disease. Toddlers may present with diarrhea, bloating, abdominal pain, poor weight gain, and irritability, while school-age children and adolescents may complain of abdominal pain; diarrhea; growth delay, including short stature; headaches; and skin rashes. Screening for celiac disease includes blood testing for celiac antibodies followed by confirmation with an upper endoscopy and biopsies for any child who has a positive screen. Treatment for celiac disease requires lifelong adherence to a gluten-free diet.

Short Bowel Syndrome (SBS)

Short bowel syndrome is a complex syndrome in which the length and function of the intestines are compromised resulting in malabsorption. The malabsorption that is associated with SBS presents as profuse watery diarrhea, poor weight gain, electrolyte imbalances, and nutritional deficiencies. The infant or child affected by SBS is unable to digest and absorb enough nutrients through the gastrointestinal tract that are necessary for normal growth and development. This malabsorption may be so severe that the child cannot survive without parenteral nutrition, which requires long-term IV access with a central line (Kaufman, 2016). Additionally, because they may not be able to digest and absorb complex foods, a gastrostomy tube (g-tube) may be used to provide supplemental enteral nutrition at a slow stable rate. Most often, this combination of parenteral and enteral nutrition is necessary to maintain fluid and electrolyte balance and to promote a normal growth pattern, allowing time for the intestinal tract to grow and adapt (Kaufman, 2016). With intestinal adaptation, infants and children can eventually be weaned off parenteral nutrition; however, this may take several years.

Pancreatitis

Pancreatitis is simply inflammation of the pancreas, an organ responsible for the production and secretion of digestive enzymes and production and secretion of insulin. The inflammation can be acute (i.e., a single isolated episode that resolves with supportive care) or chronic (i.e., progressive inflammatory changes resulting in destruction and scarring of the pancreas). Common causes of acute pancreatitis include trauma, medications, viral infections, severe systemic illness, and gallstones, and common causes of chronic pancreatitis include hereditary pancreatitis, autoimmune pancreatitis, cystic fibrosis, elevated triglycerides related to a metabolic syndrome, and congenital anomalies (Lowe, 2016). When the pancreas becomes inflamed, children may complain of pain in their upper abdomen, nausea, vomiting, and decreased appetite. Treatment of pancreatitis includes aggressive fluid management using IV fluids, pain control by IV pain medication initially followed by oral pain medications, and careful planning of nutritional intervention. At times, imaging studies (e.g., abdominal ultrasound or abdominal computed tomography) may be necessary to determine the severity of pancreatitis if the child is not improving with these supportive measures.

Inflammatory Bowel Disease (IBD)

IBD is a spectrum of diseases involving chronic inflammation of the GI tract within any segment of the intestinal tract from the mouth to the anus. Clinical symptoms, physical exam findings, and laboratory evaluation must be combined with findings of an upper endoscopy and colonoscopy with biopsies of the gastrointestinal tract to establish a diagnosis. Depending on the location and severity of the inflammation in the GI tract, IBD can be subdivided into Crohn's disease (CD), ulcerative colitis (UC), and indeterminate colitis (IC). CD typically affects the end of the small intestine (the ileum) and the beginning of the colon, but it can affect any part of the GI tract from the mouth to the anus, while UC is limited to the large intestine (colon) and the rectum. IC is suggested when the diagnosis of CD and UC is in question because the child's symptoms and clinical findings are overlapping. Children with IBD may complain of abdominal pain, diarrhea with or without blood, nausea, vomiting, weight loss, poor appetite, and/or mouth ulcers. Children may also have recurrent fever, headaches, skin rashes, and arthritis (Mamula, Markowitz, & Baldassano, 2008).

There is no cure for IBD; rather, the goal of medical management is to achieve remission to keep the disease from progressing. There are multiple forms and types of treatment ranging from oral to infused medications to nutritional therapies. Even with aggressive medical and nutritional management, IBD may be unresponsive to treatment and progress, possibly leading to uncontrolled GI bleeding, obstruction or perforation of the gastrointestinal tract, or abscess with fistula formation. In these cases, surgery may be indicated to remove the diseased part of the intestinal tract and/or placement of a temporary or permanent ostomy which may impact the child's medical and psychosocial well-being.

Engagement

Patients and families may be reluctant to receive pediatric psychological consultation and follow through on treatment recommendations if they do not understand or accept a biopsychosocial conceptualization of their GI symptoms. The biopsychosocial model is particularly relevant to GI disorders due to the overwhelming evidence for the interaction between the gut and the brain (Dovey, 2014). The model highlights that psychosocial factors *and* illness factors related to the GI disorder contribute to the child or adolescent's functioning. As such, helping the child and family cope with illness-related factors, such as symptoms, diagnostic testing and medical procedures, and prescribed treatment regimens, is essential to maintain appropriate development and optimal functioning (Cunningham & Banez, 2006). The inherent risk of not understanding or accepting the biopsychosocial model of care is that patients might not receive the type and level of intervention that has the potential to improve not only psychological functioning and quality of life for pediatric patients with GI disorders but also symptoms and perhaps even disease severity itself.

Medical providers play a crucial role in setting the stage for greater buy-in and engagement from families to integrated biopsychosocial interventions. An introduction of the psychologist as an integral member of the medical team, combined with the intentional provision of education on the brain-gut axis and the biological and psychological mechanisms of symptom presentation, can decrease the stigma that patients and their families might perceive to receiving psychology consultation. Integration of the pediatric psychologist into inpatient hospital rounds, care conferences, and clinic visits, for example, can model to families that the psychologist is embedded into the medical team and involved in all aspects of a child's care (Carter et al., 2017). Education provided by medical providers might include a discussion of known mechanisms of the brain-gut axis (e.g., gut microbiome, inflammation) as well as a stated recognition that the ongoing management of GI symptoms can be emotionally, physically, and socially taxing (Reed-Knight et al., 2017). This level of team integration and the provision of biopsychosocial education establishes the relevance of psychological assessment and intervention in the treatment of organic GI disorders. This can also clarify the role of the psychologist as a nonthreatening part of the medical team who is available to help patients identify strategies for reducing symptoms by impacting the brain-gut axis through behavioral strategies (Reed-Knight et al., 2017). In addition, providing reassurance that GI-related pain is real, is understood, and can be treated can be helpful in reducing a child's and family's anxiety about working with a pediatric psychologist.

Use of a visual aid can help guide discussions with patients about the brain-gut axis and the link to biological and psychosocial factors (Reed-Knight et al., 2017) (Appendix 1). The pediatric psychologist might further achieve engagement and buy-in from families by completing a thorough assessment of troublesome physical symptoms (e.g., abdominal pain, changes in stooling patterns, vomiting) at the first intervention. This acknowledges the family's concerns and acknowledges the child's suffering, both of which likely initiated the consultation with a GI specialist.

Formulation

In the consultation-liaison (CL) role, the pediatric psychologist is called on to assess the pediatric patient and formulate a psychosocial treatment plan in the context of the patient's primary presenting medical problem. As such, the *medical team* is the "client," a shift from more traditional therapy models (Silverman & Williams, 2014). Thus, in order to most efficiently answer the specific question or questions from the medical team, the consulting psychologist is encouraged to conduct his or her assessment in a two-staged fashion—first, by gathering information from the patient's medical record, the primary medical team, other consulting specialty services, and ancillary care team members such as Child Life and social work and, second, by meeting with the patient and his or her family members. The former is a step that ought to be carried out as thoughtfully and completely as the latter.

At the first point of contact with the medical team, it is imperative that we seek clarification from our medical colleagues about the exact nature of their question. On the surface, this may sound deceptively simple; however, it is important to consider that those consulting psychology may not share the same perspective on the psychosocial issues at hand, nor possess the expertise required to appreciate the necessary nuance involved in the timing of therapeutic assessment and intervention for our shared patients. For example, a consult question of "depression" is not nearly detailed enough to elicit the appropriate assessment methodology or intervention strategy. In this case, psychologists will need to ascertain from their medical partners if the primary concern is whether the patient meets diagnostic criteria for major depressive disorder, whether there is concern that depression is present for a patient's parent, whether down mood is preventing needed communication between the patient and medical staff, or whether depression and an associated lack of motivation are a concern for the medical team due to its likely impact on medical treatment adherence, to name just a few.

It is only once psychologists and their collaborating medical partners have settled on a specific consult question that assessment, case formulation, and intervention with the identified patient can begin. It is also at this point that the consulting psychologist will be required to triage aspects of the medical team's question that can be reasonably addressed in an inpatient setting and to postpone those that are better suited for outpatient follow-up. In general, psychologists will employ assessment strategies in a consultative role in a similar albeit more targeted fashion, than in the role of primary treatment provider. Questions for IBD patients and their families can be formulated in the following broad categories as a starting place: disease knowledge, social functioning, school, and family (Cunningham &

Banez, 2006). Additionally, and equally valuable, psychologists should assess pediatric patients' emotional and physical functioning as they, too, are frequently impacted by an acute or chronic medical condition (see Table 1).

As part of the process of gathering this information from patients and families, psychologists are encouraged to consider whether it is most appropriate to interview the patient and his/her parents together or separately and whether answers to assessment questions are obtained via interview only or through a combination of interview questions and standardized assessment tools. The determination about the format for patient and family interviews may be dictated by the patient's medical treatment and clinical status (e.g., requiring isolation, 1:1 supervision, patient being out of his/her hospital room for a procedure), the sensitivity of the information sought, and the constraints of the setting (e.g., the availability of private meeting rooms on inpatient units or in outpatient clinics). Likewise, time constraints or time sensitivity of the consultation and the primary language spoken by pediatric patients and their parents are two variables that may affect the ease and practicality of using an interview or standardized assessment tools as the preferred methods for gathering assessment information.

Table 1 Domains of assessment to aid in consultation case conceptualization

Assessment domains	Specific, sample questions
Disease knowledge	• What do patients understand about their disease? • What causes it? • How is it treated? What is the patient's/family's capacity for treatment adherence? • Is the condition life-threatening?
Social functioning	• Are the patient's friends aware of his/her GI diagnosis? • Is the patient involved in extracurricular or other school-related activities? • Does his/her GI diagnosis affect his/her ability to socialize?
School	• Has the patient missed school due to symptoms? • Can he/she maintain a full school-day schedule? • Is the school helpful with providing needed accommodation?
Family	• What do parents and caregivers understand about the GI diagnosis and its potential impact on their child's functioning—Physical, emotional, and otherwise? • Who is responsible for making sure medication is taken? • Has the diagnosis changed the parent/child dynamic, that is, have parents become overprotective, for example?
Emotional functioning	• Has the child experienced mood changes since the GI diagnosis (e.g., down mood or anxiety)? • Did the patient have emotional difficulties that predated his/her GI diagnosis? • Has the new GI diagnosis worsened these preexisting struggles?
Physical functioning	• Has the patient's physical functioning been impacted by his/her GI diagnosis? • Can he/she walk, run, and play sports as he/she used to?

Note. Adapted from Cunningham and Banez (2006)

Intervention

Psychosocial factors have been linked to disturbances in the brain-gut axis via several biological mechanisms, including alterations in pain processing, the stress response system, and gut microbiome activity (Reed-Knight et al., 2017) and, thus, are critical targets of intervention for consulting psychologists. First and foremost, clinical intervention for youth with organic GI disorders should provide anticipatory guidance and normalize patients' and families' reactions to dealing with the child's GI diagnosis and the associated treatment regimen. Second, an initial assessment as detailed in Table 1 will help identify intervention targets.

In general, youths with chronic medical conditions are at greater risk for mental health comorbidity. Data in youth with organic GI disorders suggests a greater risk for anxiety and depression, as well as internalizing disorders. Studies in youth with IBD and eosinophil-associated gastrointestinal disorders (EGID) suggest depression rates as high as two- to threefold greater compared to healthy controls (Cortina et al., 2010) or youth with other chronic medical disorders (Kappelman et al., 2014; Loftus et al., 2011). Depending on the symptom severity and impact on a patient's daily function and quality of life, a referral for cognitive-behavioral therapy (CBT) may be warranted.

CBT interventions for anxiety and depression aim to identify and change maladaptive cognitions about symptoms and pain (e.g., catastrophizing), apply cognitive reframing to improve perceived control about modifiable factors (e.g., adherence, self-care), and teach youth with GI disorders to manage pain and stress via relaxation, guided imagery, and/or self-hypnosis, have all been found to be effective (Szigethy et al., 2007, 2015). Such interventions have been shown to decrease symptoms of depression, improve disease activity, and decrease somatic symptoms (Szigethy et al., 2007, 2015) as well as improve quality of life and adaptive coping (Levy et al., 2016).

CBT can also explicitly target behavioral inactivation, a hallmark of organic GI disorders. Frequent trips to the bathroom, dietary restrictions, physical symptoms (e.g., nausea, abdominal/joint pain), and side effects of medication (e.g., swelling from steroids) can all significantly disrupt participation in normal activities and lead to activity limitations, physical deconditioning, and, ultimately, withdrawal. As such, behavioral activation is an invaluable treatment component. When normal activity is not feasible, families can be guided to modify activities (e.g., inviting friends over rather than going out, talking to a coach about remaining involved and in contact with teammates) or identify alternative activities.

GI disorders may also affect school attendance or academic performance. In fact, research in youth with IBD suggests that they incur more frequent school absences, lower grades and academic achievement, and poorer school-related quality of life compared to healthy controls (Assa, Ish-Tov, Rinawi, & Shamir, 2015; Mackner, Bickmeier, & Crandall, 2012). As such, it is essential that the school environment is supportive of a patient's psychosocial functioning and academic success, as this is likely to minimize school-related stress and encourage continued school attendance. Intervention might include contact with the school to discuss the GI diagnosis and treatment plan and the implementation of appropriate school-based services (e.g., unrestricted bathroom access, additional time to complete missed assignments), as well as a structured plan for graduated school re-entry when extended school absences have occurred (see Appendix 2). Families should also be informed about their rights for school-based accommodations in accordance with the Individuals with Disabilities Education Act (IDEA) and Section 504 of the Rehabilitation Act.

Another intervention target that has important implications for both psychosocial functioning and health outcomes is treatment nonadherence. Roughly 50–75% of children and adolescents with chronic medical conditions fail to adhere adequately to their treatments (Rapoff, 2010). This places youth with organic GI disorders at significant risk for serious complications of the disease. In IBD alone, poor adherence to medication has been linked to a *fivefold* increased risk of relapse (Kane, Huo, Aikens, & Hanauer, 2003), a 12.5% increase in annual health-care costs (Higgins, Rubin, Kaulback, Schoenfield, & Kane, 2009), and greater health-care use (i.e., hospitalizations, emergency department visits, outpatient visits) (McGrady & Hommel, 2013). Multicomponent interventions that combine empirically supported treatment components such as behavior management (e.g., behavioral contracting), guided problem-solving around adherence barriers, self-management training, and disease education have been shown to promote greater adherence among chronically ill youth (Graves, Roberts, Rapoff, & Boyer, 2010; Lemanek, Kamps, & Chung, 2001) and reflect current adherence promotion recommendations (Kahana, Drotar, & Frazier, 2008).

Adaptation

The very nature of consultative work requires that psychologists serving in this capacity consider appropriate modifications of interventions originally designed for the traditional 1-h therapy visit. The physical environment of the pediatric setting (i.e., time and the need for quick rapport, confidentiality, space/scheduling) and the developmental and cultural needs of a patient and family all bear on the type and degree of modifications to specific interventions that are needed.

With regard to the physical environment, consulting psychologists recognize that employment of an evidence-based intervention may look different depending on whether it is being executed at the bedside (i.e., on the inpatient service), in a busy medical clinic, or in a more traditional outpatient therapy clinic. In the case of the inpatient setting, in particular, the time that a provider has to spend with a patient (i.e., days until discharge) may be as little as one visit up to several visits spread over many weeks. In the context of very limited time, a psychologist has to clearly prioritize the most pressing clinical need, usually one that is affecting the current hospital admission and/or imminent discharge, as the primary target of intervention. This might mean that the "prework" that is specified in an evidence-based intervention is not able to be done at all or is done in a condensed fashion. In a medical clinic, psychology visits may need to adhere to the amount of time usually allocated to medical follow-ups (e.g., 30 min). Additionally, although not exactly a modification of the intervention itself, psychologists providing service in the context of the hospital often will need to establish patient and family buy-in and rapport much more quickly than one typically has the luxury for in other settings.

Privacy and confidentiality are also important considerations when delivering evidence-based intervention at the bedside or in a fast-paced medical clinic. Given that pediatric patients are most often joined in their hospital rooms by parents and frequently visited by other hospital staff throughout the day—nurses, janitorial and food service staff, lab techs, hospital clergy, etc.—ensuring confidentiality can be more challenging. Similarly, meeting with a psychology staff member in a medical clinic can compromise a patient's confidentiality merely by being in the same physical space as their medical providers and fellow patients. As such, psychologists will need to be especially sensitive to patients' right to confidentiality in these settings. This may require requesting no visitors or interruptions during a bedside psychology session or conducting a session in a common area on a hospital floor or, in the case of outpatient work, in an exam room at the very end of a hallway or near an entrance to decrease foot traffic during therapy visits.

Developmental level and cultural and other individual factors (e.g., age, SES, specific medical condition) also impact the type and degree of modifications to, and the delivery of, evidence-based interventions that are considered by consulting psychologists. As an example, because adolescents are known to exhibit poorer medication adherence relative to younger children, interventions for improving adherence in adolescents will necessarily have to be adapted by increasing the frequency of scheduled therapy visits and/or identifying alternatives to parent reminders for medication-taking (e.g., alarms, mobile device apps). These same sociocultural factors can serve as barriers to adherence to medical interventions (e.g., religious or cultural prohibitions against prescription medications and/or a preference for naturopathic remedies, cost of and lack of access to gluten-free foods for celiac disease, cost of and preparation time required for the simple carbohydrate diet for IBD).

Resources/Support

The work of psychologists as consultants to a medical specialty team is supported and enhanced by the clinical and practical expertise of a host of other hospital-based professionals. While the specific roles and resources available can vary greatly by institution, Child Life specialists can play critical roles in patients' preparation for procedures and pain prevention and management. Likewise, Child Life staff are responsible for delivering therapeutic groups and activities relevant to pediatric patients (e.g., movie and game nights on the inpatient unit, service animal programs, and skills building programs aimed at teaching coping skills) (Beickert & Mora, 2017). Social workers also play essential roles in supporting psychological intervention delivery. Social work staff can be key to ensuring transportation to and from appointments; coordinating multiple appointments to occur close together in time and affordable (or free) lodging for those who travel a distance to medical and psychological service visits; helping parents navigate insurance pre-authorization and/or coverage; providing support to older teens as they transition to adult health-care settings; providing food, housing, utility, and other resources for families in financial need; and supporting parents in the establishment of power of attorney, guardianship, and the like (Fonash, 2018).

Hospital volunteers are another critical resource for supporting and complementing the work of consulting psychologists. Volunteer staff can serve in the role of caregiver to a sibling while a pediatric patient and his/her parent attend appointments, help to organize holiday and birthday events to mitigate the distress associated with spending these important milestones in the hospital, and offer support to parents in getting from place to place within the hospital. Finally, hospital-based school teachers are another invaluable resource to pediatric patients and their families. Well known is the fact that chronically ill children struggle with absenteeism from school and, related to this, keeping up with academic work, and poor learning outcomes (Lum et al., 2017). Furthermore, supporting children in both academic and social activities has been hypothesized to reduce difficulties during school re-entry (Arroyos-Jurado, Paulsen, Merrell, Lindgren, & Max, 2000). As such, hospital-based teachers provide much needed services, including serving as a liaison between the patient and his/her home school, communicating with patients' school teachers to obtain needed work and/or proctor tests during hospital admissions, arranging for homebound instructors or other tutoring resources, and facilitating requests for special education services (e.g., IEPs or Section 504 Plans), as needed. Taken together, the expertise of the above professionals and environmental supports is vital to pediatric patients obtaining the frequency and quality of medical and psychological intervention needed.

Inpatient Consultation

The inpatient hospital context within which children with organic GI disorders are often initially encountered cannot be ignored or its impact underestimated. At the time of inpatient psychology consultation, many children and adolescents are either newly diagnosed with a GI disorder or have been experiencing GI symptoms for some time and are awaiting diagnosis or refinement of the treatment plan. They are likely dealing with diagnostic uncertainty and life changes incurred by symptoms, are having to learn large quantities of medical information in a relatively short period of time, and are placing their care into the hands of unfamiliar medical professionals. Understandably, stress can be quite high for patients and their family.

In addition, the hospital environment itself can impact the emotional and behavioral functioning of a patient and his/her family. Youth and their families are often in close proximity to one another for extended periods of time, with frequent visits from various medical professionals. This results in few opportunities to engage in solitary or preferred activities and little privacy. Clinical data obtained from patients with IBD and their parents suggests increased parent-child strain related to changes incurred by a new disease, including increased parental monitoring and supervision, and sharing of treatment responsibilities (Maddux, Bass, Geraghty-Sirridge, Carpenter, & Christenson, 2013). Among parents and other caregivers, the distress of having a child with a chronic medical condition can lead to overprotective parenting behaviors that conflict with the patient's attempt to assert independence and gain autonomy (Maddux et al., 2013; Mullins et al., 2007). At the same time, caregivers can experience added burden from managing competing demands of caring for their ill child in the hospital while also meeting the needs of other children in the home, with whom they might have infrequent contact while the patient is admitted. It is not uncommon for roles within a family to shift or be re-allocated when a child is admitted to the hospital. For example, if a child is hospitalized, one caregiver may need to stay with the ill child in the hospital, while the other caregiver negotiates care for siblings and household tasks (Herzer et al., 2010). Caring for a child with an organic GI disorder can also translate into extended periods of absenteeism from work, which can be taxing to a family's finances at a time when costs of medical care associated with the GI disorder are likely quite high. Sleep complaints among both patients and caregivers are also common during hospitalizations. In fact, youth and their parents have been found to experience later wake times and more night wakings, usually due to noise, pain, worry, and vital sign checks (Meltzer, Davis, & Mindell, 2012). The fatigue and sleep deprivation that ensues can render an already stressful hospitalization even more challenging.

Outpatient Consultation

As discharge nears for a pediatric inpatient, the psychologist consultant plays a key role in ensuring continuity of the psychological care provided during admission. To facilitate this, the consulting psychologist is encouraged to work with the identified discharge planning team to coordinate medical and psychological follow-up. The latter can look a number of ways, including (1) transfer from the pediatric hospital to an inpatient psychiatric facility for continued mental health treatment, (2) traditional outpatient therapy follow-up with a member of the psychology consultation team or a mental health provider in the patient's home community, or (3) behavioral health follow-up in the context of the patient's specialty medical visits. The determination of the most appropriate fit for a given patient will depend on a number of factors including the acuity of his or her mental health presentation (i.e., suicide risk and the possible need for psychotropic medication management), the distance of his or her home from the hospital, the provider availability, and the patient's insurance status.

In the case of psychological consultation in outpatient specialty and primary care settings, provision of psychological services can range from a one-time consultation (e.g., brief screening and referral), repeated psychological follow-up during a patient's specialty or primary care medical visits for continued monitoring and brief intervention, and/or traditional psychological therapy in tandem with ongoing medical follow-up. In the event that therapy is being provided by someone other than the consulting psychologist (i.e., someone in the surrounding community), a warm hand-off and continued consultation can be important factors in the success of a patient's psychological therapy. Community mental health providers may not be well versed in the nature of the patient's medical diagnosis and may need to rely on the consulting psychologist's clinical expertise as therapy gets underway in order to understand the patient's likely symptom and treatment course and potential complicating psychosocial factors. As a jumpstart to this communication, authors (MM & AD) frequently share "targets of therapy letter" with families who seek outpatient therapy in their local community for psychosocial concerns collateral to their child's GI disorder. These letters list a number of specific topics or content areas that are suggested for therapists as a resource, as addressing them is thought to support both the patient's physical and psychological well-being (see Appendix 3).

Case Example

"Jessica" is an 18-year-old Hispanic female diagnosed with UC at the age of 13, which did not respond to medical treatment and required colectomy approximately 8 months after initial diagnosis. She was able to proceed with ileostomy takedown 2 months after colectomy. Following takedown, she experienced recurrent pouchitis (i.e., inflammation that occurs in the lining of a pouch that is created during surgery to treat UC) for a period of 2 years resulting in frequent hospitalizations and multiple treatments with antibiotics. Jessica also required enteral feeds due to significant weight loss. Other symptoms experienced over this 2-year period included frequent and bloody daytime stooling, nighttime stooling, nausea and vomiting, decreased appetite, abdominal pain, and significant fatigue.

A pediatric psychologist working on the IBD team was initially consulted during one of Jessica's hospitalizations shortly before colectomy, due to concerns with sadness, and to evaluate her likely adjustment to potential surgery. During Jessica's 2-week hospital stay, the psychologist provided education about surgery and anticipatory guidance about an ostomy, evaluated Jessica's fears and worries about surgery, taught her and her parents to use positive reframing in the context of frightening medical procedures, and provided information to the family about community supports for youth with IBD. Following surgery, the psychologist provided pain management support to Jessica and her parents by teaching deep breathing techniques and guided imagery and emphasizing the use of preferred daily activities to redirect Jessica's attention away from pain.

In collaboration with the inpatient medical team, the psychologist also consulted with a social worker to assist the family with obtaining appropriate school-based accommodations given Jessica's extended absences from school, and a plan for graduated school re-entry was developed by the psychologist and social worker with input from Jessica's gastroenterologist. Child Life specialists were also consulted at the start of Jessica's hospitalization and following surgery to create a daily schedule of activities, including arts and crafts, walking around the inpatient unit, attending activities in the Teen Room, and playing board games with her parents. Throughout, the psychologist communicated regularly with the inpatient medical team to obtain frequent updates on Jessica's health status and treatment.

Following discharge from the hospital, the pediatric psychologist continued to follow Jessica on an outpatient basis, initially to evaluate her return to normal activities and management of a temporary ostomy. Over the course of these initial visits, it became apparent that Jessica's parents were struggling to give her independence and autonomy due to their own concerns with her health and well-being and their attempts to avoid additional adverse health events. Parents' heightened stress caused increased tension between them and Jessica. Jessica also struggled to return to school, and she incurred frequent absences due to ongoing gastrointestinal symptoms (e.g., abdominal pain, nausea) and anxiety about mobility and dietary restrictions during school. This caused her to fall behind in her classes and led to an increase in anxiety about her school performance. School avoidance was compounded by Jessica's perception that she was different from her peers and marginalized due to her medical diagnosis, which led to symptoms of depression and anxiety. Concerns with medication adherence were also present periodically.

Outpatient visits with the psychologist included a plan for gradually returning to normal activities, starting first with activities that posed minimal risk of illness or exacerbation or that occurred at times when Jessica's pain and GI symptoms were least bothersome. Symptoms of anxiety and depression were targeted by identifying anxious and distressing thoughts, evaluating evidence for/against those thoughts, and applying positive reframing, techniques consistent with cognitive-behavioral therapy (CBT). Adherence barriers also remained a treatment target and were addressed by setting adherence goals and applying problem-solving solutions in the family's home (e.g., using a pillbox, leaving a reminder note on her bathroom mirror). Support was also provided to parents on targeting their own distress and its impact on Jessica's overall emotional and behavioral functioning. Parents were coached on directing their concern for Jessica in a positive and developmentally appropriate manner. An outpatient social worker remained involved in Jessica's care to support the family in developing a Section 504 Plan to formalize recommended accommodations, to provide education to school personnel about her health needs, and to oversee the graduated school re-entry plan.

The psychologist also provided regular treatment updates to Jessica's primary gastroenterologist, who in turn emphasized the psychologist's role as an important adjunct to her medical treatment during routine follow-up medical visits.

Appendix 1

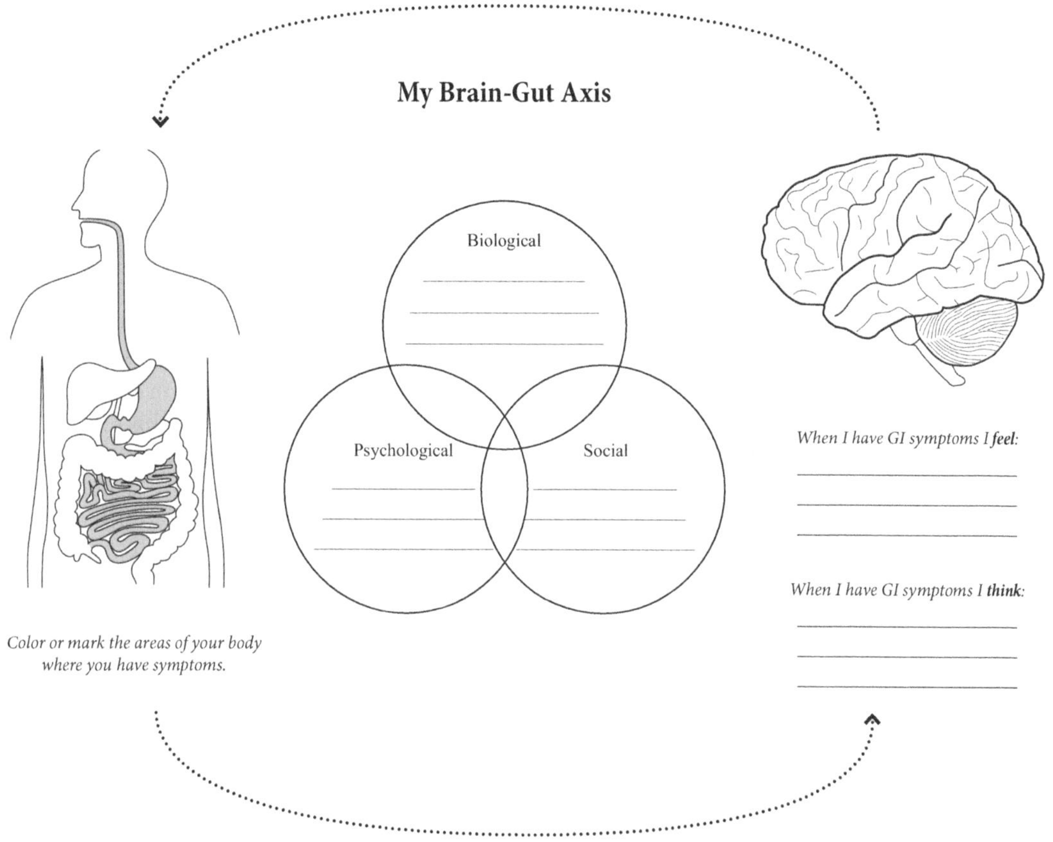

Appendix 2: Getting Back to School: A Guide for Parents

Many children with gastrointestinal (GI) disorders have school problems. They may miss school days (or even weeks!) because of symptoms, doctor's visits, being in the hospital, or school policies meant to prevent illness from spreading. They also may have a hard time paying attention in class, get behind in daily school work, or feel overwhelmed by make-up work.

Your child may require your help and support to get back to school full-time. The key to accomplishing this goal will be *creating a plan to gradually increase daily expectations*.

Graduated School Re-Entry

If your child has been out of school for a long time, he or she may need a shortened school day at first. This would be followed by longer and longer periods of attendance (as strength, stamina, and confidence increase). This gradual increase in time at school would continue until your child is back at school full time. We call this plan "graduated school re-entry." The key steps are listed below:

- Step 1. **Choose a block of class time that your child is able to attend every day without *increased* GI symptoms.** Start with a small enough amount of time to ensure your child's success and build from there. This may be as little as 1 h, a single class period, or a half day. Pay attention to what time of the day your child's symptoms tend to be the most manageable in setting up this plan. You may want to avoid starting with any classes are particularly stressful. Starting with a favorite class or activity is fine—any amount of time spent at school will increase strength, stamina, and confidence!
- Step 2. **Your child should go to school at the agreed upon time and stay at school until the scheduled ending time for that day.** This should happen regardless of pain (or other symptom) complaints. Your child should leave school at the scheduled ending time *even if he or she is feeling well.* Doing this will encourage feelings of success and help prevent symptoms from getting worse on the following day(s).
- Step 3. **Your child's progress should be reevaluated weekly (on Wednesday or Thursday, if possible).** If your child has been able to complete the plan for the previous week without increased symptoms, then class time should be increased slightly. Again, this added time may be as little as 30 min. *Remember, slow and steady is the key!*

Supporting Success and Attendance at School

There are lots of ways to support your child's success in the classroom and encourage regular school attendance. Here are a few strategies that might be helpful to your child:

- **Allow easy access to the bathroom at school.** Asking permission to leave class can be embarrassing and increase fears about not getting to the bathroom in time. It sometimes helps to work with teacher(s) to develop a private system of communication. For example, some children put a colored index card on their desk when they need to leave for the bathroom. This lets the teacher know, but allows the child to get to the bathroom quickly without disturbing the class.
- **Encourage taking brief breaks to use stress and pain management skills.** Children can help themselves feel better and stay at school by using relaxation strategies (including biofeedback), as needed. These skills can be done sitting in an office or any other place where your child's presence and activity won't bother other students. Breaks should last 10–15 min, followed by a return to class.
- **Encourage participation in clubs and sports while working on getting back to school.** Participation in these activities, even on a limited basis, may help a child stay connected with friends and improve mood. Social isolation and depression can get in the way of recovery. These feelings also can make it harder to get back to school.
- **Carefully consider make-up work.** Getting overwhelmed with schoolwork is a problem. It can increase the chance of symptoms getting worse. This can result in a cycle of missing more school, getting further behind, and getting more stressed. Sometimes it can help to reduce the amount of required schoolwork during the school re-entry process. It also can help to extend the time for completing make-up work and tests. Reducing your child's workload should be done in a thoughtful way to ensure that he or she is learning the necessary concepts while minimizing the quantity of work required (and the associated stress).
- **Set up a reasonable schedule for completing make-up work at home.** Some children have lots of make-up work to finish as they get back to school. Plus, they still have regular daily assignments and projects! We encourage parents to set up a schedule for completing

make-up work that is consistent, without being stressful or overly demanding. Set a timer for 30 min. During this time, ask your child to focus only on make-up work. After that time, have your child take a break, even if the make-up work is not fully completed. One more 30-min session can be scheduled for later in the evening, if needed. Avoid scheduling any more than these two daily 30-min periods for completing make-up work. Spending too much time on make-up work, in addition to daily assignments, may be counterproductive to recovery.

- **Consider asking for a Section 504 Plan for your child based on his or her health issues.** This plan is a written agreement between you, your child, and the school. It can help make your child's back-to-school support plan more formal and encourage participation across all school staff.

Special Situations

Homebound. In general, we discourage ongoing homebound services as a way for children to complete school requirements. For academic, social, emotional, and behavioral reasons, the best place for your child to spend his or her days is in school. If your child currently is receiving homebound services, it is important that you work with your child's medical team to help your child return to school, on a graduated basis, as part of his or her overall treatment plan. Your support and participation in this aspect of your child's treatment plan is critical.

Staying Home from School. Sometimes it can be hard to tell whether a child is sick when they have frequent abdominal pain and other GI symptoms. Parents often wonder when to let their children stay home from school. To help you navigate this tricky issue, we recommend keeping your child home from school when he or she has:

1. frequent or uncontrollable stooling through the day;
2. a temperature of 100° or higher in the last 24 h;
3. repeated vomiting and/or diarrhea in the last 24 h;
4. inability to keep down clear liquids; and/or
5. evidence of contagious infection.

If your child is too sick to go to school (using the above guide), he or she should rest quietly in bed (e.g., no TV, computer, or video games). If your child feels better before the school day ends, he or she may go to school late or work on schoolwork at home. *When in doubt, send your child to school and call your child's GI physician to discuss your child's symptoms*.

Important Reminders for Parents During the Back-to-School Process

- Return to school is *essential* for your child's physical, social, and emotional health.
- It may take several weeks for your child to return to his or her usual school routine. The key to accomplishing this goal will be to create a plan for gradually increasing daily expectations.
- Offering praise, rewards, or special activities for reaching important milestones (e.g., first full day back at school, first week at school without an absence) is encouraged.

Appendix 3

Date

Parents' address

Dear Parents,

As you know, your son/daughter, _, has a history of significant abdominal pain and other gastrointestinal (GI) issues that have greatly affected his/her daily functioning—his/her ability to attend school and spend time with friends and family, as well as his/her mood. In addition to pursuing medical care for _ through the X Clinic, we understand that you have sought psychological and behavioral support for him/her through a local mental health provider to address some of these concerns.

Individual mental health treatment is something we routinely recommend as an adjunct to our patients' medical treatment regimens. We believe that regular mental health support can help patients to regain their previous level of functioning and, in the longer term, indirectly improve their GI symptoms.

Specific therapy targets often addressed by therapists working with our patients include:

- Maintaining a consistent daily schedule that encourages functioning *with* GI symptoms
- Addressing sleep problems
- Targeting social issues that have developed secondary to lengthy absences from school and withdrawal from social activities (e.g., developing "scripts" for helping children to address peers' questions, encouraging social interaction by formalizing "play dates" or other structured social get-togethers with peers)
- Targeting academic issues that have developed secondary to prolonged school absences (e.g., coordinating with teachers to address make up work, making recommendations regarding appropriate accommodation at school)
- Encouraging active strategies (e.g., positive self-talk, deep breathing and other forms of relaxation, distraction, problem-solving) for managing physical complaints, including abdominal pain, and any known stressors
- Intervening with apparent co-morbid anxiety and depressive symptoms
- Collaborating with parents to ensure that the home environment is supportive of all the changes recommended and discussed within individual therapy visits

We appreciate your interest in working with us on behalf of _ and encourage you to share the above list with his/her current mental health practitioner. Should you have any questions regarding _'s care please contact us at 000-000-0000.

Sincerely,

References

Aronoff, S. C., & Del Vecchio, M. T. (2016). Differential diagnosis in pediatrics: A probabilistic approach. *Hospital Pediatrics, 6*(8), 504–505. https://doi.org/10.1542/hpeds.2016-0053

Arroyos-Jurado, E., Paulsen, J. S., Merrell, K. W., Lindgren, S. D., & Max, J. E. (2000). Traumatic brain injury in school-age children academic and social outcome. *Journal of School Psychology, 38*, 571–587. https://doi.org/10.1016/S0022-4405(00)00053-4

Assa, A., Ish-Tov, A., Rinawi, F., & Shamir, R. (2015). School attendance in children with functional abdominal pain and inflammatory bowel diseases. *Journal of Pediatric Gastroenterology and Nutrition, 61*(5), 553–557. https://doi.org/10.1097/MPG.0000000000000850

Beickert, K., & Mora, K. (2017). Transforming the pediatric experience: The story of child life. *Pediatric Annals, 46*(9), e345–e351. https://doi.org/10.3928/19382359-20170810-01

Carter, B., Kronenberger, W. G., Scott, E. L., Kullgren, K. A., Piazza-Waggoner, C., & Brady, C. E. (2017). Inpatient pediatric consultation-liaison. In M. C. Roberts & R. G. Steele (Eds.), *Handbook of pediatric psychology* (5th ed., pp. 105–118). New York, NY: The Guilford Press.

Cortina, S., McGraw, K., deAlarcon, A., Ahrens, A., Rothenberg, M. E., & Drotar, D. (2010). Psychological functioning of children and adolescents with eosinophil-associated gastrointestinal disorders. *Children's Health Care, 39*(4), 266–278. https://doi.org/10.1080/02739615.2010.515927

Cunningham, C., & Banez, G. (2006). *Pediatric gastrointestinal disorders: Biopsychosocial assessment and treatment*. New York, NY: Springer Science+Business Media, LLC.

Dovey, T. (2014). A biopsychosocial framework to understand children and young people with gastrointestinal problems. In C. Martin & T. Dovey (Eds.), *Paediatric gastrointestinal disorders: A psychosocial perspective* (pp. 118–133). London, UK: Radcliffe Publishing Ltd.

Fonash, A. (2018). The role of the medical social worker in a pediatric aero-digestive program. *Current Problems in Pediatric and Adolescent Health Care, 48*(4), 111–112. https://doi.org/10.1016/j.cppeds.2018.03.001

Graves, M. M., Roberts, M. C., Rapoff, M., & Boyer, A. (2010). The efficacy of adherence interventions for chronically ill children: A meta-analytic review. *Journal of Pediatric Psychology, 35*(4), 368–382. https://doi.org/10.1093/jpepsy/jsp072

Herzer, M., Godiwala, N., Hommel, K. A., Driscoll, K., Mitchell, M., Crosby, L. E., ... Modi, A. C. (2010). Family functioning in the context of pediatric chronic conditions. *Journal of Developmental and Behavioral Pediatrics, 31*(1), 26–34. https://doi.org/10.1097/DBP.0b013e3181c7226b

Higgins, P. D., Rubin, D. T., Kaulback, K., Schoenfield, P. S., & Kane, S. V. (2009). Systematic review: Impact of non-adherence to 5-aminosalicylic acid products on the frequency and cost of ulcerative colitis flares. *Alimentary Pharmacology and Therapeutics, 29*(3), 247–257. https://doi.org/10.1111/j.1365-2036.2008.03865.x

Kahana, S., Drotar, D., & Frazier, T. (2008). Meta-analysis of psychological interventions to promote adherence to treatment in pediatric chronic health conditions. *Journal of Pediatric Psychology, 33*(6), 590–611. https://doi.org/10.1093/jpepsy/jsm128

Kane, S., Huo, D., Aikens, J., & Hanauer, S. (2003). Medication nonadherence and the outcomes of patients with quiescent ulcerative colitis. *American Journal of Medicine, 114*(1), 39–43.

Kappelman, M. D., Long, M. D., Martin, C., DeWalt, D. A., Kinneer, P. M., Chen, W., ... Sandler, R. S. (2014). Evaluation of the patient-reported outcomes measurement information system in a large cohort of patients with inflammatory bowel diseases. *Clinical Gastroenterology and Hepatology, 12*(8), 1315–1323. e1312. https://doi.org/10.1016/j.cgh.2013.10.019

Kaufman, S. S. (2016). Short bowel syndrome. In R. Willie, J. S. Hyams, & M. Kay (Eds.), *Pediatric gastrointestinal and liver disease* (5th ed., pp. 405–417). Philadelphia, PA: Elsevier.

Lemanek, K. L., Kamps, J., & Chung, N. B. (2001). Empirically supported treatments in pediatric psychology: Regimen adherence. *Journal of Pediatric Psychology, 26*(5), 253–275.

Levy, R. L., van Tilburg, M. A., Langer, S. L., Romano, J. M., Walker, L. S., Mancl, L. A., ... Whitehead, W. E. (2016). Effects of a cognitive behavioral therapy intervention trial to improve disease outcomes in children with inflammatory bowel disease. *Inflammatory Bowel Disease, 22*(9), 2134–2148. https://doi.org/10.1097/MIB.0000000000000881

Loftus, E. V., Jr., Guerin, A., Yu, A. P., Wu, E. Q., Yang, M., Chao, J., & Mulani, P. M. (2011). Increased risks of developing anxiety and depression in young patients with Crohn's disease. *American Journal of Gastroenterology, 106*(9), 1670–1677. https://doi.org/10.1038/ajg.2011.142

Lowe, M. E. (2016). Pancreatitis. In R. Willie, J. S. Hyams, & M. Kay (Eds.), *Pediatric gastrointestinal and liver disease* (pp. 1016–1026). Philadelphia, PA: Elsevier.

Lum, A., Wakefield, C. E., Donnan, B., Burns, M. A., Fardell, J. E., & Marshall, G. M. (2017). Understanding the school experiences of children and adolescents with serious chronic illness: A systematic meta-review. *Child Care, Health, and Development, 43*(5), 645–662. https://doi.org/10.1111/cch.12475

Mackner, L. M., Bickmeier, R. M., & Crandall, W. V. (2012). Academic achievement, attendance, and school-related quality of life in pediatric inflammatory bowel disease. *Journal of Developmental and Behavioral Pediatrics, 33*(2), 106–111. https://doi.org/10.1097/DBP.0b013e318240cf68

Maddux, M. H., Bass, J. A., Geraghty-Sirridge, C., Carpenter, E., & Christenson, K. (2013). Assessing psychosocial functioning among youth with inflammatory bowel disease: An interdisciplinary clinic approach. *Clinical Practice in Pediatric Psychology, 1*(4), 333–343.

Mamula, P., Markowitz, J. E., & Baldassano, R. N. (2008). *Pediatric inflammatory bowel disease*. New York, NY: Springer.

Markowitz, J. E., & Liacouras, C. A. (2016). Allergic and eosinophilic gastrointestinal disease. In R. Willie, J. S. Hyams, & M. Kay (Eds.), *Pediatric gastrointestinal and liver disease* (5th ed., pp. 430–434). Philadelphia, PA: Elsevier.

McGrady, M. E., & Hommel, K. A. (2013). Medication adherence and health care utilization in pediatric chronic illness: A systematic review. *Pediatrics, 132*(4), 730–740.

Meltzer, L. J., Davis, K. F., & Mindell, J. A. (2012). Patient and parent sleep in a children's hospital. *Pediatric Nursing, 38*(2), 64–71, quiz 72.

Mullins, L. L., Wolfe-Christensen, C., Pai, A. L., Carpentier, M. Y., Gillaspy, S., Cheek, J., & Page, M. (2007). The relationship of parental overprotection, perceived child vulnerability, and parenting stress to uncertainty in youth with chronic illness. *Journal of Pediatric Psychology, 32*(8), 973–982. https://doi.org/10.1093/jpepsy/jsm044

Rapoff, M. (2010). *Adherence to pediatric medical regimens*. New York, NY: Kluwer Academic.

Reed-Knight, B., Maddux, M. H., Deacy, A. D., Lamparyk, K., Stone, A. L., & Mackner, L. (2017). Brain-gut interactions and maintenance factors in pediatric gastroenterological disorders: Recommendations for clinical care from the division 54 pediatric gastroenterology special interest group. *Clinical Practice in Pediatric Psychology, 5*(1), 93–105. https://doi.org/10.1037/cpp0000166

Rosen, R., Vandenplas, Y., Singendonk, M., Cabana, M., DiLorenzo, C., Gottrand, F., ... Tabbers, M. (2018). Pediatric gastroesophageal reflux clinical practice guidelines: Joint Recommendations of the North American Society for Pediatric Gastroenterology, Hepatology, and Nutrition and the European Society for Pediatric Gastroenterology, Hepatology, and Nutrition. *Journal of Pediatric Gastroenterology and Nutrition, 66*(3), 516–554. https://doi.org/10.1097/MPG.0000000000001889

Silverman, A., & Williams, S. (2014). Multidisciplinary team approach and the role of psychologists in gastroenterology services. In C. Martin & T. Dovey (Eds.), *Paediatric gastrointestinal disorders: A psychosocial perspective* (pp. 34–50). London, UK: Radcliffe Publishing Ltd.

Szigethy, E., Kenney, E., Carpenter, J., Hardy, D. M., Fairclough, D., Bousvaros, A., … DeMaso, D. R. (2007). Cognitive-behavioral therapy for adolescents with inflammatory bowel disease and subsyndromal depression. *Journal of the American Academy of Child and Adolescent Psychiatry, 46*(10), 1290–1298. https://doi.org/10.1097/chi.0b013e3180f6341f

Szigethy, E., Youk, A. O., Gonzalez-Heydrich, J., Bujoreanu, S. I., Weisz, J., Fairclough, D., … DeMaso, D. R. (2015). Effect of 2 psychotherapies on depression and disease activity in pediatric Crohn's disease. *Inflammatory Bowel Diseases, 21*(6), 1321–1328. https://doi.org/10.1097/MIB.0000000000000358

Eating Disorders and Avoidant/Restrictive Food Intake Disorder

Kevin K. Tsang, Lillian C. Hayes, and Chrissy Cammarata

Pediatric consultation-liaison (CL) psychologists are commonly called on to assess and support management of patients presenting with eating disorders (EDs) and feeding concerns. Outpatient consulting psychologists may be tasked to diagnose, triage, or treat patients presenting with progressive weight loss, binge eating, and/or purging behaviors. Other patients may present with restrictive feeding behaviors related to food sensitivities or fears, leading to nutritional deficiency, failure to gain weight, and family discord around eating. In the inpatient medical setting, such patients often present with severe malnutrition requiring close medical monitoring. Some patients and their families actively seek to initiate treatment, while others frankly refuse care and nutrition. Regardless of setting, it is important for the consulting psychologist to have a good working knowledge of these disorders, including differential diagnoses, treatment options and factors that inform disposition, family considerations, and strategies to effectively liaison with multidisciplinary care teams and families alike.

K. K. Tsang (✉) · L. C. Hayes
Department of Psychiatry, Boston Children's Hospital, Harvard Medical School, Boston, MA, USA
e-mail: Kevin.Tsang@childrens.harvard.edu

C. Cammarata
Department of Pediatrics, Nemours Alfred I. duPont Hospital for Children, Sidney Kimmel Medical College, Thomas Jefferson University, Wilmington, DE, USA

Diagnostic and Other Background Information

Accurate diagnosis of eating and feeding disorders requires understanding of the broad range of diagnoses within this category, as well as a number of medical concerns that may mimic these symptoms. Anorexia nervosa (AN), bulimia nervosa (BN), binge eating disorder (BED), and avoidant/restrictive food intake disorder (ARFID) are all defined within the *Diagnostic and Statistical Manual, Fifth Edition* (American Psychiatric Association [APA], 2013). AN is characterized by a restriction of nutritional intake leading to significantly low body weight. AN is commonly associated with fear of gaining weight, persistent lack of recognition of the seriousness of this low body weight, and a disturbance in the way in which one perceives one's own body weight or shape (APA, 2013). Significantly low body weight can be the result of solely restricting caloric intake or may include binge eating or purging behaviors as well. BN and BED are both characterized by episodes of binge eating, in which one eats an amount of food significantly larger than what most people would have in a discrete period and a sense of lack of control over

B. D. Carter, K. A. Kullgren (eds.), *Clinical Handbook of Psychological Consultation in Pediatric Medical Settings*, Issues in Clinical Child Psychology, https://doi.org/10.1007/978-3-030-35598-2_17

this behavior. BN includes compensatory behaviors (e.g., vomiting, laxative use) to prevent weight gain and an "unduly influence" of weight on self-evaluation, while BED is characterized by marked distress during binge eating episodes (APA, 2013). If these episodes of binge eating or purging occur with associated significantly low weight, AN would still be the appropriate diagnosis. ARFID describes an eating disturbance that results in persistent failure to meet nutritional needs and is associated with weight loss, nutritional deficiency, dependence on nutritional supplementation, or marked interference with psychosocial functioning. In ARFID, the eating disturbance is not associated with a fear of weight gain or disturbance in perception of body shape, but rather is caused by a lack of interest in eating, sensory sensitivities and aversion to food, or a concern for undesirable consequences of eating (e.g., choking, vomiting, abdominal pain; APA, 2013).

When evaluating for possible diagnosis of AN and ARFID, it is important to consider medical diagnoses that can drive weight loss, as well as psychiatric diagnoses that may impact eating. For example, a number of cancer malignancies and acquired immunodeficiency syndrome (AIDS) can contribute to significant weight loss, loss of appetite, nausea, and vomiting. Gastrointestinal diseases, including acute illnesses such as gastroenteritis and chronic disorders such as inflammatory bowel disease, eosinophilic esophagitis, or celiac disease, can contribute to weight loss, nausea, and vomiting. Medical evaluation may include blood tests, endoscopy, colonoscopy, and imaging, based on the assessment of medical providers. These presentations are, however, not usually associated with body image concerns, fears of weight gain, or persistent behaviors that interfere with weight gain (APA, 2013). That being said, the presence of one of these medical conditions is not mutually exclusive of AN or ARFID.

Similarly, depression, psychotic illness, and substance use disorders may all contribute to behaviors that limit nutritional intake, whether related to depressed mood and amotivation, atypical eating behaviors in the context of psychosis, or use of substances that decrease hunger or eating (APA, 2013). As above, these presentations are not usually associated with body image concerns or fears of weight gain. Social anxiety disorder, obsessive-compulsive disorders, and body dysmorphic disorder may also be comorbid illnesses and should be considered when these anxieties exist outside of the context of weight and eating.

In the assessment of disorders involving binge eating, a number of medical and psychiatric diagnoses should be considered. For example, neurological or genetic syndromes such as Prader-Willi and Kleine-Levin syndrome can be associated with overeating, but generally without excessive body image and weight concern (APA, 2013; Mairs & Nicholls, 2016). Obesity or overeating alone would not meet criteria for an ED either, unless compensatory behaviors (characteristic of BN) or a sense of losing control during eating episodes (characteristic of BED) is noted. Major depressive disorder (MDD) can also include diagnostic features of overeating but would not meet criteria for BN without compensatory behaviors or BED without a "sense of lack of control" during overeating episodes (APA, 2013).

Prevalence

Lifetime prevalence rates for ED by age 20 in an adolescent female community sample in the United States are estimated to be 0.8% for individuals with AN, 2.6% for those with BN, and 3.0% for BED (Stice, Marti, & Rohde, 2013). Overall ED prevalence trends for males are generally lower than the prevalence rates for females, estimated to occur at a ratio of 1:10, respectively (Muise, Stein, & Arbess, 2003). Peak age of onset is estimated to be 19–20 years for AN, 16–20 years for BN, and 18–20 years for BED (Stice et al., 2013). For ARFID, prevalence rates range from 5% to 14% in a pediatric population, and approximately 22.5% of those present to a pediatric ED day treatment setting (Norris, Spettigue, & Katzman, 2016). EDs remain challenging to treat, and mortality rates for EDs remain quite high, with estimated crude mortality rates being 5% of patients with AN and 2% for patients with BN per decade; suicide risk is also elevated in patients with AN and BN (APA, 2013).

Cultural and Social Factors

Prevalence rates also differ based on cultural and racial background. AN and BN, overall, are more prevalent for women in Western countries (e.g., United States, Canada) compared to those in China and Japan (Makino, Tsuboi, & Dennerstein, 2004). Comparing ethnic groups within the United States, lifetime prevalence rates of BED are highest, followed by rates of BN and then AN, among all ethnic groups included in the study (i.e., White non-Latino Americans, Latino Americans, African Americans, and Asian Americans; Marques et al., 2011). Rates of AN and BED do not significantly differ between ethnic groups, whereas Latinos and African Americans experience significantly higher rates of BN compared with White, non-Latino groups (Marques et al., 2011). EDs are equally common across all levels of social class (Mitchison & Hay, 2014).

In regard to family cultural factors, mother's concern for her own weight has predicted eating pathology in both boys and girls, while girls who experienced family or peer teasing about weight were 1.5 times as likely to engage in binge eating and extreme weight control behaviors (Neumark-Sztainer et al., 2007). Internalization of the "thin ideal" and body dissatisfaction also significantly contribute to the risk of BN or BED (Stice, Gau, Rohde, & Shaw, 2016). In contrast, frequent family meals, positive atmosphere at family meals, and frequent lunch intake were protective factors against binge eating and weight control behaviors (Neumark-Sztainer et al., 2007). These similar sociocultural influences do not appear to influence development or maintenance of ARFID, though additional research is still needed.

Biological/Genetic Influences

Early menarche and early pubertal development have not been consistently supported as risk factors for ED (Neumark-Sztainer et al., 2007). Twin studies have estimated shared heritability between 54% and 83% in BN, 28% and 58% in AN, and 41% and 57% in BED (Thornton, Mazzeo, & Bulik, 2013). Genetic markers have been associated with certain ED diagnoses (e.g., serotonin transporter gene associated with BN and BED, DRD4 gene associated with AN binge eating/purge type but not AN restricting type; Mitchison & Hay, 2014). As mentioned previously, being female sex may also pose a risk factor for AN, BN, and BED (Muise et al., 2003). Lower body mass index (BMI) itself also appears a risk factor for future development of AN (Stice et al., 2016). When compared to other EDs, there is a higher prevalence of males diagnosed with ARFID (21–28.6%); these individuals with ARFID are more likely to experience gastrointestinal issues and allergies than same-age peers and more likely to have a history of sensory sensitivities (Fisher et al., 2014; Norris et al., 2014). Overall, research on genetic risk factors for ARFID remains limited.

Another genetic component appears to be personal and family psychiatric history. Comorbid anxiety disorders, obsessive-compulsive disorder (OCD), and MDD are common in individuals with ED. Individuals with BN are more likely to experience self-injurious behavior, suicidal ideation, substance use, mood dysregulation, and impulsive tendencies, whereas individuals with ARFID are more likely to experience comorbid autism spectrum disorder, intellectual disabilities, and obsessive-compulsive disorders (Taljemark, Rastam, Lichtenstein, Anckarsater, & Kerekes, 2017). Anxiety disorders are also significantly more prevalent in individuals with ARFID than those with AN or BN, whereas mood disorders are more common in individuals with AN (Fisher et al., 2014). Individuals with AN have a higher likelihood of family psychiatric history when compared to individuals with ARFID (Norris et al., 2014).

Medical Basics

When evaluating for ED or ARFID, it is important to also consider medical severity. Malnutrition should be considered early in the diagnostic process given the impact of nutritional status on medical safety, treatment priorities, and individual's ability to participate in treatment. According to the Society for Adolescent Health and Medicine (SAHM, 2015), mild malnutrition can be defined by a body mass index (BMI) z-score of −1 to −1.9, loss of 10% of usual body weight, or weight at 80–90% of median BMI for age and sex. Moderate malnutrition is defined by BMI z-score of −2 to −2.9, loss of 15% of usual body weight, or weight at 70–79% median BMI for age and sex. Severe malnutrition is identified in individuals with a BMI z-score of −3 or lower, who have lost 20% of their usual body weight within 1 year or greater than 10% of body mass within 6 months, or who weight less than 70% of median BMI for age and sex. Of note, not only is malnutrition defined by current weight compared to age, sex, and height norms, but also significant weight loss must be considered. Significant weight loss can result in slowed heart rate (bradycardia) and unstable vital signs. Additionally, malnutrition can negatively impact neuropsychological functioning (Moser et al., 2003). Other medical consequences of malnutrition can include delayed or interruption of menstrual cycle in females, which can contribute to reduced bone density (Misra et al., 2008).

While chronic, progressive weight loss is typically not associated with electrolyte abnormalities, close medical monitoring may be necessary during the initial stages of restoring nutritional intake due to risks associated with refeeding syndrome, a potentially life-threatening metabolic syndrome associated with reintroduction of nutrition after starvation that can result in cardiac problems, delirium, seizures, coma, and sudden death (Garber et al., 2016). Similarly, chronic and severe purging behaviors can result in a life-threatening degradation of electrolytes, impacting cardiac functioning (Wolfe, Metzger, Levine, & Jimerson, 2001). For these reasons, it is important to collaborate with medical colleagues and consider whether acute medical stabilization is needed in an inpatient medical setting prior to starting outpatient-based care.

Engagement

Patients and their families present to care with a number of factors that may influence receptivity and readiness for treatment. Patients with ED may have limited acknowledgment or insight in the severity of their disordered eating behaviors. ED behaviors can be highly rewarding, and the prospect of reducing these behaviors may increase patient anxiety or distress. ARFID can be distressing for the competing desire to eat but feeling unable to due to fears, anxiety, or aversion. As noted above, the cognitive and affect-related symptoms associated with malnutrition may also make it difficult to engage these individuals. Families, on the other hand, frequently present at a point of distress about disordered eating behaviors that continue despite their best efforts to manage. Caregiver guilt can be present for a variety of reasons including genetic predisposition, delayed identification of illness behaviors, and feelings of ineffectiveness in curtailing the disordered eating or feeding behaviors once identified. As a result, caregivers may be highly sensitive to feeling ineffective and anxious, whether directed toward the patient or directed toward providers for any escalation of patient distress during the process of treatment.

A number of strategies can be utilized to support patients, families, and multidisciplinary providers in understanding and addressing the ED or ARFID (see Table 1). These interactions present an opportunity for the psychologist to establish a clear understanding of the disorder and realistic expectations for empirically supported treatment. Although there can be a high level of patient and family distress when first addressing feeding or eating concerns, the clinician's demonstrated capacity to tolerate this affect while bringing families onboard for the model of treatment is essential, particularly in early phases of treatment when this distress and anxiety can derail adherence to behavioral and family-based treatment models.

Table 1 Engagement and establishing treatment with patients with ED and their families

Problem	Goals	Techniques	Examples
Limited insight into eating problems or limited motivation to participate in treatment	• Focus on limiting ED behaviors • Support parental empowerment	• Emphasize life-threatening nature of ED, need for caregiver to exert parental authority to disrupt ED behaviors	• "At this point, it is clear to us that your eating disorder is making it really hard for you to take care of yourself. Your parents' job is to take care of you and so we have to do these things to help you fight your eating disorder" • "When you came to the hospital, your heart was really sick, which can sometimes happen when our bodies aren't getting enough nutrition. That was really scary for us"
Parental anxiety/ distress and guilt/ blame for who/ what caused the problem	• Address myths • Provide psychoeducation • Support parental empowerment, collaboration, and alignment	• Discuss "perfect storm" of contributing factors • Validate feelings of distress, normalizing parental reactions • Reinforcing team approach, evidence-based treatment	• "Usually, it's not one thing that caused an eating disorder to develop; it is usually many stressors or changes working together to create a 'perfect storm'" • "Many parents are surprised when they receive this diagnosis or learn more about their child's eating disorder. This happens a lot because eating disorders learn really great ways to be sneaky so they can remain undetected. The important thing is that you brought your child here for treatment so we can help treat this together"
Blaming the patient	• Externalize the illness • Ally family and patient against ED	• Use externalizing language; shift perspective to ED as cause of discord • Interview family and patient separately	• "Your child's eating disorder has a lot of control over your child right now" • "The anger, distrust, and sadness you are seeing is the eating disorder fighting against us. This means we need to keep helping your child fight this insidious illness"
Patient's anxiety	• Externalize the illness • Increase predictability and structure	• Use externalizing language to separate distress of the ED • Set up daily schedule of mealtimes and other activities.	• Name the patient's anxiety as being a response from their eating disorder (e.g., "I can tell this is really hard for your eating disorder right now") • Create a Venn diagram of patient goals (e.g., going to college, spending time with friends and family), eating disorder goals (e.g., losing weight), and shared goals. Discuss how meeting eating disorder goals affects patient's ability to meet their own goals that are important to them

Formulation

As previously noted, it is important in the context of ED and ARFID to work with medical providers in the co-management of these patients, particularly in determining level of care and urgency of medical stabilization. For example, the initial treatment goals for a child with ARFID presenting with a severely limited food palette would be different depending on their degree of caloric restriction and malnutrition. If the child is not taking in adequate calories to even maintain their weight, the priority should be to utilize preferred foods and nutritional supplementation to increase overall caloric volume before attempting to increase food variety. On the other hand, if the child is nutritionally robust, there may be more opportunity for an outpatient provider or feeding team to support stepwise increases in variety of tolerated foods. Adolescents with AN and severe malnutrition may require inpatient medical hospitalization and nasogastric (NG) feeds to allow for adequate medical stabilization and monitoring for refeeding syndrome before considering other treatment. Additionally, individuals with BN can require medical monitoring for acute cardiac risk associated with electrolyte imbalances that can occur.

The comorbid presence of agitation, suicidal ideation and self-injury, personality disorder, substance use disorders, and other psychiatric illnesses may also shape treatment decisions. Psychiatric severity may require acute management while also ensuring medical stability related to the eating or feeding disorder. Other comorbidities, such as neurodevelopmental disorders and OCD, must be accounted for. In the setting of autism spectrum disorder, olfactory or tactile sensitivities may need to be treated with repeated exposures as part of treatment. Similarly, within the setting of OCD, a more generalized approach to exposure and response prevention may be necessary in addition to repeated food exposures. Social factors that should be considered include caregiver availability, family psychiatric illness, financial stressors, housing stability, food security, cultural understanding of body image/ED, and family culture and caregiver response to distress in the setting of ED and ARFID. For example, although empirical support for family-based treatment (FBT) of AN is robust (Lock et al., 2010), families may be unable to participate for the above reasons, requiring alternative approaches.

Interventions

Within ED treatment, the strategies reviewed above in Table 1 are important components to maintain throughout intervention. Effective use of structured meal plans and consistency in care are also important to establish early in treatment. For example, findings are consistent that having a structured meal plan in place can be significantly effective in reducing need for NG feeding for individuals with AN (Couturier & Mahmood, 2009). Structured meal plans should be established in consultation with medical and nutrition providers. See Table 2 for a sample meal structure and mealtime interventions for EDs and Table 3 for a sample ARFID schedule.

Other relevant interventions for treating ED might include occupational therapy (OT) for children or adolescents with sensory issues or swallowing phobia (Manikam & Perman, 2000). Antipsychotic medications, such as olanzapine and quetiapine, have been associated with early weight gain, the reduction of rigid and obsessional thoughts, and have been safely used in children and adolescents diagnosed with AN and ARFID (Boachie, Goldfield, & Spettigue, 2003; Brewerton & D'Agostino, 2017). Selective serotonin reuptake inhibitors (SSRIs), such as fluoxetine, have been demonstrated to be variably effective in adults but not effective in adolescents with AN, effective in adults and promising in adolescents with BN, and not more effective than cognitive-behavioral therapy (CBT) in adults with BED (Golden & Attia, 2011).

There are multiple levels of care possible in the treatment of eating disorders (e.g., residential, inpatient, partial hospitalization program [PHP], intensive outpatient, outpatient). Weight restoration in AN and ARFID may be similarly effective across these levels of care (Forman et al., 2014). Noting that more severe presentations are more likely to require higher-level care placements,

Table 2 Interventions for patients with AN, BN, and BED

Meal plan	Special considerations	
• Three meals, lasting for 30 min each • Up to three snacks can be scheduled, as needed, lasting for 30 min each • Food is removed after 30 min • Parent, nurse, or other trained provider present for meals to monitor intake and support in coping • Behavioral activation between meal exposures, but avoid exercise *Sample meal plan:* 8:00–8:30 am: Breakfast 10:00–10:30 am: Snack 12:00–12:30 pm: Lunch 3:00–3:30 pm: Snack 6:00–6:30 pm: Dinner 8:00–8:30 pm: Snack	Anorexia nervosa	• Avoid discussions about food items or calories during mealtimes • Support patient in avoidance of ED behaviors including meal avoidance using skills discussed in Table 1 • Monitor patient for attempts to exercise or purge between mealtimes • Any incomplete meals should be made up with oral or nasogastric (NG) supplemental nutrition • Implementation of NG feeds varies by institution; options are to (1) immediately replace nutrition by placing NG tube and removing after supplement is given, (2) placing NG tube in the beginning of admission and allowing to remain in place until no longer needed, and (3) placing NG tube overnight and removing prior to first meal • Expectation for increasing caloric intake should be guided by medical and nutrition providers
	Bulimia nervosa	• Support patient in engaging in coping skills and externalization of the ED to help patient manage urges to binge or purge (examples in Table 1) • Consider behavioral scheduling and behavioral activation to support mood and reduce persistent attention on cognitive aspects of ED • Monitor for attempts to purge during or after meals; monitor use of laxatives and diuretics or over-exercise; restricting access to bathroom after meals may be necessary
	Binge eating disorder	• Support patient in engaging in coping skills and externalization of the ED (examples in Table 1) • Consider strategies such as mindful eating, cognitive strategies to tolerate ED ideation • Consider behavioral scheduling and behavioral activation to support mood and reduce persistent attention on cognitive aspects of ED • Monitor for attempts to binge between meals; restricting access to food items may be necessary

Table 3 Interventions for patients with ARFID

	Goal: caloric intake	Goal: diversity of feeding
Meal structure	• Three to five small meals per day, last 20–30 min each, developmentally appropriate to age of the patient • Meals should be completed sitting up in a chair with meal on a table, no significant distraction activities including TV • Utilize preferred foods to increase intake volume • Utilize planned ignoring of non-eating behaviors, minor redirection to eating task, and neutrally removing meal after time limit is reached • Provide positive reinforcement for effort during mealtimes, for any increases in meal intake; avoid punitive or critical or anxious comments for non-eating	• Three to four small meals per day, last 20–30 min each, developmentally appropriate to age of the patient; focusing on preferred food still and maintaining reasonable caloric intake. Begin by introducing one "bonus" mealtime, in which novel foods are introduced. Keep novel and preferred food exposures separate initially to reduce likelihood of avoidance of preferred foods • Meals should be completed sitting up in a chair with meal on a table, no significant distraction activities including TV • Utilize planned ignoring of non-eating behaviors, minor redirection to eating task, and neutrally removing meal after time limit is reached • Provide positive reinforcement for effort during mealtimes; avoid punitive or critical or anxious comments for non-eating
Strategies to consider	• Token reward system; earning privileges for greater percentage of meal completion • Avoid punitive strategies for non-eating behaviors	• Token reward system; earning privileges for trialing of new foods • Utilize principles of graduated exposure (touch, smell, lick, taste, small bite, big bite), reinforcing for each trial and increasing diversity utilizing similar food characteristics (look for information about food chaining for additional resources) • Avoid punitive strategies for non-eating behaviors
Nutritional supplementation	• Consider multivitamin and oral supplementation with nutritional shakes to ensure continued overall nutritional stability • If needing inpatient medical stabilization, consider role of NG feeds to support stabilization and reduce anxiety around non-eating behaviors	

Forman et al. (2014) theorized that more intensive care may compensate for more severe presentations, allowing similar rates of recuperation from low body weight. In a study examining 3-year follow-up for patients with BN, 72% of patients treated in PHP and 69% of patients treated in inpatient settings were in partial or complete remission, suggesting both levels of care may be similarly effective in the long term (Zeeck et al., 2009). It can be challenging to choose the right level of care for a patient based on clinical efficacy, and treatment planning might depend more on other clinical indications (e.g., need for constant observation, weight criteria for admission to a program). Almost 80% of individuals with AN require hospital admission for medical stability at some point, compared to 30% of individuals with ARFID (Norris et al., 2014). In any level of care, collaboration with a multidisciplinary team remains essential (Mairs & Nicholls, 2016). See Appendix 1 for additional information regarding level of care decision-making.

Adaptation

When considering empirically supported treatment approaches, individual and family factors may necessitate adaptations to care practice. Literature on high mortality rates in ED supports the need for adapting treatment approaches for individuals and families who might not be an appropriate fit for FBT, CBT, or other standardized treatment. Environmental, developmental, and cultural variables are all important to consider. Length of treatment for ED can range from several months to several years and may require repeat admissions to higher level of care, which can be a significant financial burden to families. Financial limitations might restrict access to certain effective but more expensive treatment options. Gathering support from other insurance or state-based resources may be essential in these situations, and involvement of a case manager can be quite helpful. Geographic area might also reduce access to care. Families who live in rural areas, for example, may have limited access to certain care options. In these cases, outpatient psychological treatment via telehealth with close monitoring from a primary care provider may be an option. Options to temporarily relocate to engage higher level of care or empirically supported services may be needed. Family structure is also important to consider; involvement in family-based treatment might differ depending on availability of an identified parent or guardian. Family culture, specifically beliefs about what is causing or maintaining the ED, might also differ and might require additional psychoeducation and acknowledgment of family patterns contributing to the current presentation. The developmental level of the patient and family is also important to consider. As discussed above, developmental disabilities are more prevalent in children with ARFID, and certainly children and adolescents with any type of ED may present with other developmental or learning difficulties that may impact how they learn information or implement recommendations. In these cases, any psychoeducation provided or behavior plan developed must be individualized to meet patient and caregiver needs.

A psychologist can expect their role to shift depending on patient progress. For example, if the patient's weight and medical stability declines and the patient requires medical admission, an outpatient psychologist might remain involved peripherally by communicating with the inpatient treatment team and preparing for any necessary changes in the outpatient treatment plan. In some situations, changes in patient presentation may prompt adaptations to formulation and treatment. In one longitudinal study, 12% of patients diagnosed and treated for ARFID later met criteria for a diagnosis of AN (Norris et al., 2014), highlighting the importance of flexibility in treatment planning should symptoms evolve.

Inpatient Considerations

As previously noted, a large percentage of individuals with AN and ARFID require medical hospitalization at some point in their treatment course. As noted by Norris et al. (2014), about a quarter of individuals diagnosed with ARFID and over 50% with AN needed medical hospitalization after initial evaluation. For those not needing hospitalization immediately after diagnosis, a later medical admission may represent a desperate last hope for medical stabilization and altering the future direction of care. Although there are many common factors that the knowledgeable pediatric CL psychologist will think about in the course of practice with any patient population, there are a number of logistical considerations that warrant special attention in the inpatient medical setting.

The primary goal of an inpatient medical admission for an eating or feeding disorder should generally be for medical stabilization and disposition planning. Attention should be directed to the importance of standardized approaches to management of AN, BN, and ARFID in the inpatient setting. Protocolization of management reduces variance, allows for quicker medical stabilization, and decreases bargaining and accommodation to eating or feeding disorder behaviors. Clinical pathways can vary by hospital but commonly include medical criteria for admission, clearly defined observation of patient meals and/or time after meals in which purging may occur, medical monitoring during admission, nutritional guidance regarding establishing adequate caloric intake, and (for AN and ARFID) a stepwise approach to increasing nutritional intake over time. In the case of ARFID, it may be helpful to include not only physician, nursing, nutrition, and psychology but also other disciplines to support feeding desensitization such as OT and speech and language therapy.

In working with these teams, it is also important to remember that each multidisciplinary provider exists within their own cultural context, including their own associations with weight, body image, food, and nutrition. Variance from protocol may reflect personal stigma or misattributions of blame, which warrant attention and similar support as when helping patients and their families understand the ED. While a gold standard clinical pathway has yet to be identified within the medical setting, these clinical protocols are developed to support consistency between providers and ultimately seek to provide safe, efficient medical stabilization.

In the meantime, the CL psychologist can utilize this opportunity to assess contributing and maintaining factors for the eating or feeding disorder, provide supportive guidance for use of distress tolerance skills (e.g., relaxation training), and engage patients and families in psychoeducation to understand the presenting disorder and treatment options. Establishing reasonable expectations for monitoring and recovery is essential. Whether working with patients requiring medical management for binge eating and purging or restrictive disorders, care obviously should not end with acute medical stabilization.

Outpatient Considerations

Historically, most children with an ED diagnosis were referred to higher levels of care; more recently it has been recognized that hospitalization is not a benign intervention and outpatient approaches are generally recommended, provided they meet requirements for medical stability (Madden, Hay, & Touyz, 2015). Outpatient treatment settings tend to be less disruptive and costly while also allowing for greater family support, and treatment can be of a longer duration with a continuous treatment team. With that said, outpatient treatment often requires more family involvement and does not provide 24 hour supervision as in inpatient settings.

Most youths with ED are treated in interdisciplinary outpatient settings with specialty providers working in collaboration (Rosen and The Committee on Adolescence, 2010). Ideally, a therapy team should include a mental health professional trained in providing evidence-based psychotherapies such as FBT for AN or CBT for BN, a physician specializing in ED or weight management, registered dietitians, and child and adolescent psychiatrists if pharmacological intervention is appropriate. For best results, the team should be united with an agreed-upon treatment framework and should be compassionate and firm in their recommendations with families and patients. Average treatment duration is estimated to last 6 months or longer (Espie & Eisler, 2015).

The basic agreed-upon expectation to remain in an outpatient setting is that the patient will consume sufficient calories to maintain or gain weight depending on medical needs and avoid exercising or purging at frequencies that lead to abnormal lab work or weight changes. They must also agree to meet with their treatment team regularly. In the case of youth with ED, parent or caregiver involvement is often crucial. In the event that these expectations are not met or if there is significant deterioration, a referral to a higher level of care should be considered.

Resources/Support

As with most areas of pediatric psychology, it is beneficial for CL clinicians to practice within their bounds of competence. In this case, CL psychologists should have specific clinical training and experience working with patients with ED if they are to be working with these patients. Experience can be gained in internship or fellowship settings, or with supervision and/or consultation with other psychologists, similar to developing clinical experience with any patient population. While this handbook and other evidence-based sources can be useful references (see Appendix 2), the CL psychologist or trainee unfamiliar with working with ED is encouraged to seek supervision or consultation.

As mentioned throughout this chapter, a multidisciplinary team approach is essential throughout the length of treatment (Mairs & Nicholls, 2016). CL psychologists can collaborate with other providers to ensure the patient is given an appropriate meal plan and improving or maintaining medical stability, which will give a strong foundation for the individual to work on the psychological aspects of their ED. As the patient improves in the outpatient setting, primary care providers can be quite supportive by continuing to monitor the individual's medical stability, reinforcing medical recommendations, prescribing medications, and serving as a consultant to caregivers and other providers involved. If the individual begins treatment in the outpatient setting, the primary care provider can also be helpful in recommending higher level of care based on medical necessity (Katzman, Peebles, Sawyer, Lock, & Le Grange, 2013).

Case Example: AN

Mary is a 14-year-old, Latina female, presenting with progressive weight loss over 4 months totaling 30 pounds, now with bradycardia and severe malnutrition. Medical history is unremarkable, and psychiatric history is notable for other specified anxiety disorder associated with "school stress." Parents described that she had always been a "little chubby." While they initially praised Mary for her efforts to achieve a healthier lifestyle, over the past several months, her behavior has been described as "out of control." When parents or other family members expressed concern about Mary's dieting behavior and weight loss, Mary became extremely upset and was "a completely different child." Mary denied eating concerns and stated intent to continue dieting behavior until she reached her desired weight. Mary reported that she received positive feedback from her peers for weight loss. Unknown to parents, Mary had been bullied in the past due to her weight and was also fearful of "getting fat" and being bullied again.

Due to severe malnutrition, Mary was medically hospitalized. Inpatient care was guided by a pediatric hospitalist, CL psychologist, and nutritionist in collaboration with nursing. Mary was started on a meal plan consisting of three meals and three snacks with additional fluid requirements to prevent dehydration. Mary was observably distressed for the first few meals and was difficult to engage. Mary was able to earn rewards of her choice (e.g., painting her nails with her mother, additional time on electronics) if she was able to complete meals, which led to increased meal completion. Mary was taught several coping skills, including distraction and relaxation techniques and how to externalize her ED, to manage distress before, during, and after mealtimes. Parents also received psychoeducation on strategies to support Mary, including reminding her of her motivations and goals beyond her ED and helping her to challenge distorted ED thoughts to reduce shame and guilt associated with eating. After achieving nutritional and medical stability in the hospital, her multidisciplinary team recommended ED treatment at a partial hospitalization program, where Mary and her family members participated in individual therapy, family therapy, group therapy, and continued structured mealtimes with monitoring.

Mary remained in treatment for several weeks before transitioning to outpatient care with a psychologist who provided FBT, nutritionist, and primary care provider. In therapy, Mary worked with her psychologist toward identifying and processing triggers of her ED (e.g., history of bullying), improving self-image, and addressing school anxiety. Her psychologist also helped to teach Mary's parents various ways they could support her in recovery, including encouraging her to adhere to her meal plan, reducing ED behaviors, and shifting family interactions around food (e.g., being mindful not to discuss food, weight, or calories during mealtimes). Her outpatient nutritionist continued to provide education and monitor meal planning, and several months later, Mary was able to gain some control in planning meal items with supervision from her parents. Her primary care provider continued to monitor Mary's weight and vitals and continued to reinforce recommendations from Mary's ED treatment providers.

Case Example: ARFID

Ryan is an 8-year-old, White male with history of asthma, no known psychiatric history, brought to the emergency department by his parents after 10 days of refusing solid foods and 3 days of refusing fluids. He was in his usual state of good health until 10 days prior to admission when he was eating lunch at school and choked on a mozzarella stick. Parents were desperate to help Ryan start eating again, leading to arguments at home, imploring Ryan to eat. Medical providers reported that Ryan presented with concerning symptoms of dehydration and would push away meals since being admitted for intravenous fluids.

During interview, Ryan was described as always mildly anxious, otherwise typically developing, but a "picky eater" throughout much of his life. Parents have worked to accommodate to his eating preferences, which were limited to cheese sticks, grilled cheese sandwiches, and pasta with butter. Family history was significant for paternal history of anxiety. Socially, Ryan was the youngest of three children, and the family was often driving to various basketball and dance practices during dinner time, such that meals were often in the car.

Assessing the situation, the CL psychologist, in collaboration with the medical team and nutrition, decided to prioritize increasing caloric intake. They began by initiating a daily schedule, which included three predetermined mealtimes lasting 30 min. No food or drink was available outside of these times to increase hunger and decrease satiation from grazing on snacks. Initially, only small amounts of food were presented at mealtimes and only preferred foods like pasta. Ryan sat up in a chair for all meals. Parents asked to step out during these meals due to their own anxiety, so nursing supported Ryan during these meal exposures. Over the next day, Ryan completed half of one meal and the entirety of the following meal. He was given a snack of liquid nutritional supplement, which he drank with ease, citing no fear of choking. As meals progressed, meal sizes were gradually increased, supporting Ryan in consistently eating 100% of the meal presented, after which he received verbal praise and special time with parents.

At the time of discharge, Ryan was eating a very limited variety of foods and drinking enough water by mouth to no longer need IV fluids. He continued the meal structure at home, with his family and school setting aside planned mealtimes, sitting at a table, eating preferred foods. Recognizing the importance of continuing to expand his variety of nutritious foods, Ryan continued in outpatient psychotherapy and worked with an OT while still seeing his pediatrician for medical monitoring and visits with a nutritionist in the primary care clinic. Ryan was exposed to an increasing variety of foods outside of his regular mealtimes and received stickers for successful advancement in approaching and then taking bites of new foods.

Appendix 1: Review of Levels of Care

Overview	*PCP with outpatient mental health involvement*	*Multidisciplinary outpatient*	*Intensive outpatient/partial hospitalization*	*Residential treatment center*	*Medical admission/inpatient*
	PCP management, integrated primary care psychologist or community mental health support, nutrition consult	Eating disorder specialty team with adolescent medicine physician, eating disorder mental health specialist, and nutrition support	May involve 2–5 days/week, several hours/day treatment. May be step-down from residential care	Highly structured environment for healthy eating, promoting weight gain/management, reducing destructive behaviors, and working toward effective coping skills	Medical or psychiatric admission to medically and/or psychiatrically stabilize
Medical status	Medically stable for treatment outside hospital setting				Unstable: HR near 40, orthostatic BP changes, BP <80/50 mmHg; hypokalemia, hypomagnesemia
Psychiatric status	No psych comorbidities or suicidal risk	One or more comorbid psychiatric diagnoses			Risk of danger to self or others; specific plan with lethality or intent; depression with poor impulse control or previous suicide attempt
Weight, BMI	BMI within acceptable limits for age	Persistent weight loss; BMI <18	85–90% of goal weight	75–85% of goal weight	Weight <75% of goal weight; rapid weight loss over 30 days prior to admission
			Unable to achieve prescribed weight or stop binge/purge cycle; uncontrolled symptoms		
Support	Good social support	Good social support	May have poor social support	May have poor social support	Severe family conflict or problems or absence of family or support

APA (2013) and Intermountain Healthcare (2013)

Appendix 2: Resources for Consultation-Liaison Psychologists

Organizations

- National Eating Disorders Association: www.nationaleatingdisorders.org
- Academy for Eating Disorders: www.aedweb.org
- International Association of Eating Disorders Professionals Foundation: www.iaedp.com
- National Association of Anorexia Nervosa: www.anad.org
- Binge Eating Disorder Association: www.bedaonline.com
- The Alliance for Eating Disorders Awareness: www.allianceforeatingdisorders.com
- Feeding Consortium: www.pediatricfeeding-news.com
- Feeding Matters: www.feedingmatters.org
- Residential Eating Disorders Consortium: www.residentialeatingdisorders.org
- Eating Disorders Coalition for Research, Policy, and Action: www.eatingdisordersco-alition.org

Books

- Lock, J., & Le Grange, D. (2013). *Treatment manual for Anorexia Nervosa: A family-based approach* (2nd ed.). New York: Guilford.
- Le Grange, D., & Lock, J. (2007). *Treating Bulimia in adolescents: A family-based approach* (2nd ed.). New York: Guilford.
- Thomas, J. J., & Eddy, K. T. (2018). *Cognitive-Behavioral Therapy for Avoidant/Restrictive Food Intake Disorder: Children, adolescents, and adults*. Cambridge, United Kingdom: Cambridge University Press.

Articles

Anorexia Nervosa

- Katzman, D. K., Peebles, R., Sawyer, S. M., Lock, J., & Le Grange, D. (2013). The role of the pediatrician in family-based treatment for adolescent eating disorders: Opportunities and challenges. *Journal of Adolescent Health, 53*, 433–440.
- Stiles-Shields, C., Rienecke Hoste, R., Doyle, P. M., & Le Grange, D. (2012). A review of family-based treatment for adolescents with eating disorders. *Reviews on Recent Clinical Trials, 7*, 133–140.
- Lock, J., Le Grange, D., Agras, S., Moye, A., Bryson, S. W., & Jo, B. (2010). Treatment of adolescent eating disorders: Progress and challenges. *Minerva Psichiatrica, 51*, 207–216.
- Grave, R. D, Calugi, S., Doll, H. A., & Fairburn, C. G. (2013). Enhanced cognitive behaviour therapy for adolescents with anorexia nervosa: An alternative to family therapy? *Behaviour Research and Therapy, 51*, R9–R12.

Bulimia Nervosa

- Le Grange, D. Crosby, R. D., Rathouz, P. J., & Leventhal, B. L. (2007). A randomized controlled comparison of family-based treatment and supportive psychotherapy for adolescent bulimia nervosa. *Archives of General Psychiatry, 64*, 1049–1056.
- Le Grange, D., Doyle, P., Crosby, R. D., & Chen, E. (2008). Early response to treatment in adolescent bulimia nervosa. *International Journal of Eating Disorders, 41*, 755–757.
- Linardon, J., Wade, T. D., de la Piedad Garcia, X., & Brennan, L. (2017). The efficacy of

cognitive-behavioral therapy for eating disorders: A systematic review and meta-analysis. *Journal of Consulting and Clinical Psychology, 85*, 1080–1094.

Binge Eating Disorder

- Hay, P. P., Bacaltchuk, J., Stefano, S., & Kashyap, P. (2009). Psychological treatments for bulimia nervosa and binging. *Cochrane Database of Systematic Reviews, 4.*
- Fairburn, C. G., Cooper, Z., & Shafran, R. (2003). Cognitive behaviour therapy for eating disorders: A "transdiagnostic" theory and treatment. *Behaviour Research and Therapy, 41*, 509–528.

Avoidant/Restrictive Food Intake Disorder

- Thomas, J. J., Wons, O. B., & Eddy, K. T. (2018). Cognitive–behavioral treatment of avoidant/restrictive food intake disorder. *Current Opinion in Psychiatry, 31*, 425–430.
- Manikam, R., & Perman, J. A. (2000). Pediatric feeding disorders. *Journal of Clinical Gastroenterology, 30*, 34–45.
- Zucker, N. L., LaVia, M. C., Craske, M. G., Foukal, M., Harris, A. A., Datta, N., … Maslow, G. R. (2019). Feeling and body investigators (FBI): ARFID division—An acceptance-based interoceptive exposure treatment for children with ARFID. *International Journal of Eating Disorders, 52*, 466–472.

References

American Psychiatric Association. (2013). *Diagnostic and statistical manual of mental disorders* (5th ed.). Washington, DC: American Psychiatric Association.

Boachie, A., Goldfield, G. S., & Spettigue, W. (2003). Olanzapine use as an adjunctive treatment for hospitalized children with anorexia nervosa. *International Journal of Eating Disorders, 33*, 98–103.

Brewerton, T. D., & D'Agostino, M. (2017). Adjunctive use of olanzapine in the treatment of avoidant restrictive food intake disorder in children and adolescents in an eating disorders program. *Journal of Child and Adolescent Psychopharmacology, 27*, 920–922.

Couturier, J., & Mahmood, A. (2009). Meal support therapy reduces the use of nasogastric feeding for adolescents hospitalized with anorexia nervosa. *Eating Disorders, 17*, 327–332.

Espie, J., & Eisler, I. (2015). Focus on anorexia nervosa: Modern psychological treatment and guidelines for the adolescent patient. *Adolescent Health, Medicine and Therapeutics, 6*, 9–16. https://doi.org/10.2147/AHMT.S70300

Fisher, M. M., Rosen, D. S., Ornstein, R. M., Mammel, K. A., Katzman, D. K., Rome, E. S., … Walsh, B. T. (2014). Characteristics of avoidant/restrictive food intake disorder in children and adolescents: A "new disorder" in DSM-5. *Journal of Adolescent Health, 55*, 49–52.

Forman, S. F., McKenzie, N., Hehn, R., Monge, M. C., Kapphahn, C. J., Mammel, K. A., … Woods, E. R. (2014). Predictors of outcome at 1 year in adolescents with DSM-5 restrictive eating disorders: Report of the National Eating Disorders Quality Improvement Collaborative. *Journal of Adolescent Health, 55*, 750–756.

Garber, A. K., Sawyer, S. M., Golden, N. H., Guarda, A. S., Katzman, D. K., Kohn, M. R., … Redgrave, G. W. (2016). A systematic review of approaches to refeeding in patients with anorexia nervosa. *International Journal of Eating Disorders, 49*, 293–310.

Golden, N. H., & Attia, E. (2011). Psychopharmacology of eating disorders in children and adolescents. *Pediatric Clinics of North America, 58*, 121–138.

Katzman, D. K., Peebles, R., Sawyer, S. M., Lock, J., & Le Grange, D. (2013). The role of the pediatrician in family-based treatment for adolescent eating disorders: Opportunities and challenges. *Journal of Adolescent Health, 53*, 433–440.

Lock, J., Le Grange, D., Agras, S., Moye, A., Bryson, S. W., & Jo, B. (2010). Treatment of adolescent eating disorders: Progress and challenges. *Minerva Psichiatrica, 51*, 207–216.

Madden, S., Hay, P., & Touyz, S. (2015). Systematic review of evidence for different treatment settings in anorexia nervosa. *World Journal of Psychiatry, 5*, 147–153.

Mairs, R., & Nicholls, D. (2016). Assessment and treatment of eating disorders in children and adolescents. *Archives of Disease in Childhood, 101*, 1168–1175.

Makino, M., Tsuboi, K., & Dennerstein, L. (2004). Prevalence of eating disorders: A comparison of western and non-western countries. *Medscape General Medicine, 6*, 49. Retrieved from https://www.ncbi.nlm.nih.gov/pmc/articles/PMC1435625/

Manikam, R., & Perman, J. A. (2000). Pediatric feeding disorders. *Journal of Clinical Gastroenterology, 30*, 34–45.

Marques, L., Alegria, M., Becker, A. E., Chen, C., Fang, A., Chosak, A., & Belo Diniz, J. (2011). Comparative prevalence, correlates of impairment, and service utilization for eating disorders across U.S. ethnic groups: Implications for reducing ethnic disparities in health care access for eating disorders. *International Journal of Eating Disorders, 44*, 412–420.

Misra, M., Prabhakaran, R., Miller, K. K., Goldstein, M. A., Mickley, D., Clauss, L., ... Klibanski, A. (2008). Weight gain and restoration of menses as predictors of bone mineral density change in adolescent girls with anorexia nervosa-1. *The Journal of Clinical Endocrinology & Metabolism, 93*, 1231–1237.

Mitchison, D., & Hay, P. J. (2014). The epidemiology of eating disorders: Genetic, environmental, and societal factors. *Clinical Epidemiology, 6*, 89–97.

Moser, D. J., Benjamin, M. L., Bayless, J. D., McDowell, B. D., Paulsen, J. S., Bowers, W. A., ... Andersen, A. E. (2003). Neuropsychological functioning pretreatment and posttreatment in an inpatient eating disorders program. *International Journal of Eating Disorders, 33*, 64–70.

Muise, A. M., Stein, D. G., & Arbess, G. (2003). Eating disorders in adolescent boys: A review of the adolescent and young adult literature. *Journal of Adolescent Health, 33*, 427–435.

Neumark-Sztainer, D. R., Wall, M. W., Haines, J. I., Story, M. T., Sherwood, N. E., & van den Berg, P. A. (2007). Shared risk and protective factors for overweight and disordered eating in adolescents. *American Journal of Preventive Medicine, 33*, 359–369.

Norris, M. L., Robinson, A., Obeid, N., Harrison, M., Spettigue, W., & Henderson, K. (2014). Exploring avoidant/restrictive food intake disorder in eating disordered patients: A descriptive study. *International Journal of Eating Disorders, 47*, 495–499.

Norris, M. L., Spettigue, W. J., & Katzman, D. K. (2016). Update on eating disorders: Current perspectives on avoidant/restrictive food intake disorder in children and youth. *Neuropsychiatric Disease and Treatment, 12*, 213–218.

Rosen, D. S., & The Committee on Adolescence. (2010). Clinical report: Identification and management of eating disorders in children and adolescents. *Pediatrics, 126*, 1240–1253.

Stice, E., Gau, J. M., Rohde, P., & Shaw, H. (2016). Risk factors that predict future onset of each DSM–5 eating disorder: Predictive specificity in high-risk adolescent females. *Journal of Abnormal Psychology, 126*, 38–51.

Stice, E., Marti, N. C., & Rohde, P. (2013). Prevalence, incidence, impairment, and course of the proposed DSM-5 eating disorder diagnoses in an 8-year prospective community study of young women. *Journal of Abnormal Psychology, 122*, 445–457.

Taljemark, J., Rastam, M., Lichtenstein, P., Anckarsater, H., & Kerekes, N. (2017). The coexistence of psychiatric and gastrointestinal problems in children with restrictive eating in a nationwide Swedish twin study. *Journal of Eating Disorders, 5*, 1–11.

The Society of Adolescent Health and Medicine. (2015). Position paper of the society for adolescent health and medicine: Medical management of restrictive eating disorders in adolescents and young adults. *Journal of Adolescent Health, 56*, 121–125.

Thornton, L. M., Mazzeo, S. E., & Bulik, C. M. (2013). The heritability of eating disorders: Methods and current findings. *Current Topics in Behavioral Neurosciences, 6*, 141–156.

Wolfe, B. E., Metzger, E. D., Levine, J. M., & Jimerson, D. C. (2001). Laboratory screening for electrolyte abnormalities and anemia in bulimia nervosa: A controlled study. *International Journal of Eating Disorders, 30*, 288–293.

Zeeck, A., Weber, S., Sandholz, A., Wetzler-Burmeister, E., Wirsching, M., & Hartmann, A. (2009). Inpatient versus day clinic treatment for bulimia nervosa: A randomized trial. *Psychotherapy and Psychosomatics, 78*, 152–160.

Pediatric Feeding Disorders

Melissa N. Andersen, Robert Dempster, Lauren L. Garbacz, Laura Sayers, Heather Shepard, Amy Drayton, and Rachel M. Knight

Feeding difficulties in children are common and range from mild "picky eating" to more severe food refusal. Symptoms of severe feeding difficulty may include, but are not limited to, disruptive mealtime behavior (e.g., tantruming, gagging, coughing, throwing food, vomiting, refusing to swallow, hitting, spitting, etc.), severe selectivity (limiting intake based on flavor, color, brand, or texture), reliance on supplements (e.g., formula, Pediasure), oral aversion (e.g., avoidance or fear of sensation in or around the mouth), and/or oral motor delays (Coe et al., 1997; Kerwin, 1999; Morris, Knight, Bruni, Sayers, & Drayton, 2017; Williams, Field, & Seiverling, 2010). These problems can result in inadequate weight gain, nutritional deficiencies, and feeding tube dependence (Kerwin, 1999; Morris et al., 2017; Williams et al., 2010).

M. N. Andersen (✉) · A. Drayton · R. M. Knight
L. Sayers · H. Shepard
Department of Pediatrics, C.S. Mott Children's Hospital, University of Michigan School of Medicine, Ann Arbor, MI, USA
e-mail: melandrs@med.umich.edu

R. Dempster · L. L. Garbacz
Department of Pediatric Psychology and Neuropsychology, Nationwide Children's Hospital, Columbus, OH, USA

Department of Pediatrics, The Ohio State University, Columbus, OH, USA

Diagnosis

Severe feeding problems are estimated to be experienced by 3–10% of all children, tend to worsen over time, and are often associated with negative developmental and medical outcomes (Kerwin, 1999). Prevalence rates are considerably higher for children with an autism spectrum disorder (approximately 90%; Kodak & Piazza, 2008) and children with a history of chronic medical conditions (40–70%; Lukens & Silverman, 2014). Given that feeding disorders are often impacted by medical, developmental, and behavioral factors, a multidisciplinary team should be involved in evaluation and treatment (Goday et al., 2019; Gosa, Carden, Jacks, Threadgill, & Sidlovsky, 2017; Sharp, Volkert, Scahill, McCracken, & McElhanon, 2017; Silverman, 2010).

There is a lack of consensus regarding diagnostic criteria and appropriate terminology for feeding disorders across professions. Currently, the ICD-10 code "Feeding Problems" is very broad and does not include details about the child's symptoms. It is often used by medical professionals in the field of pediatrics. The diagnosis of "dysphagia" is commonly used by speech-language pathologists (SLPs) and occupational therapists (OTs) and indicates a swallowing difficulty (Gosa et al., 2017). This diagnosis does not differentiate between oral

B. D. Carter, K. A. Kullgren (eds.), *Clinical Handbook of Psychological Consultation in Pediatric Medical Settings*, Issues in Clinical Child Psychology, https://doi.org/10.1007/978-3-030-35598-2_18

motor and behavioral difficulties in swallowing. Avoidant/restrictive food intake disorder (ARFID) was added to the *Diagnostic and Statistical Manual of Mental Disorders, Fifth Edition* (DSM-5). This provides more detailed criteria including persistent failure to meet appropriate nutritional and/or energy needs associated with one (or more) of the following: significant weight loss (or failure to achieve expected weight gain or faltering growth), significant nutritional deficiency, dependence on tube feeding or nutritional supplements, and marked interference with psychosocial functioning (American Psychiatric Association, 2013). However, even when using this diagnosis, it is essential that medical, oral motor, and nutritional areas are assessed in conjunction with feeding behavior in order to develop an appropriate and effective treatment plan (Gosa et al., 2017). Most recently, Goday et al. (2019) proposed a consensus definition and conceptual framework for a unifying diagnostic term "pediatric feeding disorder (PFD)" using the framework of the World Health Organization International Classification of Functioning, Disability, and Health in order to characterize the complex, multisystem, and multidisciplinary assessment and treatment required of PFD. The definition of PFD is "impaired oral intake that is not age-appropriate, and is associated with medical, nutritional, feeding skill, and/or psychosocial dysfunction" (Goday et al., 2019).

Medical Basics

Children with complex medical histories (e.g., constipation, gastroesophageal reflux disease, congenital heart disease, short bowel syndrome, tracheostomy/ventilator dependence, food allergies) have a higher risk of developing a PFD (Gosa et al., 2017; Hawdon, Beauregard, Slattery, & Kennedy, 2000; Lukens & Silverman, 2014), as these conditions can affect a child's ability and desire to eat. Physical discomfort stemming from medical conditions and procedures may become associated with eating (Di Lorenzo et al., 2005). When this occurs, children learn to engage in refusal behaviors (e.g., turning head, refusing to open mouth, spitting, crying, gagging, vomiting) in an effort to avoid discomfort. After medical issues are addressed, disruptive behaviors often persist (Babbitt et al., 1994; Haas, 2010).

Food refusal is largely escape-maintained (Piazza, Patel, Gulotta, Sevin, & Layer, 2003). When an aspect of eating (chewing, tasting, swallowing, digesting, etc.) is paired with pain, discomfort, or distress related to a medical condition, developmental delay, or an adverse event (e.g., choking; Seiverling et al., 2016), children are more likely to refuse food or engage in disruptive behavior to avoid pain or distress (LaRue et al., 2011; Piazza et al., 2003). Parents are then more likely to respond by delaying or removing the demand (e.g., put the spoon down, stop the meal; Borrero, Woods, Borrero, Masler, & Lesser, 2010), and children learn that refusal results in escape from eating. Behavioral interventions addressing escape behaviors are effective in treating PFDs (Morris et al., 2017; Piazza et al., 2003; Sharp et al., 2017; Sharp, Jaquess, Morton, & Herzinger, 2010; Williams et al., 2010); however, it is essential for medical factors to be evaluated before intervening to avoid causing further discomfort.

Delays in oral motor skill development, difficulties with swallowing, and aspiration (when food or liquid enters the airway rather than the esophagus) can also contribute to the development and maintenance of PFDs. An expert in oral motor issues and feeding (i.e., SLP or OT) should complete an evaluation to ensure that a child has the appropriate skills to eat efficiently and safely (Arvedson & Brodsky, 2002). Additionally, many children on tube feeds do not experience typical hunger cues, which can impact the desire to eat (Linscheid, 2006; Schauster & Dwyer, 1996).

Formulation

As noted above, a multidisciplinary evaluation is strongly recommended given the medical, nutritional, oral motor, and behavioral factors that impact feeding (Sharp et al., 2017). An SLP or OT should be involved to comprehensively assess oropharyngeal swallowing function, provide guidance on addressing oral motor deficits, provide instruction on compensatory swallowing techniques, and ensure swallowing safety with least restrictive diet textures. Many children have swallowing deficits that require patient-specific utensils, cups, positioning, textures, or bolus[1] size. It is imperative that these recommendations are consistently followed in order to prevent aspiration during treatment. SLPs or OTs can also perform instrumental assessments, such as Videofluoroscopic Swallow Studies (VFSS) and Fiberoptic Endoscopic Evaluation of Swallowing (FEES), for the subset of patients that require additional evaluation. Finally, SLPs or OTs will closely monitor the patient's progress with oral motor abilities and advance texture and bolus sizes as appropriate.

A registered dietitian (RD) assesses the anthropometrics of the child. This can include height, weight, weight for length, body mass index, mid-upper arm circumference, and hand grip strength. Nutrition-focused physical assessments are also typically performed to look for indicators of malnutrition and micronutrient deficiencies. An RD will often request a 3-day diet record to help evaluate the child's nutrient intake (Green Corkins & Teague, 2017). The goal is to provide guidance on calorie and protein requirements to promote age-appropriate growth and encourage nutritional quality of the child's diet. An RD also provides information regarding age-appropriate portion sizes, fluid requirements, and tube feeding weaning schedules if that is the goal of treatment. Adjustments of tube feeding schedules to more closely mimic mealtimes and promote hunger may be necessary (Babbitt et al., 1994; Schauster & Dwyer, 1996). More information on tube feeds can be found on the Feeding Tube Awareness Foundation's website (https://www.feedingtubeawareness.org).

From a medical standpoint, patients with PFDs will be monitored by their pediatrician or specialty care provider, often a pediatric gastroenterologist (GI). The GI often monitors and treats concerns such as constipation, gastroesophageal reflux disease, eosinophilic esophagitis, delayed gastric emptying, abdominal pain, nausea, and vomiting. Depending on medical history, patients may be followed by another specialty care provider (e.g., cardiologist, nephrologist, surgeon) regarding those concerns, which may also impact feeding. Psychologists should ensure that patients are being followed by their medical providers to rule out, monitor, and avoid discomfort while eating and to support stamina to eat.

From the behavioral perspective, assessment should include a medical record review, a clinical interview, and a feeding observation. The clinical interview should include a history of the presenting feeding concern, medical and developmental history, mealtime behaviors, caregiver response to mealtime behaviors, mealtime routines, types of food eaten consistently, additional behavioral concerns outside of feeding, mental health history, and family stressors. Feeding observation will allow for assessment of caregiver-child interactions and disruptive mealtime behaviors. Standardized rating scales are also available specifically for feeding, such as the Behavioral Pediatric Feeding Assessment Scale (Crist & Napier-Phillips, 2001) and the PediEAT (Thoyre et al., 2014). Standardized rating scales of behavioral and emotional functioning may also be useful (e.g., Child Behavior Checklist; Achenbach & Edlebrock, 1993). Given time constraints of brief consultation, these measures may be most useful in the context of consultation that will involve long-term treatment (e.g., a long inpatient admission).

Intervention

Existing research indicates that strategies used in the treatment of PFDs should be behavioral with guidance in formulating the treatment plan from other disciplines including medical providers, SLP, OT, and RD (Sharp et al., 2017). The treatment environment and format for PFDs include outpatient, intensive day treatment, and intensive inpatient (Lukens & Silverman, 2014). One of

[1] In the context of oral feeds, bolus refers to a round mass of food material, typically chewed.

the more important decisions in the context of consultation for feeding difficulties is the extent to which immediate behavioral intervention is warranted or whether referral for long-term care is more appropriate. It is crucial to ensure that the child is physically ready to proceed comfortably and safely with behavioral treatment. If a child has ongoing illness, is at risk for aspiration, or has a condition that causes discomfort, behavioral treatment is contraindicated until these symptoms are addressed.

Next, it is important to consider the time and resources necessary, including adequate training in behavioral treatment for PFDs and sufficient time to effectively implement the strategies and train caregivers. Additional materials may be needed, such as specific types of food or formula and specialized cups or utensils for safe consumption. Caregiver buy-in, readiness, and commitment are crucial for behavioral treatment to be effective. Inconsistent or improper implementation of behavioral feeding strategies can inadvertently strengthen the problem behavior or aversion. The relative risk of worsening the feeding problem should be strongly considered prior to implementing or recommending any behavioral feeding strategy (Silverman, 2015). In general, if a child has a chronic history of feeding difficulties, has never consistently eaten a developmentally appropriate variety of foods and textures, or has significant disruptive mealtime behaviors, the child will require more intensive feeding therapy than can be provided within a few encounters in the context of consultation. If a child requires intensive feeding therapy, it is not advisable to begin treatment without scheduled outpatient follow-up. The decision-making tree in Fig. 1 was crafted to assist psychology consultants with assessment and determining an appropriate direction for treatment.

Treatment Planning

Behavioral treatment for feeding problems must ultimately address the function of the behavior in order to be effective. It is well established that the primary function of food refusal and disruptive mealtime behavior is escape (Piazza et al., 2003). Therefore, a central component of behavioral feeding intervention consists of no longer allowing a child to escape or delay eating contingent on refusal or disruptive behavior (Sharp et al., 2010; Williams et al., 2010).

Treatment goals for behavioral feeding intervention in the context of consultation generally include increasing the volume and variety of food and drinks accepted and decreasing disruptive mealtime behavior. Multiple strategies exist and must be individualized to the needs of each child. The following strategies are not mutually exclusive and often used in combination (Lukens & Silverman, 2014).

Antecedent Manipulation

Antecedent manipulation often includes establishing a positive feeding environment with minimal distraction, altering the feeding schedule to promote hunger (as recommended by an RD), and modifying how food is presented. Stimulus fading is a type of antecedent manipulation that refers to systematically changing an aspect of the stimulus presented (e.g., flavor, texture, volume) to closer approximate the target stimulus. For example, if chocolate milk is a preferred drink and the goal is to increase water intake, stimulus fading would consist of slowly increasing the ratio of water to chocolate milk until the child is accepting water (Luiselli, Ricciardi, & Gilligan, 2005). Another example would include first presenting a very small bite of a nonpreferred food (e.g., turkey deli meat in the size of a grain of rice) and gradually increasing the size of the bite until it is a developmentally appropriate bite size. The nonpreferred food could also be presented on a preferred food (e.g., cracker) with the size of the preferred food systematically decreased until the child is eating just the nonpreferred food. Stimulus fading has been effectively used with other behavioral strategies (e.g., differential reinforcement and escape extinction) to increase acceptance of volume and variety (Kerwin, Ahearn, Eicher, & Burd, 1995; Williams et al., 2010).

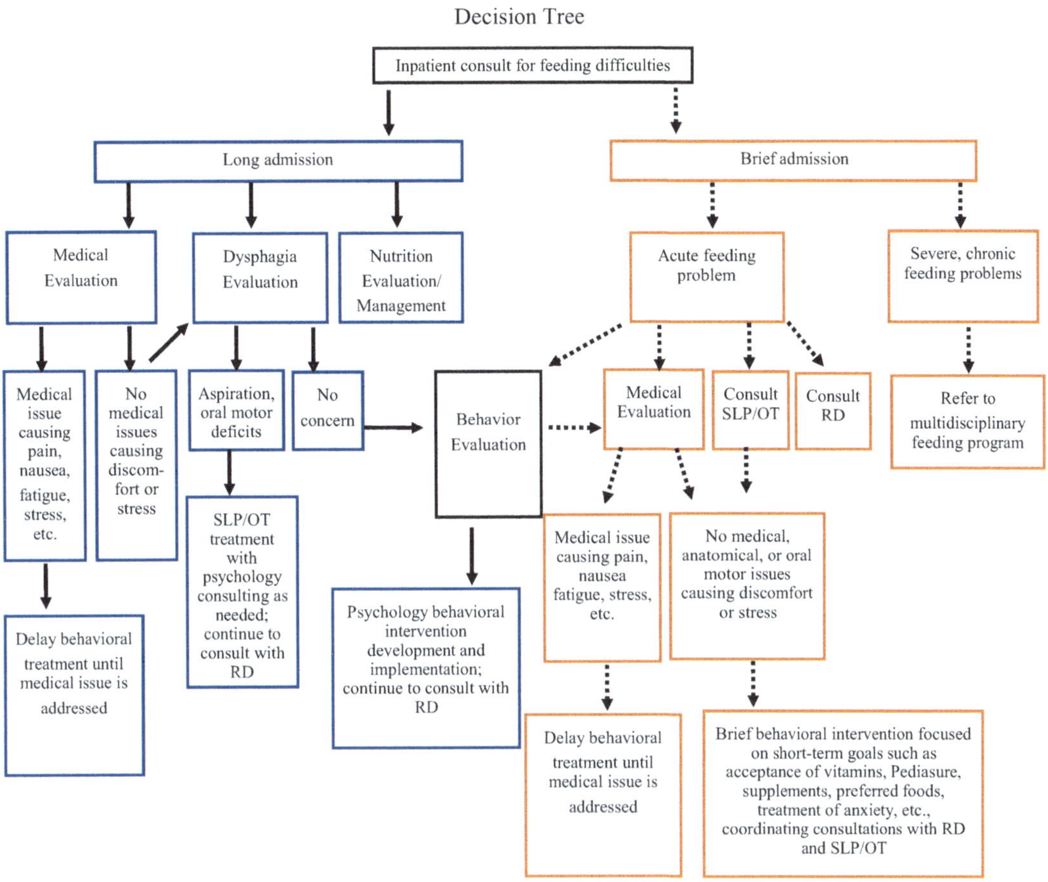

Fig. 1 Decision tree

Escape Extinction

Escape extinction (EE) consists of keeping the feeding demand in place until the child accepts the bite. In other words, refusal behaviors no longer result in escape (e.g., the spoon or cup is kept at the child's mouth until the bite or drink is accepted or expelled food is re-presented until it is swallowed; Ahearn, 1996; Penrod & VanDalen, 2010;Piazza et al., 2003; Sharp et al., 2010). EE is the most empirically validated and essential treatment component to eliminate food refusal and is often used in conjunction with other strategies such as stimulus fading, differential reinforcement, and noncontingent reinforcement in order to minimize the severity of refusal behaviors and extinction bursts (Piazza et al., 2003; Sharp et al., 2010).

Careful consideration must be made before implementing EE, as there are many situations in which it may be contraindicated in the context of consultation. Extinction bursts can be difficult for providers with little training managing the behavior and for parents who are not fully prepared and in agreement with the use of the strategy. It can require a significant amount of time to implement if the child's refusal behavior persists. Time, parent buy-in and preparation, and consistency are vital to effectively implement EE. Adequate training for all caregivers who will be implementing the strategy is also crucial, as there is a high risk that improper implementation will reinforce more intense and persistent refusal behavior.

Reinforcement Strategies

Differential reinforcement consists of providing reinforcement contingent on accepting and swallowing food (Kerwin, 2003). Reinforcers must be meaningful to the child and can be tangible (e.g., bubbles, toys, videos), attention-based (e.g., cheering, clapping, singing), and escape-based (e.g., short break from the meal). A combination of all types of reinforcers can also be used (e.g., 30 s break with a video, cheering with bubbles after each bite or sip) to increase the potency of the reinforcement. Timers can be used to establish clear expectations regarding how long a child has to take a bite to earn the reinforcer and to signal break time. Demand fading is often used in conjunction with differential reinforcement and consists of gradually increasing the volume or number of bites required in order to earn the reinforcer (Najdowski et al., 2010; Piazza et al., 2002). Differential reinforcement alone is often not enough to increase oral intake but when used in conjunction with EE can significantly reduce disruptive behavior (LaRue et al., 2011; Patel, Piazza, Martinez, Volkert, & Santana, 2002).

Noncontingent reinforcement (NCR) consists of providing attention and access to preferred items during the meal independent of the child's behavior. This strategy is largely used to decrease the aversiveness of the mealtime for the child (Reed et al., 2004). This strategy can be used as a first-line treatment approach for children with low-level feeding difficulties (e.g., otherwise healthy, developmentally appropriate diet at baseline but refusing due to an adverse event associated with eating). In children with more severe PFDs, NCR alone will not be enough to increase oral intake (Reed et al., 2004).

Systematic Desensitization

Systematic desensitization consists of repeatedly pairing the conditioned aversive stimulus (food, fluid, cup, spoon, etc.), with eating or drinking without an aversive unconditioned stimulus (e.g., swallowing without choking, eating without pain; Silverman, 2015). Graduated exposure begins with the least aversive presentation (e.g., empty spoon, bite the size of a grain of rice) and progresses along an exposure hierarchy tailored to the objective. It can be used to gradually advance volume, texture, and variety of foods, and it is often used in combination with EE and differential reinforcement (Tanner & Andreone, 2015).

Treatment Engagement

An often overlooked aspect of helping children and families with feeding difficulties is engaging parents and children from the start of treatment. Even with a solid behavior plan that incorporates a variety of disciplines, if the family does not believe in the process or collaborate in planning, they are unlikely to make lasting changes. Many families may not understand the reason for behavioral intervention and feel they need to find the medical "root cause" of the problems. Several strategies can help increase family buy-in from the beginning.

Initial Consult

Like any therapeutic alliance, engagement with the family starts at the initial meeting. Because feeding is such a basic need, families are often highly stressed when there is difficulty meeting this need. Although other disciplines may have asked about specifics related to feedings, psychologists are uniquely suited to listen to families about how feeding challenges are impacting their daily lives, family dynamics, and the guilt parents feel over not being able to feed their child. Assessing these aspects enables providers to understand the full picture and determine how feeding integrates into the families' lives. Similarly, it is important to understand which aspects of feeding are the family's primary concern. Although providers may be most concerned about tube weaning or increasing volume, a family may be more focused on increasing variety of foods. If the family does not see how a treatment plan is working toward their personal goals, then they are less likely to follow through (Kazak, Simms, & Rourke, 2002).

It is important to include the child in assessment and treatment planning. Whenever possible, assessing a child's eating in the first session shows families that recommendations are informed by direct observation and allows the opportunity to model specific strategies. Although most of the gains made with behavioral feeding therapy are made through parent training, parents are more likely to participate treatment when they believe their child has been directly assessed. In cases of ongoing therapy, establishing rapport with the child from the outset of treatment also increases the value of provider attention to help shape behavior.

Cultural Factors

During the first contact with the family and in all treatment sessions, it is important to assess how the family's culture impacts the child's life. Food and feeding are inherently intertwined with culture (Hughes et al., 2006), and integrating a family's cultural views is vital to engaging families in a feeding plan. For example, many cultures view children as the master of their domain and allow them to explore the world with few limitations aside from safety. A family with these values may have difficulty following a rigid schedule, using a high chair, and using limit setting strategies such as differential reinforcement and EE. In these situations, making 1–2 small changes at a time or identifying strategies that would fit within the family's culture is vital. Similarly, the foods chosen in treatment should fit within the family's diet and lifestyle. Cultures also vary widely in tolerance of children becoming upset, which significantly impacts the likelihood that they will follow through with a behavior plan involving EE, so all procedures should be thoughtfully explained and agreed upon in advance.

Collaborative Behavior Plans

Families will have more treatment gains when they are a partner in creating the treatment plan (Kitzmann, Dalton, & Buscemi, 2008). This can mean talking with families about initial recommendations, feasibility, and potential barriers. For example, it is often recommended to sit at the table for three meals and two snacks on a schedule. However, some families do not own dinner tables or are not home most nights of the week due to extracurricular activities. If a plan is given without considering the family's lifestyle, then the family is likely to terminate implementation prematurely or resort to modifications that may be counterproductive.

Behavior plans should be written without jargon and in a way all individuals involved can easily understand. Plans should be reviewed with all caregivers prior to implementation to problem-solve potential barriers (e.g., how the plan will work on school days versus weekends).

Small Successes

Finding ways to demonstrate small successes from the outset of treatment also helps children and families trust the strategies (Friars & Mellor, 2007). Treatment gains during an admission will depend on the child's feeding challenge, chronicity of the condition, and physical limitations. Early success can often be facilitated by setting small goals with easy or highly preferred foods to teach the child that they are rewarded for participating. Then, talking with families about how these strategies will be applied to difficult feeding challenges provides them with a map to see how treatment will help them reach their goals.

Inpatient Consultation

Inpatient consultation for feeding problems can occur for a variety of reasons. On medical units, common diagnoses and problems include failure to thrive (FTT), gastrointestinal discomfort (e.g., abdominal pain, nausea, vomiting), difficulty resuming oral intake after a medical procedure, and food refusal after a choking incident. Physicians often approach feeding cases with the task of determining whether symptoms are related to an organic, anatomical, or behavioral feeding problem (Piazza, 2008). Realistic expectations for goals and intervention success will vary widely depending on length of stay, chronicity and intensity of presenting issues, and psychologist's role as a consultant to the team.

Psychology's Role

One important distinction between outpatient treatment and inpatient consultation is that families often may not be the stakeholders initiating treatment. When children are admitted with a feeding-related or GI problem, families are often seeking medical solutions. This may present a challenge regarding how psychologists approach the consultation with the family. It is important to know who initiated the consult and what is communicated to the family about psychology involvement. Families may have varying degrees of openness to collaborate with psychologists if they do not understand how behavioral supports can help their children. Providers who initiate psychology consults also may not have a clear idea of what is needed, and psychologists must often provide this education to shape consultation questions and expectations. It may also be necessary for the psychologist to suggest involvement of other disciplines that may have yet to become involved (e.g., RD, SLP, OT).

Inpatient Treatment

Treatment on an inpatient unit often must be brief due to short length of stay. Psychologists must be realistic about what can be accomplished during the admission given multiple care providers and many competing needs. For example, it can be difficult for families to adhere to a strict meal schedule when the child is being taken away for procedures or waiting on medication delivery. It is important to communicate with all members of the care team about a realistic behavioral treatment plan. Posting written information in the patient's room and nursing orders in the chart can increase the likelihood that a plan will be followed. Given the multifaceted nature of feeding problems, it is often appropriate for psychology to co-treat with other disciplines (e.g., SLP or OT) to ensure the intervention is implemented safely (from a swallowing standpoint) and effectively (from a behavioral standpoint).

Recommendations

Typically, medical teams and families expect specific psychology recommendations to be implemented during an admission and/or as part of discharge planning (Lassen, Wu, & Roberts, 2014). Recommendations may fall short if they are not modeled and families or staff are not coached on implementation. Therefore, a critical element of inpatient consultation is the meal observation. Psychologists may only get one or two opportunities to work with a patient before discharge, so it is important to look for an immediate point of intervention. Depending on the presenting issue, a psychologist may model behavioral strategies to improve compliance with oral intake, establish a reward system to encourage participation, and educate families on use of timers, setting small goals, and improving mealtime structure. Unlike the outpatient setting, in most cases, it is not realistic to establish an elaborate treatment plan or assume there will be multiple opportunities to practice meals with families during inpatient consultations.

Planning for Success

In addition to communication with the team, inpatient feeding consults often require a great deal of logistical planning. For instance, it is often necessary to plan ahead with families and nurses to ensure the appropriate food is available at the time of consultation. Patients and families are not always available at the same time as providers. Coordination with medical staff is often necessary to ensure a patient is available and hungry when you arrive for a meal. Co-treatment may also be helpful if other providers have been consulted for feeding-related issues.

Referrals

Since many feeding issues requiring hospitalization are long-standing or severe, they cannot be fully treated before a patient is discharged. Therefore, a consulting psychologist is often tasked with referring families to local providers for ongoing outpatient feeding treatment. This requires knowledge of behavioral or multidisciplinary feeding referral options within the institution or local networks. Families who are not local to the hospital will need to be referred to providers in their own area, which may include SLP or OT when appropriate. If families are willing to travel, referral to an out-of-town intensive feeding program may also be an option.

Outpatient Consultation

When providing care in a multidisciplinary clinic, it is likely that other providers will refer to psychology for behavioral feeding issues. It is important to always keep the medical, nutritional, and oral motor factors in mind during any consultation. If a child is referred for general picky eating and is seen regularly by psychology and RD in clinic, then developing a behavior plan for incorporating new or nonpreferred foods may be appropriate. A referral to an outpatient behavioral psychologist who can collaborate with an RD may also be appropriate.

However, this chapter focuses on children with more severe PFDs. Unless psychology providers have extensive training in the assessment and treatment of PFDs, it is recommended to refer to a feeding program with a multidisciplinary team (psychology, SLP/OT, RD, MD) with a focus on behavioral intervention. Appropriate referrals may also include medical evaluation by a sub-specialist to assess possible causes of discomfort while eating, oral motor skill evaluation by an SLP or OT, evaluation by an RD to plan a nutritional diet or consolidate tube feeds, and weight checks and medical monitoring by the pediatrician.

Case Example

Gavin is a 19-month-old Nepalese boy who was admitted to the hospital for FTT and weight loss over the previous 4 months. Prior to admission, he only breastfed consistently for nutrition. The family attempted to feed him 4–5 times per day, and he typically refused all food (i.e., throwing, expelling, refusing to swallow). His family immigrated to the United States 9 months prior to his admission and did not speak English. He lived with his biological parents with no local extended family support. Upon admission, a nasogastric (NG) feeding tube was placed. He received small bolus tube feeds[2] of gradually increasing volume to monitor for re-feeding syndrome (a serious condition characterized by fluid and electrolyte imbalances that can lead to organ dysfunction when feeds are introduced after prolonged malnutrition).

Intake

Psychology and SLP were consulted to conduct a joint evaluation and create a feeding plan after tests showed no medical cause of the feeding problems. The family initially questioned the need for psychology and SLP involvement, and providers explained their respective areas of expertise and rationale for involvement. Providers obtained detailed background information, including medical and family history, barriers to participation, and cultural feeding practices. Then they observed two meals. For the first 5 min, providers observed parents feed Gavin. His mother held him on her lap and offered a graham cracker. Gavin immediately pushed it away and then turned and cried. Parents offered sips of water from a cup, from which Gavin also turned away and cried. The family noted they usually stop at this point.

[2] In the context of tube feeding, bolus refers to delivering a specified amount of fluid in a discrete period of time (e.g., 30 min).

After a brief break, providers explained the rationale for behavioral strategies and the potential for an extinction burst. The family agreed to the treatment strategies. Gavin was placed in a high chair, oriented to several potential reinforcers, and selected cartoons. Providers learned the Nepali translation for "take a bite" and used this prompt to facilitate understanding and home practice. Gavin was given bites of an empty spoon and empty straw to teach him when he takes bites, he gets a break with video access and praise. After five empty presentations, he accepted puree and small sips of apple juice. At the end of the assessment, he took 12 bites of banana puree, 5 sips of apple juice, and small bites of graham cracker. The SLP recommended offering purees and thin liquids based on his skill. Providers developed the behavior plan (Appendix) in collaboration with his family, which was posted in the room and placed in nursing orders.

Consultation Follow-Ups

Gavin was admitted for a total of 10 days. Psychology conducted three follow-up visits, and the SLP followed up twice. Visits were staggered, so Gavin was seen by one provider every weekday of admission. Over the weekend, his family practiced meals with puree and preferred drink (apple juice), with NG tube feedings scheduled after meal presentations. He worked up to full meal boluses every 3 h while awake. During the second psychology visit, parents practiced implementing the feeding plan, and the psychologist provided coaching on selective attention, simple instructions, and use of reinforcers. Gavin consistently finished 13 presentations each of the puree and drink. At this consultation, potential benefits of outpatient therapy were discussed given that he would likely be discharged with an NG tube. The family was in agreement and scheduled an outpatient follow-up visit before discharge.

At the third visit, Gavin accepted puree but completely refused a change from juice to formula. After the meal ended, the family and team decided to focus on increasing his acceptance of preferred foods and planned to gradually transition him to less preferred foods once he was eating consistently. During the final consultation, providers discussed how to integrate the behavioral strategies at home, processed potential barriers, and reviewed scheduled plans for medical and psychology follow-up, with a plan to transition to therapy once his behaviors were consistently more participatory at mealtimes.

Post-Discharge

Gavin attended a total of four outpatient psychology sessions to address behavioral feeding challenges. His disruptive behavior escalated significantly following discharge, and the team and family decided that Gavin would benefit most from an intensive treatment model. Before attending the intensive program, he was diagnosed with autism spectrum disorder as part of a developmental evaluation. He attended an 8-week intensive outpatient multidisciplinary feeding program. At the end of the program, he was eating and drinking consistently, and his NG tube was removed. His family was able to feed him consistently at home.

Summary

Gavin was admitted to the hospital for FTT and NG tube placement and to monitor for re-feeding syndrome. The goal was not to resolve feeding difficulties prior to discharge, but to stabilize him medically, establish a foundation for behavioral treatment, and facilitate outpatient referrals. Assessing family barriers and providing instruction in a culturally sensitive way were vital for establishing family buy-in to treatment.

Conclusion

Assessment and treatment of PFDs require multidisciplinary collaboration to meet the patient's physical, developmental, and behavioral needs.

Behavioral feeding strategies are the most effective, evidence-based approach for treating PFDs, but these strategies must incorporate guidance from medical providers, SLP, OT, and RD. Careful consideration should be given to cultural factors and resources (e.g., time, training) necessary for assessment and treatment when formulating the most appropriate treatment plan in the context of consultation.

Appendix: Gavin's Initial Feeding Plan

- Gavin will have tube feedings every 3 h starting at 8:00 am (8:00 am, 11:00 am, 2:00 pm, 5:00 pm, 8:00 pm). Thirty minutes before tube feedings, his family will complete a high chair meal.
- Gavin's goal is to complete five bites of food and five drinks per feeding.
- A timer will be set for 15 min at the start of each meal.
- If Gavin finishes his goal volumes at every meal for the day, increase the goal by two sips each day.
- During meals, he can watch cartoons if he is accepting bites, but if he is refusing, then this will be paused until he accepts the next bite. He gets lots of praise and attention if he is participating and no attention with simple prompt to take a bite (in Nepali) if he is refusing. He should not watch cartoons between meals, so they are more interesting when meals begin.
- If Gavin finishes his goal number of bites, he should immediately be allowed out of high chair and be able to leave. If he does not take his bites, continue to prompt him until he accepts or his timer goes off.

References

Achenbach, T. M., & Edlebrock, C. (1993). *Manual for the child behavior checklist and revised child behavior profile*. Burlington, VT: Department of Psychiatry, University of Vermont.

Ahearn, W. H. (1996). An alternating treatments comparison of two intensive interventions for food refusal. *Journal of Applied Behavior Analysis, 29*, 321–332.

American Psychiatric Association. (2013). *Diagnostic and statistical manual of mental disorders* (5th ed.). Arlington, VA: American Psychiatric Association.

Arvedson, J., & Brodsky, L. (2002). Pediatric and neurodevelopmental assessment. In *Pediatric swallowing and feeding: Assessment and management* (2nd ed., pp. 81–152). Albany, NY: Singular Publishing Group.

Babbitt, R. L., Hoch, T. A., Coe, D. A., Cataldo, M. F., Kelly, K. J., Stackhouse, C., & Perman, J. A. (1994). Behavioral assessment and treatment of pediatric feeding disorders. *Journal of Developmental and Behavioral Pediatrics, 15*, 278–291.

Borrero, C. S., Woods, J. N., Borrero, J. C., Masler, E. A., & Lesser, A. D. (2010). Descriptive analysis of pediatric food refusal and acceptance. *Journal of Applied Behavior Analysis, 43*, 71–88.

Coe, D. A., Babbitt, R. L., Williams, K. E., Hajimihalis, C., Snyder, A. M., Ballard, C., & Efron, L. A. (1997). Use of extinction and reinforcement to increase food consumption and reduce expulsion. *Journal of Applied Behavior Analysis, 30*, 581–583.

Crist, W., & Napier-Phillips, A. (2001). Mealtime behaviors of young children: A comparison of normative and clinical data. *Journal of Developmental and Behavioral Pediatrics, 22*, 279–286.

Di Lorenzo, C., Colletti, R. B., Lehmann, H. P., Boyle, J. T., Gerson, W. T., Hyams, J. S., … Walker, L. S. (2005). Chronic abdominal pain in children: A technical report of the American Academy of Pediatrics and the North American Society for Pediatric Gastroenterology, Hepatology and Nutrition. *Journal of Pediatric Gastroenterology and Nutrition, 43*, 249–261.

Friars, P. M., & Mellor, D. J. (2007). Drop out from behavioral management training programs for ADHD: A prospective study. *Journal of Child and Family Studies, 16*, 427–441.

Goday, P. S., Huh, S. Y., Silverman, A., Lukens, C. T., Dodrill, P., Cohen, S. S., et al. (2019). Pediatric feeding disorder: Consensus definition and conceptual framework. *Journal of Pediatric Gastroenterology and Nutrition, 68*, 124–129.

Gosa, M. M., Carden, H. T., Jacks, C. C., Threadgill, A. Y., & Sidlovsky, T. C. (2017). Evidence to support treatment options for children with swallowing and feeding disorders: A systematic review. *Journal of Pediatric Rehabilitation Medicine, 10*, 107–136.

Green Corkins, K., & Teague, E. E. (2017). Pediatric nutrition assessment: Anthropometrics to zinc. *Nutrition in Clinical Practice, 32*, 40–51.

Haas, A. M. (2010). Feeding disorders in food allergic children. *Current Allergy and Asthma Reports, 10*, 258–264.

Hawdon, J. M., Beauregard, N., Slattery, J., & Kennedy, G. (2000). Identification of neonates at risk of developing feeding problems in infancy. *Developmental Medicine and Child Neurology, 42*, 235–239.

Hughes, S. O., Anderson, C. B., Power, T. G., Micheli, N., Jaramillo, S., & Nicklas, T. A. (2006). Measuring feeding in low-income African-American and Hispanic parents. *Appetite, 46*, 215–223.

Kazak, A. E., Simms, S., & Rourke, M. T. (2002). Family systems practice in pediatric psychology. *Journal of Pediatric Psychology, 27*, 133–143.

Kerwin, M. E. (1999). Empirically supported treatments in pediatric psychology: Severe feeding problems. *Journal of Pediatric Psychology, 24*, 193–211.

Kerwin, M. E. (2003). Pediatric feeding problems: A behavior analytic approach to assessment and treatment. *The Behavior Analyst Today, 4*, 162–176.

Kerwin, M. E., Ahearn, W. H., Eicher, P. S., & Burd, D. M. (1995). The costs of eating: A behavioral economic analysis of food refusal. *Journal of Applied Behavior Analysis, 28*, 245–260.

Kitzmann, K. M., Dalton, W. T., & Buscemi, J. (2008). Beyond parenting practices: Family context and the treatment of pediatric obesity. *Family Relations, 57*, 13–23.

Kodak, T., & Piazza, C. C. (2008). Assessment and behavioral treatment of feeding and sleeping disorders in children with autism spectrum disorders. *Child and Adolescent Psychiatric Clinics of North America, 17*, 887–905.

LaRue, R. H., Stewart, V., Piazza, C. C., Volkert, V. M., Patel, M. R., & Zeleny, J. (2011). Escape as reinforcement and escape extinction in the treatment of feeding disorders. *Journal of Applied Behavior Analysis, 44*, 719–735.

Lassen, S., Wu, Y. P., & Roberts, M. C. (2014). Common presenting concerns and settings for pediatric psychology practice. In Y. P. Roberts, M. C. Aylward, & B. S. Wu (Eds.), *Clinical practice of pediatric psychology* (pp. 17–31). New York, NY: The Guilford Press.

Linscheid, T. R. (2006). Behavioral treatments for pediatric feeding disorders. *Behavior Modification, 30*, 6–23.

Luiselli, J. K., Ricciardi, J. N., & Gilligan, K. (2005). Liquid fading to establish milk consumption by a child with autism. *Behavioral Interventions, 20*, 155–163.

Lukens, C. T., & Silverman, A. H. (2014). Systematic review of psychological interventions for pediatric feeding problems. *Journal of Pediatric Psychology, 38*, 903–917.

Morris, N., Knight, R. M., Bruni, T., Sayers, L., & Drayton, A. (2017). Feeding disorders. *Child and Adolescent Psychiatric Clinics of North America, 26*, 571–586.

Najdowski, A. C., Wallace, M. D., Reagon, K., Penrod, B., Higbee, T. S., & Tarbox, J. (2010). Utilizing a home-based parent training approach in the treatment of food selectivity. *Behavioral Interventions, 25*, 89–107.

Patel, M. R., Piazza, C. C., Martinez, C. J., Volkert, V. M., & Santana, C. M. (2002). An evaluation of two differential reinforcement procedures with escape extinction to treat food refusal. *Journal of Applied Behavior Analysis, 35*, 363–374.

Penrod, B., & VanDalen, K. H. (2010). An evaluation of emerging preference for non-preferred foods targeted in the treatment of food selectivity. *Behavioral Interventions, 25*, 239–251.

Piazza, C. C. (2008). Feeding disorders and behavior: What have we learned? *Developmental Disabilities Research Reviews, 14*, 174–181.

Piazza, C. C., Patel, M. R., Gulotta, C. S., Sevin, B. M., & Layer, S. A. (2003). On the relative contributions of positive reinforcement and escape extinction in the treatment of food refusal. *Journal of Applied Behavior Analysis, 36*, 309–324.

Piazza, C. C., Patel, M. R., Santana, C. M., Goh, H. L., Delia, M. D., & Lancaster, B. M. (2002). An evaluation of simultaneous and sequential presentation of preferred and nonpreferred food to treat food selectivity. *Journal of Applied Behavior Analysis, 35*, 259–270.

Reed, G. K., Piazza, C. C., Patel, M. R., Layer, S. A., Bachmeyer, M. H., Bethke, S. D., & Gutshall, K. A. (2004). On the relative contributions of noncontingent reinforcement and escape extinction in the treatment of food refusal. *Journal of Applied Behavior Analysis, 37*, 27–42.

Schauster, H., & Dwyer, J. (1996). Transition from tube feedings to feedings by mouth in children: Preventing eating dysfunction. *Journal of the American Dietetic Association, 96*, 277–281.

Seiverling, L., Burns, J., Rodriguez, J., Yamazaki, H., Fernandez, A., & Yusupova, S. (2016). The effects of a brief behavioral intervention on food refusal in a child with a fear of choking. *Clinical Case Studies, 15*, 117–125.

Sharp, W. G., Jaquess, D. L., Morton, J. F., & Herzinger, C. V. (2010). Pediatric feeding disorders: A quantitative synthesis of treatment outcomes. *Clinical Child and Family Psychology Review, 13*, 348–365.

Sharp, W. G., Volkert, V. M., Scahill, L., McCracken, C. E., & McElhanon, B. (2017). A systematic review and meta-analysis of intensive multidisciplinary intervention for pediatric feeding disorders: How standard is the standard of care? *Journal of Pediatrics, 181*, 116–124.

Silverman, A. H. (2010). Interdisciplinary care for feeding problems in children. *Nutrition in Clinical Practice, 25*, 160–165.

Silverman, A. H. (2015). Behavioral management of feeding disorders of childhood. *Annals of Nutrition and Metabolism, 66*, 33–42.

Tanner, A., & Andreone, B. E. (2015). Using graduated exposure and differential reinforcement to increase food repertoire in a child with autism. *Behavior Analysis in Practice, 8*, 233–240.

Thoyre, S. M., Pados, B. F., Park, J., Estrem, H., Hodges, E. A., McComish, C., … Murdoch, K. (2014). Development and content validation of the pediatric eating assessment tool (Pedi-EAT). *American Journal of Speech-Language Pathology, 23*, 46–59.

Williams, K. E., Field, D. G., & Seiverling, L. (2010). Food refusal in children: A review of the literature. *Research in Developmental Disabilities, 31*, 625–633.

Trauma and Intensive Care

Meghan L. Marsac, Amy Meadows, Christine Kindler, and Ashley McGar

Introduction

Children with medical conditions that result in hospitalization in intensive care units (ICU) face unique potentially traumatic events (PTEs). Hospitalization brings substantial stress and challenges for patients and families. They may face new diagnoses or injuries, sudden exacerbations of existing medical conditions, high-risk treatments, emerging or worsening emotional symptoms, rotating medical teams, multiple specialists, and competing demands (e.g., school, work). Some families face difficult treatment decisions, potentially requiring an end-of-life and/or palliative care decision (Marsac, Kindler, Weiss, & Ragsdale, 2018). Thus, the PTEs and emotional responses in pediatric ICU (PICU) patients and their families fluctuate widely.

Mental health clinicians in the PICU can offer a range of services. Because the child's physical well-being may be impaired and the child and/or family may need time to adjust to the new circumstances associated with the illness or injury, many times, typical psychological treatment is not ideal during intensive care. Instead, clinicians may want to initiate rapport-building, conduct screenings or assessments of child and family emotional functioning, and focus treatment on problems related to current medical care. For example, children may have difficulty taking medication, struggle with procedure-related anxiety, and/or present challenges in cooperating with medical staff. Clinicians can also help the family in communicating with each other and with the medical team. Mental health providers can also support intensive medical care by teaching children non-pharmacological skills in pain management (e.g., diaphragmatic breathing, biofeedback; Coakley & Wihak, 2017).

In addition to directly supporting pediatric patients and their families, mental health providers have the opportunity to help to optimize patient care using a systems approach. Mental health clinicians can standardize screening and build protocols to highlight what services to offer based on screening outcomes (Kazak, Schneider, Didonato, & Pai, 2015). Mental health clinicians working in the PICU may also support the medi-

M. L. Marsac (✉)
Department of Pediatrics, Kentucky Children's Hospital, UK Health Care, University of Kentucky College of Medicine, Lexington, KY, USA
e-mail: meghan.marsac@uky.edu

A. Meadows
Department of Pediatrics, Kentucky Children's Hospital, UK Health Care, University of Kentucky College of Medicine, Lexington, KY, USA

Department of Psychiatry, Kentucky Children's Hospital, UK Health Care, University of Kentucky College of Medicine, Lexington, KY, USA

C. Kindler · A. McGar
Department of Pediatrics, Kentucky Children's Hospital, University of Kentucky School of Medicine, Lexington, KY, USA

B. D. Carter, K. A. Kullgren (eds.), *Clinical Handbook of Psychological Consultation in Pediatric Medical Settings*, Issues in Clinical Child Psychology, https://doi.org/10.1007/978-3-030-35598-2_19

cal team. Burnout in PICU physicians and nurses is high; approximately 49% of physicians and up to 65% of nurses report substantial burnout (Lawrence, Yoder, Schadler, & Shenoi, 2018; Shenoi, Kalyanaraman, Pillai, Raghava, & Day, 2018). By implementing a trauma-informed medical care approach, clinicians may be indirectly supporting families while directly supporting ICU providers (Marsac et al., 2016).

Differential Diagnoses

In considering trauma reactions in the ICU, clinicians ought to examine differential diagnoses of PTSD, anxiety, depression, and delirium. Selecting accurate diagnoses can guide evidence-based care. Children exposed to PTEs such as injury and/or illness are at risk of developing depression and anxiety disorders, sometimes comorbid with PTSD (Copeland, Keeler, Angold, & Costello, 2007). While we cannot yet fully predict which children will develop sustained emotional health symptoms following an ICU hospitalization, risk factors include ongoing exposure to PTEs, severity of illness, social factors, developmental stage, and caregiver psychological factors (e.g., maternal distress; Copeland et al., 2007).

The diagnosis of depression, anxiety, or PTSD is not clear-cut, particularly during intensive care. Approximately 35–62% of children report significant symptoms of PTSD following admission to the PICU (Nelson & Gold, 2012); rates of anxiety and depression are unknown. These disorders are often comorbid with each other and share symptoms with certain medical conditions. For example, depression, anxiety, and PTSD have many overlapping symptoms with traumatic brain injury (TBI), such as negative changes in cognition, difficulty making decisions, and irritability (American Psychiatric Association, 2013). Symptoms of delirium (e.g., sleep disturbance, apathy, agitation, emotional lability, psychosis) should also be considered in the differential diagnosis (Smith, Fuchs, Pandharipande, Barr, & Ely, 2009). Screening measures may help with diagnoses. For example, the Hospital Anxiety and Depression Scale (HADS) can be used to assess anxiety and depression in patients and caregivers of PICU patients (Samuel, Colville, Goodwin, Ryninks, & Dean, 2015). The Clinician-Administered PTSD Scale for Children and Adolescents (CAPS-CA-5) is a well-established measure of PTSD, which can be used to assess symptoms in children aged 7 and above (Pynoos et al., 2015). Tools such as the Vanderbilt Assessment for Delirium in Infants and Children can provide a structured evaluation framework for consults with concern for delirium (Gangopadhyay et al., 2017).

Suicide attempts and overdoses resulting in ICU admission require more intensive mental health evaluations, as these youth may have pre-existing psychological disorders. In the past 7 years, hospitalizations for suicidal ideation and attempts in youth has nearly doubled. About 13% of suicide attempts require admission to the ICU (Rosenberg & Mechatie, 2018). In one retrospective analysis, 8% of PICU admissions were related to poisonings, with 33% of those admissions related to suicide attempts (Even, Armsby, & Bateman, 2014). In examining the potential underlying factors for suicide attempts, clinicians should also be aware of suicide games among youth (e.g., the choking game; Andrew & Fallon, 2007), which may result from impulsivity and/or poor decision-making rather than suicidality. As opioid-related overdoses continue to rise, a significant proportion require ICU care and likely need mental health treatment post-discharge for those who survive (Kane, Colvin, Bartlett, & Hall, 2018).

The emotional health of the family should be considered in every PICU consult. Caregivers of PICU patients may experience increased rates of depression, anxiety, and PTSD compared to the general population. Nearly 84% report posttraumatic stress symptoms (PTSS) following their child's admission to the PICU, with 10.5–21% meeting criteria for PTSD (Nelson & Gold, 2012). Depression and anxiety for caregivers of children in the PICU have not been explored. However, research suggests that 4.7–36.4% of caregivers of ICU survivors experience depression and 15–24% report anxiety (van

Beusekom, Bakhshi-Raiez, de Keizer, Dongelmans, & van der Schaaf, 2016). Thus, caregivers of PICU patients may experience similar rates of depression and anxiety. Potential risk factors for caregivers include perceived severity of illness, fear of child death, length of hospitalization, child's physical appearance, and medical procedures during admission (Rees, Gledhill, Garralda, & Nadel, 2004).

Few studies have examined the emotional health of siblings of ICU patients. However, changes in parental behavior and care (e.g., switching between different caregivers, parental stress, sibling taking on parental responsibilities) may be a significant source of stress for siblings.

Additionally, siblings may experience symptoms of depression and anxiety (e.g., fear of ill sibling's safety, feelings of detachment, worry, and fear; Shudy et al., 2006). See Figure 1 for a summary of risk factors to consider when examining child and family emotional health outcomes.

Medical Basics

Critical illness in children often strikes acutely and unexpectedly. Admission criteria for the PICU generally specify life-threatening illness and/or end-organ dysfunction (Pediatrics & Medicine, 1999). Common medical conditions that result in PICU care include acute respiratory failure, injuries, sepsis, seizures, and congenital anomalies (e.g., congenital heart disease; Heron, 2017; Ibiebele, Algert, Bowen, & Roberts, 2018; Volakli et al., 2012).

Patients admitted to the PICU are often on multiple medications. Commonly used medications include opioids (e.g., fentanyl), benzodiazepines (e.g., midazolam), and dissociative agents (e.g., ketamine; Tobias, 2005). Tolerance and withdrawal can be experienced after cessation of sedation medications, especially after long-term use (Tobias, 2000). Dexmedetomidine is being used more often in pediatric sedation protocols given its safety profile and the decreased risk of delirium or withdrawal (Tobias, 2007). Recommendations for medications in a PICU setting must take into account the medical factors as well as the potential for medication interactions. For instance, even though many critically ill children may have anxiety, use of benzodiazepine or anticholinergic medications can create additional risks such as decreased respiratory drive or worsening delirium (Pandharipande et al., 2006).

Initial mortality of children admitted to a PICU remains around 10 percent and directly relates to the severity of illness (Volakli et al., 2012). Even after discharge, patients face an increased risk of mortality at 1 year (Gemke, Bonsel, & van Vught, 1995). In those who survive a critical illness, there have been concerns about neurocognitive decline and functional deficits in children after PICU admission (Bone, Feinglass, & Goodman, 2014).

Engagement

Mental health clinicians working in the PICU may want to consider how to engage the child, family, and medical team to optimize care for patients. Having a trusted medical team member introduce the clinician may help families' initial engagement in psychological services. Identifying the most stressful aspects of care with the family and offering brief interventions to start to mitigate some of this stress may help the family engage quickly.

Special considerations ought to be taken for children that have presented for care due to a non-accidental trauma (i.e., child abuse). In these cases, mental health therapists should collaborate with other team members (e.g., social workers) to work with child service agencies to prioritize child safety while developing a therapeutic relationship with the family. If no other team members can manage the child safety aspects of care, then the therapist must prioritize child safety (e.g., reporting suspected abuse, partnering with child safety agencies) while attempting to maintain a relationship with the family to support them through intensive care.

Formulation

Consistent with many arenas of pediatric psychology, consultations in the PICU frequently need to be focused and limited in scope. A thorough psychiatric assessment is often unnecessary (as emotional symptoms are typically not the reason a patient is presenting for care in the ICU) and not feasible (patients are often physically impaired; current mood is often influenced by medical condition and/or medications). Instead, focusing on the consultation question can provide the foundation for interventions during the care in the PICU. Even when a patient is being treated in the ICU following attempted harm to self or others, the primary purpose of the hospitalization is to stabilize the patient physically; thus, the clinician's role in this case may be to obtain initial information on the patient's emotional health to help determine subsequent psychiatric evaluations and placements.

As a basic process, patient care is optimized when the consulting clinician communicates directly with the medical team member who has placed the consult, gathers information from the medical record, and obtains behavioral observations and concerns from the child's nurse prior to meeting the patient and/or his or her family. With this information, the questions asked of the family can be more focused. See Table 1 for a list of possible questions to include in an initial assessment during PICU care, in addition to standard mandatory safety/abuse questions.

While in the ICU, the child remains the focus of care, even if the consult is to help a family member regulate his or her emotional reactions. If the child is substantially impaired and/or nonverbal, asking about the child's likes/dislikes and special characteristics can help engage the family. It can be helpful to learn the family's perception of how (and if) the child communicates. A clinician may also be able to help the family identify communication efforts from the child by observing child and family interactions.

Table 1 Sample questions for consultations in the pediatric intensive care unit

Question	Purpose
Children and caregivers	
What is the hardest part about the your/child's medical condition/being in the hospital?	Identify which needs to prioritize
What are you most worried about?	Identify child/family perceptions of fears that need to be addressed
Children	
Who helps you the most?	Identify existing support systems
Has there been anything good about being in the hospital?	Assess child's general perceptions/appraisals
What are you looking forward to?	Assess hope/goals
Caregivers	
Tell me about your child before this illness/injury/accident	Identify child strengths and pre-existing challenges
Have you noticed any changes in emotions or behaviors during this hospitalization?	Assess new emerging symptoms/challenges
Who supports your child? Who supports you?	Identify family support system (or lack of support)

Evidence-Based Interventions

The goal of early interventions for children in the ICU is to reduce psychological sequelae related to the illness, injury, and/or subsequent medical treatment. While some risk factors for developing persistent psychological symptoms have been identified (e.g., severity of the medical event, adverse family environment, trauma history, pre-existing anxiety, or depressive disorders; Copeland et al., 2007), only a few interventions have been developed and evaluated specifically for use in the PICU (Baker & Gledhill, 2017). See Table 2 for an overview of interventions and supporting evidence.

Table 2 Summary of interventions developed for the PICU

Intervention	Population	Method and timing	Framework	Outcomes assessed	Effectiveness
Handbook (Als, Nadel, et al., 2015)	Caregivers	Handbook given to caregiver at discharge; follow-up call 2 weeks later	Psychoeducation regarding emotional recovery, behavioral recovery, and return to normal	Caregiver anxiety, depression, and PTSS; child PTSS, emotional and behavioral difficulties, sleep	Intervention group parents reported decreased PTSS (Cohen's $d = 0.4$) and depression (Cohen's $d = 0.1$), but not anxiety; intervention group children exhibited less emotional and behavioral difficulties (Cohen's $d = 0.6$) but little differences in sleep compared to the control group
COPE intervention (Melnyk et al., 2004)	Caregivers	Audiotapes and written materials for caregiver 6–16 h after ICU admission. Booster session (audiotapes, written materials, and workbook) after transfer to the general pediatric unit. Follow-up call 2–3 days post-discharge	Educational-behavioral intervention based on self-regulation theory, control theory, and emotional contagion hypothesis	Caregiver anxiety, negative mood state, depression, stress, beliefs about and participation in the child's recovery; child adjustment (withdrawal symptoms, externalizing behaviors, negative behavioral symptoms)	COPE parents reported significantly less stress regarding their child's appearance, medical procedures, behaviors, and emotions and greater confidence in how to support child adjustment compared to the control group. Children in the intervention group experienced significantly less hyperactivity, greater adaptability, and fewer negative behavioral symptoms
Informational letter (Bouveet al., 1999)	Caregivers	Written information given to caregiver 24–48 h before the child's transfer from the PICU to the general pediatric unit	Based on the Lazarus Stress and Coping Model (i.e., sufficient preparation for changing situational factors decreases anxiety)	Caregiver anxiety	Parents who received the intervention letter reported significantly less anxiety—$F(1,47) = 18.65$, $p < 0.0005$
Follow-up clinic visit (Colville et al., 2010)	Caregivers	Appointment with PICU consultant, senior PICU nurse, and psychologist 2 months after discharge	Intended to offer families the opportunity to emotionally process their child's ICU experience	Caregiver anxiety, depression, and PTSS	Parents in the intervention group reported slightly lower (although not statistically significant) levels of anxiety, depression, and PTSS

(continued)

Table 2 (continued)

Intervention	Population	Method and timing	Framework	Outcomes assessed	Effectiveness
Follow-up clinic visit (Samuel et al., 2015)	Caregivers	Caregivers screened at discharge; those at high risk for developing psychological sequelae were invited to meet with PICU consultant, nurse, and psychologist 2 months after discharge	Opportunity to ask questions and reflect on how the admission emotionally affected caregivers	Caregiver PTSS, anxiety, and depression	No significant differences between the intervention and control groups, but small effect sizes were found for anxiety (Cohen $d = 0.21$) and depression (Cohen $d = 0.25$)

Intervention Targets

Caregiver mental health has been closely linked to child recovery (Landolt, Ystrom, Sennhauser, Gnehm, & Vollrath, 2012). Therefore, many PICU interventions are aimed at preventing and addressing parent anxiety, depression, PTSS (Als, Nadel, Cooper, Vickers, & Garralda, 2015), and negative mood state and stress (Melnyk et al., 2004). Some interventions also aim to increase caregiver knowledge of what to expect during their child's emotional and how to manage behavioral difficulties post-discharge (Als, Nadel, et al., 2015; Melnyk et al., 2004). Only a few interventions specifically target child outcomes, such as PTSS, sleep, emotional and behavioral issues, and learning difficulties (e.g., slowed information processing, problems with memory or attention; Als, Nadel, et al., 2015; Melnyk et al., 2004).

Intervention Methods and Content

PICU interventions use a variety of methods. Some interventions incorporate psychoeducation for parents about common reactions their child may experience after hospitalization and offer practical strategies for how caregivers can support the child throughout their recovery (Als, Nadel, et al., 2015; Melnyk et al., 2004). For instance, Melnyk colleagues (2004) developed a program called "Creating Opportunities for Parent Empowerment" (COPE). COPE is an educational-behavioral, three-phase intervention for children aged 2–7 years. In *phase 1* of the intervention, clinicians provide parents with audiotapes and written material regarding possible responses their child may have and how to encourage positive coping skills. In *phase 2* (after transfer to the general pediatric unit), clinicians give the child and their caregiver a workbook with activities to complete together before leaving the hospital. These activities are intended to help children express their emotions and regain a sense of control over (e.g., puppet play, reading and discussing the story of a child undergoing hospitalization). *Phase 3* involves a brief phone conversation between the clinician and caregiver a few days post-discharge, focusing on typical emotions and behaviors that the child may exhibit and how the caregiver can support positive coping. In an RCT assessing the effectiveness of the COPE intervention, parents who received the intervention, compared to those in the control group, reported significantly less stress regarding their child's appearance, medical procedures, behaviors, and emotions and expressed greater confidence in how to support their child's adjustment after discharge. COPE children, as opposed to those in the control group, experienced significantly less hyperactivity, greater adaptability, and fewer negative behavioral issues (i.e., withdrawal and externalizing behaviors) after discharge (Melnyk et al., 2004). To become trained in delivering the COPE intervention, contact intervention developers (www.cope2thrive.com).

A few interventions focused on improving caregiver mental health by facilitating communication between the family and medical team. For example, Bouve, Rozmus, and Giordano (1999) provided psychoeducation in writing and verbally to families 24 h before their child was moved from the PICU to the general pediatric unit. The letter contained information about the child's transfer, including an explanation of the decrease in intensity of care, family visitation policies, services available, and opportunities for child life and parental involvement in the recovery process. Parents who received this intervention reported significantly less anxiety about the transfer (Bouve et al., 1999).

Follow-up clinic visits have also been used to facilitate emotional processing of the ICU experience. Colville, Cream, and Kerry (2010) and Samuel and colleagues (2015) piloted interventions in which caregivers were offered an appointment with a psychologist, PICU nurse, and PICU consultant 2 months after discharge. In each of these interventions, the caregivers were encouraged to consider how they had been emotionally impacted by the hospitalization and its associated stress. Compared to those who were not offered an appointment, parents who attended the visit reported a slight (although not statistically significant) decrease in anxiety and depression (Samuel et al., 2015). Colville and colleagues (2010) also found a small decrease of PTSS in parents who participated in follow-up visits; parents who reported higher levels of stress at the time of discharge were also more likely to attend the appointment than those who had indicated lower levels of stress (Colville et al., 2010). See Table 2 and Baker and Gledhill (2017)'s systematic review for more details on potentially effective intervention components across PICU interventions (Baker & Gledhill, 2017).

Delivery and Timing of Interventions

While some interventions have been introduced during hospitalization (Bouve et al., 1999; Melnyk et al., 2004), others have been designed to take place during or shortly after discharge (Als, Nadel, et al., 2015; Colville et al., 2010; Samuel et al., 2015). Interventions designed for use in the hospital often aim to empower parents and children by providing information about changes in care (Bouve et al., 1999) and suggesting activities to help the child understand and process their hospitalization such as therapeutic medical play (Melnyk et al., 2004). Parents who experience the highest rates of stress at the time of discharge may also gain the most from the intervention, so it is an important time for the medical team to be aware of the patient and caregivers' psychological needs (Nadel, Als, & Garralda, 2015). Some interventions have been created in a format to facilitate the delivery in the home setting, such as via audiotapes and/or printed materials (Colville et al., 2010; Samuel et al., 2015). Additionally, in some circumstances, follow-up clinics can provide caregivers the opportunity to have face-to-face contact with PICU staff (Colville et al., 2010; Samuel et al., 2015).

Adaptation

Cognitive behavioral therapy (CBT) and trauma-focused cognitive behavioral therapy (TF-CBT) have a strong evidence base in treating psychological trauma reactions (Ramsdell, Smith, Hildenbrand, & Marsac, 2015). CBT focuses on changing the relationships among thoughts, emotions, and behaviors (Rothbaum, Meadows, Resick, & Foy, 2000). TF-CBT utilizes CBT strategies of psychoeducation, increasing positive coping skills, implementing exposure and cognitive restructuring, and inclusion of relapse prevention; however, it also differs from traditional CBT in that it focuses on the trauma experience and targets decreasing PTSS (Kowalik, Weller, Venter, & Drachman, 2011). While these treatments are not yet evaluated in the PICU, many of the interventions above draw from these intervention theories.

CBT and TF-CBT can be adapted for use during PICU hospitalization as well as follow-up. As noted earlier in this chapter, children and families may not be ready to engage in a full on psychological intervention during hospitalization. However, clinicians can start partnering with families to identify goal setting and to target specific challenges that families face. For example, if the child or a family member tends to catastrophize every setback, education on typical emotional reactions during intensive care as well as recognizing unhelpful thoughts may benefit the family as they move through medical care. Once a child is discharged and the child and family begins to adapt to their "new" normal, TF-CBT may help the child and family to overcome challenging emotional reactions that persist over time. In the TF-CBT trauma narrative, a child and family can each describe the parts of the ICU experience that were difficult. In turn, clinicians can facilitate reflection and integration of the experience into a coherent narrative.

In-Hospital Consultation

Before starting an evaluation, ensure that the patient and family have been informed of the rationale for the consultation. Given the nature of critical illness and injury, the patient may have limitations in communication due to mental status or medical equipment (e.g., endotracheal intubation). Therefore, clinicians may need to utilize alternative communication strategies and assistive devices in order to take a history or determine current symptoms. Thorough review of the medical chart may also yield insights about the course of illness, current medication use, and any psychiatric concerns of the primary team (DeMaso et al., 2009).

Family involvement is critical throughout the process of consultation, providing consent, determining a baseline, and providing a perspective on the course of illness. As with all consultations, logistics—where, when, and how—must be considered along with the medical specifics and consult question. Although PICUs have been moving toward more privacy, some still have an open-bay design that can complicate evaluations and family discussion.

Outpatient Consultation

Screening and Risks at the Time of Discharge

Several studies have identified risk factors for child psychological morbidity after intensive care. These include PTSS or acute stress disorder symptoms at the time of discharge, history of anxiety or depression (Stowman, 2009), younger age, higher rates of invasive procedures, feeling less in control, increased medical fears post-discharge, and type and severity of the medical event (Rennick, Johnston, Dougherty, Platt, & Ritchie, 2002). PTSS can be worsened by delusional memories from the ICU, which have been shown to manifest up to 12 months after discharge (Colville & Pierce, 2012). Children may also experience sleep disturbances during the weeks and months following a PICU admission (Als, Picouto, et al., 2015). Providers who are aware of these risk factors can incorporate screening into the discharge process and refer for follow-up services if needed.

Outpatient Treatment

Treatment post-discharge can range from brief consultation to long-term treatment. The ideal time for follow-up typically is 2 months post-discharge (Twigg, Humphris, Jones, Bramwell, & Griffiths, 2008). Focused, short-term consultations at follow-up visits may include additional screening and an opportunity to process the emotional impact of the event and provide feedback to ICU staff (Colville et al., 2010; Samuel et al., 2015). Longer-term follow-up consultations may include engaging in CBT or TF-CBT (see above) to target more persistent trauma symptoms (including PTSS, anxiety, depression; Ramsdell et al., 2015).

Case Example

Sophia was a 12-year-old female who was hospitalized in the PICU for multiple traumatic injuries following a motor vehicle collision, most notably cracked vertebrae and damage to internal organs requiring multiple surgeries. The motor vehicle crash occurred when a friend's parent was driving her with her friends to a soccer game; another car suddenly crossed center line, resulting in a head-on collision. Sophia was improperly restrained, which worsened her physical injuries.

During her PICU hospitalization, Sophia struggled with significant pain, which the medical team had difficulty controlling with medications. She was uncooperative with physical therapy and became very angry prior to each surgery. During her inpatient hospitalization in the ICU, the psychologist was consulted with a goal of increasing Sophia's cooperation with medical care. Upon completing an initial assessment, the psychologist noted that Sophia was experiencing and displaying significant anxiety. In addition, the psychologist discovered that Sophia was often at the hospital alone, due to her mother's work schedule and need to care for her siblings. The psychologist worked with Sophia on non-pharmacological pain control as well as strategies for managing her anxiety. Strategies included psychoeducation about anxiety and trauma reactions, diaphragmatic breathing, biofeedback, imagery, distraction, and modifying unhelpful thoughts. The psychologist also partnered with the medical team to create a behavioral chart to improve compliance (targeting decreased anxiety).

At discharge, the psychologist offered to help Sophia identify an outpatient therapist in her home community or to continue outpatient therapy, as she was at high risk for persistent PTSS. However, Sophia and her mother chose to terminate treatment at discharge. The psychologist provided anticipatory guidance on emotional recovery and signs and symptoms that would indicate need for additional mental health treatment.

Several months later, Sophia attended a follow-up with her back surgeon; she reported difficulties sleeping and excessive worrying. Her surgeon placed a new outpatient consult to address Sophia's newly emerged symptoms. A psychological assessment using the CAPS-CA-5 (Pynoos et al., 2015) showed elevated PTSS in each of the following domains: avoidance (of riding in the car with anyone other than her mother; of the scene of the crash), hyperarousal (difficulty settling to sleep, feelings of jumpiness), re-experiencing (intrusive thoughts about the MVC), or change in mood (increased anxiety and depressed mood).

The psychologist worked with Sophia to identify treatment goals and selected a TF-CBT approach to treatment. Sophia stated a goal of being able to tell her trauma story without distress. Over the next ten sessions (every 2 weeks per patient preference and due to long distance to travel), Sophia engaged in psychoeducation about PTSD, identified and implemented positive coping skills (diaphragmatic breathing, seeking social support), created a trauma narrative (restructuring her thoughts about the MVC), and participated in graduated exposure (viewed pictures of the accident, returned to the scene of the MVC). Sophia was able to conquer her PTSS and improve her quality of life.

Summary

Children and their families face various physical and emotional challenges following admission to the PICU, placing them at risk for trauma reactions including PTSD, anxiety, depression, and other psychological symptoms. Thus, it is important for pediatric mental health clinicians to understand their role in supporting both families and the medical team during this time. Brief screenings can help sort out psychological symptoms to inform how to best address the presenting problem/reason for the consultation. Evidence-based interventions in the PICU are in their infancy but are promising. A number of evidence-based interventions can be adapted for use in the

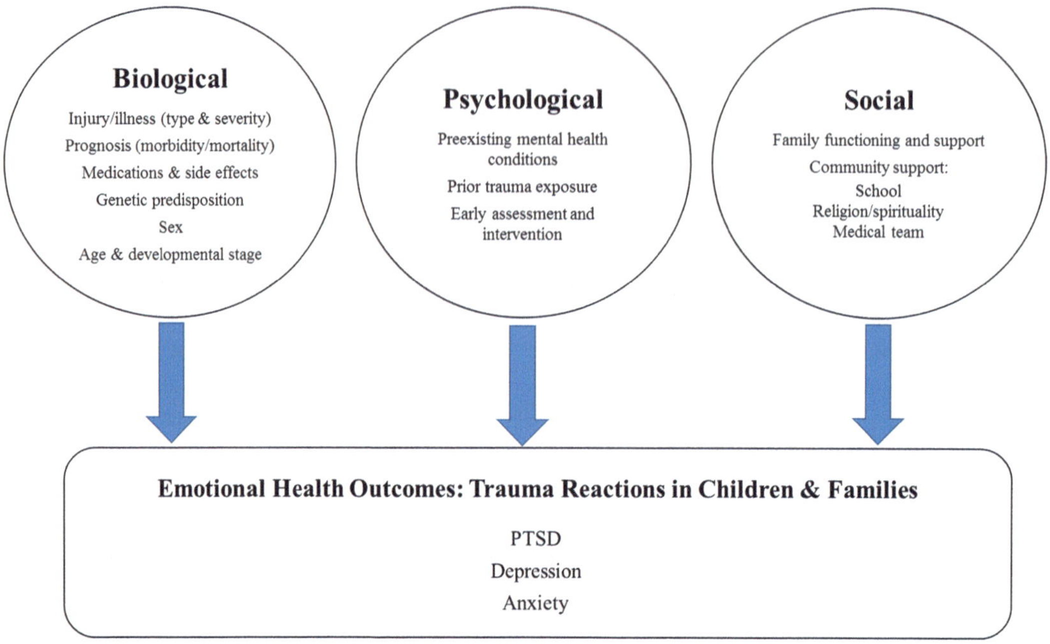

Fig. 1 Biopsychosocial theoretical framework for emotional recovery after admission to the PICU

ICU to prevent and address psychological sequelae resulting from a potentially traumatic medical event and admission to the PICU.

References

Als, L. C., Nadel, S., Cooper, M., Vickers, B., & Garralda, M. E. (2015). A supported psychoeducational intervention to improve family mental health following discharge from paediatric intensive care: Feasibility and pilot randomised controlled trial. *BMJ Open, 5*(12), e009581. https://doi.org/10.1136/bmjopen-2015-009581

Als, L. C., Picouto, M. D., Hau, S. M., Nadel, S., Cooper, M., Pierce, C. M., … Garralda, M. E. (2015). Mental and physical well-being following admission to pediatric intensive care. *Pediatric Critical Care Medicine, 16*(5), e141–e149. https://doi.org/10.1097/pcc.0000000000000424

American Academy of Pediatrics & Society of Critical Care Medicine. (1999). Guidelines for developing admission and discharge policies for the pediatric intensive care unit. *Pediatrics, 103*(4), 840–842.

American Psychiatric Association. (2013). *Diagnostic and statistical manual of mental disorders, 5th edition (DSM-5)*. Washington, DC: American Psychiatric Association.

Andrew, T. A., & Fallon, K. K. (2007). Asphyxial games in children and adolescents. *The American Journal of Forensic Medicine and Pathology, 28*(4), 303–307. https://doi.org/10.1097/PAF.0b013e318148bdb2

Baker, S. C., & Gledhill, J. A. (2017). Systematic review of interventions to reduce psychiatric morbidity in parents and children after PICU admissions. *Pediatric Critical Care Medicine, 18*(4), 343–348. https://doi.org/10.1097/pcc.0000000000001096

Bone, M. F., Feinglass, J. M., & Goodman, D. M. (2014). Risk factors for acquiring functional and cognitive disabilities during admission to a PICU. *Pediatric Critical Care Medicine, 15*(7), 640–648. https://doi.org/10.1097/pcc.0000000000000199

Bouve, L. R., Rozmus, C. L., & Giordano, P. (1999). Preparing parents for their child's transfer from the PICU to the pediatric floor. *Applied Nursing Research, 12*(3), 114–120.

Coakley, R., & Wihak, T. (2017). Evidence-based psychological interventions for the management of pediatric chronic pain: New directions in research and clinical practice. *Children, 4*(2), 9. https://doi.org/10.3390/children4020009

Colville, G., & Pierce, C. (2012). Patterns of post-traumatic stress symptoms in families after paediatric intensive care. *Intensive Care Medicine, 38*(9), 1523–1531. https://doi.org/10.1007/s00134-012-2612-2

Colville, G. A., Cream, P. R., & Kerry, S. M. (2010). Do parents benefit from the offer of a follow-up appointment after their child's admission to intensive care? An exploratory randomised controlled trial. *Intensive and Critical Care Nursing, 26*, 146–153. doi: 10.1016/j.iccn.2010.02.005

Copeland, W., Keeler, G., Angold, A., & Costello, E. (2007). Traumatic events and posttraumatic stress in childhood. *Archives of General Psychiatry, 64*(5), 577–584.

DeMaso, D. R., Martini, D. R., Cahen, L. A., Bukstein, O., Walter, H. J., Benson, S., … Medicus, J. (2009). Practice parameter for the psychiatric assessment and management of physically ill children and adolescents. *Journal of the American Academy of Child and Adolescent Psychiatry, 48*(2), 213–233. https://doi.org/10.1097/CHI.0b013e3181908bf4

Even, K., Armsby, C., & Bateman, S. (2014). Poisonings requiring admission to the pediatric intensive care unit: A 5-year review. *Clinical Toxicology, 52*(5), 519–524.

Gangopadhyay, M., Smith, H., Pao, M., Silver, G., Deepmala, D., De Souza, C., … Fuchs, C. (2017). Development of the Vanderbilt assessment for delirium in infants and children to standardize pediatric delirium assessment by psychiatrists. *Psychosomatics, 58*(4), 355–363.

Gemke, R. J., Bonsel, G. J., & van Vught, A. J. (1995). Long-term survival and state of health after paediatric intensive care. *Archives of Disease in Childhood, 73*(3), 196–201.

Heron, M. P. (2017). Deaths: Leading causes for 2015. National Vital Statistics Report, Editor.

Ibiebele, I., Algert, C. S., Bowen, J. R., & Roberts, C. L. (2018). Pediatric admissions that include intensive care: A population-based study. *BMC Health Services Research, 18*(1), 519–524.

Kane, J. M., Colvin, J. D., Bartlett, A. H., & Hall, M. (2018). Opioid-related critical care resource use in US Children's Hospitals. *Pediatrics, 141*(4), e20173335.

Kazak, A. E., Schneider, S., Didonato, S., & Pai, A. L. (2015). Family psychosocial risk screening guided by the Pediatric Psychosocial Preventative Health Model (PPPHM) using the Psychosocial Assessment Tool (PAT). *Acta Oncologica, 54*(5), 574–580. https://doi.org/10.3109/0284186X.2014.995774

Kowalik, J., Weller, J., Venter, J., & Drachman, D. (2011). Cognitive behavioral therapy for the treatment of pediatric posttraumatic stress disorder: A review and meta-analysis. *Journal of Behavior Therapy and Experimental Psychiatry, 42*(3), 405–413. https://doi.org/10.1016/j.jbtep.2011.02.002

Landolt, M. A., Ystrom, E., Sennhauser, F. H., Gnehm, H. E., & Vollrath, M. E. (2012). The mutual prospective influence of child and parental post-traumatic stress symptoms in pediatric patients. *Journal of Child Psychology and Psychiatry, 53*(7), 767–774. https://doi.org/10.1111/j.1469-7610.2011.02520.x

Lawrence, J., Yoder, K., Schadler, A., & Shenoi, A. (2018). 1285: Burnout among nurses in the pediatric intensive care unit in the United States. *Critical Care Medicine, 46*(1), 626. https://doi.org/10.1097/01.ccm.0000529288.96145.13

Marsac, M. L., Kassam-Adams, N., Hildenbrand, A. K., Nicholls, E., Winston, F. K., Leff, S. S., & Fein, J. (2016). Implementing a trauma-informed approach in pediatric health care networks. *JAMA Pediatrics, 170*(1), 70–77.

Marsac, M. L., Kindler, C., Weiss, D., & Ragsdale, L. (2018). Let's talk about it: Supporting family communication during end-of-life care of pediatric patients. *Journal of Palliative Medicine, 21*(6), 862–878. https://doi.org/10.1089/jpm.2017.0307

Melnyk, B., Alpert-Gillis, L., Feinstein, N., Crean, H., Johnson, J., Fairbanks, E., … Corbo-Richert, B. (2004). Creating opportunities for parent empowerment: Program effects on the mental health/coping outcomes of critically ill young children and their mothers. *Pediatrics, 113*(6), e597–e607.

Nadel, S., Als, L. C., & Garralda, M. E. (2015). Treatment of parental post-traumatic stress disorder after PICU admission: Who, what, where, when? *Pediatric Critical Care Medicine, 16*(9), 877–878. https://doi.org/10.1097/pcc.0000000000000502

Nelson, L. P., & Gold, J. I. (2012). Posttraumatic stress disorder in children and their parents following admission to the pediatric intensive care unit: A review. *Pediatric Critical Care Medicine, 13*(3), 338–347. https://doi.org/10.1097/PCC.0b013e3182196a8f

Pandharipande, P., Shintani, A., Peterson, J., Pun, B. T., Wilkinson, G. R., Dittus, R. S., … Ely, E. W. (2006). Lorazepam is an independent risk factor for transitioning to delirium in intensive care unit patients. *Anesthesiology, 104*(1), 21–26.

Pynoos, R., Weathers, F., Steinberg, A., Marx, B., Layne, C., Kaloupek, D., … Kriegler, J. (2015). Clinician-administered PTSD scale for DSM-5—Child/adolescent version. Scale available from the National Center for PTSD at www.ptsd.va.gov.

Ramsdell, K. D., Smith, A. J., Hildenbrand, A. K., & Marsac, M. L. (2015). Posttraumatic stress in school-age children and adolescents: Medical providers' role from diagnosis to optimal management. *Pediatric Health, Medicine and Therapeutics, 6*, 167–180. https://doi.org/10.2147/phmt.S68984

Rees, G., Gledhill, J., Garralda, M. E., & Nadel, S. (2004). Psychiatric outcome following paediatric intensive care unit (PICU) admission: A cohort study. *Intensive Care Medicine, 30*(8), 1607–1614.

Rennick, J., Johnston, C., Dougherty, G., Platt, R., & Ritchie, J. (2002). Children's psychological responses after critical illness and exposure to invasive technology. *Developmental and Behavioral Pediatrics, 23*(3), 133–144.

Rosenberg, K., & Mechatie, E. (2018). Youth hospitalizations for suicidal ideation and attempts have steadily increased. *AJN: The American Journal of Nursing, 118*(8), 64. https://doi.org/10.1097/01.naj.0000544170.38854.03

Rothbaum, B. O., Meadows, E. A., Resick, P. A., & Foy, D. W. (2000). Cognitive-behavioral therapy. In E. Foa, T. M. Keane, & M. J. Friedman (Eds.), *Effective treatments for PTSD: Practice guidelines from the international society for traumatic stress studies* (pp. 320–325). New York, NY: Guilford Press.

Samuel, V. M., Colville, G. A., Goodwin, S., Ryninks, K., & Dean, S. (2015). The value of screening parents for their risk of developing psychological symptoms after PICU: A feasibility study evaluating a pediatric intensive care follow-up clinic. *Pediatric Critical Care Medicine, 16*(9), 808–813. https://doi.org/10.1097/pcc.0000000000000488

Shenoi, A. N., Kalyanaraman, M., Pillai, A., Raghava, P. S., & Day, S. (2018). Burnout and psychological distress among pediatric critical care physicians in the United States. *Critical Care Medicine, 46*(1), 116–122. https://doi.org/10.1097/ccm.0000000000002751

Shudy, M., de Almeida, M. L., Ly, S., Landon, C., Groft, S., Jenkins, T. L., & Nicholson, C. E. (2006). Impact of pediatric critical illness and injury on families: A systematic literature review. *Pediatrics, 118*(Suppl 3), S203–S218. https://doi.org/10.1542/peds.2006-0951B

Smith, H. A. B., Fuchs, D. C., Pandharipande, P. P., Barr, F. E., & Ely, E. W. (2009). Delirium: An emerging frontier in management of critically ill children. *Critical Care Clinics, 25*(3), 593–614. https://doi.org/10.1016/j.ccc.2009.05.002

Stowman, S. A. (2009). Posttraumatic stress disorder and other consequences of a PICU admission. UNLV theses, dissertations, professional papers, and capstones, p. 88.

Tobias, J. D. (2000). Tolerance, withdrawal, and physical dependency after long-term sedation and analgesia of children in the pediatric intensive care unit. *Critical Care Medicine, 28*(6), 2122–2132.

Tobias, J. D. (2005). Sedation and analgesia in the pediatric intensive care unit. *Pediatric Annals, 34*(8), 636–645.

Tobias, J. D. (2007). Dexmedetomidine: Applications in pediatric critical care and pediatric anesthesiology. *Pediatric Critical Care Medicine, 8*(2), 115–131. https://doi.org/10.1097/01.pcc.0000257100.31779.41

Twigg, E., Humphris, G., Jones, C., Bramwell, R., & Griffiths, R. D. (2008). Use of a screening questionnaire for post-traumatic stress disorder (PTSD) on a sample of UK ICU patients. *Acta Anaesthesiologica Scandinavica, 52*(2), 202–208. https://doi.org/10.1111/j.1399-6576.2007.01531.x

van Beusekom, I., Bakhshi-Raiez, F., de Keizer, N. F., Dongelmans, D. A., & van der Schaaf, M. (2016). Reported burden on informal caregivers of ICU survivors: A literature review. *Critical Care, 20*, 16. https://doi.org/10.1186/s13054-016-1185-9

Volakli, E. A., Sdougka, M., Drossou-Agakidou, V., Emporiadou, M., Reizoglou, M., & Giala, M. (2012). Short-term and long-term mortality following pediatric intensive care. *Pediatrics International, 54*(2), 248–255. https://doi.org/10.1111/j.1442-200X.2011.03545.x

Pediatric Rehabilitation Psychology

Jacqueline N. Kaufman and Sarah Lahey

Psychological care in the rehabilitation setting is unique relative to many other healthcare settings in that it is, by design, a highly multi-specialist care environment. The rehabilitation context is one in which there are naturally occurring routine interactions between physical, occupational, and speech therapists, physicians, psychologists, nurses, and social workers, among others.

Pediatric Rehabilitation Psychology: An Evolving Subspecialty

While pediatric rehabilitation psychology is not currently a recognized subspecialty within the American Psychological Association (APA), many psychologists have chosen this as a formal area of practice, focusing on the rehabilitation needs of the full range of pediatric health conditions seen in inpatient and outpatient rehabilitation settings. For the sake of consistency, we will refer to the psychologist provider in a pediatric rehabilitation setting as a "pediatric rehabilitation psychologist," although this is often defined variably by site and provider as will be described below. While there are multiple pathways to providing pediatric rehabilitation care, there are two primary pathways followed by most rehabilitation-focused pediatric psychologists.

J. N. Kaufman (✉)
Department of Physical Medicine and Rehabilitation, University of Michigan Medical School, Ann Arbor, MI, USA
e-mail: jaqk@med.umich.edu

S. Lahey
Clinical Neuropsychologist, Brain Injury and Pediatric Programs, Brooks Rehabilitation, Jacksonville, FL, USA

Pathways for Rehabilitation Training

The first pathway, which we will refer to as the "medical pathway," is one whereby the individual is trained largely as a pediatric psychologist who treats patients with a wide range of pediatric medical conditions. During pre-doctoral internship training, the psychologist typically has one or more rotations on a rehabilitation unit as his/her first formal exposure to the setting and various types of disability. Psychologists in this track may have more foundational training in behavioral interventions including applied behavior analysis, pain management, coping strategies training, and cognitively oriented psychotherapy techniques (e.g., cognitive behavioral therapy; see Spirito et al. (2003) for a review). For providers in pediatric psychology, care is commonly organized around the target condition or classes of conditions (e.g., diabetes, cystic fibrosis, cancer, gastrointestinal conditions). In contrast,

B. D. Carter, K. A. Kullgren (eds.), *Clinical Handbook of Psychological Consultation in Pediatric Medical Settings*, Issues in Clinical Child Psychology, https://doi.org/10.1007/978-3-030-35598-2_20

pediatric rehabilitation psychology is less organized around the specific health conditions treated and more focused on a rehabilitation philosophy of multi-specialty care, facilitating patient and family adjustment to disability, and re-entry/participation in activities of daily living, regardless of the presenting condition. Pediatric rehabilitation psychologists benefit from pediatric medical/health psychology training (typically found within more structured pediatric psychology programs) with subsequent choice of internship and fellowship training that is primarily in inpatient and outpatient rehabilitation care facilities.

In the second pathway, which we will call the "neuro-focused pathway," training is largely as a pediatric neuropsychology provider, with training experience focusing on the assessment of congenital and acquired neurocognitive disorders. Providers in this track generally have more foundational training in the neuroanatomical, neurophysiological, and medical underpinnings of neuro-behavioral and neurocognitive dysfunction. This distinct path typically targets common injuries and illnesses associated with pediatric neurorehabilitation, including acquired brain injury (traumatic brain injury (TBI), anoxia, stroke) and congenital neurodevelopmental disabilities such as cerebral palsy, spina bifida, and genetic syndromes with their associated primary habilitation (helping individuals acquire new skills) needs. Unique for neuro-focused track providers in pediatric rehabilitation psychology (relative to exclusively neuropsychology-focused work) is a tendency to also have an interest in topics of disability, multi-/interdisciplinary care, and optimization of participation for patients.

Scope of Practice: Aligning with Training Expertise

Importantly, because of the unique expertise and training requirements for conducting quality psychotherapy and interventions, as well as conducting informed neuropsychological testing and interpretation, it is essential that psychologists who work in rehabilitation settings are fully cognizant of the proficiencies and training necessary to conduct the many potential elements of their work and to maintain a practice that is entirely within the parameters of their personal competencies, depending upon their training track. As such, some providers without formal neuropsychology training may limit their cognitive assessment practice primarily to screening tools rather than conducting comprehensive neuropsychological testing, and others with less intervention and behavioral therapy training may limit their intervention and psychotherapy work to a smaller subset of basic behavioral strategies rather than more complex psychotherapeutic interventions. When skill demands exceed training, consultation with psychology colleagues with appropriate specialized expertise is essential. Although habilitation is an element of care provided by pediatric rehabilitation psychologists, this chapter will focus primarily on rehabilitation and patient transition to outpatient rehabilitative care. Practice of the pediatric rehabilitation psychologist will be illustrated by first providing two cases that typify care demands for these providers and then following these cases through the different elements of consultative care in the inpatient and outpatient settings.

Case Examples

Case 1: Traumatic Brain Injury (TBI)

Ray was a 10-year-old boy who was traveling with his family after a little league game. The van carrying Ray, his father, and older sister was "T-boned" by another vehicle traveling at 45 mph. The sister, who was sitting in the front passenger seat, died immediately in the accident. Ray's father was injured with a broken femur, while Ray sustained a severe traumatic brain injury (TBI) as well as several severe orthopedic injuries. There was a prolonged extraction from the vehicle during which time the patient was largely non-responsive, though he reported hearing his father screaming for his sister. Ray and his father were transported to a local hospital where Ray was treated surgically for an intracerebral hemorrhage and depressed skull fracture. He underwent multiple surgeries for his orthopedic injuries and required a tracheostomy and ventilator support. After 5 weeks in the PICU, he was transferred to an inpatient pediatric rehabilitation unit for intensive rehabilitation care.

Case 2: Congenital Cerebral Palsy (CCP)

Zaniya was a 13-year-old girl with a diagnosis of cerebral palsy (CCP) secondary to premature triplet birth (25 weeks' gestation), a history of very low birth weight, retinopathy of prematurity, grade IV intraventricular hemorrhage, and quadriplegia requiring assistance with all areas of activities of daily living. The patient was well known to the rehabilitation unit as she had been admitted previously for multiple procedures to manage her chronic severe spasticity, and the family was generally comfortable with the hospital given her many procedures and hospitalizations. This admission was for a selective dorsal rhizotomy (SDR) to treat spasticity, and the family expressed their expectation of significant functional gains post the surgery. In contrast, the neurosurgeon felt that it had been clearly explained to the family that the patient's improvements would be relatively modest, largely limited to improving her ability to sit in her wheelchair comfortably for longer periods of time and improvement in her ability to maneuver her power chair. Due to her chronic medical issues and hospitalizations, the family had been fairly indulgent and permissive with Zaniya, contributing to her poor behavior and non-compliance with efforts to engage her in therapies. Following her SDR, steady progress in physical and occupational therapies were key to maximizing Zaniya's potential benefit from the procedure. Unfortunately, she expressed dislike for her therapists and often refused participation in therapy sessions. Further complicating treatment was the fact that the parents were reluctant to do anything that might upset Zaniya as this tended to cause them to feel guilty, with the result that they became dissatisfied with the team for "pushing" their daughter in rehabilitation.

Formulation

Over the past three decades, the biopsychosocial model has evolved as perhaps the most endorsed model for case formulation in mental health and also has been widely adopted throughout medicine, including the rehabilitation setting. In rehabilitation, it is important to consider the interacting role of biological, psychological, and social factors as they impact functional outcome and psychological adaptation (Wright, 1960). Both the World Health Organization (WHO) International Classification of Impairment, Disability, and Handicap (1980) and the WHO International Classification of Functioning, Disability and Health (ICF) (2001) correspond closely with the biopsychosocial model of rehabilitation in their focus on promoting patient functional independence and maximal participation in society, all within the context of the environment in which the individual lives. The ICF framework conceptualizes the complex interplay between health condition and environmental and personal factors that impact one's ability to participate in society. Figure 1 illustrates how this model can be employed to identify the influencing factors affecting participation for patients with conditions like TBI and CCP.

The pediatric rehabilitation psychologist is often consulted to address specific behaviors or problems occurring in the rehabilitation setting that are interfering with the individual's participation in rehabilitation therapies, nursing, and/or medical care. In Case 1—TBI, the consultation may have been for assistance in managing the patient's agitation and restlessness secondary to his specific level of recovery, i.e., Ranchos Los Amigos Coma Scale level IV (RLAS IV). These potentially self- and other injurious behaviors were negatively impacting Ray's participation in rehabilitation therapies. The inpatient neurorehabilitation setting can often provide the psychologist with ready access to resources for assessment and treatment planning. Relevant history can typi-

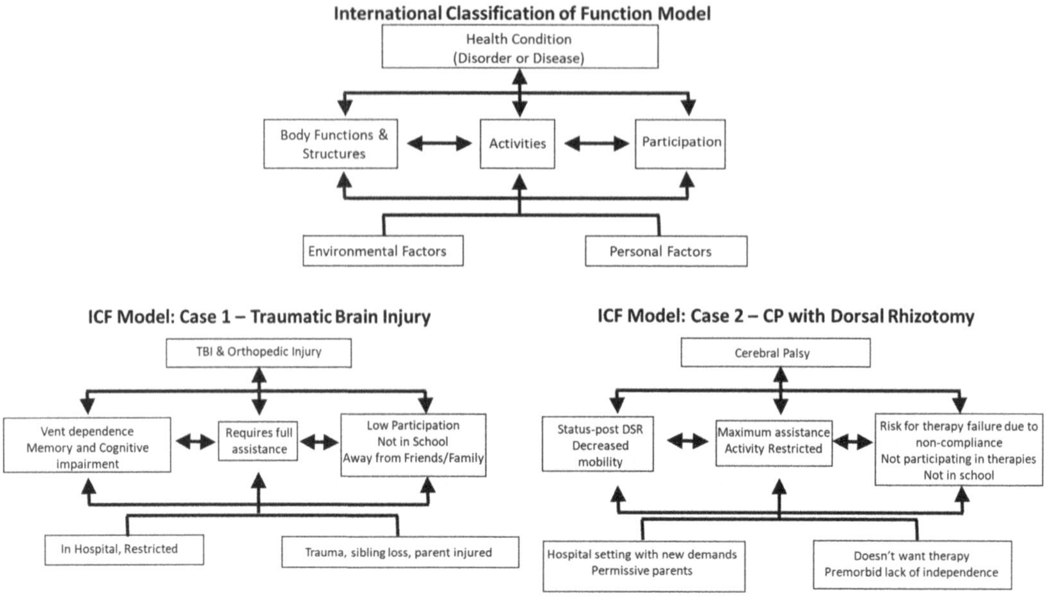

Fig. 1 International Classification of Function. Conceptualization of functioning for Case 1 and Case 2 using the International Classification of Functioning, Disability and Health

cally be found within the patient's medical records and obtained through interviews and observations with the patient and/or family over multiple brief occurrences (i.e., needn't be carefully scheduled). Collateral data can be gathered from rehabilitation staff, as well as observers of premorbid functioning such as teachers and primary care providers. The patient can be observed in a variety of settings in order to obtain a full spectrum of functioning and interaction with various environments. For instance, the level of stimulation that a patient can tolerate can be trialed across the individual and quiet setting to more challenging and complex settings (such as the therapy gym) in order to test out or practice strategies to maintain attention and focus in preparation for discharge and return to the community.

Consultation services may also be provided to assist the patient and family members' coping and adjustment to the child's injury/illness. This is particularly common for new-onset or acute medical conditions, such as a TBI or stroke. Attending to family functioning is important given the role the child's family plays in moderating the emotional and behavioral effects of the injury or illness. For instance, family dysfunction has been linked to increased child disruptive behaviors and functioning following TBI and may negatively impact behavioral and functional outcomes over time (Anderson et al., 2013; Yeates et al., 1997, 2004; Yeates, Taylor, Walz, Stancin, & Wade, 2010). Conversely, the family may serve as a resiliency support for the child, acting as a protective factor when considering long-term psychosocial outcome.

Given that many patients are in a state of recovery during the rehabilitation course, ongoing assessment and updating of the treatment plan are essential. For instance, as the child with TBI emerges from an agitated stage into a more confused (but appropriate) state, awareness of functional impairments may emerge, and with that, it increases frustration or sadness in reaction to their functional losses. Therefore, the clinician's role may require shifting from a focus primarily on behavioral management to increased focus on teaching coping skills and adjustment to injury.

Medical and Rehabilitation Basics

Rehabilitation Settings

Once the patient has been medically stabilized and/or has been transferred out of the intensive care unit, there are several different paths on which the patient can continue to recover (Fig. 2). Often the patient will receive rehabilitation therapies in the acute hospital setting, while at other times, rehabilitation services may not be initiated until the patient is transferred to a freestanding inpatient rehabilitation hospital. If the level of medical necessity does not warrant a hospital setting, the patient may transfer home and receive outpatient or home health rehabilitation therapies. Many decisions regarding the preferred setting for rehabilitation care involve a combination of medical necessity, insurance guidelines/limits, as well as some consideration of the psychosocial milieu factors.

The inpatient rehabilitation setting ideally offers a comprehensive, multidisciplinary, or interdisciplinary team approach that includes high-intensity physical, occupational, and speech and language therapies (Singh, Küçükdeveci, Grabljevec, & Gray, 2018). As needed, the patient can continue to receive medical and nursing care while participating in more rigorous therapies. The pediatric rehabilitation psychologist is actively involved in care at the patient, family, and system level in this setting.

Outpatient rehabilitation programs also provide ongoing rehabilitation interventions, generally at a lower intensity and frequency than seen in the inpatient setting. The pediatric rehabilitation psychologists often serve a vital role at this type of program in addressing the patient's transition to the home and community environment and the increased likelihood of adaptation and coping difficulties as they reintegrate into their roles within their family, peer network, school, and community.

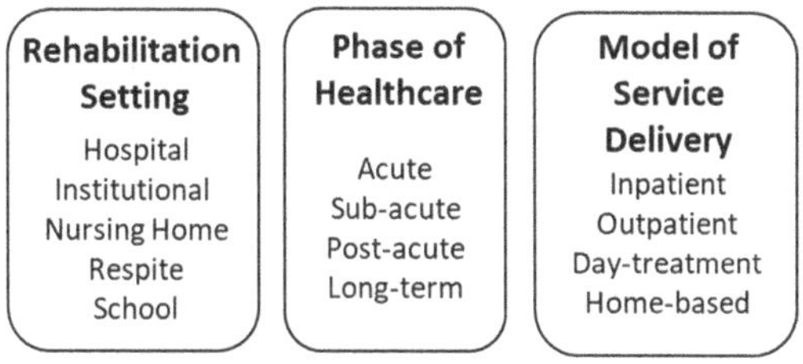

Fig. 2 Pathways of recovery. (Adapted from the World Health Organization Rehabilitation Guidelines Matrix, a matrix of rehabilitation settings, phases of healthcare, and models of service delivery)

Rehabilitation Metrics

The rehabilitation setting utilizes several scales, or metrics, in order to more easily classify and communicate an individual's level of functioning or severity of injury. For the pediatric rehabilitation psychologist, it is important to have a familiarity with these scales in order to maximize efficiency in patient care. The most common scales used in the rehabilitation setting are touched on below.

Glasgow Coma Scale

The Glasgow Coma Scale (GCS) is a neurological scale which aims to give a reliable and objective way of recording the conscious state of a person for initial as well as subsequent assessment (Teasdale & Jennett, 1974). A patient is assessed against the criteria of the scale in the domains of eye, verbal, and motor responding. The resulting points give a patient score between 3 (indicating deep unconsciousness) and 15 (fully conscious).

Rancho Los Amigos Scale/Levels of Cognitive Functioning Scale

The Rancho Los Amigos Scale (RLAS), aka the Rancho Los Amigos Levels of Cognitive Functioning Scale (LOCF) or Rancho Scale, is a medical scale used to classify individuals after a closed head injury, including traumatic brain injury, based on cognitive and behavioral presentations as they emerge from coma (Bushnik, 2000). An individual may be given a score from one to eight. A score of one represents nonresponsive cognitive functioning, whereas a score of eight represents purposeful and appropriate functioning (Fulk, 2007). The eight levels represent the typical sequential progression of recovery from TBI. However, individuals progress at different rates and may plateau at any stage of recovery. Patients are scored based on combinations of criteria in domains including responsiveness to stimuli, ability to follow commands, presence of non-purposeful behavior, and orientation, among others. The Ranchos Los Amigos Scale—Revised (RLAS-R) is an updated measure used in some facilities which employs a 10-point descriptive measurement of cognitive and behavioral functioning in individuals with brain injury, with an expansion of granularity at the upper levels of cognitive function and recovery (Lin & Wroten, 2019).

WeeFIM/FIM

The pediatric version of the Functional Independence Measure (FIM) can be administered through observation, direct interview, or both. The WeeFIM instrument consists of a minimal data set of 18 items that measure functional performance in 3 domains: self-care, mobility, and cognition. Performance of the patient on each of the items is assigned to one of seven levels of an ordinal scale that represents the range of function from complete and modified independence (levels VII and VI) without a helping person to modified and complete dependence (levels V to I) with a helping person.

Rehabilitation Team Members

The core team members that make up the rehabilitation team in the inpatient setting typically include an attending physiatrist (a physician that specializes in rehabilitation needs), a case manager, nursing staff, and the rehabilitation therapy team which includes the occupational therapist (OT), physical therapist (PT), and speech-language pathologist (SLP). The OT is responsible for helping patients regain their ability to perform daily living and work activities (e.g., grooming, dressing, bathing). The PT supports improving mobility and restoration of physical function. The SLP helps restore function for patients with problems related to cognitive, communication, or swallowing issues. Most inpatient rehabilitation settings also include a clinical neuropsychologist to assist with diagnostics, evaluation, and treatment of neurocognitive, emotional, and behavioral issues that may arise as a result of the injury or illness. Additional team members may include child life, music therapists, and a school representative or liaison.

Multidisciplinary, Interdisciplinary, and Transdisciplinary Teams

Teamwork is commonplace in many areas of psychology and perhaps even more so in rehabilitation psychology. Multidisciplinary team members learn from other fields and disciplines but remain solidly within the boundary of the identified primary field. In interdisciplinary care, there is often an overlap between disciplines and, at times, a blurring of professional boundaries (Körner, 2010). For example, a psychologist and speech pathologist may partner to assess strategies for using augmentative communication devices rather than considering cognitive and speech strategies separately. In transdisciplinary care, disciplinary boundaries are transcended, care is person centered, and cross-fertilizing occurs to maximize solutions to problems (Choi & Pak, 2007; Karol, 2014). Pediatric rehabilitation psychologists commonly adopt an interdisciplinary or transdisciplinary approach, in which practitioners transcend boundaries of specialization and integrate information, goals, and approaches across specialties with a common treatment goal. In Case 1—TBI, the physiatrist focused on evaluating current medications to determine whether the patient was overly sedated due to his/her pain medication, speech therapy focused on improving feeding so that he/she had more energy to stay alert throughout the day, and the pediatric rehabilitation psychologist, occupational therapy (OT), and physical therapy (PT) providers teamed up to provide co-therapy to reduce fatigue through behavioral activation and identify possible causes of disengagement and potential motivators for participation. The psychologist served as a communication liaison to ensure behavioral strategies were consistent across all team members. Each team member had a determined pathway to contribute and employed their expertise to work with the team in a unified way.

Engagement

The concept of the stakeholder is important in rehabilitation. It refers to the people (e.g., patients, parents, teachers, friends) and support systems (e.g., schools, employers, hospitals, insurance companies) that have an interest in the outcome of the target patient. This interest can be physical, psychological, logistical, and financial, but all stakeholders play a role in determining care pathways in rehabilitation. The role of the pediatric rehabilitation psychologist on the rehabilitation team often includes facilitating "buy-in" and commitment to integrated interventions with the goal of optimizing outcomes for the patient. In the case of our patient with TBI, the pediatric rehabilitation psychologist worked with a patient's school teacher to have homework sent to the hospital in part to help the teacher and school continue to see the patient as a child who could return to the classroom and participate again in learning after a serious injury. This served as a sign to the parents that the team had hope in the ability of the child to improve. In the case of our child with CP, the pediatric rehabilitation psychologist developed a functional tracking sheet that could capture subtle signs of improvement in engagement that could be used to support ongoing coverage for stay at the hospital under the patient's insurance. This buy-in at the school, family, and insurance level is commonplace work for the psychologist in the rehabilitation setting.

Engagement: Case 1—TBI

In the example of our patient with TBI, the parents became disengaged from therapies and stopped therapy sessions because they wanted to focus on tracheostomy tube removal and thought that this didn't appear to be a priority of the treating team. The pediatric rehabilitation psychologist was able to bring the pulmonology team, physiatrist, and physical therapist together with the family for a meeting to explain that while the patient's progress in increasing his duration of standing provided encouragement that he may begin walking, it was also increasing debilitating fatigue and interfering with his ability to maintain arousal throughout the day. By maintaining his tracheostomy and providing light ventilator support at night, the team found that Ray had better oxygenation and energy during the day to participate in therapies. By bringing members of the care team together to identify these barriers and then exploring solutions to reach a shared goal, the meeting facilitated the family's understanding that the continued tracheostomy tube and ventilation support was in fact needed because the patient was improving, and thus not a sign of a lack of progress. This team approach to family education helped maximize patient and family engagement as collaborators with mutually shared treatment goals and desired outcomes.

Engagement: Context and Intensity

Strategies for patient and family engagement tend to vary for the rehabilitation psychologist dependent on whether the child's condition is congenital or acquired, the acuity of the child's condition, and/or the phase of rehabilitation.

Context and Intensity: Case 1—TBI

The pediatric rehabilitation psychologist first engaged acutely in the ICU, while the patient was in a more tenuous medical state with frequent monitoring of the patient's arousal/awareness. While contact with the patient's family focused almost exclusively on trauma-based interventions, including coping with the uncertainty of the child's condition, cognitive-behavioral therapy was also helpful in managing stress and parental irrational beliefs (e.g., "self-care is not a priority") associated with the new caregiver role. The pediatric rehabilitation psychologist also provided psychoeducation, which included handouts and discussion of the patient's medical condition and associated sequelae. As the patient stabilized, more directed conversations were held addressing longer-term outcomes, including discussion of post-discharge services. Following transfer to the inpatient neurorehabilitation unit, caregiver education was targeted on preparation for discharge to home with decreased support from the medical treatment team. Finally, the patient's cognitive improvement allowed him to participate in more insight-oriented therapy with the rehabilitation psychologist to better address acceptance and coping with his injury. For the qualified rehabilitation psychologist, neuropsychological evaluation with liaison work between the medical providers, therapists, and schools may be the point of their engagement with the patient. In all of these instances, the rehabilitation psychologist is core to the unified messaging of the rehabilitation team and serves in the role of keeping communication across all stakeholders open and consistent.

Interventions and Adaptations to Intervention

In the inpatient setting, the most common referrals to the pediatric rehabilitation psychologist include (in accordance with competencies as noted earlier) supportive psychotherapy to assist with adjustment and coping, cognitive monitoring, participation in rehabilitation therapies, pain management, and psychoeducation regarding the injury and recovery trajectory. In the inpatient setting, there are often rapid changes in patient functional status, and, consequently, therapeutic intervention goals and strategies tend to be short term (e.g., for days rather than unchanging over the course of the full hospitalization) and are subject to frequent revision in the service of addressing recovery of function. Assessment and treatment can frequently be complicated by deficits in patient mobility, cognitive and speech impairments, medical equipment factors (e.g., ventilator support), medication effects (e.g., sedation for acute pain, agitation, and/or seizure), and challenges with sufficient arousal to participate in treatment (e.g., coma status, acutely or chronically altered cognitive functioning).

Adaptation of Interventions

When working with patients with more severe deficits, it is important to establish the child's ability to engage in basic dichotomous choice making. Even at more severe levels of impairment, strategies can be developed for assessing the quality of choice making (Van Tubbergen, Warschausky, Birnholz, & Baker, 2008), as well as methods for training in choice making (Dew, Collings, Dillon Savage, Gentle, & Dowse, 2018). Another early intervention is to modify the patient's environment to optimize orientation and participation and to minimize agitation. This may include utilization of visible references (e.g., walker blocking exit from bed as a reminder to use walker outside of bed). Orientation calendars and pictures of rehabilitation team members are commonly used, as are memory books to document daily activities, and written therapy goals and homework employed as a reference and resource throughout the day.

For children able to engage in more directed intervention for cognitive impairment, there are a number of cognitive rehabilitation strategy approaches. Early on, strategies such as errorless learning are commonly employed to facilitate higher rates of correct practice while reducing the opportunities to integrate erroneous approaches (Baddeley, 1992). In this method, expectations are made clear, and errors are anticipated, and the patient prompted to avoid them, with reinforcement specifically for successful errorless completion. Errorless learning is particularly helpful for individuals with severe TBI and/or memory impairments where there is more difficulty utilizing the feedback from errors and developing a deeper understanding of the material. Within this learning approach, the teacher works to ensure that large numbers of correct trials are achieved to facilitate proceduralization of each step. The TEACH-M method (Ehlhardt, Sohlberg, Glang, & Albin, 2005; Ehlhardt et al., 2008) integrates errorless learning with the addition of higher-order cognitive training. Another common approach to be used separately or in tandem with a cognitive approach involves the direct teaching/training of specific skills and/

or direct drilling in cognitive processes designed to advance capacity (Sohlberg, Ehlhardt, & Kennedy, 2005). Since considerable drilling and repetition are required, likely extending well past the period of acute hospitalization, this approach is best reserved for patients admitted for extended stay on the rehabilitation unit and/or where continuity of intervention can be assured with the transition to outpatient care.

Case 1: TBI

Due to the severity of his brain injury, Ray's cognitive status was too altered at the time of transfer to the rehabilitation service to participate in insight-oriented therapies. In fact, as he was transferred, his status was improving slightly (moving from Ranchos levels III to IV), resulting in *increased* agitation and confusion. Therapeutically, the primary intervention target was to reduce agitation, provide orientation cues, and initiate a team schedule to ensure the patient had optimal structure. In parallel to the patient's care, considerable work was done with the family via the provision of supportive insight-oriented therapy as well as psychoeducation to help with coping with the emergence of what appeared subjectively to be worsening symptoms (physical acting out, child behaving in ways not congruent with family values, swearing, etc.).

As the patient became increasingly stable with his transfer to rehabilitation, more practical issues of grief and bereavement over the loss of his older sister became relevant, and interventions included a focus on trauma and grief for the parent and patient, as well as other more peripheral family members. In some instances, brief cognitive assessment with accessible measures may further inform the approach for interventions.

In-Hospital Consultation

Points of Contact

For pediatric rehabilitation psychologists providing in-hospital consultation, the points of contact vary dependent upon the specific expertise of the provider and circumstances of the patient. For the neuro-focused pathway provider, the pediatric rehabilitation psychologist may make first contact in the pediatric intensive care setting for the purpose of facilitating tracking of cognitive status as a predictor of longer-term functional outcomes. Providers equipped to conduct bedside cognitive assessment may be asked to provide the primary rehabilitation team with opinions regarding behavioral and cognitive readiness for a transfer to a rehabilitation service. It is quite common for rehabilitation teams to initiate some rehabilitation services (e.g., PT, OT, SLP) with the patient while still in the PICU and prior to their formal admission to the inpatient rehabilitation service, and this would likely include the pediatric rehabilitation psychologist. However, other patients may still be under the care of medical providers (surgery, intensivists, orthopedists, etc.) in the pediatric medical hospital, with the rehabilitation team deferring involvement until the patient is transferred to the primary rehabilitation service.

Finally, some patients will be admitted for procedures that are completed acutely with a planned admission to rehabilitation, and in this scenario, the pediatric psychologist providing rehabilitation care is often among the first providers to initiate care. There are other circumstances where the point of contact may be with other care providers on the team, more than the identified patient or their family. We will use our case illustrations to describe the wide range of variability for care contact for the pediatric rehabilitation psychologist.

Points of Contact: Case 1—TBI

In the case of our 10-year-old patient with TBI, there was considerable contact prior to the formal rehabilitation service admission due to the complexity of the projected rehabilitation needs. A common rehabilitation concern for individuals with more severe TBI is related to the need for ventilation support. The pediatric rehabilitation psychologist facilitated anxiety reduction and coping with acute onset needs for ventilator support even while Ray was in the PICU. Because tracking of neurological status is essential to prognostic determination, the pediatric rehabilitation psychologist assumed the responsibility of tracking arousal and responsiveness and communicated these findings with the PICU and rehabilitation teams, as well as the family as appropriate. As noted previously, not all pediatric rehabilitation psychologists are sufficiently trained in neuropsychological and cognitive assessment, and care must be taken to ensure that boundaries of competency are not violated when determining duty allocation. Because regular assessment of coping and adjustment are often addressed by a PICU psychologist and/or PICU social worker, the pediatric rehabilitation psychologist may have a very restricted role in this instance limited to tracking and monitoring, and to some degree psychoeducation, of TBI if appropriate. For instances where the PICU does not have a pediatric psychologist or where social work does not provide this support, the pediatric rehabilitation psychologist may provide some or all of those services, and this can vary widely by the staffing structure of the hospital/service.

Once transferred to the rehabilitation floor, points of contact are frequent and differ from the more consultative and monitoring role on the PICU service. The role often shifts to facilitating patient and family adjustment and coping with the circumstances of the accident, mourning the loss of loved ones, participation in rehabilitation, facilitation of productive rehabilitation team dynamics, psychoeducation, cognitive testing, and cognitive rehabilitation. Contacts may be limited to one-on-one interactions, though often contacts expand out to include co-treatments with other clinicians, as well as family-system-based contacts or outreach to post-discharge care partners (e.g., outpatient therapists, schools, additional caregivers).

Points of Contact: Case 2—CCP

In the case of our patient with CCP, Zaniya's presentation to the rehabilitation service came immediately after a very short postoperative stay on the surgical unit following her surgery to reduce spasticity. In this instance, the pediatric rehabilitation psychologist does not necessarily initiate contact after admission to the rehabilitation service as the physical and occupational therapy team have a standing protocol for post-selective dorsal rhizotomy care that has consistently worked well. Here, the first point of contact was in the context of team rounds when the physical therapist raised concerns about difficulty with the patient's non-compliance in the therapy setting. The physical therapists expressed frustration over the parents and their role in the non-compliance, and the pediatric rehabilitation psychologist served as a provider of psychoeducation for the rehabilitation team, explaining common family system dynamics that can contribute to and reinforce the problem. The first point of contact with the patient came after the rehabilitation team was unable to engage the child in necessary therapies to continue justifying the inpatient stay with her insurance providers. This contact was a co-treat therapy session with physical therapy to observe the patient behavior in vivo, as well as the parent response to the therapy session. Care was brief and focused on patient engagement and parent education about optimal supportive parenting strategies to facilitate patient engagement and participation, such as positive reinforcement for preferred behaviors and planned ignoring for non-preferred or disruptive behaviors. Contacts were frequent and included co-treat contacts initially and rapidly faded after engagement was established.

Points of Contact: Discharge to Outpatient Care and Home

Discharge from the inpatient rehabilitation setting occurs when several criteria have been met. Generally, the patient must no longer require around-the-clock medical care, and the next level of care, whether home with family or another healthcare setting, is equipped to safely manage the needs of the patient. Often, the patient will continue to receive outpatient therapies in the community. Outpatient rehabilitation services mirror those in the inpatient setting regarding the key therapy team members, though unlike the interdisciplinary inpatient environment, not all therapies may be included. The most prominent role of the pediatric rehabilitation psychologist in this setting is to identify and ameliorate barriers to participation in therapies and to support ongoing adaptation to injury/illness and integration into the community. Common barriers include pain symptoms, mood difficulties impacting motivation or adjustment, or the direct sequelae of the injury including behavioral dysregulation or cognitive deficits and their effect on daily functioning and social relationships.

For acquired conditions, medical acuity has typically decreased prior to the transition to the lower level of care or home setting. The focus shifts to adaptation to the injury as the child navigates this new context of home and community. As the patient's awareness of their deficits increases, it is crucial to monitor for new mood symptoms and intervene accordingly. Indeed, the rates of new-onset psychiatric conditions following impairment associated with pediatric TBI and other conditions requiring outpatient rehabilitation services are significantly higher than those found in the general population (Laliberte Durish, Pereverseff, & Yeates, 2018). Modifications to psychotherapeutic interventions are often needed due to cognitive, emotional, and interpersonal changes following injury (Gallagher, McLeod, & McMillan, 2016). For instance, the clinician may need to incorporate memory aids into the consultation in order to support carryover and increase the likelihood of generalization to other areas (i.e., home, school).

The transition home for pediatric patients with a congenital condition will often look different than that for an acute injury or acquired injury. The patient and family typically have an already established team of healthcare professionals with whom they will resume services. The child with a congenital condition will likely have established specialized educational services (typically in the form of an Individualized Education Program (IEP)) or accommodations to support physical, cognitive, developmental learning differences in the academic setting. Any new recommendations for academic instruction that have arisen from changes in functioning can be incorporated into their existing plan accordingly.

Pediatric Rehabilitation: A Multifaceted Care Setting

The field of pediatric rehabilitation psychology is unique and complex due to the wide range of conditions treated as well as the often large number of healthcare and community specialists that are part of the treatment team and community reintegration process. For the pediatric psychologist providing consultation in a rehabilitation facility, the path to providing care is often multifaceted, and thus the scope of practice consequently may vary considerably across providers, ranging from the fast-paced and heavily interdisciplinary or transdisciplinary practice exemplified by inpatient acute care settings to outpatient care settings characterized by longer-term interactions and care provision. The unifying factor in the provision of rehabilitation services to children and their families is the organization of care designed to optimize recovery of function and a return of the child (and their family) to maximal participation in the activities of daily living. Going forward, there is an ongoing need to better delineate the competency areas for those specializing in pediatric rehabilitation psychology in the neurorehabilitation setting and understanding that the pediatric realm is unique and distinct from the adult care setting, and partnerships with the full range of pediatric psychology specialists offer many opportunities for collaboration.

References

Anderson, V., Beauchamp, M. H., Crossley, L., Hearps, S. J. C., Catroppa, C., & Yeates, K. O. (2013). Social competence at 6 months following childhood traumatic brain injury. *Journal of the International Neuropsychological Society, 19*(5), 539–550.

Baddeley, A. D. (1992). Implicit memory and errorless learning: A link between cognitive theory and neuropsychological rehabilitation? In L. R. Squire & N. Butters (Eds.), *Neuropsychology of memory* (2nd ed., pp. 309–314). New York, NY: Guilford Press.

Bushnik, T. (2000). The level of cognitive functioning scale. *The Center for Outcome Measurement in Brain Injury*. Retrieved from http://www.tbims.org/combi/lcfs

Choi, B. C., & Pak, A. W. (2007). Multidisciplinarity, interdisciplinarity and transdisciplinarity in health research, services, education and policy: 1. Definitions, objectives, and evidence of effectiveness. *Clinical and Investigative Medicine, 29*, 351–364.

Dew, A., Collings, S., Dillon Savage, I., Gentle, E., & Dowse, L. (2018). "Living the life I want": A framework for planning engagement with people with intellectual disability and complex support needs. *Journal of Applied Research of Intellectual Disabilities, 32*(2), 401–412.

Ehlhardt, L. A., Sohlberg, M. M., Glang, A., & Albin, R. (2005). TEACH-M: A pilot study evaluating an instructional sequence for persons with impaired memory and executive functions. *Brain Injury, 19*(8), 569–583. https://doi.org/10.1080/00269905040001 3550

Ehlhardt, L. A., Sohlberg, M. M., Kennedy, M., Coelho, C., Ylvisaker, M., Turkstra, L., & Yorkston, K. (2008). Evidence-based practice guidelines for instructing individuals with neurogenic memory impairments: What have we learned in the past 20 years? *Neuropsychological Rehabilitation, 18*(3), 300–342. https://doi.org/10.1080/09602010701733190

Fulk, G. D. (2007). Traumatic brain injury. In S. B. O'Sullivan & T. J. Schmitz (Eds.), *Physical rehabilitation* (5th ed., pp. 895–935). Philadelphia, PA: F. A. Davis Company.

Gallagher, M., McLeod, H. J., & McMillan, T. M. (2016). A systematic review of recommended modifications of CBT for people with cognitive impairments following brain injury. *Neuropsychological Rehabilitation, 29*(1), 1–21. https://doi.org/10.1080/09602011.2016.1258367

Karol, R. L. (2014). Team models in neurorehabilitation: structure, function, and culture change. *NeuroRehabilitation, 34*(4), 655–69. https://doi.org/10.3233/NRE-141080

Körner, M. (2010). Interprofessional teamwork in medical rehabilitation: A comparison of multidisciplinary and interdisciplinary team approach. *Clinical Rehabilitation, 24*(8), 745–755. https://doi.org/10.1177/0269215510367538

Laliberte Durish, C., Pereverseff, R., & Yeates, K. (2018). Depression and depressive symptoms in pediatric traumatic brain injury: A scoping review. *Journal of Head Trauma Rehabilitation, 33*(3), 18–30. https://doi.org/10.1097/HTR.0000000000000343

Lin, K., & Wroten, M. (2019). Ranchos Los Amigos. [Updated January 19, 2019]. In StatPearls [Internet]. Treasure Island, FL: StatPearls Publishing. Retrieved from https://www.ncbi.nlm.nih.gov/books/NBK448151/

Singh, R., Küçükdeveci, A. A., Grabljevec, K., & Gray, A. (2018). The role of interdisciplinary teams in physical and rehabilitation medicine. *Journal of Rehabilitation Medicine, 50*(8), 673–678. https://doi.org/10.2340/16501977-2364

Spirito, A., Brown, R.T., D'Angelo, E., Delamater, A., Rodrigue, J., & Siegel, L. (2003). Society of pediatric psychology task force report: Recommendations for the training of pediatric psychologists. *Journal of Pediatric Psychology, 28*(2), 85–98.

Sohlberg, M. M., Ehlhardt, L., & Kennedy, M. (2005). Instructional techniques in cognitive rehabilitation: A preliminary report. *Seminars in Speech and Language, 26*(4), 268–279. https://doi.org/10.1055/s-2005-922105

Teasdale, G., & Jennett, B. (1974). Assessment of coma and impaired consciousness: A practical scale. *Lancet, 2*, 81–84.

Van Tubbergen, M., Warschausky, S., Birnholz, J., & Baker, S. (2008). Choice beyond preference: Conceptualization and assessment of choice-making skills in children with significant impairments. *Rehabilitation Psychology, 53*(1), 93–100.

World Health Organization. (1980). *International classification of impairments, disabilities, and handicaps: A manual of classification relating to the consequences of disease, published in accordance with resolution WHA29.35 of the twenty-ninth World Health Assembly, May 1976*. Geneva, Switzerland: World Health Organization. Retrieved from http://www.who.int/iris/handle/10665/41003

World Health Organization. (2001). *International classification of functioning, disability and health: ICF*. Geneva, Switzerland: World Health Organization. http://www.who.int/iris/handle/10665/42407

Wright, B. A. (1960). *Physical disability: A psychological approach*. New York, NY: Harper & Row.

Yeates, K., Taylor, H., Drotar, D., Wade, S., Klein, S., Stancin, T., & Schatschneider, C. (1997). Preinjury family environment as a determinant of recovery from traumatic brain injuries in school-age children. *Journal of the International Neuropsychological Society, 3*(6), 617–630.

Yeates, K., Taylor, H., Walz, N., Stancin, T., & Wade, S. (2010). The family environment as a moderator of psychosocial outcomes following traumatic brain injury in young children. *Neuropsychology, 24*(3), 345–356.

Yeates, K. O., Swift, E., Taylor, H. G., Wade, S. L., Drotar, D., Stancin, T., & Minich, N. (2004). Short- and long-term social outcomes following pediatric traumatic brain injury. *Journal of the International Neuropsychological Society, 10*(3), 412–426.

Burn Injuries

Janelle M. Mentrikoski, Carisa Parrish,
Ariel M. Aballay, and Christina L. Duncan

Diagnosis and Medical Basics

Burns are one of the most traumatic and painful injuries that children experience. There are a variety of causes (e.g., hot surfaces, friction, chemicals, cold surfaces/frostbite, electricity), though scalds are the most common (e.g., D'Souza, Nelson, & McKenzie, 2009). Sociodemographic factors, such as age, gender, socioeconomic status, and ethnicity, have been associated with risk for burn injury. Indeed, the majority of pediatric burn injuries occur in children below the age of 5 years (Sheridan, 2018). Relatedly, the cause of burn injury varies as a function of age (Krishnamoorthy, Ramaiah, & Bhananker, 2012), with scalds occurring most often in younger children, while thermal injuries are most prevalent in older children (Sheridan, 2018). Boys generally have higher rates of burn injuries than girls (D'Souza et al., 2009). In addition, lower family income, living in deprived neighborhoods, having young or single parents, being part of a larger family, and having lower education in parents have all been linked to increased incidence of pediatric burn injuries (Alnababtah, Khan, & Ashford, 2016). In some cases, child abuse and neglect need to be considered as a possible causative factor (Krishnamoorthy et al., 2012; Latenser & Kowal-Vern, 2002).

Burns are classified by depth of injury and by total body surface area (TBSA) or percentage of the patient's body that is impacted by the burn. Systemic effects of burn injuries are minimal when TBSA is less than about 10%, while large or extensive burns can result in multi-organ dysfunction or failure (Sheridan, 2018). The depth of the burn or layers of skin and tissue affected, in particular, defines wound management approach. Depth classifications, in order of increasing depth, are superficial (first degree), superficial

J. M. Mentrikoski (✉)
Children's Mercy Kansas City, Kansas City, MO, USA

Department of Pediatrics, University of Missouri-Kansas City, Kansas City, MO, USA
e-mail: jmmentrikoski@cmh.edu

C. Parrish
Johns Hopkins Medicine, Baltimore, MD, USA

Department of Psychiatry and Behavioral Sciences, Johns Hopkins School of Medicine, Baltimore, MD, USA

A. M. Aballay
Department of Surgery, West Penn Hospital Burn Center, Allegheny Health Network, Pittsburgh, PA, USA

Temple University, Philadelphia, PA, USA

C. L. Duncan
Department of Psychology, West Virginia University, Morgantown, WV, USA

Department of Pediatrics, West Virginia University School of Medicine, Morgantown, WV, USA

B. D. Carter, K. A. Kullgren (eds.), *Clinical Handbook of Psychological Consultation in Pediatric Medical Settings*, Issues in Clinical Child Psychology, https://doi.org/10.1007/978-3-030-35598-2_21

partial-thickness (second degree), deep partial-thickness (second degree), full-thickness (third degree), and fourth degree (involving muscles and bones) (Yin, 2017). Superficial and superficial partial-thickness burns typically are treated fully on an outpatient basis when they involve small TBSA; otherwise, this depth of a burn can require hospitalization when it covers a large TBSA (e.g., sunburns or burns from tanning beds). Burn wound management for superficial partial-thickness burns involves cleansing, debriding [i.e., removal of devitalized and necrotic tissue with scalpel or blunt (i.e., scrub brush) instrument], and applying topical antimicrobial agents. Regular dressing changes are required, with frequency (e.g., daily, weekly) varying by type of dressing used (e.g., standard mesh gauze, silver-containing dressings, biologic dressings) (Krishnamoorthy et al., 2012). Selection of dressing depends on several injury and wound factors (Rowan et al., 2015); however, when feasible, dressings that require fewer dressing changes are preferred to reduce painful impact of this routine care on children (Krishnamoorthy et al., 2012). For burns that are deep partial-thickness or deeper, inpatient hospital stays are usually required, along with surgical excision (removal of devitalized or necrotic tissue) and, in some cases, full- or split-thickness skin grafting surgery or use of engineered skin tissue to promote effective healing (Krishnamoorthy et al., 2012). Split-thickness skin grafting involves transferring portions of healthy skin (donor site) to cover the debrided wound. This surgery is intended to restore physical function and improve future scar appearance (Rowan et al., 2015). Depending upon the size of the injury (i.e., TBSA) and the availability of healthy skin tissue for grafting (Krishnamoorthy et al., 2012), surgeries may be staged across time.

Beyond covering the wound, pediatric burn care involves fluid resuscitation, nutrition support (due to increased caloric demands from hypermetabolic state), burn-specific physical (PT) and occupational therapy (OT), respiratory management (if inhalation injury occurs), and pain management (Rowan et al., 2015). Pain management is a key component of burn care. Patients often experience procedure-related acute pain, which can be excruciating and typically is more severe than the background, chronic pain they may have (Krishnamoorthy et al., 2012). As a result, anticipatory anxiety with painful medical procedures is common and can exacerbate the pain experience. Pharmacological agents (e.g., opioids, adjunct anxiolytics) are a standard part of pediatric burn care, though tolerance and withdrawal are key concerns to consider when devising a pain medication plan (Krishnamoorthy et al., 2012). As a result, dressing changes under anesthesia are becoming more commonplace in the treatment of children with burns.

Once the wound is closed, the patient's care shifts to the rehabilitation phase. Depending upon the depth of the wound, children may be prescribed compression garments to prevent hypertrophic scarring, thereby enhancing scar appearance (Latenser & Kowal-Vern, 2002). Hypertrophic scars arise from a protracted healing process and appear thicker, redder, and firmer in appearance when compared to normal scars. Compression garments are fitted carefully to the patient, are worn at all hours except during bathing, and are typically prescribed for at least a year (Rowley-Conwy, 2014). In addition, when a burn injury crosses a joint, PT and OT exercises may be required to optimize range of movement and function (Sheridan, 2018). Reconstructive surgery and staged surgical revisions, especially in growing children, may be required (Sheridan, 2018), and thus patients can be followed long term for their burn care.

Engagement

Not surprisingly, childhood burn injuries and their care are stressful to children and their families, as well as to healthcare providers in burn care. Consequently, pediatric psychologists are valued colleagues in the multidisciplinary team for inpatient and outpatient burn care. Generally speaking, families understand the need for and readily engage in biopsychosocial interventions, recognizing that the child's and family's short- and long-term emotional well-being will be optimized by care that extends beyond medicine. If possible, it is often a good idea to introduce the role of psychologists during the inpatient hospitalization or at the initial outpatient appointment, regardless of psychosocial needs. This approach facilitates psychologists being viewed as part of routine burn care, and as such, psychologists can provide support and therapy when needed throughout the child's burn care, rather than providing therapy only when there are significant concerns.

Formulation

Not only do patients and their families have to cope with the traumatic nature of their burn injuries (i.e., the circumstances surrounding its cause); they may be faced with medical traumatic stress related to the care of these injuries. Therefore, when completing consultations for children with burn injuries, it may be beneficial for pediatric psychologists to utilize a conceptual framework, which takes into consideration medical traumatic stress, to guide their psychological assessment, case formulation, and treatment. Medical traumatic stress is defined in the pediatric literature as "a set of psychological and physiological responses of children and their families to pain, injury, serious illness, medical procedures, and invasive or frightening treatment experiences" (Kazak et al., 2006; National Child Traumatic Stress Network, 2003; Price, Kassam-Adams, Alderfer, Christofferson, & Kazak, 2015). A conceptual framework that takes into consideration medical traumatic stress is the Integrative Model of Pediatric Medical Traumatic Stress (Kazak et al., 2006; Price et al., 2015). In this model, stress responses are not presumed to comprise a diagnosis of formal stress psychiatric disorders, such as acute stress disorder or posttraumatic stress disorder. Although these disorders and others (e.g., anxiety, depression) may evolve in pediatric burn survivors over time, the pediatric medical stress model provides a few points that are relevant for conceptualizing emotional impact of burn injuries in children and their parents (Kazak et al., 2006; Price et al., 2015). First, a range of normative emotional and behavioral reactions to medical events is expected. Such stress reactions do not necessarily imply presence of a pathological response. Second, a social contextual approach is ideal for intervention. Children are not only individuals; rather, they exist within multiple social contexts (e.g., family, dyadic relationship, community). Thus, optimal interventions are likely to take parental and familial relationships and reactions into account. Finally, the medical stress model describes child and parent responses across time, in light of premorbid functioning and the child's developmental status. The varying needs of children and their parents across time can be used to guide and tailor supportive and preventive interventions, including the goals to change the potentially stressful experience, prevent posttraumatic stress symptoms and/or other adjustment difficulties, and reduce psychological distress when present (Price et al., 2015). Indeed, effective problem-focused interventions should be tailored to the needs of the individual patient and their families and will need to consider the family unit as a whole to be fully effective. Using the medical stress model as a guiding framework, the next section reviews appropriate assessment and treatment approaches for consulting pediatric psychologists.

Interventions in the Inpatient Setting/In-Hospital Consultation

Pediatric psychologists may be called to consult on patients when they are initially admitted to the hospital for their burn injuries. Psychological services (e.g., supportive, direct intervention) will vary across the inpatient setting as a function of the patient's medical status (e.g., severity of the burn injuries) and resulting care. Pediatric psychologists consulting during inpatient hospitalizations are likely working alongside the medical team (e.g., nurses, surgeons) as well as other psychosocial team members (e.g., child life specialists, social workers). As in other pediatric consultation-liaison (CL) roles, it is helpful to clarify the role of all team members. Pediatric psychologists meet with the pediatric patient, parents, and other family members to evaluate how the child and family interpret the child's injuries and treatments, including wound debridement and dressing changes. Normalization of emotional responses begins during this initial phase to reassure parents and patients that stress is common and tends to be time-limited. This emotional validation strategy is employed to decrease parent and child anxiety and build optimism for the resilience of the child and family.

Please see Table 1 for a summary of parent and child interventions in inpatient and outpatient burn settings. The role of the psychologist at this initial stage begins with a targeted assessment of the child's developmental level, pre-existing psychological symptoms/disorders (e.g., anxiety, disruptive behavior), child's initial coping

Table 1 Summary of parent and child interventions in the inpatient and outpatient burn settings

Parent	Child
Inpatient	*Inpatient*
• Evaluate coping/understanding of medical care	• Evaluate coping/understanding of medical care
• Targeted assessment of relevant background information (e.g., pre-existing psychological symptoms)	• Targeted assessment of relevant background information (e.g., pre-existing psychological symptoms)
• Normalization of emotional reactions and supportive counseling	• Normalization of emotional reactions and supportive counseling
• Coaching of appropriate emotional/behavioral management strategies during child's dressing changes (e.g., modeling positive coping, praising brave behavior during dressing change)	• Create routine/structure for hospitalization to facilitate adjustment
• Prepare for transition home (e.g., problem-solve how to effectively complete dressing changes, establishing behavioral plans)	• Teach/practice active coping strategies (e.g., relaxation, distraction, virtual reality)
• Referrals for outpatient services as needed (e.g., family therapy)	• Brief interventions (e.g., behavioral plans)
	• Assist staff with providing appropriate control/choices to children
	• Prepare for transition home (e.g., sleep hygiene)
	• Referrals for outpatient services as needed (e.g., individual therapy)
Outpatient	*Outpatient*
• Evaluate coping/understanding of medical care	• Evaluate coping/understanding of medical care
• Targeted assessment of relevant background information (e.g., pre-existing psychological symptoms)	• Targeted assessment of relevant background information (e.g., pre-existing psychological symptoms)
• Normalization of emotional reactions and supportive counseling	• Normalization of emotional reactions and supportive counseling
• Coaching of appropriate emotional/behavioral management strategies during child's dressing changes (e.g., modeling positive coping, praising brave behavior during dressing change)	• Teach/practice active coping strategies (e.g., relaxation, distraction, virtual reality)
• Brief interventions (e.g., graduated exposure tasks, sleep hygiene, behavioral plans) for common adjustment difficulties (e.g., bathing or sleep difficulties, general behavioral concerns)	• Brief interventions (e.g., developing coping menus, response prevention) for common adjustment difficulties (e.g., itching)
• Assist with contacting child's teachers and school to prepare for school reintegration	• Assist with school/social reintegration (e.g., rehearse appropriate responses to questions)
• Referrals for outpatient services as needed (e.g., family therapy)	• Address concerns with teasing/bullying
	• Referrals for outpatient services as needed (e.g., individual therapy)

responses to the injury and subsequent pain, and parental responses. Given the nature of the hospital stay, child-focused interventions tend to focus on promoting effective coping with medical procedures and therapies and ultimately preparing children and parents for the transition home. Evidence-based strategies include relaxation, distraction during medical procedures, and establishing age-appropriate routines for sleep. Research also supports the use of virtual reality as a way for children to reduce pain associated with burn dressing changes and associated procedures (Malloy & Milling, 2010). Additionally, psychologists may help with devising behavioral plans to improve adherence to burn care, such as increasing nutritional intake or cooperation with PT or OT. Psychologists may also assist with creating a normal routine/schedule for patients with longer hospitalizations, including scheduled time for completing school work and time for recreational activities as appropriate. Furthermore, psychologists can guide hospital staff in giving children appropriate choices during their hospital stay when feasible (e.g., completing vitals before or after breakfast) or providing children with age-appropriate control (e.g., having children participate in dressing changes by removing outer dressings).

For parents displaying anxiety or avoidance related to their child's burn injury or its care, cognitive-behavioral and acceptance-based modes of emotional validation and normalization may assist them in engaging appropriately in their child's treatment. Depending on the hospital's procedures, some parents may be asked to actively participate in their child's dressing changes during a hospitalization. Other hospitals may not involve parents in dressing changes until just prior to the child's discharge. Regardless of the timing of their involvement during dressing changes, parents may benefit from coaching to ensure effective management of understandable discomfort related to their child's injury and associated pain and distress behaviors. Indeed, research indicates that parental attention to child distress during painful medical procedures reduces adaptive coping in children, whereas differential attention to children's positive behaviors (e.g., cooperation with the procedure) is associated with improved child coping (Blount, Devine, Cheng, Simons, & Hayutin, 2008). Consequently, parent coaching should include directing parents' attention toward the child's positive coping, modeling labeled praise for adaptive child and parent behavior, and suggesting what aspects of their child's distress to ignore during the dressing change (Blount et al., 2008). In particular, parents are instead encouraged to provide verbal prompts and positive attention for the child's positive coping (e.g., engaging in distraction or deep breathing) and cooperative behavior. Parents can be further guided to attend to other positive behaviors (e.g., sharing thoughts and feelings calmly) once the dressing change has ended to promote the child's emotion regulation. Like in vivo coaching models of behavioral parent training (e.g., Parent-Child Interaction Therapy; Bagner, Fernandez, & Eyberg, 2004), some parents may find it useful to have the psychologist modeling and providing directive feedback, including praise, differential attention, and emotional support during initial parent-led dressing changes (Blount et al., 2008). This level of emotional and cognitive support may serve to facilitate exposure sessions to alleviate parental anxiety that could otherwise hamper optimal adherence to the medical care of their child's burn injury. In addition, pediatric psychologists can prompt parents to problem-solve how to effectively complete dressing changes at home, if medically indicated. For example, one parent/caregiver can focus on the dressing change, while the other parent/caregiver assists with distraction and praises the child's cooperative and brave behavior. Moreover, special rewarding activities (e.g., access to a particular television program) can be saved to use only during dressing changes.

Besides providing guidance and support during dressing changes, psychologists may be called upon to support parents/caregivers and extended family members during the inpatient hospitalization due to the circumstances of the burn injury. While relatively understudied, burn injuries may cause significant disruptions in family relationships (e.g., Bakker, Maertens, Van Son, & Van Loey, 2013). For example, a child may have sustained the injury while under the care of a family member or older sibling, which may result in significant parent/caregiver self-blame and guilt. In addition, parents or caregivers may have witnessed the burn injury and subsequently may experience their own trauma reactions. Fortunately, parent distress tends to decrease with time (Bakker, Van Loey, Van Son, & Van der Heijden, 2010; Parrish et al., 2019), as the child's health improves. Nonetheless, parental trauma, guilt, and self-blame should be assessed, as these negative emotions have been shown to interact with burn severity to increase maternal risk for posttraumatic stress symptoms (Bakker et al., 2010) and may represent malleable factors to reduce psychological risk in caregivers. There may be other factors that contribute to parent distress following a child's burn injury, and pediatric psychologists are encouraged to cast a wide net to ensure best supports to parents. For instance, some parents express concern about changes in skin tone and pigmentation, and this concern can be particularly relevant to parents of ethnic minority youth (Parrish et al., 2019). In conjunction with the medical team, pediatric psychologists can foster parental understanding of accurate medical information to appropriately calibrate their expectations. Parents may further benefit from support in identifying their reactions as normative and use cognitive and mindfulness strategies to reduce maladaptive rumination; however, no research has examined the benefits of these interventions for parents of children with burn injuries. Overall, providing appropriate supports to parents is crucial, as studies highlight the importance of parent adjustment in predicting children's emotional adjustment to burn injuries (De Young, Hendrikz, Kenardy, Cobham, & Kimble, 2014).

Unfortunately, there are instances of abuse and non-accidental burn injuries that result in involvement from child protective services (CPS) and/or the local police. Ongoing CPS and police investigations, and supervised visitation and/or possible removal of children from a family's home, can be very stressful and difficult for families and will likely require some sort of psychological support during the pediatric hospitalization. If necessary, families may require appropriate referrals for family therapy or adult outpatient providers upon discharge.

Challenges in Inpatient Consultation Psychologists may face a number of challenges when completing in-hospital consultations for children with burn injuries. Some common challenges include completing consultations within the confines of the patient's medical treatments in the acute setting, adjusting psychosocial care to shorter lengths of inpatient stays, defining or re-defining the referral question(s), and having availability of psychologists during medical procedures (Yu, Wier, & Elixhauser, 2011). In particular, one of the more common challenges is implementing treatment recommendations in an acute setting, especially for children with extended hospital stays due to more severe burn injuries or children with pre-existing/acute behavioral concerns (e.g., defiance, tantrums) that impact completion of medical tasks. For some staff and families, ignoring tantrums and child distress is counterintuitive to compassionate care that they believe should be provided in a hospital setting. For instance, maintaining consistency in routines and responses to misbehaviors (e.g., selective attention) on the inpatient unit is often beneficial for the child because it provides a sense of structure and predictability, thereby facilitating adjustment; however, medical teams and staff might find it difficult to appropriately discipline a misbehaving patient who they perceive as suffering from a burn injury.

Another challenge of working in an inpatient setting is variability with length of hospital stays. Depending on the hospital and its admission protocols, some children with smaller and/or partial-thickness burns may be hospitalized briefly (e.g., <3 days), while children with more severe burns tend to have longer hospital stays due to the need for skin graft surgery and associated PT and OT. Some youth with extensive, deep burns may also be transferred to an inpatient rehabilitation facility after hospital discharge to regain optimum functioning prior to returning home. In other instances, hospitals may discharge patients in between staged, successive skin grafting surgeries. Consequently, pediatric psychologists may find it difficult to fully implement treatment plans or recommendations during brief hospital stays and, as such, may have to rely on providing general psychoeducation on effective coping strategies and resources for outpatient services as needed.

In addition, psychologists may have to redefine the referral question if medical staff express a desire for psychologists to "debrief" and/or process the burn wound (and/or its etiology) with the patient prior to discharge. In particular, some staff may request a psychologist's assistance in showing the patient his/her wounds. As previous research has suggested, debriefing, in itself, after a traumatic event is often not beneficial for children (e.g., Sijbrandij, Oliff, Reitsma, Carlier, & Gersons, 2006). On the other hand, having psychological support as part of desensitization may be appropriate. Thus, psychologists may find themselves having to provide psychoeducation and guidance to medical staff on trauma-informed care (see the National Traumatic Stress Network website for resources) to foster appropriate referral requests.

Not unlike care procedures with other pediatric populations (e.g., port access during chemotherapy in pediatric oncology patients), another common challenge facing psychologists providing inpatient burn consultations is clinician availability during burn dressing changes. As mentioned previously, burn dressing changes are often painful and distressing for patients and their families. Having psychologists present can facilitate coping via providing distraction, reinforcing emotional regulation, and teaching other active coping strategies to assist with pain management. However, due to other time or scheduling constraints, psychologists may not be available during these painful procedures but could offer guidance to other clinical staff with greater availability (e.g., child life specialists, nurses).

Finally, providing care for children with burn injuries can be difficult for medical providers, and as such, it is important for all burn providers to be cognizant of provider burnout and seek appropriate self-care as warranted.

Interventions in the Outpatient Setting/Outpatient Consultation

Burn care has shifted over the past several years and is characterized by briefer hospital stays followed by at-home care with outpatient management (American Burn Association, 2017). As a result, much of the wound care burden has moved from trained medical staff to parents and caregivers. Many parents find pediatric burn wound care quite stressful, with rates of 20–50% of parents displaying symptoms of stress in response to their child's burn injury (Bakker, Van der Heijden, Van Son, & Van Loey, 2013; De Young et al., 2014; Parrish et al., 2019), especially during the first few weeks after the injury. Some studies found higher levels of distress in parents of children with larger burns (Hall et al., 2006; Parrish et al., 2019), and other studies have suggested that parents of girls and older children display more distress (Bakker, Van Loey, Van der Heijden, & Van Son, 2012). Not unlike inpatient hospitalizations, interventions employed during outpatient treatment should address both parent and child coping given the dynamic interplay between parent and child adjustment.

Similar to recommendations for inpatient dressing changes, pediatric psychologists can help to coach parents to nurture their child's positive coping (e.g., taking deep breaths, engaging in guided imagery) rather than providing excessive reassurance for the child's distress verbalizations and behaviors during outpatient dressing changes. Besides dressing changes, pediatric psychologists may assist with other difficulties during outpatient follow-up visits, including the child's anxiety with bathing (given its association with dressing changes) and sleep disturbances. Hence, it may be useful to employ exposure-based activities (e.g., graduated exposure to aspects of medical care) and consider reward schedules to ensure return to usual behavior to help children who may be anxious during bathing. In addition, sleep disturbances such as nightmares, bed-wetting, sleepwalking, and bedtime problems (e.g., bedtime stalling) may occur in pediatric burn patients (e.g., Rose, Sanford,

Thomas, & Opp, 2001), although this is a relatively understudied area. Sleep hygiene, stimulus control, and sleep restriction are all possible interventions that can be addressed during outpatient burn follow-up (e.g., Meltzer & Crabtree, 2015) to assist with sleep disturbances.

In addition to the stresses of ongoing outpatient medical treatment, children at this time are often asked to return to their typical routines (e.g., daycare, school, social activities). For school-age children, preparation for school reintegration is useful, as peers are often curious about their classmate's absence from school or inquire about the child's injury if dressings or compression garments are visible. Pediatric psychologists can help rehearse appropriate responses to peer inquiries and coach children how to share any social challenges with parents and teachers should concerns emerge upon return to school (e.g., Phoenix Society for Burn Survivors, 2016). Parents are encouraged to contact teachers prior to their child's return to school to ensure maximum adult support during the transition. For parents of young children, there may be particular anxiety about allowing children to return to regular daytime care and concerns about sufficient protection from further injury. Interventions include helping parents understand medical and physical needs of their child and guidance from the medical team about appropriate timeframe of return to the child's usual schedule and activities.

To assist with targeting outpatient behavioral health concerns, pediatric psychologists may consider the use of psychological screeners to assess needs. These screeners might include measures of quality of life (e.g., physical adjustment, sleep, body image, coping with medical treatment, peer relationships), anxiety, depression, and posttraumatic stress symptoms. Their results can be useful in guiding the psychologist's approach to psychosocial treatment within outpatient burn care or suggest the possible need for referral for more extensive psychotherapy. Pediatric burn survivors (and their family) with significant emotional and mood problems that persist or develop after wound healing may benefit from a referral for parent training, family therapy, and/or cognitive-behavioral therapy. Persistence or development of behavioral concerns 1 month or more after the child's injury is often a good time guideline for psychologists when determining the necessity for outpatient services, as most DSM-5 diagnosable disorders require the presence of clinical symptoms for at least 1 month, with the exception of acute stress disorder. If parents continue to express elevated distress or excessive guilt, they also may benefit from a referral to see an adult mental health provider.

Adaptation

Regardless of the setting where the pediatric psychologist provides consultation for the pediatric burn patient (i.e., inpatient, outpatient specialty clinic, primary care), cognitive-behavioral treatment elements can be used for a range of situations, including shaping understanding of the injury and its subsequent effects, teaching and promoting effective coping skills for medical procedures, and supporting parents in playing an active role in their child's burn care. In the acute inpatient setting, the pediatric psychologist will likely focus on brief interventions to target acute emotional and behavioral changes that are impacting delivery of medical treatment. In addition, the pediatric psychologist may provide supportive therapy services to both the patient and the family, as the acute setting is often not the ideal time to begin in-depth processing of the traumatic injury. Rather, the psychologist is more often focusing on managing acute adjustment difficulties. Indeed, previous research suggests that a significant portion of psychological consultations in hospitals is focused on providing supportive therapy, rather than specific interventions (Carter et al., 2003). In contrast, in the outpatient setting, the pediatric psychologist may spend more time on addressing chronic concerns, such as dealing with teasing/bullying, school re-entry, and posttraumatic stress symptoms. If the pediatric psychologist serves only as a consultant within this outpatient setting or if the family resides some distance from the burn care center, the pediatric psychologist may choose to refer the patient to a more traditional outpatient therapy venue.

Some of the psychological interventions mentioned previously can be adapted based on the developmental level of the patient. For example, distraction techniques for pain management can range from comfort holds or breastfeeding for infants, to the use of loud and engaging toys for preschoolers, to guided imagery, cognitive distraction activities (e.g., alphabet games, books with hidden images), or virtual reality for school-aged children and teenagers (Dise-Lewis, 2001). For children of all ages, it is often recommended to teach and practice these behavioral distraction strategies prior to the acute medical procedure, when the child is calm. In addition, youth of all ages typically benefit from maintaining a consistent sleep/wake cycle, visual and daily schedules that include upcoming procedures, isolating painful procedures to a specific room (e.g., treatment room), and scheduling preferred activities throughout the day (Dise-Lewis, 2001). Younger children are more concrete and tend to respond well to preparation before medical procedures or before seeing their burn wounds for the first time in language that fits their developmental level (Dise-Lewis, 2001). For older children and adolescents, providing education and preparation often gives them a sense of control (Dise-Lewis, 2001), as does allowing them to participate in dressing changes when appropriate (e.g., assisting staff with removing outer bandages) and allowing them to establish their daily schedule and routines during their inpatient hospitalization and when they return home.

As with all evidence-based treatments, cultural awareness is important. One of the more common barriers to implementing culturally competent care is the stigma often felt by families of various cultural backgrounds when meeting with psychologists. This may often result in minimizing emotional and behavior concerns that may present during a hospitalization (e.g., Victor, Hamoda, & Tsang, 2018). Prior to modifying evidence-based treatment to fit a family's cultural needs, the culturally competent psychologist will need to establish a relationship with the patient and family, as well as develop a language to explain evidence-based treatment that aligns with the patient's cultural values. While some families may be supportive of relaxation and distraction techniques, incentive-based approaches may be challenging. For example, typical behavior plans that reinforce positive behaviors and selectively ignore minor misbehaviors may be in conflict with a patient's cultural values and traditional forms of discipline and limit setting (e.g., Victor et al., 2018). Working jointly with the patient and his/her family to develop an effective behavioral plan is often necessary to be mindful of cultural values (Victor et al., 2018).

Resources and Support

A pediatric psychologist must have clinical expertise and flexibility in adapting evidence-based, brief interventions to address the emotional and behavioral concerns of youth who are being treated for burn injuries, as well as providing assistance to parents. It has been suggested that psychologists working in acute settings such as the PICU or a burn unit should maintain a skill set that includes being calm and thinking clearly to provide guidance for the "chronically acute" patient and families (Tunick, Gavin, DeMaso, & Meyer, 2013). For example, because not all burn units may have child life specialists, a pediatric psychologist should be prepared to provide in vivo distraction during dressing changes and come prepared with a variety of distraction tools (e.g., bubbles, tablet computers with games, music) that are engaging for children of different ages.

Coordinating psychological interventions across the varied professionals involved on burn care teams can be challenging for a pediatric psychologist. Often times, psychologists will need to communicate recommendations to the medical team (e.g., nurse practitioners, nursing staff), as well as coordinate services with social work and child life who may have overlapping care responsibilities. As noted earlier, the pediatric psychologist may work with nutrition and/or PT/OT to develop behavioral plans to address adherence to dietary and PT/OT tasks, respectively. Participating in weekly/biweekly medical rounds often is a useful forum to explain psychosocial interventions to all members of the treatment team. Likewise, holding family conferences with representatives from the burn team can ensure that the patient/family and the medical team understand the treatment plan and goals. Finally, not only are pediatric psychologists providing services directly to children and their families; they might also need to provide support to the medical team, particularly when patients and/or families are displaying challenging behaviors or when patients are critically ill.

Summary

Recent estimates suggest that nearly 300 children are treated for burn injuries every day across the United States (Centers for Disease Control, 2016). The acute treatment and potential long-term management of burn injuries are often distressful for the pediatric patients and their families. Pediatric psychologists can help facilitate positive adjustment in youth with burn injuries, starting with the initial inpatient hospitalization and continuing through long-term outpatient follow-up. Commonly, pediatric psychologists can provide a variety of psychological services, ranging from supportive care to active distraction or modeling of effective coping strategies, as well as assisting with reintegration into society after the burn is healed. Given the painful and often traumatic nature of burn injuries, as well as the variety of services that psychologists can offer, pediatric psychologists can be invaluable members of a multidisciplinary burn care team. Two case examples are presented below that help illustrate the role of pediatric psychologists when working with youth with burn injuries.

Case Examples

Case 1 "Logan" is a 4-year-old male who was admitted to a burn center after sustaining partial-thickness scald burns to his bilateral hands. His burn injury was ruled non-accidental and deliberately caused by someone taking care of him (non-relative). Logan's medical course included bilateral skin grafts to assist with wound healing and pressure garment and laser therapy to assist with scar management and functionality. Psychology was consulted during Logan's inpatient admission to assist with post-injury adjustment. The initial consultation during Logan's hospitalization focused on providing Logan and his parents with support, as his parents reported significant guilt associated with Logan's injuries. Logan's parents were encouraged to engage in self-care during his hospitalization and utilize social supports as necessary. Logan's parents revealed some minor behavioral difficulties prior to his burn injury, including non-compliance at meal times and bedtime, as well some instances of tantrums and physical aggression directed toward his mother. During his inpatient admission, it was felt that Logan and his family were coping within normal expectations, although it was felt that pain and decreased hand functioning might impact Logan's mood and behaviors. Logan and his parents were provided with psychoeducation about normal expectations after burn injuries, including changes in mood and behavior. Active coping and relaxation skills (e.g., bubble breathing, distraction) were reviewed and encouraged to assist with pain and behavior management. Due to Logan's prior history of behavioral concerns, it was recommended that Logan's parents continue to set limits and address behavioral concerns as warranted during his hospitalization. Over the course of Logan's hospitalization, his parents' feelings of guilt impacted their ability to engage in self-care (e.g., take breaks from Logan's hospital room), which in turn increased their frustration and impacted their ability to console and provide care for Logan. As a result, Logan became difficult to comfort when his parents attempted to separate, and his parents noticed an increase in irritability and sadness in Logan. After his skin graft surgery, developmentally appropriate communication strategies were reviewed with Logan's family in regard to how to talk with him about his skin grafts. For example, Logan was told that some skin from his leg was going to be used as a "band-aid" or glove to cover his injuries on his hands to help his hands heal and get better.

Psychology continued to follow Logan and his family in the outpatient setting. As Logan transitioned home, additional concerns became evident, including increased itching to hands and skin graft donor sites, increased fear around water and bath time, sleep initiation difficulties, increased irritability and anger toward his younger siblings, and increased defiant behavior and physical aggression toward others. Brief behavioral interventions were conducted with Logan and his family in the outpatient setting, including parental management strategies (e.g., selective attention, behavioral plan to reinforce positive behavior), graduated exposure to water and the use of distraction during bath time, distraction and active coping strategies to assist with itching, and sleep hygiene. Ultimately, Logan and his family were referred for outpatient behavioral health services to continue addressing his emotional and behavioral concerns.

Case 2 "Megan" is a 9-year-old female who was admitted to a burn center after sustaining a flame burn injury. Her burn injuries occurred when her dress was enflamed while sitting around a campfire, resulting in full-thickness burns to her left leg (12% TBSA). Psychology was consulted during Megan's inpatient admission to assist with post-burn adjustment. The initial consultation during Megan's hospitalization focused on providing psychoeducation on normal expectations after burn injury, including changes in mood and behaviors. During her inpatient admission, Megan was taught a variety of active coping and relaxation skills (e.g., diaphragmatic breathing, guided imagery) to assist with mood and pain management. Megan coped well during her hospitalization, and she denied concerns with acute stress or pain management. She was subsequently discharged home with follow-up in the outpatient burn clinic; however, Megan's burns required additional skin graft surgery, which resulted in a second inpatient admission. During her second admission, Megan endorsed anxiety about procedures due to fear of pain and increased worries about her mother taking care of her burns at home. Brief cognitive-behavioral strategies were implemented during Megan's second hospitalization and included teaching self-regulation and active coping strategies for pain management (e.g., diaphragmatic breathing, distraction, behavioral plan for reinforcing brave behavior during dressing changes) as well as devising a "coping bag" with items (e.g., bubbles, pinwheels) to assist her in coping during dressing changes. Megan continued to deny acute stress symptoms during the second hospitalization.

After Megan was discharged from the hospital, she experienced significant procedural anxiety during her outpatient dressing changes. To address these concerns, Megan was prepared prior to her dressing changes, and effective coping strategies were elicited. Megan reported that she responded best with distraction strategies, so guided imagery was reviewed and utilized during her dressing changes. Moreover, she was provided with a sense of control by allowing her to take off some of her dressings; however, Megan began engaging in stalling behaviors (e.g., asking for more time), which only increased her anxiety and fear. Megan ultimately benefited from limited reassurance, breaking her dressing changes into small goals, and using active distraction. Besides Megan's procedural anxiety, she denied adjustment difficulties at home, and she was able to return to baseline functioning after her burns were healed. During her 6-month follow-up, Megan denied concerns with teasing or bullying related to her burn injury.

Attachments/Additional Resources

The following websites provide excellent resources for pediatric psychologists working with pediatric burn survivors, in addition to handouts that can be shared with these patients and their families.

National Traumatic Stress Network (https://www.nctsn.org/). This website provides resources and handouts on trauma-informed care and medical traumatic stress (e.g., typical expectations after a traumatic injury). Patient handouts are also available in Spanish.

Phoenix Society for Burn Survivors (https://www.phoenix-society.org/). This website shares resources and handouts on a large variety of topics, including traumatic loss, advocating for educational needs, sibling adjustment, teasing and bullying, dealing with staring, managing feelings of guilt, helping children cope during hospitalizations, and school reentry. A sample handout for staring and teasing that summarizes some relevant materials from this website is displayed in the Appendix.

Appendix: When People Stare, Tease, and Ask Questions

When your body is changed by an injury or an illness, social situations often can lead to other people staring or asking questions. At first, the reaction of others can be difficult. However, you can learn new behavioral skills to help you respond to others' reactions. The good news is that most people learn to accept the changes in their body image. This acceptance takes time, support from others, and a willingness to learn new social survival skills. Here are some tips to help you along the way:

1. **How to cope with staring**
   - Most people stare because they are curious or concerned
   - Only a few people stare because they are rude
   - **What to *do and say*—Some options are:**
     Stand up straight, look directly at the person, and smile. Say something like "How's it going?" or "Hi, I'm (your name)"
     Offer a brief response such as "I got burned by fireworks, but I'm fine now" or "I got hurt in a car wreck but I'm doing much better"
     Address the staring person directly—"Please do not stare at me."
     Use humor or sarcasm—"Do I have something on my face?" Or "I'm having a bad hair day!"
     Ignore the person who is staring
   - **Practice your favorite response or responses**
     In front of a mirror
     With a parent or close friend
   - **Be proactive**
     Give your classmates information before you come to school, so they can be prepared for your new appearance.
     Be a part of an assembly before returning to school to give your classmates information. You can do a presentation, or you can have your healthcare worker, school nurse, or parent do this.
2. **How to cope with teasing**
   - Unfortunately, many children who have been burned or injured get teased.
   - It is important to have a plan for handling teasing before it starts.
   - **What to *do* —Some options are:**
     Look strong and confident, stand up straight, keep your head up, make eye contact, and use a strong voice when speaking.
     Use "I" statements such as "I want you to stop staring at me." Or "I want you to stop calling me names."
     Respond with "You might be right" each time someone teases you.
     Shrug your shoulders and respond with a casual statement such as "Oh well, I don't care."
     Use humor or sarcasm. Examples include: "Thank you for the compliment!" "You are being so nice to me!"
     Walk away if the person teasing you becomes dangerous or threatening. Talk to a trusted adult or parent.
   - **What *not* to do:**
     Show the teaser that he/she has upset you by getting mad or crying because that will only increase teasing.
     Offer to fight the person.
     Always ignore the teasing (unless the person teasing is dangerous).

Tell an adult as a first step. Try to resolve the conflict by yourself if you can.

3. **How to cope with questions**
   - Although people usually ask questions because they are curious or concerned, it may get really annoying when people keep asking you the same questions *over and over again* or when people you do not know ask you personal questions.
   - **What to *do and say*—Some options are:**
     Take a deep breath before responding.
     Remind yourself that people are not asking questions to be mean or nosy.
     Ending your responses with "Thanks for asking" is a nice way to let people know that you do not want to talk about your injury anymore.
     Practice a *short answer* for people you do not know. "I got burned while I was trying to cook. Thanks for asking"
     Practice a *long answer* for people you want to share a little bit more information with. "I lost my leg in a car accident last summer. I'm still getting used to walking with crutches, but I'm getting really fast. What would you like to know about my situation?"
     If you feel uncomfortable with someone's question, you can always say "I really don't feel like talking about my injury."

Adapted from Qualye, B.H. (2001) "Tools to handle questions and teasing" and "When people stare" *Burn Support News*

References

Alnababtah, K., Khan, S., & Ashford, R. (2016). Socio-demographic factors and the prevalence of burns in children: An overview of the literature. *Paediatrics and International Child Health, 36*(1), 45–51. https://doi.org/10.1179/2046905514Y.0000000157

American Burn Association. (2017). *National burn repository 2017 update: Report of data from 2008–2017*. Retrieved from http://ameriburn.org/quality-care/2017-national-burn-repository-annual-report/

Bagner, D. M., Fernandez, M. A., & Eyberg, S. M. (2004). Parent-child interaction therapy and chronic illness: A case study. *Journal of Clinical Psychology in Medical Settings, 11*(1), 1–6. https://doi.org/10.1023/B:JOCS.0000016264.02407.fd

Bakker, A., Maertens, K. J., Van Son, M. J., & Van Loey, N. E. (2013). Psychological consequences of pediatric burns from a child and family perspective: A review of the empirical literature. *Clinical Psychology Review, 33*(3), 361–371. https://doi.org/10.1016/j.cpr.2012.12.006

Bakker, A., Van der Heijden, P. G., Van Son, M. J., & Van Loey, N. E. (2013). Course of traumatic stress reactions in couples after a burn event to their young child. *Health Psychology, 32*(10), 1076. https://doi.org/10.1037/a0033983

Bakker, A., Van Loey, N. E., Van der Heijden, P. M., & Van Son, M. M. (2012). Acute stress reactions in couples after a burn event to their young child. *Journal of Pediatric Psychology, 37*(10), 1127–1135. https://doi.org/10.1093/jpepsy/jss083

Bakker, A., Van Loey, N. E., Van Son, M. J., & Van der Heijden, P. G. (2010). Brief report: Mothers' long-term posttraumatic stress symptoms following a burn event of their child. *Journal of Pediatric Psychology, 35*(6), 656–661. https://doi.org/10.1093/jpepsy/jsp090

Blount, R. L., Devine, K. A., Cheng, P. S., Simons, L. E., & Hayutin, L. (2008). The impact of adult behaviors and vocalizations on infant distress during immunizations. *Journal of Pediatric Psychology, 33*(10), 1163–1174.

Carter, B. D., Kronenberger, W. G., Baker, J., Grimes, L. M., Crabtree, V. M., Smith, C., & McGraw, K. (2003). Inpatient pediatric consultation-liaison: A case-controlled study. *Journal of Pediatric Psychology, 28*(6), 423–432. https://doi.org/10.1093/jpepsy/jsg032

Centers for Disease Control. (2016). Burn prevention. Retrieved from https://www.cdc.gov/safechild/burns/index.html

D'Souza, A. L., Nelson, N. G., & McKenzie, L. B. (2009). Pediatric burn injuries treated in US emergency departments between 1990 and 2006. *Pediatrics, 124*(5), 1424–1430. https://doi.org/10.1542/peds.2008-2802

De Young, A. C., Hendrikz, J., Kenardy, J. A., Cobham, V. E., & Kimble, R. M. (2014). Prospective evaluation of parent distress following pediatric burns and identification of risk factors for young child and parent posttraumatic stress disorder. *Journal of Child and Adolescent Psychopharmacology, 24*(1), 9–17. https://doi.org/10.1089/cap.2013.0066

Dise-Lewis, J. E. (2001). A developmental perspective on psychological principles of burn care. *Journal of Burn Care and Rehabilitation, 22*, 255–260.

Hall, E., Saxe, G., Stoddard, F., Kaplow, J., Koenen, K., Chawla, N., … King, D. (2006). Posttraumatic stress symptoms in parents of children with acute burns. *Journal of Pediatric Psychology, 31*(4), 403–412. https://doi.org/10.1093/jpepsy/jsj016

Kazak, A. E., Kassam-Adams, N., Schneider, S., Zelikovsky, N., Alderfer, M. A., & Rourke, M. (2006). An integrative model of pediatric medical traumatic stress. *Journal of Pediatric Psychology, 31*, 343–355.

Krishnamoorthy, V., Ramaiah, R., & Bhananker, S. M. (2012). Pediatric burn injuries. *International Journal of Critical Illness and Injury Science, 2*(3), 128–134. https://doi.org/10.4103/2229-5151.100889
Latenser, B. A., & Kowal-Vern, A. (2002). Paediatric burn rehabilitation. *Pediatric Rehabilitation, 5*(1), 3–10.
Malloy, K. M., & Milling, L. S. (2010). The effectiveness of virtual reality distraction for pain reduction: A systematic review. *Clinical Psychology Review, 30*, 1011–1018. https://doi.org/10.1016/j.cpr.2010.07.001
Meltzer, L. J., & Crabtree, V. M. (2015). *Pediatric sleep problems: A clinician's guide to behavioral interventions*. Washington, DC: American Psychological Association.
National Traumatic Stress Network. (2003). *Medical traumatic stress*. Retrieved from https://www.nctsn.org/
Parrish, C., Shields, A., Morris, A., George, A., Reynolds, E., Borden, L., ... Ostrander, R. (2019). Parent distress following pediatric burn injuries. *Journal of Burn Care and Research, 40*(1), 79–84. https://doi.org/10.1093/jbcr/iry048
Phoenix Society for Burn Survivors. (2016). *How do I handle myself when someone stares (at my burn scars)?* Retrieved from https://www.phoenix-society.org/blog/entry/how-do-I-handle-when-someone-stares-at-my-burn-scars
Price, J., Kassam-Adams, N., Alderfer, M. A., Christofferson, J., & Kazak, A. E. (2015). Systematic review: A reevaluation and update of the integrative (trajectory) model of pediatric medical traumatic stress. *Journal of Pediatric Psychology, 41*(1), 86–97.
Rose, M., Sanford, A., Thomas, C., & Opp, M. R. (2001). Factors altering the sleep of burned children. *Sleep, 24*(1), 45–51.
Rowan, M. P., Cancio, L. C., Elster, E. A., Burmeister, D. M., Rose, L. F., Natesan, S., ... Chung, K. K. (2015). Burn wound healing and treatment: Review and advancements. *Critical Care, 19*, 243. https://doi.org/10.1186/s13054-015-0961-2
Rowley-Conwy, G. (2014). Management of major burns: Rehabilitation and recovery. *Nursing Standard, 28*(25), 65–70.
Sheridan, R. (2018). Burn care for children. *Pediatrics in Review, 39*(6), 273–284.
Sijbrandij, M., Oliff, M., Reitsma, J. B., Carlier, I. V. E., & Gersons, B. P. R. (2006). Emotional or educational debriefing after psychological trauma: Randomized controlled trial. *Journal of Psychiatry, 189*, 150–155. https://doi.org/10.1192/bjp.bp.105.021121
Tunick, R. A., Gavin, J. A., DeMaso, D. R., & Meyer, E. C. (2013). Pediatric psychology critical care consultation: An emerging subspecialty. *Clinical Practice in Pediatric Psychology, 1*(1), 42–54. https://doi.org/10.1037/cpp0000006
Victor, E. C., Hamoda, H. M., & Tsang, K. K. (2018). Implementation of a behavioral intervention in consultation-liaison with an international family. *Clinical Practice in Pediatric Psychology, 6*(1), 42–50. https://doi.org/10.1037/cpp0000203
Yin, S. (2017). Chemical and common burns in children. *Clinical Pediatrics, 56*(5S), 8S–12S. https://doi.org/10.1177/0009922817706975
Yu, H., Wier, L.M., & Elixhauser, A. (2011). Hospital stays for children, 2009 (Healthcare Cost and Utilization Project Statistical Brief No. 118). Retrieved from http://www.hcup-us.ahrq.gov/reports/statbriefs/sb118.pdf

Neonatal Intensive Care

Casey Hoffman, Michelle M. Greene,
and Amy E. Baughcum

Consultation to the neonatal intensive care unit (NICU) is unique in that the primary focus of clinical concern is often the parent rather than the identified pediatric patient. However, the parent-infant dyad, family, or individual infant may also be the focus of clinical attention. In each case, the consulting psychologist must differentiate between normative coping responses which require general support and elevated clinical presentations that require more targeted interventions. Therefore, this work requires a diverse set of knowledge, including understanding the impact of the perinatal period on parents, the impact of having an ill infant on parents and siblings, and the impact of being an ill infant on the neonate's experiences and development.

C. Hoffman (✉)
The Children's Hospital of Philadelphia, Philadelphia, PA, USA

Department of Child and Adolescent Psychiatry and Behavioral Sciences, The Children's Hospital of Philadelphia, Philadelphia, PA, USA
e-mail: HOFFMANC@email.chop.edu

M. M. Greene
Rush University Children's Hospital, Chicago, IL, USA

Department of Pediatrics, Rush University Medical Center, Chicago, IL, USA

A. E. Baughcum
Nationwide Children's Hospital, Columbus, OH, USA

Department of Pediatrics, The Ohio State University College of Medicine, Columbus, OH, USA

Differential Diagnosis

Parent Functioning

The postpartum period is an emotionally vulnerable period for parents associated with an increased incidence of mental health conditions for both mothers and fathers, referred to as postpartum mood and anxiety disorders (PMADs) (Hoffman, Dunn, & Njoroge, 2017). Infant hospitalization confers further risk, with rates of depression and post-traumatic stress disorder (PTSD) ranging from a quarter to a third of parents of NICU infants (Roque, Lasiuk, Radünz, & Hegadoren, 2017) and rates of suicidal ideation of up to 30% among NICU mothers (Lefkowitz, Baxt, & Evans, 2010). At NICU admission, parents can experience a range of emotional reactions including intense fear, anxiety, helplessness, guilt, loss, and sadness (Hynan, Mounts, & Vanderbilt, 2013). There is often an adjustment period for parents as they make sense of an unfamiliar, intense medical setting and rules governing their interactions with their new infant. Traumatic events are numerous and include both threats to their own infant's survival and potentially other infants in the unit. Parents may also

B. D. Carter, K. A. Kullgren (eds.), *Clinical Handbook of Psychological Consultation in Pediatric Medical Settings*, Issues in Clinical Child Psychology, https://doi.org/10.1007/978-3-030-35598-2_22

learn their infant has a diagnosis that will be chronic or life limiting. In addition, parents may have the stress of making decisions about whether to continue the infant's life-sustaining treatments in the face of a poor prognosis. Further, parents' emotional reactions may occur in the context of a history of infertility, miscarriage, stillbirth, or infant loss (including the twin/triplet sibling of the current NICU patient), further exacerbating and complicating stress reactions (Totapally, Youngblut, Cantwell, Moral, & Brooten, 2013).

A significant challenge for the consulting psychologist is distinguishing between the stress reactions commonly experienced by parents of NICU infants and symptoms representing a greater level of clinical concern (see Table 1). Parental responses must be evaluated in relation to cultural considerations, individual differences, prior mental health history, and family context.

Dyadic Functioning

Disruption in the emerging parent-infant relationship is also a focus of clinical attention in the NICU. Hospitalization of infants results in an unnatural separation of parent and infant and a lack of early parental autonomy in infant care. This may result in a delay in the process of parent-infant bonding, which provides the foundation for a secure parent-infant attachment. The consulting psychologist must differentiate between the expected delay in bonding and concerns that may reflect an emerging pattern of maladaptive parent-infant interactions (see Table 2).

Infant Functioning

The infant as an individual may also be the focus of clinical attention for the psychologist, particularly for infants with extended hospitalizations. Reasons for referral may include concern for developmental delay or sleep disruption. Many medical conditions in the neonatal period place infants at increased risk for developmental delay. However, clinicians must be aware of the limits of developmental assessment in the intensive care setting and distinguish between temporary delays and more lasting impairment (see section "Assessment and formulation").

Table 1 Considerations in NICU parent differential diagnosis

NICU stressor	Normative parent responses	Potential clinical concern
NICU admission and course	Range of emotions Emotions rise and fall with infant's progress and setbacks (description of an "emotional roller coaster") Worry, fearfulness, and anxiety that waxes and wanes Periodic tearfulness Altered or reduced sleep, eating, and self-care Engages in conversations with NICU providers, may not understand or remember medical details, and needs repetition	Restricted range of affect Negative emotions dominate despite infant's progress Continuous anxiety that does not even temporarily lessen; hypervigilance at bedside or in phone calls Uncontrollable crying past the first 2 weeks postpartum Insufficient sleep, eating, and self-care Conversations with NICU providers are repeatedly strained, require much more time than is typical, and are confusing/unsatisfying
Loss of normative pregnancy, delivery, and neonatal period at home	Feelings of sadness/grief related to loss of enjoyable pregnancy, planned labor and delivery, expected transition to parenthood	Traumatic responses, including flashbacks to delivery, difficulty processing loss of control regarding birth plan, cannot enjoy infant's progress and milestones
Pumping breast milk for an infant who is not yet feeding by mouth	Worry about adequacy of milk supply Fatigue related to sleep disruption	Perseveration about milk supply Does not feel rested even when there are opportunities to sleep

Table 2 Considerations in dyadic functioning in the NICU

NICU stressor	Normative parent responses	Potential clinical concern
Physical separation of parent and infant	Delay in transition to parental identity Regular visitation balanced with other obligations Makes efforts to call for updates when not present	Detachment or disinterest Avoidance of visitation, or refuses to leave the bedside Does not call regularly when not able to be present
Critically ill infant with medical support	Anxiety regarding holding, touching, and caring for infant but attempts these tasks with support Builds feelings of parental competence with increasing exposure to infant care; improves in ability to understand infant cues Builds perception of infant as a "fighter" and assigns positive personality characteristics to infant	Persistent avoidance of interactions with the infant, either through decreased visitation or avoidance during visitation Continues to feel ineffective in infant care despite opportunities to learn; observed to over- or under-stimulate infant; feels disliked by baby Assigns negative characteristics to infant; says infant resembles a person with whom the parent has a conflicted relationship

Family Functioning

Infant hospitalization can also affect the broader family system. Parents may have increased conflict with each other due to different coping styles, grandparents may struggle to both support their children and worry about their grandchild, and siblings can have difficulty coping as they adjust to having a new sibling while also being separated from the sibling and sometimes also from parents. Psychologists may be called upon to determine whether family members' reactions constitute normative adjustment or a potential adjustment disorder. Due to their expertise in co-parenting and couple functioning, family systems, and child development, psychologists can play a vital role in helping to mitigate stress for family members and determining whether community-based treatment or supports are warranted.

Medical Basics

Infants are admitted to the NICU with a large array of diagnoses. Most, though not all, NICU conditions fall into one of the following four broad categories: prematurity, perinatal asphyxia, congenital anomalies and/or genetic diagnoses, and neonatal abstinence syndrome.

The Center for Disease Control vital statistics indicates in the United States approximately one in ten infants are born *premature* (<37-week gestation). The majority (72%) are late preterm births (34–36 weeks) (Martin & Osterman, 2018). The remaining infants are moderately preterm (32–33 weeks, 12%), very preterm (VPT <32 weeks, 10%), and extremely preterm (EPT <28, 6%). Survival rates in the United States have improved over the past few decades, including for those born at the border of viability: 36% at 23 weeks, 59% at 24 weeks, and 77% at 25 weeks (Patel et al. 2017). Lower gestational age is related to increased medical complications, mortality, and neurodevelopmental disabilities including cerebral palsy, intellectual disability, autism spectrum disorder, and vision and hearing impairment (Stephens & Vohr, 2009).

Due to the timing of fetal lung development, respiratory distress is nearly ubiquitous in preterm infants. Many VPT and EPT infants have difficulty breathing on their own and require invasive mechanical ventilation. Continuous positive airway pressure (CPAP) is also commonly used and transitioned to supplemental oxygen delivered via nasal cannula. Bronchopulmonary dysplasia (BPD), or the continued need for respiratory support after 36-week gestational age, occurs in nearly 25% of VPT infants (Lemons et al., 2001). Apnea (breath holding) and bradycardia (slow heart rate) are common (As and Bs) and lead to desaturation (decreased blood oxygen level). Other common comorbidities include sepsis (blood-borne infection), necrotizing enterocolitis (NEC, infection of the intestine), retinopathy of prematurity (ROP, eye disease with abnormal vascularization of the retina), neurological injury (brain bleeding known as intraventricular hemorrhage [IVH], post-hemorrhagic hydrocephalus requiring a brain [VP] shunt, or white matter injury known as periventricular leukomalacia [PVL]), and patent ductus arteriosus (PDA, an unclosed hole in the aorta of the heart).

VPT infants initially require total parenteral nutrition (TPN), intravenous nutrients. Infants gradually transition to enteral feeds with human milk or formula through a nasogastric (NG) or orogastric (OG) tube and then transition to feeding by breast or bottle. When gastric feeds are not tolerated, a nasoduodenal (ND) or nasojejunal (NJ) tube may be used. A surgically placed gastrostomy tube (G-tube) may be needed when eating by mouth is significantly delayed.

Perinatal asphyxia is the result of insufficient pulmonary or placental gas exchange and can result in hypoxia and organ injury. Knotting of the umbilical cord around the infant's neck, placental insufficiency, severe maternal hypotension, or traumatic delivery can be the cause. Hypoxic-ischemic encephalopathy (HIE) refers to brain injury related to perinatal asphyxia. Therapeutic hypothermia (i.e., "cooling," lowering body temperature to 91.4–95.0 degrees F) occurs within the first few hours after birth and may mitigate injury to the brain and other organs. Infants with HIE receive electroencephalogram (EEG) to monitor for seizures and a magnetic resonance imaging (MRI) to evaluate brain injury. Neurodevelopmental prognoses vary according to the severity of HIE and use of cooling (McAdams & Juul, 2016).

Infants with *congenital anomalies*, or structural differences present at birth, and *genetic syndromes* are often admitted to the NICU. Some infants have been diagnosed in utero allowing family preparation, while others are diagnosed after birth. Congenital heart defects or disorders (CHDs, 1 in 100 live births) and Down syndrome (DS, 1 in 700 live births), respectively, are the most common type of congenital anomaly and the most common chromosomal abnormality among live-born infants (Gilboa et al., 2016). Most CHDs involve the interior walls of the heart, valves of the heart, or large blood vessels. CHDs may require no intervention, medicine and cardiac catheterization procedures, or substantial and serial surgical corrections. Children with DS have specific physical features and often have hypotonia, speech delay, mild-moderate intellectual disability, heart defects, sleep apnea, hearing loss, and eye diseases. Neural tube defects, including myelomeningocele (spina bifida) which impacts the central nervous system (Wilson, 2014), and defects causing pulmonary hypoplasia, such as congenital diaphragmatic hernia (McGivern et al., 2015), require surgical intervention and necessitate NICU care.

Infants born to mothers with opioid and/or other substance use disorders are at risk for withdrawal, referred to as *neonatal abstinence syndrome* (NAS) (Tolia et al., 2015). NAS is associated with infant irritability, feeding problems, altered muscle tone, sleep-wake disturbances, and autonomic dysregulation. Management of NAS is driven by serial administration of scoring systems for symptoms. NAS is treated through supportive care including developmentally sensitive handling and pharmacologic therapy, which frequently involves opioid therapy and subsequent controlled opioid weaning.

Engagement

Family engagement with psychology support in the NICU starts with a strong foundation of support for psychology from neonatology, nursing, and the hospital administration. Psychologists should educate staff about the benefits of including them on the healthcare team (e.g., greater parental compliance with the infant's medical plan, increased parental collaboration with the bedside nurse). Psychologists' training in scientific methods should also be highlighted as beneficial to NICU research initiatives as well as quality improvement projects.

Parents in the NICU may benefit from psychology services, yet several barriers can impact

Table 3 Strategies to promote parental engagement with psychology services in the NICU

Barriers to engagement	NICU team strategies	Psychologist strategies
• Parent concern about stigma of meeting with a psychologist, worry it means they are "crazy" • Parent worry about being judged to be an inadequate parent • Parent concern about confidentiality • Parent perception of not having enough time to meet with a psychologist • Parent concern for discussing emotions when already feeling vulnerable • Parent preference for focusing on time with infant during visit • Prior experience with psychologists that was not perceived as helpful	• Social work or other personnel can make parents aware of the availability of psychology early in the admission to normalize accessing this support • Bedside nurse can look for opportunities to promote the role of psychology during conversations with parents • Medical team can explain to parents that the psychologist is part of the team and define the goals of the consult • NICU administration can ensure that there are private meeting rooms for the psychologist to meet with a parent • Bedside nurse can reassure parent that they are available to hold/tend to the infant while parent is meeting with the psychologist	• Normalize stress, difficult emotions, and thoughts for NICU parents • Distinguish between psychology services in the NICU and outpatient individual services • Discuss confidentiality including communication with the NICU team, charting, and billing • Tell parents that they can stop services at any time • Be willing to meet with parents at the bedside if they prefer • Identify an initial "port of entry" based on the parent's biggest priority, such as communicating with the team, concerns about the infant or sibling, or their own sleep difficulties • Provide explicit education about the benefit for the infant when parents are well-supported

their willingness to engage with this support. Both the psychologist and the broader NICU team can employ strategies to maximize parental engagement as summarized in Table 3.

Assessment and Formulation

Having a new baby is a significant transition and requires adjustment for the family in terms of negotiating new roles and routines. This is further complicated by medical complications and displacement of infant in the hospital rather than home. Understanding the family's pre-existing strengths and challenges as well as the impact of this new infant within the broader family system is critical in formulating a support plan.

When conducting an initial interview with families, it is important to consider issues impacting parental availability to their infant as well as overall psychological adjustment (see Table 4). Direct observations of functioning combined with reports from bedside staff and multidisciplinary team members are also essential to identify targets for intervention.

In addition to a thorough clinical interview, mental health screening instruments can be administered to NICU parents to gather information about symptoms of depression or posttraumatic stress (see Appendix 1 for summary). Parents whose scores are elevated will require timely follow-up to determine the most appropriate next steps, and when a suicidal ideation question is endorsed, an immediate safety assessment should be conducted. Embedded NICU psychologists may wish to consider implementing a universal screening program for NICU parents, which requires several additional considerations (Hynan et al., 2013).

Psychologists may also be consulted for neurodevelopmental assessments of the hospitalized infant. Assessment tools vary based on infant gestational age and require specific training in infant assessment (for summary, see Appendix 2). Developmental scores are based on corrected age for infants born <37 weeks (D'Agostino et al., 2013). Developmental delays should be identified as targets for intervention rather than considered prognostic of later developmental functioning. Interpretation of testing findings should include attention to several medical and environmental factors, which are summarized in Table 5 (Noble & Boyd, 2012).

Table 4 Assessment of family functioning in the neonatal intensive care unit

Family background	Current self-report of functioning	Clinician and staff observations of current functioning
• Family composition • Language preferences • Religious and cultural affiliations (including implications for infant's medical course or treatment) • Support network • Financial resources and employment (including any challenges related to the infant's hospital) • Housing • Legal history, including substance abuse or child protection involvement • Educational history, literacy, learning differences • Prior preferred coping strategies • Past trauma history • Parent mental health history, including postpartum mood and anxiety disorders, suicidal ideation/attempts, or hospitalizations • Past sibling behavioral or emotional concerns • Previous pregnancy or infant losses • History of infertility • Previous experience with the NICU • Current pregnancy history	• Perception of labor and delivery experience • Expressed understanding of infant's medical issues, treatment plan, and prognosis • Perception of parenting role • Expressed interest and comfort with infant care • Perception of infant and attributions for infant behavior • Self-care and routines including sleep, eating, respite, and managing pumping/breastfeeding • Use of coping strategies • Postpartum mood including symptoms of anxiety, depression, and traumatic stress • Current suicidal ideation, intent, or plan • Signs of alterations in reality testing • Relationship dynamics with support persons • Current work arrangements • Current life stressors • Current sibling behavioral and emotional concerns, including adjustment to new baby	• Frequency of parent visitation • Frequency of telephone contact with staff • Comfort of communication and engagement with staff • Reactions to medical information • Reactions to support offered • Demonstration of appropriate boundaries • Willingness to be involved in infant's care • Presentation at the bedside including affect, anxiety, and any signs of altered mental status • Interaction style with infant including sensitivity, interest, nurturing, and signs of bonding • Co-parenting behaviors • Signs of conflict between family members/relationship dynamics • Observed difficulties in sibling coping or adjustment

Table 5 Influences on hospitalized infants' developmental progression

Medical conditions	Equipment/medications	Sensorimotor opportunities/experiences
• Chronic lung disease • Pulmonary hypertension • Cardiac conditions • Gastroesophageal reflux • Neurological immaturity/abnormalities/conditions • Congenital anomalies • Genetic conditions • Surgical conditions • Hearing impairment • Visual impairment	• Respiratory support • Feeding tube • Lines/IVs with immobilizer • Chest tubes • Drains • Mittens to prevent tube pulling • Tight swaddling • Casting • Splints • Helmet for head shaping • Sedating medications (especially the impact on alertness and visual skills)	• Contact with parents • Frequency of being held and touched • Position restrictions/opportunities for movement • Opportunities for non-nutritive sucking • Auditory input, including infant-directed speech • Visual input, including crib attaching toys • Cycled lighting • Sleep disruption for nursing or medical intervention

Interventions for Inpatient Consultation

Mental health interventions in the NICU can focus on alleviating parental distress, improving family functioning, enhancing the parent-infant relationship, and/or increasing the developmental competence of the infant. Due to the inextricable links between the functioning of the parent, infant, and broader family system, interventions often overlap these areas in their focus or impact. Psychologists provide direct services as well as consultation to the multi-disciplinary team. Competency in liaison work is as important in the NICU as it is in other hospital units. Psychologists take an active role with the coordination of psychosocial care with other disciplines such as social work, chaplaincy, child life, developmental therapists, and lactation consultants and liaison with the medical and nursing teams. Despite inevitable overlap between roles, with coordination, the team can work toward shared goals. Psychologists often benefit from gathering additional information to enhance their expertise (see Appendix 3).

Parent Interventions

Intervention studies for parents of NICU infants to date are limited with restricted generalizability. Most focus on preterm infants only, exclude fathers and non-fluent English speakers, have a non-representative range of ethnicities, and have high rates of participant refusal (up to 45%). A recent meta-analysis of NICU-based interventions for mothers using a randomized controlled design found fewer than ten eligible studies assessing depressive or anxiety symptoms (Mendelson, Cluxton-Keller, Vullo, Tandon, & Noazin, 2017). Approaches that have been shown to be effective or have promising pilot data are summarized in Table 6.

As a complement to interventions administered by psychologists, peer-to-peer support should be considered to optimize parent adjustment in the NICU (Hall, Ryan, Beatty, & Grubbs, 2015). These programs vary in how they are administered but include a veteran NICU parent who provides peer support to the current NICU parent. Trained former NICU parents can support current NICU family functioning through a variety of roles (Bourque et al., 2018).

Dyadic Interventions

Dyadic interventions focus on increasing parents' understanding of their infant's cues and care needs, as well as increasing physical contact between the parent and infant as a means of decreasing parental stress and increasing parent sensitivity in interactions (see Table 7). Promoting parental sensitivity and responsiveness are crucial to promoting secure parent-infant attachment, which in turn has direct implications for infant health and child development (Hoffman et al., 2017). In the NICU, parents often lack understanding of their medically fragile infant's cues and have more difficulty establishing their parental role, although education is related to increased sensitivity during interactions and decreased parenting stress (Browne & Talmi, 2005). Increasing positive physical interactions between parent and infant has been found to decrease maternal anxiety and depression (Welch et al., 2016), and kangaroo care (KC), or skin-to-skin mother-infant holding, is a well-studied intervention with numerous benefits to infant regulation and health indicators (Boundy et al., 2016) as well as parental mood and role for both mothers (Athanasopoulou & Fox, 2014) and fathers (Cong et al., 2015; Varela, Tessier, Tarabulsy, & Pierce, 2018). These approaches require coordination with nursing and developmental therapists, who are critical for implementation.

Infant Interventions

Hospitalized infants are unique among pediatric patients in that they endure a multitude of atypical sensory experiences, including painful and intrusive sensations, at a time when their sensory systems are undergoing rapid development. Both

Table 6 Treatment approaches for NICU parents

Treatment	Common NICU targets	Special considerations
Cognitive behavioral therapy/acceptance and commitment therapy	*Cognitive targets*: • Perseveration about infant's risk of not surviving • Sense of responsibility/guilt for infant's condition • Thoughts that the infant's course reflects the parent being "punished" for prior behavior/decisions • Viewing self as a "bad," "irrelevant," or "unnecessary" parent • Irrational thoughts about hospital/provider role in infant's illness • Perseveration on a specific aspect of infant's care/management • Concern sibling will be emotionally harmed due to less parent attention • Expectations that the parent's partner will utilize the same coping strategies *Behavioral targets*: • Decrease avoidance of the hospital or infant • Decrease avoidance of support system/build additional supports • Decrease excessive hygiene behaviors designed to avoid germ exposure • Build self-care, including eating, sleeping, exposure to sunlight, light exercise, and medical follow-up • Establishing an adaptive daily routine • Build engagement in pleasurable activities • Build effective communication with partner, supports, and NICU teams	• Fears for infant survival may be rational as medical acuity can shift suddenly • Likewise, infection is a real threat for ill infants, but preventative behaviors can be out of proportion to the threat • For some parents, behaviors during pregnancy or genetic contributions may be known factors in the infant's illness or hospitalization • The traumatic pregnancy/birth/NICU experience can increase automatic negative thoughts • Parents' perseverative or irrational thoughts related to infant care often have a foundation in an actual event or a breakdown in communication with providers • NICU parents have difficulty utilizing their pre-existing support network as they feel their friends and family cannot relate to NICU life • NICU parents have limited time for self-care, further truncated by pumping • Access to healthy meals decreases in the hospital • Postpartum mothers may have movement restrictions
Relaxation techniques	• Deep breathing • Progressive muscle relaxation • Mindfulness • Guided imagery • Use of music therapy • Use of yoga	• Teach away from bedside to avoid distractions • Guide in implementing techniques at bedside • Be aware of body sensitivity among postpartum mothers
Trauma-informed CBT	• Include the development of a trauma narrative using journaling or scrapbooking	• Although prior unrelated traumatic experiences should be acknowledged, the NICU setting is insufficient to provide adequate treatment to fully address them • Crisis intervention may be more appropriate in the height of ongoing traumatic experiences
Psychoeducation	• Knowledge of preterm/ill infant's appearance, behaviors, development, and competencies • Knowledge of mental health diagnoses including PMADs and PTSD	• Consider providing a group format to provide opportunities for parent-to-parent support. • See Appendix 4 for parent educational resources
Bereavement support	• Support for processing prior pregnancy/infant losses • Support for coping with loss of twin or triplet sibling	• Parent may be able to process some aspects of the loss(es), although other aspects may be too difficult to address until after the discharge of the current NICU patient

Table 7 Treatment approaches for NICU parent-infant dyads

Intervention	Special considerations
Kangaroo care/ skin-to-skin care/ holding infant	• Parents can safely hold intubated infants if the NICU team judges medically appropriate • Preterm infants should be held for at least 1 h to maximize the benefit given the stress of the transitions
Developmentally supportive touch	• Psychologists guide parents, along with nursing and developmental therapists, in providing containment touch, facilitating tucking, hand-holding, and pacifier access • Parents can physically support infants during painful/intrusive procedures to promote infant regulation and improve parental confidence
Participation in routine care	• Parents should be encouraged to participate in diaper changes, mouth care, taking infant's temperature, etc. as early as possible to promote parental confidence
Infant massage	• Typically used for more stable, older preterm infants • Requires training in infant massage to teach parents
Use of scent cloths	• Parents and infants exchange cloths with their scents to promote bonding (can also be used with siblings)
Infant-directed speech	• Storybook reading, singing, and speaking to infants create routines and opportunities for positive parent-infant interactions
Parent psychoeducation	• Providing education regarding infant's reflexes, cues, competencies, and sleep-wake patterns enhances parents' abilities to respond sensitively to their needs
Use of pictures and videoconferencing	• Parents who are unable to visit the NICU on a regular basis should be provided with pictures of their infant to facilitate a sense of connectedness and bonding • Web cameras or videoconferencing approaches can also help parents connect from afar but should not be considered a substitute for in-person visits

over- and under-sensory stimulations can confer additional risk for these patients who are at the highest at risk for poor neurodevelopmental outcomes (Rein, 2008). A recent review of sensory-based interventions found that KC and language/music stimulation administered to the infant, as well as multimodal sensory interventions, were the most effective for improving infant development (Pineda et al., 2017).

Although sleep is known to be important for neurodevelopment and learning across the lifespan, sleep disruption is common in the hospital setting. A systematic review of sleep interventions in the NICU concluded that more research is needed to make empirically based recommendations in this area (van den Hoogen et al., 2017). However, psychologists can help promote appropriate infant sleep patterns by recommending (1) clustered nursing care to avoid repeated disruption; (2) cycled lighting for infants who do not require an isolette cover; (3) avoidance of unneeded nighttime interventions; (4) a simple but consistent bedtime routine once an infant is about 2 months of age and sedating medications are minimized; and (5) tracking of sleep patterns with a simple sleep log if difficulties persist to identify targets for intervention.

Nursing Support

The professional with the largest role in the daily care of the infant and family in the NICU is the bedside nurse. Due to the emotionally demanding nature of this work, the consulting psychologist will undoubtedly be asked to provide support to nurses caring for families (Hall, Cross, et al., 2015). As many as half of NICU nurses have been found to report moderate-severe levels of secondary traumatic stress, and over a third met criteria for PTSD (Beck, Cusson, & Gable, 2017), which is a level similar to NICU parents themselves. The ability to debrief and seek assistance from a mental health professional were listed by nurses as helpful in coping with trauma. Another potentially beneficial model of delivering support to NICU nurses lies in establishing an ongoing reflective supervision group lead by a mental health professional (Lorrain, 2016). Administration must support this work by protecting nurses' time to participate.

Adaptation

It is important to acknowledge that despite attempts to deliver evidence-based treatments to parents of NICU infants, challenges exist to providing treatment in the consistent, sequential, and comprehensive manner tested in empirical studies. Changes in the medical disposition of the infant from week to week can influence parental distress as well as interest in engaging with treatment. The infant may also be discharged or transferred prior to meeting treatment goals with parents. Therefore, therapeutic approaches must have the flexibility to be delivered in various sequences that are most sensitive to the family's changing needs, and brief interventions may be advantageous (Mendelson et al., 2017). It is also helpful if interventions can be delivered either away from or at the bedside depending on parental preference and the NICU environment. Treatment in a group setting may offer the advantage of providing peer-to-peer support along with access to a trained mental health professional. Digital health approaches may offer greater accessibility for parents who cannot be at the hospital during typical work hours due to their own work responsibilities, transportation challenges, or caregiving for other children.

Clinicians must also be sensitive to individual differences in parents' physical and emotional resources, family structures, cultures, fertility/loss history, and beliefs about their infants and parenting roles. Parents may hold different beliefs about the role of the mother, father, and grandparents in the physical care of the infant, which impacts strategies used to enhance parent-infant attachment. The clinician must take care not to make assumptions about these roles but rather determine these factors for each family as part of treatment planning.

Resources/Support

Psychologists in the NICU are required to have a diverse set of clinical skills. Experience with adult and child psychopathology, family systems, health psychology, and child development are essential for appropriate psychological conceptualization, assessment, and intervention in the NICU (Hynan et al., 2015). Pediatric psychologists must consider their scope of practice as their training will likely vary in delivering a full range of interventions to parents, infants, and dyads. Pediatric psychologists are essential in promoting parental coping with infant hospitalization, which will necessarily involve intervening with parent symptoms such as depressed mood, anxiety, traumatic responses, and poor sleep. They may also be called upon to provide safety and risk assessment and crisis intervention. When parents demonstrate clinical level of psychiatric symptoms, pediatric psychologists play a key role in educating parents about adult mental health providers and facilitating referrals to them. In these cases, pediatric and adult clinicians play complementary roles in providing comprehensive care for NICU parents. If parents are willing to sign a release of information form, communication between providers can further enhance care.

To successfully provide services in the NICU, psychologists benefit from the support of the multi-disciplinary team for their role, physical resources such as space, and a plan for financial sustainability. To gain the necessary support, psychologists should not only engage neonatology leadership in understanding the value of their role but also spend time gathering information from other NICU staff who have potentially overlapping roles, such as social workers, nurse specialists, or developmental specialists. These partnerships are critical in order to identify ways for psychologists to complement rather than conflict with existing supports.

Physically, it can be difficult for psychologists to find space to meet with a family privately. Although this is changing, many NICUs do not have private rooms, and patients are in an "open bay" with several patients in the same space. If the infant is in a shared space, offering to meet privately in a room with a door respects the family's right to confidentiality and allows for sharing of sensitive information. Stepping away from the bedside can also be quite helpful to avoid distractions from the infant's monitors and avoid interruptions. However, when it is appropriate, meeting at bedside can help minimize parental separation from the infant, which may be very important, particularly for parents with limited time to visit.

Financial support of psychologists' time in the NICU is another important consideration. Given recent recognition of psychological distress among families of hospitalized infants, there is a growing trend for psychologists to have time dedicated to the NICU. A portion of the psychologist's salary may be supported by the institution or through grant funding. For psychologists who bill for services, health and behavior codes may potentially be used for assessment and intervention services, as services are provided in relation to the infant's medical diagnosis (Lines, Douglas, Angalet, & Pendley, 2012). Developmental or psychological testing codes can also be used for assessment of the infant. However, payment for these codes likely varies by state and insurance carrier. Therefore, psychologists need to work closely with the hospital billing and compliance departments to determine the most appropriate codes. These departments also provide guidance about required elements so that psychologists comply while documenting in the infant's chart yet avoid divulging details that will unnecessarily compromise parental privacy.

Outpatient Consultation

It is widely recognized that hospitalized infants and their families are at risk for ongoing challenges after NICU discharge. NICU follow-up clinics are multi-disciplinary and provide a range of medical, developmental, and psychosocial services over the first few years of life (Bockli, Andrews, Pellerite, & Meadow, 2014; Kuppala, Tabangin, Haberman, Steichen, & Yolton, 2012). Psychologists are well positioned to provide comprehensive assessment of NICU graduates beginning in infancy and extending throughout childhood. However, given the specialization required to assess neurodevelopment in infants and young children, most clinics include an embedded psychologist rather than utilizing a member of the consultation-liaison team. NICU graduates are known to be at risk for developmental delay, intellectual disability, learning disabilities, autism spectrum disorder, cerebral palsy, attention-deficit/hyperactivity disorder, sensory processing difficulties, social skill deficits, feeding disorders, anxiety disorders, and depression (Nosarti, Murray, & Hack, 2010). Therefore, assessment of all developmental domains is important, including: cognition and learning; play; language; motor; social; emotional; behavior; adaptive skills; and relationships. Early identification and diagnosis are important for access to early interventions and improved outcomes. Results from assessments facilitate anticipatory guidance with parents to promote developmental progress and prompt advocacy for their child's needs with early intervention programs, school systems, and outpatient providers. Assessment results also aid in decision-making about needed diagnostic workups (e.g., neurologic imaging or genetic testing) or specialist referrals (e.g., audiology, ophthalmology, and sleep or feeding clinics).

Psychologists further assess family functioning in follow-up clinics, including parental adjustment to their infant/child's medical needs and conduct parent mental health screening. Results of family screening and assessments allow for psychoeducation about the presence of concerns, the importance of parents' own mental health in their child's health and well-being, and the role that parent mental health treatment can have in improving outcomes.

Case Example

Sam Jones is a former 24-week preterm infant and surviving twin. His twin sister died suddenly in the NICU at 3 months of age from an infection. Sam has a 5-year-old brother. Sam required a several months NICU stay due to complications of extreme prematurity, including severe chronic lung disease, pulmonary hypertension, and reflux. He needed prolonged ventilator support and was several weeks post-term age when he was successfully extubated to CPAP and gradually weaned to oxygen via nasal cannula. Sam's continued feeding difficulties resulted in surgery to have a G-tube placed. The nurses caring for Sam noticed that Mrs. Jones was frequently mentioning the strain of managing Sam's long hospitalization along with her older son's needs and the impact of these factors on her relationship with

Mr. Jones. The nurses were unsure how to support Mrs. Jones and asked the unit social worker to consult psychology. The psychologist conducted an initial assessment and provided weekly intervention for the remainder of Sam's stay in the NICU and step-down unit. Mrs. Jones expressed difficulty sleeping due to waking with anxiety and trouble remembering to eat meals. Her range of affect was restricted, and she reported limited engagement in enjoyable activities. Mrs. Jones denied suicidal or homicidal ideation and reported a hopeful future orientation regarding bringing Sam home. She expressed a clear emotional investment in Sam, describing him as "strong" and a "fighter." She read to him and spoke to him often. She presented to the hospital appropriately groomed and dressed each day and participated in her son's care. Mrs. Jones was initially avoidant of discussing Sam's twin sister, stating that she "tried not to think about her" and refused to take the keepsakes that the nurses had made for her. Mrs. Jones reported stressors in her support system, with feedback from her family that perpetuated her feelings of self-blame for the loss of Sam's twin and feeling that she was not a "good mother" to Sam or his older brother. She reported no mental health history and reported that she used to be a "happy person."

The psychologist conceptualized Mrs. Jones's presentation as related to bereavement, with features of post-traumatic stress, and family relationship problems. Initial therapy approaches focused on improving self-care through cognitive behavioral approaches including anxiety reduction techniques for sleep and setting reminders for meals. It was difficult for Mrs. Jones to prioritize engaging in enjoyable activities, although some activities such as eating lunch outside for 20 minutes and listening to music were incorporated. Cognitive restructuring was used to identify automatic thoughts about her parenting and examining the evidence that she was a good mother. After this initial phase of treatment, trauma-informed approaches were utilized to help Mrs. Jones stop avoiding thoughts and feelings about her deceased daughter. Scrapbooking was offered to help Mrs. Jones create a narrative of her daughter's life, and she was encouraged to begin to discuss her feelings of loss, as well as how to help her older son process the loss through participation in grief therapy. After discharge, Sam was seen in the neonatal follow-up clinic. Testing revealed mild global developmental delays in infancy and toddlerhood but with progress toward catch-up. Mrs. Jones was counseled about early intervention and outpatient developmental intervention services that would benefit Sam, as well as how to facilitate his skills at home. Mental health screening for Mrs. Jones revealed continued clinically significant post-traumatic stress symptoms. Mrs. Jones was counseled about the importance of seeking further mental health evaluation and treatment. She acknowledged distress but expressed she did not have time to pursue her own therapy due to Sam's medical follow-up appointments. The psychologist helped to engage Mrs. Jones in problem-solving about how she might be able to find time and emphasizing the benefit to Sam of her own self-care. The social worker was enlisted to help identify insurance-compatible mental health providers in her community.

Conclusions

In sum, consultation to the NICU requires knowledge of both typical parent and infant adjustment in the perinatal period, as well as an understanding of the challenges that infant hospitalization poses at these times of great transition. While parents play a critical role with all pediatric patients, a focus on parents is especially critical in the NICU given that parents and infants have not yet had a chance to establish their relationship and that infants are entirely reliant on others to recognize and respond to their needs through their nonverbal cues. Pediatric psychologists are well suited to provide consultation services in the NICU due to their knowledge of child development, parenting, family systems, hospital systems, and emotional distress. Psychologists can provide direct interventions to improve coping an adaptation of individual families, as well as support the multi-disciplinary teams that care for critically ill infants to improve the families' experience at each stage of the NICU journey.

Appendix 1: Mental Health Screening Instruments Commonly Used for Parents of Infants

Screening tool	Domain assessed	Number of items	Public domain	Notes
Edinburgh Postpartum Depression Scale (EPDS)[a]	Postpartum depression	10	Yes	Available in several languages, contains suicidal ideation question
Postpartum Depression Screening Scale (PDSS)[b]	Postpartum depression	35	No	Contains suicidal ideation question, has total score and seven subscores
Public Health Questionnaire (PHQ-2, PHQ-9)[c]	Depression in the general population	2, 9	Yes	PHQ-2 uses the first two items of the PHQ-9. Lower specificity than others, available in several languages
Center for Epidemiological Studies Depression Scale (CES-D)[d]	Depression in the general population	20	Yes	Original does not have suicidal ideation question, revised version does
Columbia Suicide Severity Rating Scale (C-SSRS) lifetime/recent[e]	Suicide risk assessment	2–6, structured interview	Yes	Spanish versions available. Full-scale version also available for those who are trained
Impact of Events Scale—Revised (IES-R)[f]	Post-traumatic stress	22	Yes	Four symptom clusters
Davidson Trauma Scale[g]	Post-traumatic stress	17	No	Three symptom clusters
PTSD checklist for DSM-V (PCL-5)[h]	Post-traumatic stress	20	Yes	Items map onto DSM-V diagnostic criteria
Modified Perinatal Post-Traumatic Stress Disorder Questionnaire (Modified PPQ)	Perinatal specific post-traumatic stress	14	Yes	Maps onto three symptom clusters

[a]https://www.aap.org/en-us/advocacy-and-policy/aap-health-initiatives/practicing-safety/Documents/Postnatal%20Depression%20Scale.pdf
[b]https://www.wpspublish.com/store/p/2902/pdss-postpartum-depression-screening-scale
[c]https://www.phqscreeners.com/
[d]http://www.chcr.brown.edu/pcoc/cesdscale.pdf; http://cesd-r.com/
[e]http://cssrs.columbia.edu/the-columbia-scale-c-ssrs/about-the-scale/
[f]http://www.emdrhap.org/content/wp-content/uploads/2014/07/VIII E_Impact_of_Events_Scale_Revised.pdf
[g]https://www.mhs.com/MHS-Assessment?prodname=dts
[h]https://www.ptsd.va.gov/professional/assessment/adult-sr/ptsd-checklist.asp
[i](Callahan, Borja, & Hynan, 2006)

Appendix 2: Sample of Neurobehavioral and Developmental Assessment Measures for NICU Infants

Measure	Age range	Domains assessed
NICU Network Neurobehavioral Scale (NNNs)[a]	28–46-week gestational age	Neurological integrity Behavioral functioning Stress/abstinence
Neurobehavioral Assessment of the Preterm Infant (NAPI)[b]	32–40-week gestational age	Motor development Alertness and orientation Irritability
Assessment of Preterm Infants' Behavior (APIB)[c]	Birth–44-week gestation age	Autonomic Motor State organization Attention Self-regulation
Bayley Scales of Infant Development, Fourth edition[d]	1–42 months	Cognition Language (receptive and expressive) Motor (fine and gross) Social-emotional Adaptive
Mullen scales of early Learning[d]	1–68 months	Visual reception Fine motor Gross motor Receptive language Expressive language

[a]https://www.brown.edu/research/projects/children-at-risk/about
[b]http://med.stanford.edu/NAPI/methods.html
[c]https://nidcap.org/en/programs-and-certifications/apib-training/overview-3/
[d]https://www.pearsonassessments.com

Appendix 3: Suggested Resources for Psychologists Working with Families in the NICU

Source	Description
http://support4NICUparents.org	National Perinatal Association Clinician resources for working in the NICU (see "for professionals" section)
http://postpartum.net	Postpartum support international Provides resources and training for clinicians in perinatal mood and anxiety disorders
https://www.zerotothree.org	Zero to three Resources and training for professionals working with young children
Handbook of Infant Mental Health, 4th Edition, by Charles H Zeanah Jr. (2019)	Definitive text on the impact of early influences on young child mental health, including information about assessment, interventions, and systems
Neurodevelopmental Outcomes of Preterm Birth by Chiara Nosarti, Robin Murray, and Maureen Hack (2010)	Summarizes the literature on the impact of prematurity on children from infancy to adulthood
Cognitive Behavioral Therapy for Perinatal Distress by Amy Wenzel and Karen Kleiman (2014)	Provides clinicians with guidance on the use of CBT for emotional distress in the prenatal and postpartum periods
Trauma Informed Care in the Perinatal Period by Julia Seng and Julie Taylor (2015)	Provides guidance on infusing trauma-informed care into perinatal work

Appendix 4: Suggested Resources for Families in the NICU

Source	Description
http://marchofdimes.org	March of Dimes Resources and support for NICU families
http://support4NICUparents.org	National Perinatal Association Resources and tools for NICU parents (see "For Parents" section)
http://postpartum.net	Postpartum Support International Resources for parents about perinatal mood and anxiety disorders
http://www.p2pusa.org/	Parent to Parent USA Emotional support and information for families of children with special health needs through creating a match with an experienced mentor parent
http://www.unitegriefsupport.org/	Unite Inc. Grief support for miscarriage, stillbirth, and infant death
Understanding the NICU: What Parents of Preemies and other Hospitalized Newborns Need to Know by The American Academy of Pediatrics, edited by Jeanette Zaichkin, Gary Weiner, and David Loren (2016)	Comprehensive text to help families understand NICU medical terms and technology, major medical conditions and complications, and impact on parenting of having a hospitalized infant
NICU Journal: A Parent's Journey by the American Academy of Pediatrics (2017)	Practical parent education about hospitalized infants with places to record week-to-week milestones and progress
Preemies: The Essential Guide for Parents of Premature Babies, 2nd Edition, by Dana Wechsler Linden, Emma Trenti Paroli, and Mia Wechsler Doron (2010)	Information provided by parents and a neonatologist about prematurity, from risks for prematurity through considerations for discharge
Parenting Your Premature Baby and Child: The Emotional Journey by Deborah L. Davis and Mara Tesler Stein (2004)	Focuses on the range of emotional reactions that parents experience when dealing with their child's premature birth from prior to delivery through life after discharge, and provides considerations for ways to cope along the way

References

Athanasopoulou, E., & Fox, J. R. E. (2014). Effects of kangaroo mother care on maternal mood and interaction patterns between parents and their preterm, low birth weight infants: A systematic review: Kangaroo mother care, maternal mood, and parent–infant interact. *Infant Mental Health Journal, 35*(3), 245–262. https://doi.org/10.1002/imhj.21444

Beck, C. T., Cusson, R. M., & Gable, R. K. (2017). Secondary traumatic stress in NICU nurses: A mixed-methods study. *Advances in Neonatal Care, 17*(6), 478–488. https://doi.org/10.1097/ANC.0000000000000428

Bockli, K., Andrews, B., Pellerite, M., & Meadow, W. (2014). Trends and challenges in United States neonatal intensive care units follow-up clinics. *Journal of Perinatology, 34*(1), 71–74. https://doi.org/10.1038/jp.2013.136

Boundy, E. O., Dastjerdi, R., Spiegelman, D., Fawzi, W. W., Missmer, S. A., Lieberman, E., … Chan, G. J. (2016). Kangaroo mother care and neonatal outcomes: A meta-analysis. *Pediatrics, 137*(1), e20152238. https://doi.org/10.1542/peds.2015-2238

Bourque, C. J., Dahan, S., Mantha, G., Robson, K., Reichherzer, M., & Janvier, A. (2018). Improving neonatal care with the help of veteran resource parents: An overview of current practices. *Seminars in Fetal and Neonatal Medicine, 23*(1), 44–51. https://doi.org/10.1016/j.siny.2017.10.005

Browne, J. V., & Talmi, A. (2005). Family-based intervention to enhance infant-parent relationships in the neonatal intensive care unit. *Journal of Pediatric Psychology, 30*(8), 667–677. https://doi.org/10.1093/jpepsy/jsi053

Callahan, J. L., Borja, S. E., & Hynan, M. T. (2006). Modification of the Perinatal PTSD Questionnaire to enhance clinical utility. *Journal of Perinatology, 26*, 533–539.

Cong, X., Ludington-Hoe, S. M., Hussain, N., Cusson, R. M., Walsh, S., Vazquez, V., … Vittner, D. (2015). Parental oxytocin responses during skin-to-skin contact in pre-term infants. *Early Human Development, 91*(7), 401–406. https://doi.org/10.1016/j.earlhumdev.2015.04.012

D'Agostino, J. A., Gerdes, M., Hoffman, C., Manning, M. L., Phalen, A., & Bernbaum, J. (2013). Provider use of corrected age during health supervision visits for premature infants. *Journal of Pediatric Health Care, 27*(3), 172–179. https://doi.org/10.1016/j.pedhc.2011.09.001

Gilboa, S. M., Devine, O. J., Kucik, J. E., Oster, M. E., Riehle-Colarusso, T., Nembhard, W. N., … Marelli, A. J. (2016). Congenital heart defects in the United States: Estimating the magnitude of the affected population in 2010. *Circulation, 134*(2), 101–109. https://doi.org/10.1161/CIRCULATIONAHA.115.019307

Hall, S. L., Cross, J., Selix, N. W., Patterson, C., Segre, L., Chuffo-Siewert, R., … Martin, M. L. (2015). Recommendations for enhancing psychosocial support of NICU parents through staff education and support. *Journal of Perinatology, 35*(Suppl. 1), S29–S36. https://doi.org/10.1038/jp.2015.147

Hall, S. L., Ryan, D. J., Beatty, J., & Grubbs, L. (2015). Recommendations for peer-to-peer support for NICU parents. *Journal of Perinatology, 35*(Suppl 1), S9–S13. https://doi.org/10.1038/jp.2015.143

Hoffman, C., Dunn, D. M., & Njoroge, W. F. M. (2017). Impact of postpartum mental illness upon infant development. *Current Psychiatry Reports, 19*(12), 100. https://doi.org/10.1007/s11920-017-0857-8

Hynan, M. T., Mounts, K. O., & Vanderbilt, D. L. (2013). Screening parents of high-risk infants for emotional distress: Rationale and recommendations. *Journal of Perinatology, 33*(10), 748–753. https://doi.org/10.1038/jp.2013.72

Hynan, M. T., Steinberg, Z., Baker, L., Cicco, R., Geller, P. A., Lassen, S., … Stuebe, A. (2015). Recommendations for mental health professionals in the NICU. *Journal of Perinatology, 35*(1), S14–S18. https://doi.org/10.1038/jp.2015.144

Kuppala, V. S., Tabangin, M., Haberman, B., Steichen, J., & Yolton, K. (2012). Current state of high-risk infant follow-up care in the United States: Results of a national survey of academic follow-up programs. *Journal of Perinatology, 32*(4), 293–298. https://doi.org/10.1038/jp.2011.97

Lefkowitz, D. S., Baxt, C., & Evans, J. R. (2010). Prevalence and correlates of posttraumatic stress and postpartum depression in parents of infants in the neonatal intensive care unit (NICU). *Journal of Clinical Psychology in Medical Settings, 17*(3), 230–237. https://doi.org/10.1007/s10880-010-9202-7

Lemons, J., Bauer, C. R., Oh, W., Korones, S., Papile, L., Stoll, B., … Stevenson, D. (2001). Very low birth weight outcomes of the National Institute of child health and human development neonatal research network, January 1995 through December 1996. NICHD Neonatal Research Network. *Pediatrics, 107*(1), E1.

Lines, M. M. T., Douglas, W., Angalet, G. B., & Pendley, J. S. (2012). Commentary: The use of health and behavior codes in pediatric psychology: Where are we now? *Journal of Pediatric Psychology, 37*(5), 486–490. https://doi.org/10.1093/jpepsy/jss045

Lorrain, B. (2016). Reflective peer consultation as an intervention for staff support in the NICU. *Newborn and Infant Nursing Reviews, 16*(4), 289–292. https://doi.org/10.1053/j.nainr.2016.09.022

Martin, J. A., & Osterman, M. J. K. (2018). Describing the increase in preterm births in the United States, 2014–2016. *NCHS Data Brief, 312*, 1–8.

McAdams, R. M., & Juul, S. E. (2016). Neonatal encephalopathy: Update on therapeutic hypothermia and other novel therapeutics. *Clinics in Perinatology, 43*(3), 485–500. https://doi.org/10.1016/j.clp.2016.04.007

McGivern, M. R., Best, K. E., Rankin, J., Wellesley, D., Greenlees, R., Addor, M.-C., ... Martos, C. (2015). Epidemiology of congenital diaphragmatic hernia in Europe: A register-based study. *Archives of Disease in Childhood-Fetal and Neonatal Edition, 100*(2), F137–F144. https://doi.org/10.1136/archdischild-2014-306174

Mendelson, T., Cluxton-Keller, F., Vullo, G. C., Tandon, S. D., & Noazin, S. (2017). NICU-based interventions to reduce maternal depressive and anxiety symptoms: A meta-analysis. *Pediatrics, 139*(3), e20161870. https://doi.org/10.1542/peds.2016-1870

Noble, Y., & Boyd, R. (2012). Neonatal assessments for the preterm infant up to 4 months corrected age: A systematic review. *Developmental Medicine & Child Neurology, 54*(2), 129–139. https://doi.org/10.1111/j.1469-8749.2010.03903.x

Nosarti, C., Murray, R. M., & Hack, M. (2010). Neurodevelopmental *outcomes of preterm birth: From childhood to adult life*. Cambridge: Cambridge University Press; 2010.

Patel, R. M., Rysavy, M. A., Bell, E. F., & Tyson, J. E. (2017). Survival of infants born at periviable gestational ages. *Clinical Perinatology, 44*, 287–303.

Pineda, R., Guth, R., Herring, A., Reynolds, L., Oberle, S., & Smith, J. (2017). Enhancing sensory experiences for very preterm infants in the NICU: An integrative review. *Journal of Perinatology, 37*(4), 323–332. https://doi.org/10.1038/jp.2016.179

Rein, C. (2008). In D. M. Teti (Ed.), *NICU-based interventions for high-risk infants* (pp. 295–315). Oxford: Blackwell Publishing Ltd.

Roque, A. T. F., Lasiuk, G. C., Radünz, V., & Hegadoren, K. (2017). Scoping review of the mental health of parents of infants in the NICU. *Journal of Obstetric, Gynecologic & Neonatal Nursing, 46*(4), 576–587. https://doi.org/10.1016/j.jogn.2017.02.005

Stephens, B. E., & Vohr, B. R. (2009). Neurodevelopmental outcome of the premature infant. *Pediatric Clinics of North America, 56*(3), 631–646. https://doi.org/10.1016/j.pcl.2009.03.005

Tolia, V. N., Patrick, S. W., Bennett, M. M., Murthy, K., Sousa, J., Smith, P. B., ... Spitzer, A. R. (2015). Increasing incidence of the neonatal abstinence syndrome in US neonatal ICUs. *The New England Journal of Medicine, 372*(22), 2118–2126. https://doi.org/10.1056/NEJMsa1500439

Totapally, B., Youngblut, J. M., Cantwell, G. P., Moral, T. d., & Brooten, D. (2013). Parent health and functioning 13 months after infant or child NICU/PICU death (neonatal intensive care unit/pediatric intensive care unit). *Pediatrics, 132*(5), e1295.

van den Hoogen, A., Teunis, C. J., Shellhaas, R. A., Pillen, S., Benders, M., & Dudink, J. (2017). How to improve sleep in a neonatal intensive care unit: A systematic review. *Early Human Development, 113*, 78–86.

Varela, N., Tessier, R., Tarabulsy, G., & Pierce, T. (2018). Cortisol and blood pressure levels decreased in fathers during the first hour of skin-to-skin contact with their premature babies. *Acta Paediatrica, 107*(4), 628–632. https://doi.org/10.1111/apa.14184

Welch, M. G., Halperin, M. S., Austin, J., Stark, R. I., Hofer, M. A., Hane, A. A., & Myers, M. M. (2016). Depression and anxiety symptoms of mothers of preterm infants are decreased at 4 months corrected age with Family Nurture Intervention in the NICU. *Archives of Women's Mental Health, 19*(1), 51–61. https://doi.org/10.1007/s00737-015-0502-7

Wilson, R. D. M. D. (2014). Prenatal screening, diagnosis, and pregnancy management of fetal neural tube defects. *Journal of Obstetrics and Gynaecology Canada (JOGC), 36*(10), 927–939. https://doi.org/10.1016/S1701-2163(15)30444-8

Pediatric Oncology

Stacy R. Flowers, Aimee K. Hildenbrand, and Jennifer A. Hansen-Moore

A remarkable advancement in evidence-based psychosocial oncology care occurred when the Standards for Psychosocial Care for Children with Cancer and Their Families were published (Wiener, Kazak, Noll, Patenaude, & Kupst, 2015). With support from the Mattie Miracle Cancer Foundation (www.mattiemiracle.com), pediatric oncology psychosocial professionals collaboratively developed 15 standards for services considered essential for *all* youth with cancer and their families. These universal standards can help guide psychosocial oncology clinical practice, and readers are strongly encouraged to review them in conjunction with this chapter.

S. R. Flowers (✉)
Family Medicine Residency, Dayton, OH, USA

Department of Family Medicine, Boonshoft School of Medicine, Dayton, OH, USA

Wright State University, Dayton, OH, USA
e-mail: stacy.flowers@wright.edu

A. K. Hildenbrand
Nemours/AI duPont Hospital for Children, Wilmington, DE, USA

Division of Behavioral Health, Center for Healthcare Delivery Science, New York, NY, USA

J. A. Hansen-Moore
Department of Pediatric Psychology and Neuropsychology, Nationwide Children's Hospital, Columbus, OH, USA

Department of Pediatrics, The Ohio State University College of Medicine, Columbus, OH, USA

Diagnosis

Cancer is an umbrella term for a group of diseases involving abnormal cells that continuously divide and spread, sometimes forming tumors and invading nearby tissues. Cancer is relatively rare in youth, with approximately 16,000 diagnosed annually in the United States. Among children from birth to age 14, common cancers include leukemias, central nervous system (CNS) tumors, lymphomas and reticuloendothelial neoplasms, sarcomas, and neuroblastoma. For youth ages 15–19, frequently occurring cancers include lymphomas, CNS tumors, leukemias, germ cell and gonadal tumors, and thyroid cancer. Despite its low incidence, pediatric cancer is the leading cause of disease-related mortality among youth in the United States.

Presenting symptoms of pediatric cancer are typically nonspecific and mimic common childhood conditions; these symptoms can include fever, fatigue, headaches, bone, joint, muscle, or abdominal pain, nausea, vomiting, diarrhea, constipation, sore throat, bruising, and nosebleeds. As a result of its rarity and the ambiguity of initial symptoms, childhood cancer is often challenging to diagnose in its early stages. Unfortunately, delays in diagnosis can result in

B. D. Carter, K. A. Kullgren (eds.), *Clinical Handbook of Psychological Consultation in Pediatric Medical Settings*, Issues in Clinical Child Psychology, https://doi.org/10.1007/978-3-030-35598-2_23

poorer prognosis, increased therapy intensity, and greater risk of medical complications. Once a cancer diagnosis is suspected, youth are typically referred to pediatric cancer centers, which offer multidisciplinary resources to provide the most accurate diagnosis, appropriate therapies, supportive care, and long-term follow-up. Diagnostic workup can include clinical, laboratory, and specialized imaging studies. However, a definitive cancer diagnosis can only be made via pathologic confirmation.

Many families describe the initial evaluation of symptoms, referral to a pediatric cancer center, and further diagnostic workup as a frightening, confusing, and overwhelming process. Particularly when symptoms have persisted for weeks or months, families report feelings of guilt, regret, anger, frustration, and desperation (Evans, Wakefield, McLoone, & Cohn, 2015). Experiences of misdiagnosis and diagnostic delays may contribute to family distrust in clinicians. When receiving the definitive diagnosis, parents frequently report emotional turmoil (e.g., disbelief, grief, fear), which can hinder their ability to process and retain important diagnostic, prognostic, and treatment information and make complex medical decisions.

Medical Basics

Most childhood cancers are treated using a multimodal approach, with specific treatments (e.g., surgery, radiation, chemotherapy, hematopoietic stem cell transplantation (HSCT)) selected based on cancer type and stage. Treatment frequently occurs in specialized cancer centers, where many youth participate in multicenter clinical trials that involve standardized treatment protocols. Duration, frequency, and intensity of treatment varies based on the type of cancer. Due to advancements in pediatric cancer care, survival rates in the United States have risen considerably over the past three decades. Currently, over 80% of youth survive at least 5 years following diagnosis, although there is significant variability based on cancer type and age at diagnosis with adolescents generally experiencing poorer survival rates than children.

Youth undergoing cancer treatment may experience numerous disease complications and treatment side effects. These can include pain, nausea, vomiting, diarrhea, constipation, anorexia and malnutrition, fatigue, hair loss, myelosuppression (i.e., decreased bone marrow activity, resulting in fewer platelets and blood cells) and associated infections, bleeding, sleep disturbances, and respiratory distress. These symptoms and complications are associated with impaired quality of life for youth with cancer.

Childhood cancer survivors may experience treatment-related complications long after active therapy ends. Physical late effects can include cataracts, hearing loss, dental abnormalities, obesity, hypothyroidism, cardiovascular, pulmonary, hepatic, and renal dysfunction, infertility, musculoskeletal growth problems, and secondary cancers. In fact, 75% of survivors have at least one chronic health condition, and 40% experience a severe, disabling, or fatal late effect by 30 years post diagnosis (Landier, Armenian, Meadows, & Bhatia, 2015). Additionally, survivors may experience neurocognitive sequelae such as impairments in learning, attention, processing speed, memory, executive functioning, and verbal, visual spatial, and perceptual skills, particularly those who received chemotherapy and/or cranial radiation early in childhood. A subset of survivors also experience long-term psychosocial challenges, including anxiety, depression, posttraumatic stress, and compromised social functioning (Bitsko et al., 2016). As a result, survivors frequently receive oncology follow-up care in the years after treatment termination to monitor potential recurrent and secondary cancers, assess short- and long-term complications, and receive health maintenance counseling and treatment for late effects.

Engagement

Engaging children with cancer and their families in psychosocial interventions can be challenging, particularly around the time of diagnosis and early treatment stages when parents endorse elevated distress, significant scheduling demands, and a singular focus on "survival" and the immediate needs of the child (Hocking et al., 2014). However, many families also report a need for psychosocial support within the first several months after a child's diagnosis (Hocking et al., 2014). Early initiation of psychological consultation can reduce family resistance, aid in developing rapport and trust between the clinician and family, and address or prevent psychological factors from impeding medical treatment. Clinicians can enhance family engagement in psychosocial interventions in the early phase after diagnosis by adopting a flexible, value-based approach, which allows patients and families to identify areas of concern or priority. In particular, early consultation efforts should seek to normalize families' emotional experiences, provide psychoeducation, and offer concrete and practical strategies focused on reducing immediate distress and facilitating adaptive coping.

Youth and family buy-in for psychological consultation may also be enhanced when psychologists are integrated members of the oncology care team and psychosocial supports are presented as components of standard care. This can help reduce stigma associated with mental health services. In addition, such integration enables psychologists to communicate and collaborate more effectively with other members of the care team and to provide multimodal interventions that are tailored to the child and family's needs throughout the course of treatment.

Case Formulation

The initial consultation serves as an opportunity to build rapport, efficiently gather information about a patient and family's history and current functioning across domains, and address emerging or ongoing concerns. See Table 1 (Appendix) for suggested domains to assess with sample questions. Ongoing systematic assessment and consultation across the treatment trajectory is recommended as patients and families are dynamic and constantly changing.

Providers should complete a thorough chart review prior to meeting the family to ensure understanding of significant medical results, diagnosis, prognosis, and treatment plan. Consulting with the medical team prior to meeting with the family may also inform providers about how to best approach patients and families. For example, if a patient or caregiver is slow to warm up, is reluctant to engage with new providers, or is wary of unexpected visitors, providers may wish to stop in briefly to introduce themselves and schedule a time to return based on family preference. These families may also benefit from warm handoffs or joint sessions with familiar providers.

When beginning a consultation, it is important for psychologists to introduce themselves, provide information about their role, and discuss the psychosocial services available. Clinicians should also convey that the consultation involves gathering information about current and past functioning across various domains. Patients and families are often open to sharing their stories of how the child came to be diagnosed with cancer. Allowing patients and families to share their experience is frequently an effective way to build rapport and communicate empathy. From there, it is a natural transition to engage in a conversation about other suggested domains (detailed below). In the oncology setting, a thorough consult may take a few sessions to complete; rarely is all information gathered in one meeting.

It is important to note that the goal of the consult should not be to get as much information from the patient and family as possible. Rather, the ultimate purpose of the initial consult is to begin building a relationship infused with rapport, trust, value, and meaning that will enable the multidisciplinary team to provide high-quality oncology care for the child and family. When a consult is placed, it is often during a time of great vulnerability for families. The interactions between providers and families in the initial consult can set the tone for ongoing treatment. Deciding what information is of highest priority to obtain in an initial consultation can assist clinicians to appropriately balance rapport building with information gathering.

Demographic Data Knowing the patient's age and developmental level will help prepare the provider for the most likely areas of concern.

Table 1 Specific domains to assess with sample questions

Domains to assess	Specific content	Sample questions for parent	Sample questions for child or AYA
Demographic	Age Gender Race and ethnicity Language Disability status	What do you prefer to be called? What does your child prefer to be called? Are you more comfortable speaking in English or another language?	What do you prefer to be called? Do you have any nicknames that you want us to use? Are you more comfortable speaking in English or another language?
Medical history	Previous/chronic illnesses Injuries Surgeries Medications Family medical history	Tell me about your child's medical history. Any previous health problems? Chronic illnesses? Serious injuries? Surgeries? Does your child take any medications? If so, how does your child do with taking medication? What aspects are most challenging? How does your child do with treatment, hospitalization, and providers? Has anyone in the family ever been diagnosed with cancer? Does the patient know anyone who has been diagnosed with cancer? If so, what was the outcome? Tell me about your family medical history, both maternal and paternal sides of the family.	Are you generally healthy or have you been sick a lot? Have you been hurt or injured so badly that you had to go to the hospital? What happened? Have you ever spent the night in the hospital before? What for? How was that? Do you take any medicine? If no, have you in the past? What for? What is the hardest part of taking medicine for you?
Current medical	Diagnosis Location Results of physical exam/vitals Lab results Medications Symptoms Treatment plan Treatment modalities Staging/prognosis Coping with hospitalization Late effects	What is your understanding of why your child is in the hospital? What information do you know? What information are you waiting for? What has your child been told? What have other family members been told? Where is your child's cancer? What type of cancer is it? Has the team talked to you about treatment? How long will it last? What will it involve? (chemotherapy, surgery, radiation, transplant) Have you talked to the team about your child's prognosis? What have they said?	Why are you in the hospital? What have you been told? Do you know what it is called? Where is your (cancer, tumor, bump)? What is the plan for treatment? What do you think will happen? What questions do you have for your team? What do you wish you had more information about? How are you dealing with being in the hospital?

Physical	Current physical functioning Past physical functioning Ability for Self-Care/ADLs Changes Since Onset of Diagnosis Side effects Appetite Sleep Energy Pain Nausea/vomiting Symptom management Physical appearance changes Sex drive (if appropriate) Fertility	What physical changes have you noticed since your child has been diagnosed? What does your child do independently? Has any of that changed recently? How is s/he sleeping? Eating/drinking? How has his/her energy level been? What side effects has your child experienced? Have you noticed any changes in your child's physical appearance?	What has changed since you've been diagnosed? How are you sleeping? Eating/drinking? How has your energy level been? Have you had any physical problems since being in the hospital?
Family	Primary caregiver Family size Family members Family dynamics Financial resources Parent dyad Parent coping and adjustment Sibling coping and adjustment Changes in roles and responsibilities Family communication Family stressors Current or past intimate partner violence Involvement of children's services Substance misuse Incarcerations	Who do you live with? Who else lives at home? Are there other important caregivers or family members who reside outside of the home? How would you describe your relationship with partner/patient/other children? How would you describe your family? How would you describe the home environment? How have family roles changed since diagnosis? What changes in family roles do you anticipate? Are there any extended family members or friends who will provide support during treatment? Any other ongoing stressors for your family? e.g., poor support system, low health literacy, substance misuse, unstable housing, Children's Services involvement, previous traumatic experiences, current/past abuse, unreliable transportation, divorce, new sibling, financial issues, distance from hospital, insurance issues, death/grief, family member medical issues, recent move, legal issues, untreated mental health issues, unemployment	Who lives at your house? Who mostly takes care of you? Who do you like to take care of you when you don't feel well? How do you get along with your parent(s)? Brothers/sisters? Others who live in the home? How do your parents get along with each other? Do you like being at home? Why or why not? What's the best thing about your family? What do you like least about your family? What about your family makes you happy? Sad? Mad? Scared? Excited? If you are feeling angry, mad, sad, or happy who do you want to tell first? Do people in your family keep a lot to themselves or do they tell each other everything? What has been stressful at home?

(continued)

Table 1 (continued)

Domains to assess	Specific content	Sample questions for parent	Sample questions for child or AYA
Emotional	Current/past mental health history Family mental health history (current/past diagnosis, treatment, management) Changes to mood (state and trait) Coping with diagnosis, treatment, prognosis Coping with physical functioning, side effects, physical appearance changes Comfort with disclosure of diagnosis Coping of patient and caregivers Personality Substance misuse Current/past suicide ideation, plans, attempts Self-harm Current/past trauma Current stressors	Tell me about your family mental health history, both maternal and paternal sides of your family. Anxiety? Depression? Alcohol or drug use? Trauma? How have you coped with your child's diagnosis? How has your child coped? How have siblings coped? How have other caregivers coped with diagnosis? What has been the hardest thing for you? For your child? For others in the family? Who do you think is having the most difficulty coping? How do you deal with stress? Do you tend to talk about things or keep things to yourself? Do you have someone you can talk to about how you are feeling? What are you most worried about? What do you think your child is most worried about? What has been the hardest thing for you since your child was diagnosed? Has anything good come from your child's diagnosis?	Are you a worrier? If yes, What do you worry most about? Do you tend to keep your feelings inside or do you talk to others? Who do you talk to? How have you coped with your diagnosis? Have you told anyone? What did you say? What do you think your parents are most worried about? Who has this been the hardest for? How would you describe your mood? Have you been feeling down/blue/sad recently? What about in the past? What kinds of things make you feel happy? Sad? Mad? Scared? Has anything good come from your cancer? Have things ever been so bad that you thought of hurting yourself or tried to hurt yourself?
Cognitive	Thought content Understanding of disease Health beliefs Attitudes and expectations (illness, treatment, health care providers) Meaning of illness Philosophy of life Intelligence Information preferences	What kinds of things do you find yourself thinking about your child's diagnosis, treatment, or prognosis? Tell me your understanding of the disease, treatment, and prognosis. How do you think your child came to be diagnosed with this disease? What do you expect will happen? Do you tend to be an optimist or pessimist? How much control do you think you have over your child's treatment and prognosis? What is your attitude towards treatment? Towards your child's oncology team? Towards the hospital? Have you been able to make any meaning of why your child was diagnosed with cancer? What is your highest level of education? Was school difficult for you? Did you ever have any struggles with reading or writing? Are you someone who likes to have all the information or would you rather be told just what you need to understand the "big picture?" How do you prefer to have information given to you (written, spoken, visual)? Who do you want information shared with? Who do you want present during discussions with the medical team?	When you think about your cancer, what kinds of things do you wonder about? What do you know about cancer? What do you know about why kids get cancer? Why do you think kids get cancer? What kinds of things do you have control over? What do you think will happen after treatment? Do you like to know all the information or would you rather have just a little bit at a time? Do you tend to remember things really easily or does it help to have information repeated? Do you remember information better if it is written down, spoken, or visual? Do you feel comfortable asking the doctors questions? Sometimes kids like to talk to the doctors alone because they are worried they will upset their parents if they ask certain questions or have things they want to talk about in private. Have you ever wanted to talk to the doctors alone? Do you like to get updates from the doctors or from your parents?

Social	Support system Peer relationships History of teasing/bullying Intimate relationships Disclosure/increased attention Social media involvement Hobbies/interests Extracurricular activities Relationship with treatment team	Tell me about your support system. Who do you go to for support? Do you have people who you can tell everything or do you tend to keep things to yourself? Tell me about your child's support system. Has your child been teased/bullied? Is your teen/young adult involved in a romantic relationship? How open are you in discussing your child's diagnosis, side effects, prognosis with others? How has your child coped with increased attention? What kinds of extracurricular activities is your child involved in? What hobbies/interests does your child have? What do they like to do for fun? How are you getting along with your child's treatment team?	Tell me about your friends. How many do you have? Can you tell them anything or do you tend to keep things to yourself? Have you been teased/bullied? Are you in a romantic relationship? Have you told your friends/partner about your diagnosis? How has it been getting increased attention? What kinds of sports/clubs/groups/activities are you involved in? What are your hobbies/interests? What do you like to do for fun? How are you getting along with your medical team?
Developmental	Attainment of milestones Coping with transitions Separations Language Motor skills Maturity Independence/autonomy Regressive behaviors Temperament	Tell me about your child's development. Did s/he meet her/his milestones as expected? Do you remember having any concerns about your child's development? How does your child cope with transitions? How does your child cope with separations? Have you noticed any regressive behaviors (i.e., bed wetting, thumb sucking, baby talk, wanting you to do things they were previously doing independently)? Tell me about your child's personality. What words best describe your child?	How do you do with changes in routines? How do you do when mom/dad leave the room or when you are alone? Tell me 5 words that describe you best.
Behavioral	Adherence Behavioral difficulties Approach to treatment Demands Agreeableness Impulsivity	How does your child do taking medications? About how many doses do they miss per week? Is it a struggle to get your child to follow the treatment plan? What have you tried to help with this? How would you describe your child's behavior? What has been the most challenging aspect of parenting your child? How do you typically discipline your child when s/he misbehaves?	How do you do taking medicine? What is the hardest thing about taking your medications? What gets in the way of you taking your medicine? What kinds of things do you get in trouble for? What happens when you get in trouble? What do your parents do? Time out Spank Take away a privilege Talk it out Yell How often do you get in trouble?

(continued)

Table 1 (continued)

Domains to assess	Specific content	Sample questions for parent	Sample questions for child or AYA
Academic	Grade level School name Type of school Academic performance Previous retainment Special services/supports (IEP/504) Previous testing Contacts and communication with school Plan for remediation of school work Plans for future	Tell me about your child's schooling: Grade level Type of school Typical attendance and grades Has your child ever been held back or repeated a grade? Has your child ever had psychoeducational testing completed? Have you ever been told your child has a learning disability? If yes, what supports does s/he receive? Does s/he have an IEP or 504 Plan? If yes, what does this provide? Who on your child's academic team should we communicate with about school issues? Is the school aware of the current situation? What was their response? What is your plan for getting schoolwork completed while your child is in the hospital/being treated?	What grade are you in? What school do you go to? Is that a private or public school? What kind of grades do you get? What is your favorite thing about school? What do you like least about school? What are your plans after you finish school?
Occupational	Past employment Current employment	Are you currently employed? Have you ever been employed? What kind of work have you done? What does your employer know about the current situation? How have they responded? Are other caregivers employed? What kind of work do they do?	Have you ever had a job? What kind of work is it? What do you enjoy about it? What is the most difficult part of your job? Do they know about your diagnosis? If so, how have they responded? (If appropriate) What kind of work do you hope to do in the future?
Socio-cultural	SES Access to health insurance Access to treatment Policies, rules, and regulations Cultural view of diagnosis, treatment, prognosis Religious beliefs Health care system FMLA Cultural values Biases (providers, health care system)	Do you have health insurance? Have you had any challenges related to coverage? Are finances a stressor? Is there anything about your culture, beliefs, or religious practices that would be important for your child's medical team to know? Are you/is your family religious/spiritual? Please tell me about your beliefs. What values are important to your family? How does your culture view cancer and medical treatment for cancer? Is there anything you feel the staff does not understand about your culture that would be helpful for them to know? Who in your family is involved in making medical decisions about your child? Is there anyone outside of your family who helps to make these decisions?	Are you religious/spiritual? Please tell me about your beliefs. What things are the most important to your family? Is there anything you wish your doctors/nurses knew about your or your family's background that they don't know or understand?

For example, toddlers may be most distressed by having new providers or being without a familiar caregiver. School-aged children may be most distressed by fear of pain and procedures and missing school and peer interactions. Adolescents often present with concerns related to changes in physical appearance (e.g., hair loss), limited peer interactions, feeling left out, and increased unwanted attention (Hedstrom, Ljungman, & von Essen, 2005; Kupst & Patenaude, 2015). Basic information regarding gender and sexual identity will also be helpful to the provider and multidisciplinary oncology care team.

Medical History Obtaining information about medical history will provide insight into a child's previous experiences with the medical system. For children who have been in the hospital before or have followed a medical regimen, understanding their ability to cope with these demands may provide insight into how they will adjust to current challenges. With regard to the child's current cancer diagnosis, providers should first inquire what the child knows and determine whether the family is comfortable discussing the diagnosis with the child present. One of the greatest harms to rapport would be for the clinician to be the first to mention "cancer" in front of the child without parent consent. Providers should gather information regarding the type of cancer, as well as presenting and current symptoms. It is helpful to be familiar with current medications, significant labs, scan results, and any upcoming procedures. Inquiring about the treatment plan provides useful information about the patient's anticipated treatment trajectory. Providers may also inquire about staging and prognosis, which can reveal important information regarding the family's understanding of diagnosis, treatment, and prognosis. Assessing any previous experiences that families have had with cancer provides an opportunity to offer psychoeducation regarding the differences between childhood and adult cancers and help the family process how prior experiences may be impacting current adjustment.

Physical Functioning Patients and caregivers are often open to discussing how the child's cancer diagnosis and treatment have impacted physical functioning. For patients and families that are reluctant to engage, discussing physical concerns first may be less threatening. Providers should assess common side effects such as nausea, vomiting, loss of appetite, fatigue, sleep problems, and pain as unmanaged symptoms can significantly impair quality of life.

Family Functioning While many domains of functioning are important to assess, understanding the family system, including family risk and resiliency, is essential. Indeed, the family system is among the most important domains predictive of child adjustment to cancer (Kazak & Barakat, 1997). It is not uncommon for families to experience significant changes in functioning following a child's cancer diagnosis (e.g., increased marital strain/conflict). Important aspects of the family system to evaluate include the quality of parent–child relationships, relational dynamics between family members, communication styles, family roles and responsibilities, and areas of tension and cohesion. Assessing how parents are coping generally provides a reasonable predictor of how the child may ultimately cope. Additionally, siblings of children with cancer are an at-risk group with unique vulnerabilities and needs (e.g., concerns about the ill sibling, disruptions in routine, increased caretaking role; Gerhardt, Lehmann, Long, & Alderfer, 2015). Ongoing systematic psychosocial assessment should be completed as part of the standard care for youth with cancer and their families (Kazak et al., 2015).

In addition to broader aspects of family functioning, clinicians should assess family-level risk and protective factors in order to tailor interventions and engage appropriate members of the multidisciplinary team. Risk factors include current and significant prior stressors such as domestic violence, abuse or neglect, financial strain, unemployment, unstable housing, substance misuse, legal problems, and untreated or severe mental health issues. Additional family stressors that can complicate coping include single or lone parenting, a limited support system, poor coping skills, low health literacy, cognitive deficits, unreliable transportation, changes in family composition (e.g., birth, death, separation/ divorce), and family member medical issues. Assessing current sources of family stress allows providers to coordinate care to reduce the impact of these stressors on child and family adjustment. During the consult, clinicians should also assess resiliency factors that may help offset or mediate risk factors such as strong support system, openness to support/resources, financial security, open communication style, and adaptive coping with prior adversities.

Emotional Functioning Families vary in the ways in which they cope with a cancer diagnosis. Gathering information about prediagnosis child and family emotional functioning can provide insight into anticipated coping or concerns that a patient or family member may experience while undergoing cancer treatment. It is beneficial to obtain information about past and current mental health diagnoses and treatment for youth with cancer and their family members. When baseline emotional and behavioral concerns are identified, psychologists should seek to provide early and ongoing assessment and plan for continued management during treatment (Kearney, Salley, & Muriel, 2015). Cancer diagnosis and treatment involve significant challenges for families, and many youth and caregivers report increased distress. In general, it is also useful to assess current and past suicidal ideation, intent, or attempts and self-injurious behavior.

Cognitive Functioning Various complex demands are placed on families of children with cancer. Understanding patient and caregiver cognitive functioning allows the multidisciplinary team to tailor education and provide support as necessary. Identifying cognitive limitations can assist providers in selecting and using communication strategies to ensure that patients and families are able to fully consent to treatment, understand diagnosis and prognosis, and comprehend and adhere to treatment regimens. Cognitive assessment also involves assessment of health beliefs, attitudes, and expectations. Neurocognitive assessment allows for monitoring and intervention recommendations for cognitive late effects. In addition, the initial consult should gather family information preferences. Some patients and family members prefer all the information available, while others may be easily overwhelmed when too much information is presented at once. In addition to discussions with providers, many families benefit from receiving education in multiple formats (e.g., visual demonstrations, handouts, books, videos, online resources).

Social Functioning The innate need for belongingness and social relationships may be challenged when a child is undergoing cancer treatment. Many children with cancer endure lengthy separations from peers due to risk of exposure and compromised immune system functioning. Maintaining social relationships is important to many patients (Christiansen et al., 2015). Obtaining information about the child and their family's support system, peer relationships, and romantic relationships can reveal targets for psychosocial support and intervention. Inquiring about the patient's comfort in discussing their cancer diagnosis with others can be an indicator of how they are coping. It is often beneficial to provide anticipatory guidance about ways to disclose their diagnosis and prepare for reintegration to school and social activities. Included in the domain of social functioning is assessment of experiences with bullying, social media use, extracurricular activities, and general interests/ hobbies.

Developmental History Developmental history should include the attainment of milestones (e.g., motor skills, language, social, emotional, and behavioral development), as well as insights into child temperament. Gathering a thorough developmental history can provide key information regarding developmental challenges, coping strategies, ability to self-soothe, tolerance of transitions and separations, and general personality traits. Assessing autonomy and any developmental regression since diagnosis can facilitate specialized interventions. Gathering information related to parents' understanding of typical development is also helpful as caregivers who have unrealistic expectations of their child's responses to cancer diagnosis and treatment may create undue stress for their child.

Behavioral Functioning Hospitalization is not a typical experience for most children. Behavioral challenges are not uncommon when children are faced with an overstimulating environment with unfamiliar providers and expected to comply with new, frightening, and/or painful treatments. Many children undergoing cancer treatment experience significant disruption to their daily routines and miss the comfort of home, family, and pets. Adding to this stress is physical discomfort due to cancer and its treatment. As such, it is important to gather information regarding a child's current behavior at home, in school, and in the hospital. It is also critical to assess preexisting behavioral functioning, including how caregivers typically manage common behavioral challenges. Some parents become more overprotective or permissive when a child has cancer. Understanding past and current parental discipline strategies allows clinicians to tailor behavior management interventions and provide important education to parents (e.g., dangers of spanking in the context of low platelets). Providers should also gather information on the child's ability to listen, comprehend, and follow directions, as well as their activity level, impulsivity, attention-seeking behaviors, and limit testing, which may predict how the child will adhere to treatment. Assessment of adherence to treatment is also recommended.

Academic Functioning For school-aged children, school comprises a large part of their identity. Obtaining information about prior academic performance is useful to anticipate learning needs during cancer treatment. Clinicians should assess patient grade level, name and type of school, attendance and performance, previous retention, specialized services or support (IEP/504), and any previous academic or intellectual testing. For adolescents and young adults, it is useful to gather information regarding plans following high school. It is also helpful to obtain school contacts, inquire about what the educational team has been told, discuss plans for academic continuity during treatment, and prepare for school reentry (Thompson et al., 2015).

Socio-cultural Factors Consultation for children with cancer should assess socio-cultural factors such as family socio-economic status, social determinants of health, and access to healthcare. It is imperative to gather information about cultural identification, beliefs, communication, and views of how cultural values impact the individual and family system. For many families, religious or spiritual beliefs are a particularly important aspect of identity, core values, and traditions, which may strongly influence coping with adversity and meaning making. Understanding a family's cultural values provides a perspective on how they approach their child's treatment and how they interact with the medical team. It may also be beneficial to assess the family's experience with or perception of any biases within the healthcare setting.

Intervention

The consultation process should inform case conceptualization and provision of targeted intervention. Common clinical issues may include patient and family coping and adjustment, behavioral concerns, medical traumatic stress, procedural pain and distress, symptom management, decision making (e.g., clinical trial enrollment, fertility preservation), and adherence issues. Psychosocial needs may emerge at any time throughout the cancer trajectory, though some concerns may be more prominent at critical junctures (i.e., initial diagnosis, survivorship, relapse, end of life). Individual, family, and marital cognitive-behavioral (CBT) and acceptance-based therapy (ACT) approaches tend to be the most widely utilized.

Coping and Adjustment Many approaches to treatment begin with psychoeducation and the provision of anticipatory guidance. Providing patients and families with developmentally appropriate information regarding the disease, anticipated treatment, side effects, and long-term late effects aids in decision making; reduces worry, anxiety, and distress; and helps build trust and rapport (Thompson & Young-Saleme, 2015).

General CBT strategies may be used by clinicians to encourage emotional expression and aid in the development of adaptive coping strategies. Several evidence-based interventions can be helpful in the management of anxiety (e.g., Coping Cat, exposure therapy, trauma-focused CBT, ACT) and depression (e.g., interpersonal therapy, CBT, ACT) among youth with cancer. In addition, several interventions have been developed specifically for youth with cancer, including games (e.g., Shop Talk; Wiener, Battles, Mamalian, & Zadeh, 2011), coping kits (Marsac et al., 2012), journals (e.g., This Is My World workbook; ccr.cancer.gov/Pediatric-Oncology-Branch/psychosocial/education), and books for bibliotherapy. In addition to promoting adaptive coping, clinicians may help foster posttraumatic growth. The Promoting Resilience In Stress Management (PRISM) protocol is a four-session individual intervention for adolescents and young adults that aims to promote adaptive cognitive coping, posttraumatic growth, and benefit finding (Rosenberg et al., 2018). Some patients experience depression or anxiety at a level that may warrant the addition of psychopharmacological intervention.

Children with cancer undergo profound changes to their social lives during treatment. They miss out on school, sports, extracurricular activities and may be occasionally isolated from family and friends while immunosuppressed. Opportunities to meet with other pediatric cancer patients and survivors through hospital-based groups, camps, social events, and peer mentoring can help provide a sense of normalcy and promote positive coping (Christiansen et al., 2015). These may be especially helpful for youth at risk of poorer social functioning after treatment (e.g., brain tumor patients and those who received CNS-directed treatment or HCST).

Psychosocial support for families during treatment is likewise an important component of care. Typical interventions include normalization of the family's experience, problem-solving skills training, coping with illness uncertainty, and focusing on resiliency (Kearney et al., 2015). In addition, several cancer-specific interventions have been developed to address parent coping and distress, including the Surviving Cancer Competently Intervention Program (SCCIP; Kazak et al., 2005), Bright IDEAS Problem-Solving Skills Training (PSST; Sahler et al., 2002), PRISM for Parents (PRISM-P; Yi-Frazier et al., 2017), a clinic-based interdisciplinary illness uncertainty intervention at initial diagnosis (Mullins et al., 2012), and the Parent-Social Cognitive Intervention Program for HSCT (Manne, Mee, Bartell, Sands, & Kashy, 2016).

Siblings of children with cancer also experience significant life disruption. Younger children may experience increased separation anxiety and disruptive behaviors as primary caregivers spend more time away from home. School-aged children often struggle with loss of parental attention, disruption in extracurricular activities, and anxiety about the cancer and prognosis, particularly when they are unable to visit the hospital regularly (Gerhardt et al., 2015). Siblings often benefit from developmentally appropriate information about diagnosis and treatment and an opportunity for open dialogue and questions. SuperSibs (www.alexslemonade.org/campaign/supersibs) provides various resources for siblings of children with cancer. In addition, the Siblings Coping Together (SibCT) intervention promotes adaptive problem-solving and coping skills (Barrera, Neville, Purdon, & Hancock, 2018).

Behavioral Concerns Parents often have many questions and concerns regarding how to parent a child with cancer. Providing normalization, psychoeducation, and anticipatory guidance can facilitate the navigation of new parenting roles. However, a subset of patients have significant behavioral concerns that warrant additional intervention. Children who receive corticosteroids have increased risk of externalizing difficulties and may experience steroid-induced psychosis. Parent training and maintaining consistent expectations for behavior, along with education that these changes may be treatment driven and time limited, are important behavioral interventions. The development of structure and routine and use of praise and rewards, redirection, and distraction are most effective. When needed, parents can implement age-appropriate consequences such as time out or loss of privileges. Neuroleptic medications may also be useful in situations where behavioral difficulties are not sufficiently managed through behavioral interventions alone.

Adherence Adherence to medications, immunosuppression or treatment restrictions, and clinic attendance are critically important when a child has cancer as adherence has significant implications for treatment efficacy and relapse prevention (Bhatia et al., 2014; Pai & McGrady, 2015). Pediatric psychologists play a critical role in addressing the often-multifaceted challenges of adherence. While the most frequently cited reason for nonadherence is forgetting, additional factors may play a role. Depression can decrease motivation to engage in self-care or child care. Cognitive difficulties may increase challenges with planning and executing medication management and treatment adherence. Financial or social responsibilities may conflict with the treatment plan. Finally, side effects may deter patients from optimal adherence. Interventions such as increasing structure around medication administration, caregiver monitoring, reducing barriers (e.g., teaching pill swallowing techniques), motivational interviewing, and instituting reward systems can be helpful in promoting adherence. New interventions have great potential to increase adherence with equipment (e.g., MEMs caps), technology (e.g., video diaries, smartphone apps), and games (e.g., "Re-Mission"; Kato, Cole, Bradlyn, & Pollock, 2008).

Physical Symptoms Patients with cancer may experience multiple symptoms, including acute or chronic pain, nausea, vomiting, fatigue, appetite loss, and sleep difficulty. Those who are sexually active may experience sexual dysfunction. Psychologists are skilled at providing nonpharmacological symptom management strategies. These can include distraction, relaxation (e.g., deep breathing, hypnosis, biofeedback), and other CBT and ACT techniques. In regard to acute or procedural pain, it is important for providers to engage in procedural preparation that is well timed, is developmentally appropriate, and describes the sequence of events that will occur and what pain or other sensations to expect (Flowers & Birnie, 2015). Youth may also benefit from rehearsal, modeling, and/or medical play. Parent-based interventions can be used to decrease attending behaviors and augment communication patterns that contribute to a child's pain experience (Caes et al., 2014). For patients with phantom limb pain after amputation, mirror box therapy may be helpful in decreasing pain (Anghelescu et al., 2016).

End-of-Life Issues Advanced care planning, including desired location of death and code status, is a critical component of optimal end-of-life care. Psychologists can be integral in facilitating these difficult conversations. Research suggests that many bereaved parents do not regret having had these discussions with their child, whereas a subset does express regret over not doing so before their child's death (Kreicbergs, Valdimarsdottir, Onelov, Henter, & Steineck, 2004). Tools exist for children (e.g., My Wishes) and adolescents (e.g., Voicing My Choices) to express their preferences for end-of-life care (Wiener et al., 2012). Tailored interventions can assist with the family's understanding and promotion of wishes at end of life (Lyon, Jacobs, Briggs, Cheng, & Wang, 2013). Religious and cultural considerations should be discussed with the family to help the team navigate conversations in a sensitive and respectful manner (Wiener, McConnell, Latella, & Ludi, 2013). Contact with the family following the patient's death is strongly recommended in order to assess coping and provide resources (Lichtenthal et al., 2015).

Adaptation

Clinicians should consider the need to modify an intervention based on the environment in which services are delivered. Within the inpatient setting, medical treatments and procedures often take precedence and patients may be unavailable during daytime hours, have less privacy due to a shared room or the presence of visitors, and often experience frequent interruptions by providers and staff. Consultation in medical clinics can pose similar challenges, with the added barrier of time constraints. Despite the challenges of adapting care, providing families with continuity of care across the treatment trajectory and settings can be helpful.

Developmental needs of the patient may also warrant a modification of evidence-based intervention. Younger patients may have increased difficulty with stamina, may be out of their routine, or generally do not feel well enough to meet typical developmental expectations (i.e., feeding self, toileting, brushing teeth, completing schoolwork). The patient may experience significant frustration as a result of increased limitations (functional and/or imposed by the care team). Additionally, children may be on food restrictions, sleep deprived, anxious, or irritable. Clinicians should offer developmentally appropriate choices and opportunities for children to assume control when possible, encourage independence in those tasks that they are able to complete, and provide anticipatory guidance to parents regarding the differences between age-appropriate behavior (e.g., testing limits), stress reactions (e.g., tantrums, hyperarousal, withdrawal), and symptom-driven behaviors (e.g., increased crying/lethargy due to feeling unwell). Additionally, the clinician will need to use judgment in determining which adaptations will work best for each patient (e.g., consultation broken into shorter, smaller segments over time, or a more intensive approach for time-sensitive issues such as pill swallowing). Clinicians should take special care in using developmentally appropriate language that children can understand (see Breyer, 2015, for examples of developmentally appropriate language).

Families may experience increased difficulty in coordinating multiple appointments and complex medical regimens. Families frequently encounter appointment, lab, and pharmacy delays, as well as changes in treatment plans and unanticipated intervention or hospital admissions. These unexpected and/or uncontrollable situations may increase frustration and reduce openness to psychological consultation. Clinicians should be prepared to see patients and families at their worst. As such, it is ideal for the psychologist to accommodate youth and their families whenever feasible and incorporate flexibility into their practice.

Efforts should be made to ensure that every patient and caregiver understands information provided by the care team. When there is a low health literacy, institutions should ensure a variety of modalities, including written, verbal, video-delivered, and online methods to accommodate different learning styles, preferences, and abilities. Providers are encouraged to use teach-back methods to ensure patient/family understanding. Similarly, families that do not speak the same language as the care team need access to professional interpretive services and should not rely on children or other family members for interpretation.

Training/Resources

Clinicians who are best prepared to work with the pediatric oncology population are those trained in clinical psychology and, more specifically, those with training and supervised experiences in child clinical, health, and/or pediatric psychology. Essential to working with children with cancer is a solid understanding and application of child development. Providers must understand child social, emotional, and cognitive growth and development in typically and atypically developing children. Further expertise comes from exposure and training in working with children who have serious chronic illness, experience practicing within a medical setting and with multidisciplinary teams, familiarity with medical terminology, and understanding of childhood cancers, cancer treatments, and their impact on children and families. Trainees can be more fully immersed by working with supervisors who practice in pediatric oncology. Providers should develop core competencies and training in developmental, behavioral, and psychological assessment and intervention; pain management; adherence; and grief and bereavement (Patenaude, Pelletier, & Bingen, 2015).

Providers working with children with cancer and their families often experience differences in the delivery of services that are uncommon in traditional psychotherapy. For example, psychologists working in pediatric oncology rarely adhere to working within a 50-minute weekly session framework with patients and families. Instead, the duration and frequency of sessions often fluctuate depending on patient needs and circumstances. For example, clinicians may meet with a patient or their family daily for extended amounts of time or may briefly check in weekly or monthly depending on the patient's needs. In addition, psychosocial oncology providers will often encounter differences in boundaries that are atypical of traditional therapy, such as being in the presence of bodily excretions (e.g., blood, vomit, feces, urine) and significant changes to the body (e.g., amputation, disfigurement, colostomy), as well as psychological experiences such as terminal illness, uncertainty, threats to bodily integrity, and patient bodily exposure (e.g., nudity for procedures/exams). Clinicians who are flexible, open-minded, and compassionate; have high distress tolerance; and are good communicators are most well suited for this context.

Providers benefit from access to resources such as technology (e.g., tablets, video games, virtual reality), toys, arts and crafts, games, books, and activities to help provide distraction and normalization. There are also many oncology-specific resources available, including journals, therapeutic board games, books, dolls, stuffed animals, and coping kits. The greatest resources and support to psychologists are often other psychosocial oncology team providers.

Inpatient Consultation

The hospital setting presents multiple logistical issues related to assessing and intervening on psychological concerns. There are often issues related to privacy, and medical procedures and treatments often take precedence, which may make it challenging to find time to meet with patients and families. Additional barriers can include the child not feeling well and parents being primarily focused on caring for or entertaining the child. It is not uncommon for a parent to want to discuss a sensitive topic but feel unable to step away from bedside. Likewise, caregivers may be unavailable to participate in the consultation while they are at work, caring for other children, or getting much-needed respite.

Inpatient hospitalization also presents challenges in communication. Ensuring that families' concerns are expressed and communicated accurately and efficiently is essential as breakdowns in communication (e.g., due to shift changes, transitions in care, involvement of multiple providers and teams) are often a source of anxiety and frustration for parents. It is often helpful to provide families with information about how the inpatient unit operates (e.g., hierarchy of medical staff, rounding process, patient/parent groups, meals, roles and responsibilities of different care team members), along with a tour of the inpatient unit and outpatient clinic. While open communication between members of the care team can facilitate optimal care delivery, psychologists should be mindful about issues of confidentiality and refrain from holding conversations in public areas within the hospital. Additionally, psychologists often become trusted providers, and families may disclose sensitive patient or family information unrelated to cancer care. Caution should be used in sharing this information, and psychologists should obtain patient/parent permission or discuss the rationale for sharing sensitive, nonmedical information.

Outpatient Oncology Clinic Consultation

Youth with cancer often have many oncology clinic visits for labs, tests, physical exams, scan results, and outpatient chemotherapy. They are also often seen in the outpatient clinic for sick visits or when there are additional concerns. Some visits are relatively brief, and others may last all day depending on treatment needs. Initial oncology clinic visits may be challenging for children given the unfamiliar space, as well as new expectations and providers. However, families are often less stressed in the outpatient setting, and these visits provide the opportunity for psychologists to observe how the child more typically presents relative to the inpatient setting. While meeting a patient/family in clinic can be challenging as children often undergo procedures (blood draw, port access, dressing changes) and may need to meet with multiple medical providers, psychology follow-up during these visits often strengthens rapport and enables clinicians to provide continuity of care between the inpatient and outpatient settings. Increased collaboration and coordination with other providers is often needed due to time and space constraints to ensure that patient and family needs are met. The oncology clinic setting may present additional privacy concerns as waiting rooms and clinics may not offer individual spaces. Psychologists should be mindful of what information is communicated in shared spaces and should request access to private room if sensitive information will be discussed.

Outpatient Psychology Clinic Consultation

Treatment for pediatric cancer can be very intensive and place significant demands on families. It is therefore recommended that providers remain flexible and accommodating with regard to patients' treatment schedules and needs. For example, clinicians can attempt to meet with patients when they are admitted or during oncology clinic visits. However, there are some circumstances in which consultation and intervention cannot wait to be completed during scheduled inpatient admissions or clinic visits. Situations that are time sensitive (e.g., difficulties with pill swallowing), intensive (e.g., need for procedural support and rehearsal), pervasive (e.g., behavioral concerns at home, school, or the hospital in need of parent training), or a high priority for the family may require psychological outpatient treatment.

There are special considerations when a child is seen in an outpatient behavioral health setting. Children with compromised immune functioning should be instructed to wear a mask or be given a separate waiting area and should have access to sanitized surfaces and minimized contact with sick individuals to reduce infection risk. Additionally, for children using ambulating supports (e.g., walker, wheelchair), there should be level walkways that are clear of obstacles or narrowed hallways, consistent with ADA standards. Depending on a child's specific needs, thought should be given to medication schedule, strong smells, need for drinks or snacks, and access and distance to restrooms and parents in the waiting room. Additionally, youth should be prepared to visit a nononcology clinic setting where others may be present and unaccustomed to seeing a child without hair, in a wheelchair, wearing a mask, or with a limb amputated.

Case Example

An 8 year-old girl, Mae, presented to the emergency department following one week of increased fatigue, fever, leg pain, and bruising. In the emergency department, her mother was informed of abnormal labs indicative of acute lymphoblastic leukemia (ALL). Mae's mother became upset and tearful, left the room, and immediately called family and friends to disclose Mae's cancer diagnosis. Mae sat frightened as medical personnel entered and exited the room.

Psychology was consulted on the third day of admission to help the family cope and adjust to new onset ALL. After consulting with Mae's nurse, it was discovered that there were also concerns for regressive behaviors such as bed wetting, resistance to taking medications, and increased difficulty separating from her mother. Most challenging for medical staff was difficulty in completing exams and procedures given Mae's intense level of distress. Additional background information obtained from the chart indicated that Mae lives at home with her 10 year-old brother and biological mother and father. Mae's mother works part-time as a school bus driver, while her father works full-time in manufacturing. Mae is in the second grade and is doing well academically with no concerns. Socially, she has many friends and plays soccer and swims.

After reviewing the medical record and consulting with Mae's nurse, the psychologist approached the family and introduced her role as part of the oncology care team. Mae's mother expressed openness to the consultation; however, Mae was reluctant to engage. Her mother was tearful and expressed worry about how Mae has been coping. She whispered that Mae had not yet been informed of her diagnosis because she did not want to worry Mae. Her mother also noted that Mae was previously healthy and has never been admitted to the hospital before. Whereas Mae was previously full of energy and very independent, her mother commented that now she is wetting the bed and is resistant to out-of-bed activities and self-care tasks. She expressed embarrassment and frustration with regard to Mae's regression and anxious reactions when medical providers enter the room and a sense of helplessness in comforting Mae.

In addition, Mae's mother reported several ongoing family stressors, including financial strain, behavioral difficulties in Mae's older brother, poor communication and increased tension in her relationship with Mae's father, and maternal history of depression. Resiliency factors included a strong support system, stable housing, openness to support and resources from providers, and strong mother–child attachment. Mae's mother noted that she has overcome many challenges in the past and has learned helpful coping strategies from her therapist.

As the visit progressed, Mae slowly began to participate and share her perspectives. She described many aspects of the hospital that she strongly dislikes: being awoken in the middle of the night; inability to move her arm due to the IV; missing school, family, friends, and pets; not being able to play outside or participate in sports; boredom; and unfamiliar food. Mae reported that she had not gotten out of bed to use the restroom due to uncontrolled leg pain and had been refusing medication due to difficulties swallowing pills. Most significantly, she expressed anxiety and fear about pain and being hurt by medical providers. She acknowledged worries about her mother leaving the bedside for fear of something bad happening to her (Mae) while her mother is away. She also endorsed feeling frustrated about only being told that she is "sick" and not understanding why she needs to be in the hospital or undergo painful procedures.

Interventions

Psychoeducation During the initial consult, the psychologist validated and normalized Mae's mother's concerns while also providing psychoeducation on (1) the benefits of open, honest, developmentally appropriate communication with Mae about her diagnosis and treatment plan to foster trust and engagement in her treatment and (2) the negative impact of withholding information on children's emotional functioning as youth often understand that something is wrong and may feel confused, frightened, and/or angry at their parents' lack of disclosure. The psychologist also reassured Mae's mother that children often cope well and tend to be very resilient. The psychologist also discussed the importance of reassuring youth, especially young children, that they did not cause their cancer, that they could not have prevented it, and that it is not contagious.

Afterward, Mae's mother felt reassured and confident in her ability to inform Mae of her diagnosis and treatment. The family was provided with a cancer workbook, stuffed animal, and book to help explain cancer and treatment. By openly discussing Mae's cancer diagnosis, her mother was able to explore Mae's concerns and worries, answer questions and provide reassurance, and discuss anticipated side effects of treatment (e.g., hair loss) and Mae's preferences for how to prepare and cope with these upcoming challenges. In addition, the psychologist met with Mae to provide reassurance that she did not cause or contribute to her diagnosis, normalize and validate emotions and worries, and provide anticipatory guidance regarding treatment trajectory and procedures. Mae subsequently became more interactive with staff and was able to ask questions and express concerns.

Procedure Preparation Mae was provided with honest, age-appropriate information about what would happen during procedures, including sensations to expect, as well as opportunities to rehearse new procedures. Whenever possible, she was offered choices with regard to how procedures were conducted in order to enhance her sense of control. Mae expressed desire to learn distraction and relaxation techniques to cope with procedural anxiety. As a result of these interventions, she exhibited decreased distress during exams and procedures.

Pill Swallowing The psychologist engaged Mae in pill swallowing practice to facilitate oral medication administration. The psychologist brought a pill swallowing kit to the room, played videos about pill swallowing, and modeled the steps. With encouragement, praise, and rewards, Mae was able to learn how to swallow pills efficiently within two days of practicing, which increased her confidence and sense of control.

Pain Management The psychologist introduced nonpharmacological pain management strategies for Mae to use in combination with medication management. Specifically, psychoeducation was provided on the autonomic nervous system, gate control theory, and mind–body connection. Next, the psychologist instructed Mae in relaxation using portable biofeedback equipment. Mae especially enjoyed imagery and often chose to imagine curling up with her dog at home. Relaxation apps were recommended to facilitate continued practice. Goal setting and problem-solving around healthy habits (e.g., maintaining a consistent sleep schedule, adequate hydration, and diet) were also provided to enhance symptom management.

Anxiety Management Mae often became anxious around medical procedures and about separations from her mother. With support from the psychologist, she was able to identify relationships between anxious thoughts, feelings, and behaviors. She was instructed in the use of cognitive reframing, positive self-talk, and calming statements to reduce anxiety. In vivo exposures were conducted to reduce anxiety about separations. As Mae became more comfortable with hospital staff and felt more in control, her anxiety gradually improved.

Psychoeducation/Anticipatory Guidance for Parents Sessions were primarily completed with Mae and her mother. When possible, Mae's brother and father were also included. Parents were provided with psychoeducation on parenting a child with cancer and promoting sibling coping and adjustment. The psychologist also discussed the importance of parent self-care and assisted Mae's mother and father in setting goals and problem-solving barriers to engaging in self-care activities.

Parent Coping To support parent adjustment, the psychologist delivered components of the SCCIP intervention (e.g., identifying relationships between adversities, beliefs, and consequences, reframing maladaptive thoughts, enhancing communication between parents). By processing together the role of cancer within the family and the impact of their beliefs about cancer on emotions, behaviors, and relationships, Mae's parents were able to better communicate their needs and demonstrated reduced distress.

References

Anghelescu, D. L., Kelly, C. N., Steen, B. D., Wu, J., Wu, H., DeFeo, B. M., … Burgoyne, L. (2016). Mirror therapy for phantom limb pain at a pediatric oncology institution. *Rehabil Oncol, 34*(3), 104–110.

Barrera, M., Neville, A., Purdon, L., & Hancock, K. (2018). "It's just for us!" perceived benefits of participation in a group intervention for siblings of children with cancer. *Journal of Pediatric Psychology, 43*(9), 995–1003.

Bhatia, S., Landier, W., Hageman, L., Kim, H., Chen, Y., Crews, K. R., ... Relling, M. V. (2014). Adherence to oral 6-mercaptopurine in African American and Asian children with acute lymphoblastic leukemia: a Children's Oncology Group study. *Blood, 124*(15), 2345–2353. https://doi.org/10.1182/blood-2014-01-552166

Bitsko, M. J., Cohen, D., Dillon, R., Harvey, J., Krull, K., & Klosky, J. L. (2016). Psychosocial late effects in pediatric cancer survivors: A report from the Children's Oncology Group. *Pediatric Blood & Cancer, 63*(2), 337–343.

Breyer, J. (2015). Talking to children and adolescents about cancer. In L. Wiener, M. Pao, A. E. Kazak, M. J. Kupst, A. F. Patenaude, & R. J. Arceci (Eds.), *Pediatric psycho-oncology: A quick reference on the psychosocial dimensions of cancer symptom management* (2nd ed., pp. 221–239). New York, NY: Oxford Press.

Caes, L., Vervoort, T., Devos, P., Verlooy, J., Benoit, Y., & Goubert, L. (2014). Parental distress and catastrophic thoughts about child pain: Implications for parental protective behavior in the context of child leukemia-related medical procedures. *The Clinical Journal of Pain, 30*(9), 787–799.

Christiansen, H. L., Bingen, K., Hoag, J. A., Karst, J. S., Velazquez-Martin, B., & Barakat, L. P. (2015). Providing children and adolescents opportunities for social interaction as a standard of care in pediatric oncology. *Pediatric Blood & Cancer, 62*(Suppl 5), S724–S749.

Evans, N. T., Wakefield, C. E., McLoone, J. K., & Cohn, R. J. (2015). Familial diagnostic experiences in paediatric oncology. *British Journal of Cancer, 112*(1), 20–23.

Flowers, S. R., & Birnie, K. A. (2015). Procedural preparation and support as a standard of care in pediatric oncology. *Pediatric Blood & Cancer, 62*(Suppl 5), S694–S723.

Gerhardt, C. A., Lehmann, V., Long, K. A., & Alderfer, M. A. (2015). Supporting siblings as a standard of care in pediatric oncology. *Pediatric Blood & Cancer, 62*(Suppl 5), S750–S804.

Hedstrom, M., Ljungman, G., & von Essen, L. (2005). Perceptions of distress among adolescents recently diagnosed with cancer. *Journal of Pediatric Hematology/Oncology, 27*(1), 15–22.

Hocking, M. C., Kazak, A. E., Schneider, S., Barkman, D., Barakat, L. P., & Deatrick, J. A. (2014). Parent perspectives on family-based psychosocial interventions in pediatric cancer: A mixed-methods approach. *Support Care Cancer, 22*(5), 1287–1294.

Kato, P. M., Cole, S. W., Bradlyn, A. S., & Pollock, B. H. (2008). A video game improves behavioral outcomes in adolescents and young adults with cancer: A randomized trial. *Pediatrics, 122*(2), e305–e317.

Kazak, A. E., Abrams, A. N., Banks, J., Christofferson, J., DiDonato, S., Grootenhuis, M. A., ... Kupst, M. J. (2015). Psychosocial assessment as a standard of care in pediatric cancer. *Pediatric Blood & Cancer, 62*(Suppl 5), S426–S459.

Kazak, A. E., & Barakat, L. P. (1997). Brief report: Parenting stress and quality of life during treatment for childhood leukemia predicts child and parent adjustment after treatment ends. *Journal of Pediatric Psychology, 22*(5), 749–758.

Kazak, A. E., Simms, S., Alderfer, M. A., Rourke, M. T., Crump, T., McClure, K., ... Reilly, A. (2005). Feasibility and preliminary outcomes from a pilot study of a brief psychological intervention for families of children newly diagnosed with cancer. *Journal of Pediatric Psychology, 30*(8), 644–655.

Kearney, J. A., Salley, C. G., & Muriel, A. C. (2015). Standards of psychosocial care for parents of children with cancer. *Pediatric Blood & Cancer, 62*(Suppl 5), S632–S683.

Kreicbergs, U., Valdimarsdottir, U., Onelov, E., Henter, J. I., & Steineck, G. (2004). Talking about death with children who have severe malignant disease. *The New England Journal of Medicine, 351*(12), 1175–1186.

Kupst, M. J., & Patenaude, A. F. (2015). Coping with pediatric cancer. In L. S. Wiener, M. Pao, A. E. Kazak, M. J. Kupst, & A. F. Patenaude (Eds.), *Pediatric psycho-oncology: A quick reference on the psychosocial dimensions of cancer symptom management* (pp. 241–250). New York, NY: Oxford University Press.

Landier, W., Armenian, S. H., Meadows, A. T., & Bhatia, S. (2015). Late effects of childhood cancer and its treatment. In P. A. Pizzo & D. G. Poplack (Eds.), *Principles and practice of pediatric oncology* (Vol. 62, 7th ed., p. 275). Philadelphia, PA: Wolters Kluwer Health.

Lichtenthal, W. G., Sweeney, C. R., Roberts, K. E., Corner, G. W., Donovan, L. A., Prigerson, H. G., & Wiener, L. (2015). Bereavement follow-up after the death of a child as a standard of care in pediatric oncology. *Pediatric Blood & Cancer, 62*(Suppl 5), S834–S869.

Lyon, M. E., Jacobs, S., Briggs, L., Cheng, Y. I., & Wang, J. (2013). Family-centered advance care planning for teens with cancer. *JAMA Pediatrics, 167*(5), 460–467.

Manne, S., Mee, L., Bartell, A., Sands, S., & Kashy, D. A. (2016). A randomized clinical trial of a parent-focused social-cognitive processing intervention for caregivers of children undergoing hematopoetic stem cell transplantation. *Journal of Consulting and Clinical Psychology, 84*(5), 389–401.

Marsac, M. L., Hildenbrand, A. K., Clawson, K., Jackson, L., Kohser, K., Barakat, L., ... Alderfer, M. A. (2012). Acceptability and feasibility of family use of The Cellie Cancer Coping Kit. *Support Care Cancer, 20*(12), 3315–3324.

Mullins, L. L., Fedele, D. A., Chaffin, M., Hullmann, S. E., Kenner, C., Eddington, A. R., ... McNall-Knapp, R. Y. (2012). A clinic-based interdisciplinary intervention for mothers of children newly diagnosed with cancer: A pilot study. *Journal of Pediatric Psychology, 37*(10), 1104–1115.

Pai, A. L., & McGrady, M. E. (2015). Assessing medication adherence as a standard of care in pediatric oncology. *Pediatric Blood & Cancer, 62*(Suppl 5), S818–S828.

Patenaude, A. F., Pelletier, W., & Bingen, K. (2015). Communication, documentation, and training standards in pediatric psychosocial oncology. *Pediatric Blood & Cancer, 62*(Suppl 5), S870–S895.

Rosenberg, A. R., Bradford, M. C., Barton, K. S., Etsekson, N., McCauley, E., Curtis, J. R., … Yi-Frazier, J. P. (2018). Hope and benefit finding: Results from the PRISM randomized controlled trial. *Pediatric Blood & Cancer, 66*, e27485.

Sahler, O. J., Varni, J. W., Fairclough, D. L., Butler, R. W., Noll, R. B., Dolgin, M. J., … Mulhern, R. K. (2002). Problem-solving skills training for mothers of children with newly diagnosed cancer: A randomized trial. *Journal of Developmental and Behavioral Pediatrics, 23*(2), 77–86.

Thompson, A. L., Christiansen, H. L., Elam, M., Hoag, J., Irwin, M. K., Pao, M., … Kelly, K. P. (2015). Academic continuity and school reentry support as a standard of care in pediatric oncology. *Pediatric Blood & Cancer, 62*(Suppl 5), S805–S817.

Thompson, A. L., & Young-Saleme, T. K. (2015). Anticipatory guidance and psychoeducation as a standard of care in pediatric oncology. *Pediatric Blood & Cancer, 62*(Suppl 5), S684–S693.

Wiener, L., Battles, H., Mamalian, C., & Zadeh, S. (2011). ShopTalk: A pilot study of the feasibility and utility of a therapeutic board game for youth living with cancer. *Support Care Cancer, 19*(7), 1049–1054.

Wiener, L., Kazak, A. E., Noll, R. B., Patenaude, A. F., & Kupst, M. J. (2015). Standards for the psychosocial care of children with cancer and their families: An introduction to the special issue. *Pediatric Blood & Cancer, 62*(Suppl 5), S419–S424.

Wiener, L., McConnell, D. G., Latella, L., & Ludi, E. (2013). Cultural and religious considerations in pediatric palliative care. *Palliative & Supportive Care, 11*(1), 47–67.

Wiener, L., Zadeh, S., Battles, H., Baird, K., Ballard, E., Osherow, J., & Pao, M. (2012). Allowing adolescents and young adults to plan their end-of-life care. *Pediatrics, 130*(5), 897–905.

Yi-Frazier, J. P., Fladeboe, K., Klein, V., Eaton, L., Wharton, C., McCauley, E., & Rosenberg, A. R. (2017). Promoting Resilience in Stress Management for Parents (PRISM-P): An intervention for caregivers of youth with serious illness. *Families, Systems & Health, 35*(3), 341–351.

Diabetes

Jessica C. Kichler and Katherine Bedard-Thomas

The increasing role of the pediatric psychologist in working with children and adolescents with type 1 diabetes (T1D) has been outlined in the literature (Kichler, Harris, & Weissberg-Benchell, 2015) and often involves multidisciplinary care with a medical team. Much is known about different outpatient treatment approaches that can occur in a variety of settings within this population (Hilliard, Powell, & Anderson, 2016), but more specifics about recommended clinical practices for inpatient T1D care is warranted. The inpatient CL psychologist has a unique role in providing evidence-based assessments and brief interventions, which can positively impact the course of the child's T1D treatment long term.

J. C. Kichler (✉)
Behavioral Medicine and Clinical Psychology, Cincinnati Children's Hospital Medical Center, Cincinnati, OH, USA

Department of Pediatrics, University of Cincinnati School of Medicine, Cincinnati, OH, USA
e-mail: Jessica.Kichler@cchmc.org

K. Bedard-Thomas
Behavioral Medicine and Clinical Psychology, Cincinnati Children's Hospital Medical Center, Cincinnati, OH, USA

Diagnosis

In T1D, an autoimmune response in the body causes islet beta cell destruction in the pancreas, which ultimately leads to the body no longer being able to produce endogenous insulin (a hormone that processes carbohydrates needed to sustain life). It is unclear why an autoimmune response occurs, but it is theorized to be related to genetic vulnerability and potentially even an environmental trigger (Christoffersson, Rodriguez-Calvo, & von Herrath, 2016). There is typically a "honeymoon period" after the initial diagnosis of T1D, in which some remaining islet beta cells still function in the pancreas. During this time, some insulin production may still occur for typically around 6–12 months post diagnosis. However, virtually all patients with T1D still start on at least some exogenous insulin at the time of diagnosis. Eventually, the remaining islet beta cell functioning is fully depleted by the immune system, and the person with T1D relies completely on external insulin to maintain in-target glycemic levels.

Although the primary focus of this chapter is T1D (formerly known as juvenile-onset diabetes), it is also important to separate out the medical differences between T1D versus type 2 diabetes (T2D) as there are many misconceptions between these two distinct, but related, diagnoses. In T2D (formerly known as adult-onset diabetes),

B. D. Carter, K. A. Kullgren (eds.), *Clinical Handbook of Psychological Consultation in Pediatric Medical Settings*, Issues in Clinical Child Psychology, https://doi.org/10.1007/978-3-030-35598-2_24

the body becomes increasingly resistant to effectively using the endogenous insulin that is produced by the islet beta cells in the pancreas. This occurs for a variety of reasons, including factors such as increased weight, genetic vulnerability, elevated stress hormones, lack of exercise, etc. Over time, if the islet beta cells in the pancreas are not able to keep up with the body's demands for insulin, these patients may have to also take exogenous insulin to keep their glycemic levels on target. Unlike individuals with T1D, there is no evidence of islet cell antibodies in the blood stream for those with T2D, indicating an absence of an autoimmune attack on the islet beta cells in the pancreas. Depending on how far the T2D symptoms have progressed, the initial interventions at diagnosis are primarily focused on lifestyle changes (e.g., diet, exercise), oral medications to improve insulin sensitivity, and/or initiation of exogenous insulin.

For many, the presenting symptoms prior to making a diagnosis of T1D can often be vague and misleading (e.g., polyuria, polydipsia, fatigue, nausea, weight loss). Patients can go months with symptoms in the outpatient primary care setting before a diagnosis is made (typically through a blood or urine test), so there is often feelings of guilt or anger around missing the initial signs of T1D either by the family or toward the medical teams that may have initially misdiagnosed the symptoms. The average age of onset is about 10 years of age, with an increase in incidence rates for those in the 5–15-year-old range (Lawrence et al., 2014). Some patients with newly diagnosed T1D are hospitalized at diagnosis as a standard of care, and others have a day hospital or outpatient treatment model for initial T1D education and support. In addition, a smaller portion of the patients require hospitalization in the intensive care unit (ICU) regardless of the typical protocol for patients newly diagnosed with T1D due to their initial clinical presentation being severe enough to warrant more intensive medical stabilization. For some, the circumstances around the initial diagnosis of T1D can lead to long-standing adjustment and coping issues that persist over time as patients and families learn to manage this chronic condition.

In addition to the diagnosis of T1D, there are often concurrent, clinically significant emotional issues that may develop over time for patients with T1D that warrant diagnosis and treatment. These most often include but are not limited to depression, anxiety, adjustment disorders, disordered eating behaviors, attention deficit hyperactivity disorder (ADHD), and disruptive behavioral disorders (Corathers et al., 2013; Kovacs, Goldston, Obrosky, & Bonar, 1997; Young-Hyman et al., 2016). Additionally, premorbid psychosocial stressors increase the risk of these symptoms and may lead to difficulties immediately after the initial diagnosis of T1D. Separate from diagnosable mental health conditions (e.g., depression, anxiety), diabetes-specific distress and burnout are also very common symptoms that many individuals with T1D experience throughout their lifetime at varying degrees (Shapiro et al., 2017; Weissberg-Benchell & Antisdel-Lomaglio, 2011). These distress/burnout symptoms are defined as an uncomfortable emotional state in response to T1D self-management and are not typically viewed as pathological in nature. They are often limited to diabetes-related areas and considered part of the normative experience of long-term coping related to a complex medical condition. Given this, when making clinical diagnoses for psychosocial symptoms, it is important to remember that although there is some overlap in the differential diagnosis of depression, adjustment disorder, and T1D distress/burnout (e.g., all are related to negative emotions), there are also important distinctions to make, such as functional impairment, severity of symptoms, and impact of the negative emotions on specific areas of life (Snoek, Bremmer, & Hermanns, 2015).

Medical Basics

The T1D medical regimen is very complex and requires three primary tasks: (1) frequent glucose monitoring multiple times a day (recommended six to eight checks) either through a glucometer (finger prick) or a continuous glucose monitor (inserted into the skin), (2) precise carbohydrate counting (in grams) of all food/drinks consumed, and (3) intensive insulin dosing throughout the day using either a syringe/pen injection device or a subcutaneous insulin pump (a cannula is placed under the skin for 2–3 days at a time to deliver the insulin). There are two types of insulin given daily: bolus and basal. Bolus dosing is done through giving fast-acting insulin (average length of action is 2–3 h) to correct in the moment for carbohydrates consumed and current blood glucose levels. Basal insulin is a consistent amount of background insulin given within a 24-hour period regardless of the amount of carbohydrates consumed or the blood glucose levels throughout the day. This basal dose is administered either through a once daily injection or by continuously giving small doses throughout the day via the subcutaneous insulin pump. These T1D self-management tasks may appear to be deceptively simple; however, individuals with T1D have to complete these tasks within the context of energy expenditure (activity/exercise), stress, puberty, and other factors that all impact glycemic levels (Hood, Hilliard, Piatt, & Ievers-Landis, 2015). Average blood glucose levels over the previous 2–3 months is routinely measured though a lab test, called hemoglobin A1c (HbA1c), with a goal HbA1c of <7.0% for children (DiMeglio et al., 2018).

The technologies available to assist with T1D self-management are constantly changing, including new versions of subcutaneous insulin pumps, continuous glucose monitors that assess blood glucose levels every few minutes for 7–10 days at a time, and hybrid closed-loop systems that work to both measure blood glucose levels and subsequently dose insulin based on these levels in near-real time. Despite these technological advances, the nuances of T1D self-management for each person with T1D is multifaceted and requires active participation by the individual and their family/caregivers regardless of the device they use to administer insulin or check glucose levels. Therefore, it is important for all providers working with an individual with T1D to appreciate not only the complexity of their medical regimen but also the complexity of the behavioral management of T1D within individuals' unpredictable daily lives, especially for children and adolescents (Hood et al., 2015). Similarly, the way in which providers discuss how closely a patient follows their recommended medical regimen needs to be as nonjudgmental as possible. Given this, for the purposes of this chapter, the term "self-management," as opposed to "compliance" or "adherence," will be used when referencing the construct of managing one's T1D care within the context of multiple influences and factors.

Engagement

The CL psychologist has the unique opportunity to serve as one of the first providers to introduce the biopsychosocial model to patients and families, effectively setting the stage for potential outpatient work with a psychologist as an integrated part of their diabetes team. One of the ways CL psychologists work to promote trust and engagement as a means to facilitate the "buy in" for psychological services is by reflecting their appreciation for common barriers to change that are faced by patients and their families (e.g., recognizing the complexity of their medical regimen, acknowledging competing demands for time, identifying apprehension for needle injections). Further, in order to build a therapeutic alliance that demonstrates compassion and supportiveness, it is imperative that CL psychologists use a language that is encouraging, have an overall empathetic tone, ask open-ended questions, and collaboratively develop goals with the patient and family. Interactions that are blaming, induce guilt, and/or use scare tactics rarely work for sustaining behavior changes for anyone, but these approaches have been shown to be especially detrimental in T1D care (Hood et al., 2015). Dickenson and colleagues (Dickinson et al., 2017) outlined in detail how we, as providers, can use more effective communication with patients with T1D in order to minimize shame, disapproval, and discouragement. For example, they suggest the use of a person-first language (e.g., person with diabetes instead of diabetic as a noun), language that does not imply judgment (e.g., declined instead of refused), and strength-based language (e.g., checked blood glucose instead of tested blood glucose).

In order to be successful at engaging patients, the CL psychologist providing services to inpatients with T1D during hospitalizations needs to not only use inclusive language but also be able to interact with individuals from varying developmental levels, ranging from very young children to young adults who may be working to transition to adult care. CL psychologists may be asked to provide their services for myriad reasons, including adjustment to initial T1D diagnosis, improving self-management after an episode of diabetes ketoacidosis (DKA) (when blood ketones build up in the body due to not having enough insulin available that leads to the body's acidity to increase to dangerous levels, which can eventually cause coma or death), or for an unrelated, comorbid admission (e.g., surgical intervention, infection, or any procedure or surgery requiring being without food for a significant period of time). During these consultations, CL psychologists work to build a therapeutic alliance with the patient and family while taking into account the patient's age, sex, ethnic background, community infrastructure, health literacy, level of independence, and any previously established beliefs or judgments of people with T1D (Hood et al., 2015). An important way for CL psychologists to build rapport and facilitate engagement is to focus on the assessment of the baseline coping skills and adjustment strategies that the patient and their family have established prior to coming into the hospital, as well as to roll with any resistance that the family may have in needing to be hospitalized. Overall, the CL psychologist aims to serve as an integral part of the multidisciplinary team through their expertise in child development, family systems, psychosocial and behavioral aspects of complex medical conditions in youth, and empirically supported interventions for people with T1D. By promoting child and family health during their interactions with patients and family members, CL psychologists can effectively demystify the biopsychosocial approach and potentially impact the family's willingness and readiness to accept mental health support services throughout their child's lifetime with T1D.

Formulation

Although there is a large body of literature that supports a pediatric psychologist in conducting assessments and developing treatment plans for patients with T1D in outpatient care settings, much less information is available to assist CL psychologists with best formulating a problem-focused intervention during inpatient care (Kichler et al., 2015). During the period of initial diagnosis, the CL psychologist will want to explore the child and family's understanding of T1D and expectations for their medical care going forward, assess for typical expressions of distress or discomfort, identify different ways that family members cope and communicate during times of adversity, and determine any additional strengths and/or barriers to their medical management. Another role of the CL psychologist is to normalize adjustment issues, especially by providing anticipatory guidance for the first 1–2 years post diagnosis, when there is some evidence that initial depressive symptoms may persist over time (Grey, Whittemore, & Tamborlane, 2002; Kovacs et al., 1997; McGill et al., 2018). There may only be limited time for the CL psychologist to administer formal questionnaires during an inpatient admission; however, by taking a brief mental health history, one can identify any premorbid psychosocial functioning issues (e.g., ADHD, depression, anxiety, needle phobia, math learning disabilities) that may impact the patient's success with future T1D self-management. Finally, the CL psychologist can assess the impact of the T1D diagnosis on the larger family system's functioning (e.g., parental depression and/or anxiety), as well as get a general sense of the family's health literacy and numeracy skills, i.e., ability to interpret readings from the glucometer, calculate the number of grams of carbohydrates consumed, and perform calculations for adjusting insulin accordingly (Hood et al., 2015). This clinical data will be beneficial to the multidisciplinary team in their ability to implement treatment plans over time.

The CL psychologists may also be consulted to provide inpatient evaluation and formulation of a treatment plan in situations other than initial diagnosis. One of the most typical reasons is a child/adolescent who was admitted for DKA. Approximately one DKA occurs for every 14 patients in the United States per year after diagnosis (Maahs et al., 2015); therefore, this often leads to the subsequent consultation of a CL psychologist for services. In these cases, the CL psychologist can contribute to the formulation of the post-discharge treatment plan by quickly assessing for the following factors in the patient and family: (1) motivation and other indicators of one's readiness for behavior change, such as evidence of learned helplessness, avoidant coping, secondary gain from maladaptive behaviors, and negative health beliefs; (2) behavioral management of T1D, such as the level of parental supervision and monitoring, whether the child has developmentally appropriate levels of self-care behaviors within the context of their social and emotional maturity, and their ability to use problem-solving skills; and, (3) emotional concerns, such as symptoms of depression (including passive or active suicidal ideation), anxiety, disordered eating, ADHD, and diabetes distress/burnout. Patients and families are frequently under significant stress during their hospital stay; however, spending time gathering this information about the biopsychosocial factors that led to an inpatient admission for DKA allows the CL psychologist to accurately formulate a comprehensive understanding of the situation and provide recommendations to the team that can be implemented more in depth after discharge.

Intervention

Evidence-based interventions are utilized when working with common clinical referral issues for patients with T1D, such as difficulties with self-management, adjustment/coping issues, family conflict, depression, diabetes burnout, and anxiety. For CL psychologists, these are typically brief and targeted interventions (Hilliard et al., 2016) regardless of whether they are addressed inpatient during an admission or outpatient in clinic. The goal of these interventions is to improve the child's functioning through improving family collaboration and communication, as well as shared parent-child responsibility for self-management (family teamwork). Interventions that include behavioral strategies (e.g., increased knowledge, problem-solving skills), organizational tools to increase structure and routines, and motivational interviewing techniques to increase readiness to change behaviors have all been shown to help facilitate the self-management of T1D through improving self-management and glycemic control. Additionally, to enhance general adjustment and coping in children with T1D, coping skill training that focuses on extinguishing high-risk behaviors and decreasing clinical distress has also been found to be effective.

Goal setting is critical when working with patients with T1D. The SMART framework (specific, measurable, achievable, realistic, and time based) for goal-setting strategies is recommended to be used with every encounter when establishing self-management goals (Hood et al., 2015). For interventions to be as effective as possible and maintained, it is important to have patients implement their goals as soon as possible after the recommendation is made. Ways that this can be encouraged may include having them pair their planned behavioral changes with an existing routine, identify an upcoming event that they would like to receive as a reinforcement that can help them sustain their motivation (e.g., obtaining a driver's license or going on a sleepover), brainstorm how the parent may be able to support the child to maintain their efforts to change, and identify a way to ask the T1D provider for feedback on their progress between specialty care clinic visits (Hood et al., 2015).

Adaptation

As outlined above, most of the theories on interventions for children and families with T1D come from social cognitive therapy, family system theory, and social ecological models. The systemic reviews on the best available research evidence suggest that these interventions all have a modest but meaningful (small- to medium-effect sizes) impact on quality of life, T1D self-management, and glycemic levels (Hood et al., 2015). In order to achieve larger effect sizes, interventions need to have multiple components to their intervention (rather than those that are strictly educationally based), address modifiable diabetes-related and family processes (rather than only self-management behavioral outcomes), and be delivered sooner (rather than later) after the diagnosis of T1D (Hood et al., 2015). Even with a strong literature base for T1D interventions, in general, CL psychologists still need to utilize the evidence-base process when making decisions about how to best implement interventions (Spring, Craighead, & Hitchcock, 2009). It is important to consider individual child and/or family characteristics within the larger context of each child's environment, as well as other available resources such as the practitioner's own expertise in T1D.

When adapting interventions to meet the context and needs of the child and family's characteristics, the CL psychologist aims to tailor the expectations or goals of the intervention on multiple levels. As mentioned previously, the CL psychologist should consider the family's readiness for change, any functional aspects of present maladaptive behaviors, other structural demands on the family's time and energy (including household chaos), and the family's competing demands and priorities (Levin, Kichler, & Polfuss, 2013). In addition, the CL psychologist needs to be able to quickly identify if there are any other comorbid issues that may impact the patient and family's organizational abilities and success with completing self-management effectively, such as ADHD, executive dysfunction (e.g., planning, initiation of tasks, inhibition of behaviors), or learning disorders (including numeracy issues; Goethals et al., 2018; Mulvaney, Lilley, Cavanaugh, Pittel, & Rothman, 2013). Based on this assessment, the CL psychologist may need to adapt interventions to be more in line with the needs of the patient and family at the time of the consult, such as focusing on support during inpatient hospitalization, readiness or "buy in" to the idea of engaging in outpatient long-term follow-up, and/or setting more attainable SMART goals that are individualized for that patient/family. These goals likely will not result in the immediate achievement of what the American Diabetes Association ideally recommends for optimal self-management goals; however, an acknowledgement of these small, but important, first steps toward readiness to change is vitally important to build sustained change over time. From a family system perspective, CL psychologists may need to identify and address salient family conflict issues, such as miscarried helping (Duke, Wagner, Ulrich, Freeman, & Harris, 2016), where the parent/caregiver is trying to be helpful and supportive but does so in a manner that is shame inducing and paradoxically decreases the patient's likelihood of completing self-management in the long run.

When making decisions about adapting interventions, factors such as practitioner expertise in working with children and families with T1D also need to be considered. The CL psychologist not only needs to be trained in pediatric psychology but should also be able to implement behavioral interventions from the best available research evidence and be at least modestly well versed in T1D physiology. The CL psychologist does not have to rise to the level of being an expert in T1D, nor do they have to replace the role of the diabetes educator, diabetes social worker, or diabetes medical provider. Conversely, the services provided by the other diabetes team members should also aim to augment the assessment and brief intervention work that the CL psychologist provides.

Resources/Support Given that T1D is a chronic condition that is primarily managed on an outpatient basis by a large multidisciplinary team, it is essential that the CL psychologist collaborate with the diabetes team members in order to obtain a wide range of resources and support for the patient/family. This includes endocrinology providers (medical doctors and/or nurse practitioners), social workers, dieticians, and certified diabetes educators from the outpatient team. The outpatient multidisciplinary team is often very knowledgable of the history of each of their patients, as well as the general behavioral/emotional impact of T1D on their families. However, since the inpatient multidisciplinary team (e.g., social worker, nursing staff, child life specialists) may not be as familiar with the patient/family as the outpatient team is, the role of the CL psychologist can be helpful in coordinating inpatient and outpatient care and providing a unique perspective. Additionally, the CL psychologist may be able to connect with the patient/family as a "new" member to the medical team—someone with fresh ideas, perspective, and possibly distance from preconceived biases or judgments perceived by the patient/family.

In addition to the CL psychologists' role in providing inpatient treatment directly to the patients and their families, they may also have to provide support and interventions to the multidisciplinary diabetes team to help them most effectively engage with their patients and families. For example, the CL psychologist may need to remind the diabetes team members that readiness to change is a state not a trait, help set up boundaries of what the CL psychologist can and cannot do during a brief interaction with the patient and their family, remind the team of patient and family autonomy in making decisions about their treatment, and model the art of rolling with resistance when interacting with patients and families. Rollnick, Miller, and Butler (2008) outlined recommendations to help health care providers use the "spirit" of motivational interviewing in their interactions with the family (e.g., reflective listening, exploring ambivalence, open-ended questioning). Similarly, the CL psychologist can provide feedback and model for the diabetes team member strategies for using guidance rather than direct advice giving, employ collaborative problem-solving to remove barriers to self-management rather than provide/prescribe solutions to the family, and engage in family communication in a way that honors the patient's perspective rather than inadvertently induce more shame and guilt about the patient's T1D self-management.

From a system perspective, the CL psychologist can provide support at the health care delivery system level, including providing training and education to medical providers and allied health professionals (e.g., certified diabetes educators, social workers, nurses) about how they can deliver brief, clinic-integrated behavioral interventions independently, even when no psychologist is available for consultation. This kind of integrated approach can be very cost-effective and help yield more efficacious health outcomes by integrating behavioral interventions more readily into already demanding and time-intensive medical visits. The American Diabetes Association provides recommendations for providing routine psychosocial assessments and T1D self-management and support education to patients with T1D (Young-Hyman et al., 2016). The CL psychologist can integrate these recommendations along with psychosocially minded, evidence-based interventions to disseminate to the larger health system and thus impact the overall work with children with T1D and their families.

In-Hospital Consultation

Inpatient psychology consultation for patients with T1D is typically sought at the time of initial diagnosis and for DKA admissions. Under both circumstances, consults are inherently faced with several barriers: patients typically feel very sick, leading up to admission due to their bodies having literally been starved of energy and nutrients; admissions tend to only be a couple of days in length, so there is not a lot of time for multiple follow-ups; most care will be provided through outpatient follow-up, so it is not always possible to complete extensive inpatient interventions; and patients and families often feel shamed and blamed for being admitted for DKA or are overwhelmed with trying to understand and accept a new diagnosis while also absorbing the complex information provided from diabetes education. Given this, the CL psychologist's assessment will need to be brief, focused, and targeted at getting patient and family's "buy-in" for outpatient care follow-up. During the admission, the CL psychologist should capitalize on setting the stage for increasing motivation and readiness to change while realizing that most change will still need to occur after discharge and with the involvement of the diabetes team.

Typical inpatient CL interventions for newly diagnosed patients will focus on what needs to be acutely completed during the admission. Of top priority is assuring that the T1D self-management information provided to the patient and family is heard, understood, and retained and especially that home medical care can be competently conducted (e.g., insulin administration, blood glucose checking). Some families will require considerable intervention to be ready for discharge home, while others will acclimate relatively quickly. Potential interventions may include support around the new diagnosis, adjustment to the medical situation/expectations, psychoeducation about T1D, problem-solving around the expected medical regimen with the transition to home, and potential needle fears. Of note, needle fears may be present at the time of the new diagnosis, develop with the in-hospital introduction of insulin injections, or occur well after initial diagnosis and the introduction of injections. This can be of great concern as avoidance of needles can lead to difficulties completing self-management behaviors and lead to suboptimal care (e.g., insistence on using the same injection site, reluctance to completing lab draws, time-consuming/procrastinating rituals during the injections, and/or the child not allowing others to do any injections for them, which can lead to caregiver burnout).

When involved with inpatient admissions for DKA, CL psychologists will often employ therapeutic strategies similar to behavioral family system therapy for diabetes (BFST-D) interventions (Wysocki et al., 2007). This type of approach helps clinicians combine aspects of motivational interviewing, family system interventions, and cognitive behavioral therapy approaches, but in a briefer and more targeted manner. For example, CL psychologists may want to use contingency management strategies to focus on increasing one specific self-management behavior (e.g., frequency of blood glucose checks), identify immediate barriers for the self-management of T1D prior to discharge, highlight various coping strategies that can be used to deal with caregiver burnout/distress, and focus on obtaining ongoing outpatient treatment for sustained improvements in glycemic control over time. Just as in the outpatient setting, the CL psychologist can quickly teach problem-solving strategies during an inpatient consultation. Specifically, they should provide a clear, simplified message that focuses on a single, focused recommendation (as opposed to many) with small amounts of information and provide this information in multiple formats (e.g., verbal, visual, written) at the literacy level of the patient and family (Hood et al., 2015). An effective approach is to include a "teach me back" method, where the CL psychologist has the child teach the parent what they just learned. Despite the evidence base for such interventions in adolescents, more research is needed to better understand their utility within the various clinical settings and with child and young adult populations (Hilliard et al., 2016).

The inpatient CL psychologist is often called upon to provide safety assessments and planning for high-risk behaviors in patients with T1D, including suicidality and self-harm (Matlock, Yayah Jones, Corathers, & Kichler, 2017). This could involve determining whether the patient is experiencing active versus passive suicidal ideation and/or self-harm behaviors (especially as it relates to the potentially lethal misuse of insulin) and determining the type and level of psychological/psychiatric intervention needed. When there is active suicidal ideation (e.g., the patient expresses a specific plan, implies intent to harm oneself, has had a previous attempt, has access to means), then the CL psychologist needs to collaborate with inpatient psychiatry/crisis team colleagues to determine whether or not the patient requires an inpatient psychiatric hospitalization, 1:1 sitters at the hospital bedside, and/or removal of access to insulin so that caregivers have full control. The CL psychologist may be asked to help work with the family and the care team to develop a graduated reintroduction of insulin access over time as patients demonstrate safe use of insulin in less and less restrictive environments.

If the CL psychologist's assessment demonstrates more passive suicidal ideation (e.g., has no specific plan, denies intent, has no prior known attempt, but does have thoughts/ideation about not wanting to live anymore), then the CL psychologist can work with the family to help them develop a safety plan that includes, but is not limited to, increasing supervision by caregivers, limiting full access to high-risk objects (e.g., insulin, other medications, weapons) as appropriate, exploring alternative coping strategies to deal with the distress in a healthier manner, facilitating open communication with patient and support network at home, and providing safety contact information and resources if symptoms escalate in the future. Similarly, self-harm behaviors (i.e., cutting/harming their body for emotional coping/regulation purposes) can manifest through passively declining to care for T1D or actively engaging in physical injury behaviors (e.g., using insulin needles to cut skin). Like interventions for passive suicidal ideation, the CL psychologist can work with caregivers to make environmental changes (e.g., remove objects from the patient's immediate area that can be used for self-harm and increase visual monitoring for further physical injuries on the body), as well as increase open and honest communication about emotions by making one's private distress into a more open and nonjudgmental conversation, provide alternative coping strategies when the patient has the urge to self-harm (e.g., distraction, self-soothing), and identify safety contacts to rely upon for support when triggered.

Outpatient Consultation

As mentioned previously, if an inpatient hospitalization occurs for a patient with T1D (other than at initial diagnosis), there is almost always going to be a recommendation by the CL psychologist for the family to seek outpatient therapy follow-up to help address the longer term goals of improving self-management, cope with comorbid mental health issues and/or diabetes burnout, or address any family-conflict about T1D care. Being admitted for diabetes-related complications (such as DKA) as a child is relatively rare, and most DKA admissions stem from significant self-management issues over an extended period. Given this, the CL psychologist can help the family recognize that the status quo cannot be maintained once discharged as there will need to be behavioral and family system changes over time. Many of the families will need longer term outpatient follow-up services that use individual, family, and group-based interventions with providers familiar with the intersection of T1D and psychosocial issues. However, even though outpatient services are often recommended, not all families will be able to immediately go into traditional outpatient individual/family therapy because of myriad barriers (e.g., transportation, finances, schedules, and waitlists). Sometimes bridge care (i.e., brief, supportive care) may be provided by the CL psychologist in the outpatient setting in order to provide ongoing care until the family can secure outpatient treatment.

Another outpatient consultation model that may be relevant for CL psychologists is providing clinical services in the outpatient multidisciplinary clinic setting. These psychologists are embedded directly into the clinic to provide brief, targeted strategies to improve adjustment, adherence, and coping (Kichler et al., 2015). The psychologists involved in this type of consultative model may also be asked to do real-time psychosocial screening and follow-up, such as through standardized interviews, parent-proxy questionnaires, and child/adolescent self-report measures. For example, depression and suicidal ideation can be routinely assessed and addressed during clinic visits (Corathers et al., 2013). Similar to the CL consultations provided within an inpatient setting, brief behavioral, organizational, and motivational interviewing techniques provided by a psychologist in the outpatient clinic setting have been found to be helpful in improving adherence, coping, and distress while decreasing high-risk behaviors (Kichler et al., 2015).

There are also new and innovative extensions to the CL consultative model that have recently been used in T1D populations. For example, the Novel Interventions in Children's Healthcare (NICH) program is an intervention that uses a wide variety of mental health services with the families who have high rates of repeated DKA hospitalizations to improve health outcomes using care coordination and case management (Harris et al., 2013). The interventions are provided by multiple types of mental health providers and across many systems (e.g., family, school, and hospital) and yielded some positive initial results (Wagner, Barry, Stoeckel, Teplitsky, & Harris, 2017). Despite not having strong empirical evidence yet, another future extension to consultative work for children with T1D and their families will likely involve telehealth follow-up options, such as videoconferencing, phone contacts, remote glucose downloads through websites, and web-based education (Giani & Laffel, 2016; Lee, Ooi, & Lai, 2017). Specifically, telemedicine has the potential to decrease barriers for families of children with T1D to receive mental health support for T1D self-management (e.g., distance, time, and financial), but there remain many obstacles to making these telehealth options a standard method of care (e.g., insurance reimbursement, licensure guidelines across state lines). Therefore, work is needed to better understand if a telehealth consultative approach can have a positive impact on health outcomes, such as improved glycemic levels, reduced frequency of hospitalizations for DKA, and promotion of a higher quality of life for children with T1D and their families.

Case Example

"Stephen" was an 11-year-old male who was diagnosed with T1D 3 years prior and had a history of ADHD. He lived at home with his single mother and 13-year-old brother. After diagnosis, Stephen was followed closely by an outpatient multidisciplinary team, consisting of a primary physician, nurse practitioner, dietician, and social worker, as well as a psychologist both through clinic consultation and the more traditional outpatient therapy. His involvement with the psychologist waxed and waned over a 2-year period, depending on psychosocial stressors (e.g., finances, changes in living situations, and inconsistent transportation to appointments). In the outpatient setting, therapeutic goals focused on increasing Stephen's willingness to complete his T1D tasks without behavioral outbursts, as well as increase Mother's parenting abilities to effectively manage Stephen's behaviors while not giving him too much responsibility for his T1D self-management for which he is not developmentally ready. Medically, Stephen typically was able to remain more stable (i.e., more in-target glycemic levels with an HbA1c range = 8–10%) when supports were in place (e.g., regular sessions with the psychologist, consistent medical clinic appointments, assistance with his medical regimen at school from the nurse); however, despite best efforts, he required several admissions to the hospital for DKA—sometimes for stabilization on the general medical floor and other times emergently to the intensive care unit (ICU).

Once, Stephen required admission for severe hyperglycemia following his refusal to follow rules and expectations at home, his loss of consistent support from a school nurse during a break, and a limited follow-up with outpatient psychology due to transportation issues. During his admission, inpatient CL psychology was asked to provide support with the stress of hospitalization, a discussion of barriers to self-management at home, and a discussion of reengaging with the outpatient psychologist. The CL psychologist initially met with Stephen alone and spent time building rapport by watching a few minutes of the television program he had on in the room and then learning about his hobbies, likes/dislikes, school situation, friendships, and family makeup. As comfort increased, the CL psychologist was able to gradually work up to "harder" questions about his understanding of his medical history, current admission, medical expectations/regimen, and barriers to self-management. Questions were framed by the CL psychologist in developmentally appropriate ways in order to meet Stephen at his level (e.g., what's your understanding of why you're in the hospital? All kids miss their medications sometimes—how often would you say you miss your insulin? What makes it hard to take your insulin? Sometimes kids tell me that they don't want their friends to know they have diabetes—is that the case for you?).

With this information, the CL psychologist facilitated a discussion between Stephen and his mother, highlighting areas where Stephen is struggling and would benefit from additional support, as well as concerns that his mother had about his choices. The CL psychologist utilized acceptance-based strategies to identify Stephen and his mother's goals and values (e.g., staying out of the hospital, improved family relationships), motivational interviewing techniques to identify areas of change and readiness for change (e.g., limited T1D understanding, improving routines), as well as problem-solving (e.g., how to logistically get back into outpatient therapy). Additionally, the CL psychologist further facilitated a discussion between Stephen and his mother as both were emotional when his mother shared her worry for Stephen's health and safety both in the short term and long term. Prior to completing the consult, the goals for moving forward were reviewed by the CL psychologist: (1) speak with the medical team about focusing education efforts directly with Stephen to increase his understand of *why* he is being asked to do the things he is asked; (2) focus on improved communication at home, specifically listening to one another and maintaining calm voices within a discussion; (3) reestablish a school routine for insulin management with the school nurse; (4) set up regular follow-up with outpatient psychologist; and (5) follow up with outpatient psychiatry for medication management for Stephen's ADHD. Stephen and his mother agreed with these goals and expressed gratitude for the consult to help them communicate, organize themselves, and plan for moving forward after discharge.

Following discharge from the above admission, Stephen reengaged with outpatient psychology, and with support from his school nurse, routine and expectations were again established for Stephen and his mother using behavioral interventions and problem-solving strategies. Stephen also restarted psychotropic medications for his ADHD symptoms. Ultimately, Stephen was able to have some more developmentally appropriate independence around his medical regimen, and his mother knew more about when and how to give him opportunities to take ownership for his role in his T1D care while also providing supportive direct supervision and monitoring to assure that he was accurately caring for himself. She and the school nurse also communicated more often than before, and the school nurse felt more empowered to make T1D self-management decisions even when she did not have regular communication with his mother. At the same time, additional supports were put in place in the community to help him secure in-home therapy services to address real-time behavioral issues, identify a recreation center that he could attend after school, and be engaged in prosocial activities, and a community health worker from the hospital was assigned to Stephen's case to help with managing health care logistics (e.g., transportation, medication refills, appointment scheduling).

Unfortunately, as is not uncommon for many patients and families, life changes and events occur, routines fade, and the acuity of medical admissions diminishes. For example, several months after the DKA admission mentioned above, Stephen's mother was out of town on a planned trip (during another school break) and arranged for Stephen to be supervised by a trusted adult, who had minimal T1D experience/training. Even though Stephen had some independence in his care and knew, in general, what was supposed to be done for his self-management, he had been recently started on a new insulin pump and too much trust was placed in the technology to help monitor Stephen's T1D care. During this time that his mother was away, Stephen engaged in eating without dosing insulin and his technology failed; therefore, his blood glucose levels were not properly monitored/supported despite the trusted adult's reported best efforts. He ultimately required an ICU admission following severe DKA and the need for resuscitation upon admission.

Unfortunately, the CL psychologist was not consulted during this admission; however, the inpatient team utilized the assistance of the inpatient social worker in order to determine whether there was a need for child protective service (CPS) involvement and safe discharge planning. A report was ultimately made to CPS for follow-up; however, Stephen was deemed safe to be discharged into the care of his mother and the outpatient multidisciplinary team to reestablish effective T1D self-management skills again, especially over school breaks, when one of the major support team members (e.g., school nurse) was not able to provide regular support. This back and forth between inpatient and outpatient settings for some patients is common and requires strong communication between providers in each setting to maximize the utilization of appropriate resources.

Appendix: Attachments: Resources for Patients and Families (∗Note: Not an Exhaustive list∗)

On-line Resources

American Diabetes Association® (ADA)—http://www.diabetes.org/

- Including Diabetes Camps, the Safe At School Program, and Know Your Rights Campaign

JDRF©—https://www.jdrf.org/

- Including local chapters, support groups, parent mentoring programs, advocacy, and fundraisers
- Type One Nation Summit: http://jdrfsummit.org/

Children with Diabetes® (CWD)—http://www.childrenwithdiabetes.com/

- Including the Friends for Life® conferences

College Diabetes Network© (CDN)—https://collegediabetesnetwork.org/

- Including local chapters to support students at universities/colleges

Beyond Type 1©—https://beyondtype1.org/

dLife©—https://dlife.com/

diaTribe©—https://diatribe.org/

Glu©—https://myglu.org/

Blogs (e.g., Six Until Me™, A Sweet Life™) and Facebook Groups

Podcasts (e.g., TypeNone—Type 1 Diabetes (and more!)©, The Bravest Life©, Juicebox Podcast: Type 1 Diabetes©)

Apps (e.g., CalorieKing®, Blue Loop®, mySugr®)

Books

Children's Diabetes Foundation©: https://www.childrensdiabetesfoundation.org/books/

Raising Teens with Diabetes: A Survival Guide for Parents by Moira McCarthy

Cheating Destiny: Living with Diabetes, America's Biggest Epidemic by James S. Hirsch

Type 1 Teens: A Guide to Managing Your Life with Diabetes by Korey K. Hood, PhD

Diabetes Burnout: What to Do When You Can't Take It Anymore by William H. Polonsky, PhD, CDE

Transitions in Care: The Challenges of Diabetes In Young Adults by Howard Wolport, MD, Barbara Anderson, PhD, CDE, and Jill Weissberg-Benchell, PhD, CDE

Bright Spots and Landmines: The Diabetes Guide I Wish Someone Had Handed Me by Adam Brown

Think Like a Pancreas: A Practical Guide to Managing Diabetes with Insulin by Gary Scheiner, MS, CDE

References

Christoffersson, G., Rodriguez-Calvo, T., & von Herrath, M. (2016). Recent advances in understanding Type 1 Diabetes. *F1000Res, 5*. https://doi.org/10.12688/f1000research.7356.1

Corathers, S. D., Kichler, J., Jones, N. H., Houchen, A., Jolly, M., Morwessel, N., … Hood, K. K. (2013). Improving depression screening for adolescents with type 1 diabetes. *Pediatrics, 132*(5), e1395–e1402. https://doi.org/10.1542/peds.2013-0681

Dickinson, J. K., Guzman, S. J., Maryniuk, M. D., O'Brian, C. A., Kadohiro, J. K., Jackson, R. A., … Funnell, M. M. (2017). The use of language in diabetes care and education. *Diabetes Care, 40*(12), 1790–1799. https://doi.org/10.2337/dci17-0041

DiMeglio, L. A., Acerini, C. L., Codner, E., Craig, M. E., Hofer, S. E., Pillay, K., & Maahs, D. M. (2018).

ISPAD Clinical Practice Consensus Guidelines 2018: Glycemic control targets and glucose monitoring for children, adolescents, and young adults with diabetes. *Pediatric Diabetes, 19*(Suppl 27), 105–114. https://doi.org/10.1111/pedi.12737

Duke, D. C., Wagner, D. V., Ulrich, J., Freeman, K. A., & Harris, M. A. (2016). Videoconferencing for teens with diabetes: Family matters. *Journal of Diabetes Science and Technology, 10*(4), 816–823. https://doi.org/10.1177/1932296816642577

Giani, E., & Laffel, L. (2016). Opportunities and challenges of telemedicine: Observations from the wild west in pediatric type 1 diabetes. *Diabetes Technology & Therapeutics, 18*(1), 1–3. https://doi.org/10.1089/dia.2015.0360

Goethals, E. R., de Wit, M., Van Broeck, N., Lemiere, J., Van Liefferinge, D., Bohler, S., … Luyckx, K. (2018). Child and parental executive functioning in type 1 diabetes: Their unique and interactive role toward treatment adherence and glycemic control. *Pediatric Diabetes, 19*(3), 520–526. https://doi.org/10.1111/pedi.12552

Grey, M., Whittemore, R., & Tamborlane, W. (2002). Depression in type 1 diabetes in children: Natural history and correlates. *Journal of Psychosomatic Research, 53*(4), 907–911.

Harris, M.A., Spiro, K., Heywood, M., et al. (2013). Novel interventions in children's health care (NICH): innovative treatment for youth with complex medical conditions. *Clin Pract Pediatr Psychol. 1*(2), 137–145.

Hilliard, M. E., Powell, P. W., & Anderson, B. J. (2016). Evidence-based behavioral interventions to promote diabetes management in children, adolescents, and families. *American Psychologist, 71*(7), 590–601. https://doi.org/10.1037/a0040359

Hood, K. K., Hilliard, M., Piatt, G., & Ievers-Landis, C. E. (2015). Effective strategies for encouraging behavior change in people with diabetes. *Diabetes Management (London), 5*(6), 499–413.

Kichler, J. C., Harris, M. A., & Weissberg-Benchell, J. (2015). Contemporary roles of the pediatric psychologist in diabetes care. *Current Diabetes Reviews, 11*(4), 210–221.

Kovacs, M., Goldston, D., Obrosky, D. S., & Bonar, L. K. (1997). Psychiatric disorders in youths with IDDM: Rates and risk factors. *Diabetes Care, 20*(1), 36–44.

Lawrence, J. M., Imperatore, G., Dabelea, D., Mayer-Davis, E. J., Linder, B., Saydah, S., & D'Agostino, R. B., Jr. (2014). Trends in incidence of type 1 diabetes among non-Hispanic white youth in the U.S., 2002–2009. *Diabetes, 63*(11), 3938–3945. https://doi.org/10.2337/db13-1891

Lee, S. W. H., Ooi, L., & Lai, Y. K. (2017). Telemedicine for the management of glycemic control and clinical outcomes of Type 1 Diabetes mellitus: A systematic review and meta-analysis of randomized controlled studies. *Frontiers in Pharmacology, 8*, 330. https://doi.org/10.3389/fphar.2017.00330

Levin, L., Kichler, J. C., & Polfuss, M. (2013). The relationship between hemoglobin A1C in youth with type 1 diabetes and chaos in the family household. *The Diabetes Educator, 39*(5), 696–704. https://doi.org/10.1177/0145721713496872

Maahs, D. M., Hermann, J. M., Holman, N., Foster, N. C., Kapellen, T. M., Allgrove, J., … Holl, R. W. (2015). Rates of diabetic ketoacidosis: International comparison with 49,859 pediatric patients with type 1 diabetes from England, Wales, the U.S., Austria, and Germany. *Diabetes Care, 38*(10), 1876–1882. https://doi.org/10.2337/dc15-0780

Matlock, K. A., Yayah Jones, N. H., Corathers, S. D., & Kichler, J. C. (2017). Clinical and psychosocial factors associated with suicidal ideation in adolescents with type 1 diabetes. *The Journal of Adolescent Health, 61*(4), 471–477. https://doi.org/10.1016/j.jadohealth.2017.05.004

McGill, D. E., Volkening, L. K., Pober, D. M., Muir, A. B., Young-Hyman, D. L., & Laffel, L. M. (2018). Depressive symptoms at critical times in youth with type 1 diabetes: Following type 1 diabetes diagnosis and insulin pump initiation. *The Journal of Adolescent Health, 62*(2), 219–225. https://doi.org/10.1016/j.jadohealth.2017.09.017

Mulvaney, S. A., Lilley, J. S., Cavanaugh, K. L., Pittel, E. J., & Rothman, R. L. (2013). Validation of the diabetes numeracy test with adolescents with type 1 diabetes. *Journal of Health Communication, 18*(7), 795–804. https://doi.org/10.1080/10810730.2012.757394

Rollnick, S., Miller, W. R., & Butler, C. (2008). *Motivational interviewing in health care: helping patients change behavior*. New York: Guilford Press.

Shapiro, J. B., Vesco, A. T., Weil, L. E. G., Evans, M. A., Hood, K. K., & Weissberg-Benchell, J. (2017). Psychometric properties of the problem areas in diabetes: Teen and parent of teen versions. *Journal of Pediatric Psychology, 43*, 561. https://doi.org/10.1093/jpepsy/jsx146

Snoek, F. J., Bremmer, M. A., & Hermanns, N. (2015). Constructs of depression and distress in diabetes: Time for an appraisal. *The Lancet Diabetes and Endocrinology, 3*(6), 450–460. https://doi.org/10.1016/s2213-8587(15)00135-7

Spring, B., Craighead, W. E., & Hitchcock, K. (2009). Evidence-based practice in psychology. In *Corsini's encyclopedia of psychology* (4th ed., pp. 603–607). New York: Wiley.

Wagner, D. V., Barry, S. A., Stoeckel, M., Teplitsky, L., & Harris, M. A. (2017). NICH at its best for diabetes at its worst: texting teens and their caregivers for better outcomes. *Journal of Diabetes Science and Technology, 11*(3), 468–475. https://doi.org/10.1177/1932296817695337

Weissberg-Benchell, J., & Antisdel-Lomaglio, J. (2011). Diabetes-specific emotional distress among adolescents: Feasibility, reliability, and validity of the problem areas in diabetes-teen version. *Pediatric Diabetes, 12*(4 Pt 1), 341–344. https://doi.org/10.1111/j.1399-5448.2010.00720.x

Wysocki, T., Harris, M. A., Buckloh, L. M., Mertlich, D., Lochrie, A. S., Mauras, N., & White, N. H. (2007). Randomized trial of behavioral family systems therapy for diabetes maintenance of effects on diabetes outcomes in adolescents. *Diabetes Care, 30*(3), 555–560.

Young-Hyman, D., de Groot, M., Hill-Briggs, F., Gonzalez, J. S., Hood, K., & Peyrot, M. (2016). Psychosocial care for people with diabetes: A position statement of the American Diabetes Association. *Diabetes Care, 39*(12), 2126–2140. https://doi.org/10.2337/dc16-2053

Cystic Fibrosis

Adrienne P. Borschuk and Stephanie S. Filigno

Diagnosis and Medical Basics

Cystic fibrosis (CF) is a progressive genetic disease that results in the overproduction of thick, sticky mucus throughout the body. Individuals with CF have two copies of a defective gene called CF transmembrane regulator (CFTR), and there are over 1000 varieties of these CF-causing mutations (CFF, 2018b). CF is often diagnosed at birth through newborn screening, which is performed by all 50 states (Comeau et al., 2007); however, given the large number of mutations, some individuals with rarer mutations are "missed" and diagnosed later in life. Late diagnoses may also occur for children born before the state newborn screening guidelines started. Newborn screening can result in false positives, which can be highly stressful for parents (Tluczek, Orland, & Cavanagh, 2011). Children with CF who are not diagnosed and treated appropriately will continue to struggle with growth and weight gain, GI manifestations, and frequent respiratory infections (Sanders, Zhang, Farrell, Lai, & Wisconsin, 2018; VanDevanter, Kahle, O'Sullivan, Sikirica, & Hodgkins, 2016). A suspected CF diagnosis is confirmed via a sweat test, an indepth genetic testing, and a clinical evaluation (Cystic Fibrosis Foundation, 2018b).

Given the wide range of genetic mutations that cause cystic fibrosis, there is a spectrum of presentation, with great individual variation in phenotypic expression. Generally, primary organ systems affected include the respiratory system and gastrointestinal (GI) system. Individuals with cystic fibrosis often have a recurrent cough, which is exacerbated when they have an illness. A decline in pulmonary function over the lifespan, and during the time of acute illness, is to be expected and attributed to the cycle of infection leading to inflammation and ultimately irreversible tissue damage. The GI system is affected specifically with difficulty in absorbing nutrients and poor growth, which is addressed through taking pancreatic enzymes (85% of individuals will need these) with fat-containing meals and beverages. In addition, problems with constipation (and in severe cases distal intestinal obstruction syndrome (DIOS)) and/or diarrhea and gassiness are common, with some individuals developing CF-related liver disease. Having cystic fibrosis can also affect the sinuses, including recurrent

A. P. Borschuk · S. S. Filigno (✉)
Cincinnati Children's Hospital Medical Center, Cincinnati, OH, USA

Behavioral Medicine and Clinical Psychology, Cincinnati Children's Hospital Medical Center, Cincinnati, OH, USA

University of Cincinnati College of Medicine, Cincinnati, OH, USA
e-mail: Stephanie.Filigno@cchmc.org

B. D. Carter, K. A. Kullgren (eds.), *Clinical Handbook of Psychological Consultation in Pediatric Medical Settings*, Issues in Clinical Child Psychology, https://doi.org/10.1007/978-3-030-35598-2_25

sinusitis and the potential need to see subspecialists for sinus surgery. The blockage of the reproductive organs with mucus can also lead to difficulties with conception for females, and most males with CF (approximately 97%) are sterile due to agenesis of the vas deferens. Over time, approximately 20% of teens and 50% of adults with CF will develop cystic-fibrosis-related diabetes (Cystic Fibrosis Foundation, 2018b) and need to interface with endocrinology.

When free of respiratory symptoms, individuals with CF are recommended to follow their intensive daily health routine. Airway clearance therapy (ACT), the most time-consuming CF treatment, typically lasts 1 h and is done two to three times per day. Individuals with CF also take oral medications, including medications targeting the underlying CFTR defect (CFTR modulators), and nebulized medications. This treatment regimen is preventative and is recommended regardless of how physically well a person feels. One type of ACT is chest physiotherapy (CPT) and is performed manually by another person. Other forms of ACT provide increased flexibility and independence, such as high-frequency oscillating vests (including a recent portable vest option) or oscillating positive expiratory pressure. Many individuals are also expected to do daily sinus rinses with hypertonic saline. With such an involved and time-consuming treatment regimen, strict adherence to these treatments is generally poor (Modi et al., 2006).

During episodes of acute illness, the number of recommended treatments is increased in order to move mucus and expectorate it to prevent the further development of symptoms, requiring more time and energy when that individual is already not feeling physically well. When they have an acute respiratory infection, they will likely be prescribed oral antibiotics to treat the infection. If oral antibiotics do not sufficiently resolve symptoms, they may be admitted to the hospital for up to 2 weeks to receive intravenous (IV) antibiotics and more aggressive airway clearance to treat the pulmonary exacerbation. They also may receive physical therapy to aid in moving mucus and allow it to be cleared more easily. Throat cultures are routinely obtained to determine what pathogens the individual is growing in order to identify appropriate antibiotics to eradicate the organism(s). During hospital stays, ideally a hospital bedside teacher is available to aid students in their ability to receive some instruction and stay as caught up on schoolwork as possible. Child life services are also an important aspect of the admission, to provide access to pleasant activities and supportive and preventative interventions, such as relaxation and distraction during painful medical procedures.

The ultimate goal of the hospital admission is to restore health. Occasionally, admissions will be "planned" to occur at a time that is more convenient for the individual and/or family while still occurring at the appropriate time to address the exacerbation and may be "expected" based on failure of other treatments to improve health. However, many times the need to have a hospital admission is unexpected and, therefore, especially stressful given its interference with family routines, school, and other important activities. And while the decision to admit is often a shared goal between the medical team, family, and individual with CF, there are many factors for the CL provider to be aware of that make admissions inconvenient, stressful, and even distressing. First, being away from home and away from caregivers, siblings, and pets can be very upsetting. The need for an admission can occur at the same time as big life events, such as birthdays, holidays, and family and/or school events, such as sports tournaments, dances, and even planned family vacations. Second, due to infection control recommendations, individuals with CF are not allowed to interact face to face in order to prevent the sharing of illness-causing organisms that can be highly isolating. Third, the hospital environment and frequent monitoring by hospital staff can have a negative impact on sleep, with equipment alarms going off and lights not being sufficiently dimmed during sleep hours. Individuals with CF are also often more sedentary and confined to their hospital room during the admission, which is much different than their life at home. Fourth, there can be stress on the caregiver and family system during admissions as the family attempts to balance visiting and caring for the individual in the hospital with the co-occurring demands and responsibilities at home and at work. Admissions can also trigger an individual or family's fear of worsening the disease. Along these lines, the CL provider may hear the term lung function "baseline," which refers to a general range or goal, referencing the highest lung function observed in a specific period of time that is the target to reach prior to discharge.

Infection control procedures are institution specific but require care providers to wear some form of personal protective equipment (PPE) upon entering the room, which typically includes a gown, gloves, and sometimes a mask. Depending on the hospital regulations, the mask may cover both the provider's mouth and eyes to avoid droplet transmission. Individuals with CF are also strongly recommended to wear a mask upon entering the hospital environment through the course of the visit until they leave the hospital, which can bring upon some self-consciousness as other people observe them wearing the mask.

Given the medical complexities (i.e., navigating the medical system and insurance system), illness uncertainties, and burden of daily care, individuals and their support systems can be significantly affected emotionally, behaviorally, and cognitively. While many individuals and systems may be resilient throughout the lifespan (Ernst, Johnson, & Stark, 2010) and are able to balance daily care demands with optimizing quality of life, being proactive in providing anticipatory guidance, conducting clinical assessment, and delivering brief interventions to address areas of need is ideal to promote wellness (Boat, Filigno, & Amin, 2017) in parent–child interactions, sibling interactions, and patient–provider interactions.

Engagement

Once the CL provider has a comprehensive understanding of the potential wide range of impact that having CF, and specifically a pulmonary exacerbation, can have on various aspects of quality of life (including physical, emotional, behavioral, and social functioning), the provider is able to bring a perspective to interdisciplinary care that is highly focused on the emotional and behavioral health and needs of the individual with CF and the support system. The CL provider can elevate relevant psychosocial factors that impact wellness, healthy coping, and adherence promotion so that other care team members are aware of these factors and can consider them in the overall biopsychosocial model to best understand the health promotion landscape.

Ultimately, the hospital admission will restore health and equip the individual with CF with the skills to optimize the management of CF daily care once they return home. CL providers are intermittently involved in interdisciplinary CF care team and may not know the individual and/or family background, as well as the medical team; therefore, communicating with the team about relevant historical and current biopsychosocial factors is essential. It is also important for the CL provider to be mindful of potential bias that team members may have developed in their interactions with the individual and/or family and to approach assessment and need for intervention with openness and flexibility. Depending on individuals' past experiences with mental health care providers, the CL provider may need to introduce psychosocial care benefits, focus on brief assessment and intervention, and educate people about the role of CL and the potential advantages of including this service within the overall CF health care model. Specifically, the CL provider can be familiar with the mental health guidelines (Quittner et al., 2014) that recommend annual screening for anxiety and depression and the best practice treatment recommendations, as well as some of the literature that has linked mental health with adherence and physical health outcomes (Barker & Quittner, 2016; Smith, Modi, Quittner, & Wood, 2010).

The CL provider can normalize the impact of stressors that occur during an admission and during the life of an individual with CF and both the support system and the health care team. This critical task is accomplished via frequent communication between interdisciplinary inpatient care providers about treatment targets, progress with interventions, and ongoing needs. CL psychologists can also significantly aid in the development of residents and fellows in teaching hospitals, who typically play a key role in the care of individuals during an admission stay. CL psychologists can provide education about how psychosocial factors are impacting current functioning and how communication and/or approach to medical care can be adapted to fit the needs of the individual with cystic fibrosis.

Formulation

There are many resources available to inpatient clinicians that allow them to gather comprehensive background information on their patient. Individuals with CF have frequent, well-documented contact with their CF care team that can serve as a reference for psychologists starting to work with the patient and/or family. These records include medical information and social work notes and should also include annual anxiety and depression screenings of patients *and sometimes caregivers*. Finally, some CF centers may use a comprehensive psychosocial screener of the family system, using adapted assessments like the Psychosocial Assessment Tool (Kazak et al., 2012).

Often, the referral reason identified by the medical team is not the only or primary challenge for the individual with CF and their family. Stressful medical experiences, like weight checks, pulmonary function tests (PFTs), blood draws, and peripheral inserted central catheter (PICC) placement are all opportunities for anticipatory preparation and in vivo support. Psychologists can liaise with child life specialists to comprehensively assist individuals and their families in these situations. Therapies and treatments in a child's daily medical regimen, such as airway clearance or diabetes management tasks, can also be addressed during hospitalizations. Clinicians should be prepared to assess barriers to adherence, collaboratively generate and test solutions, and engage in role play or practice during these care tasks. If present, family members should be included in the treatment. There are other common areas of impairment occurring outside of the hospital for patients with CF. The impact of missing school and school needs specific to CF are an emerging area of research. Studies indicate that children with CF have frequent school absences (Filigno et al., 2018) due to hospitalizations, clinic visits, and sick days (as well as significant need for parents to get support advocating for their child in the school environment (Filigno et al., 2017, 2018). Clinicians should assess for symptoms of school avoidance, experiences of bullying, or academic disengagement. Sleep can also be disrupted both in and outside of the hospital. Psychologists can conduct a baseline assessment of sleep habits for the patient and family members, specifically attending to physical symptoms causing disruption (e.g., shortness of breath, cough, GI symptoms) and the impact of the child's treatment schedule on sleep.

Intervention

One key role of CL providers is to normalize the reactions to the experience of having CF, or caring for an individual with CF, given the highly complex regimen and unpredictability associated with the chronic condition. A pioneering multinational study conducted in nine countries, including the US, revealed that individuals with CF and their families had elevated rates of anxiety and depressive symptoms two to three times greater than observed in the general population (Quittner et al., 2014).

A CL provider's clinical assessment will identify targets for intervention and provide evidence-based interventions to help individuals and families to optimize wellness and decrease impairment. Certainly, a common focus is on teaching coping skills that aid in promoting optimal quality of life and management of the disease. The stressors addressed by a CL psychologist may be directly related, or unrelated, to the daily management of CF. For example, strategies to cope with painful medical procedures may be a frequent target given children with CF are at greater risk for experiencing medically traumatic events such as throat cultures, blood draws, or PICC placements (Blackwell & Quittner, 2015). Anxiety reduction strategies, such as exposure and response prevention for procedural distress, and relaxation and distraction techniques are used to address these concerns. On the other hand, the CL provider may be working with an individual on how to cope with a difficult relationship breakup or academic stress. In order to promote improved adherence to prescribed regimens, the CL provider can help develop strategies for promoting daily routines, set and monitor progress toward goals, and engage in collaborative problem-solving (Modi et al., 2012). An overarching approach is how to explore an individual's goals and values in order to enhance motivation to consistently engage in the completion of the complex regimen given the many barriers.

In terms of early childhood, CL providers can aid patients and families by teaching parents skills to help them establish a warm, nurturing, authoritative relationship with their child. Parent training interventions, including parent management training, teach parents how to use parent attention (verbal and physical) to encourage infants and toddlers to cooperate with daily treatments. Establishing a consistent daily care routine (Grossoehme, Filigno, & Bishop, 2014) supported by caregiver persistence and a positive and supportive approach to completion of care can be modeled. Moreover, there is a strong literature demonstrating that behavioral interventions are effective in increasing calorie intake and improving parent–child interactions at mealtime (Powers et al., 2015; Stark et al., 2009), which can be uniquely affected in CF given the increased calorie needs and concomitant parent pressure to feed, as well as the effects of gastrointestinal symptoms on appetite. Using family therapy strategies to promote positive sibling relationships may also be warranted.

Thoughts and feelings about self-acceptance are strongly developing during school age and adolescence. It is around this time typically that children notice that they are doing different things during the day, including taking CF medications and doing daily treatments. In addition, being excluded or missing out on peer activities may increase feelings of isolation, especially during periods of illness and hospitalization (Jamieson et al., 2014). A natural response is to feel different, embarrassed, and ashamed of having CF. Body image concerns may also start at this age when there is shorter stature, a distended belly, and/or a gastrostomy tube. CL providers may therefore provide interventions to address disordered body image and/or weight-related behavior.

In young adulthood, there are ever-increasing expectations for independent responsibility for CF care. In order to prepare for the effective transfer of treatment responsibility, helping patients and families to build the skills and confidence in self-management prior to independent living (Madan, Alpern, & Quittner, 2014) using a gradual, planned, and supportive shift of treatment responsibility can aid in managing CF more effectively and independently (Gravelle, Paone, Davidson, & Chilvers, 2015). An additional area that CL providers can be prepared to address are the unique challenges of whether or not to disclose their disease at work, to friends, and to intimate partners. Although the decision-making process around self-disclosure is nuanced, CL providers can help identify if there may be benefits in terms of better social support and self-efficacy (Borschuk et al., 2016) and promote assertiveness and effective communication through disclosure. Notably, individuals with CF often have the same goals as non-CF peers in terms of family planning. Sharing this information with medical providers to promote the empathetic conceptualization of these individuals as complete people, with aspiration and desires for their future, is another opportunity.

The CL provider can also be involved in exploring thoughts and feelings about pursuing or not pursuing lung transplant as individuals with CF start to experience severe difficulty breathing associated with progressive lung damage. Depending on disease severity, this may occur as early as adolescence or in young adulthood and can involve the expertise of child life and palliative care services when available.

Adaptation

It may be necessary to modify some aspects of psychological intervention in response to patient factors. Diaphragmatic breathing may be challenging, cause physical discomfort, or cue feelings of anxiety or panic. Breathing exercises can be modified to instead focus on the rate and rhythm of breaths. Worries or experiences that may qualify as thinking errors in other groups, such as shortened lifespan, may be realistic in CF. Medical information about prognostic factors, such as life expectancy, should be shared in developmentally sensitive ways, which may be done with parents only and away from the youth with CF. The CL provider also can play a crucial role in helping CF care teams balance the presentation of treatment options to individuals and their families in a way that promotes shared decision-making and reduces pressure to express the "socially desirable" response. For example, while ambivalence about pursuing lung transplantation is to be expected given the complexities associated with surgery and pre-and post-surgical processes, it may be difficult to for the individual with CF to discuss this ambivalence honestly in the context of a long-standing patient-provider relationship.

Individuals with CF often express worries related to disease progression. Specific bacteria (e.g., burkholderia cepacia) have been identified as highly damaging, and a history of these bacteria can exclude individuals from lung transplant programs due to research indicating low survival rates post transplant (Li et al., 2018). A variety of medication-related concerns also exist in individuals with CF. Side effects related to a typical daily regimen are not insignificant and can include mood or behavioral changes (Cystic Fibrosis Foundation, 2018a). Medication interactions (Talwalkar et al., 2017) are also of concern and are difficult to identify given the volume of medications prescribed. A balance must be achieved among the individual, their family, and the care team around maximizing treatment effectiveness, as well as quality of life. While rare, some antibiotics used to treat exacerbations carry the risk of serious side effects, such as skin color changes, vision or hearing loss, and injury to organs. Individuals with CF may also harbor a *realistic* fear of developing antibiotic resistance, which reduces the likelihood of effectively treating future infections. This is of particular concern to providers of individuals engaging in high-risk sexual behaviors, who may require repeated treatment of sexually transmitted infections with antibiotics.

CF-specific adaptations have been made to cognitive behavioral therapy (CBT) manuals (Friedman et al., 2018) and acceptance and commitment therapy (ACT) manuals (O'Hayer et al., 2018). These changes specifically assess the impact of CF on an individuals' life, its involvement in their mental health concerns, and the impact of their mental health concerns on their ability to sustain daily self-management and live a life worth living in accordance with personal values (O'Hayer et al., 2018). These adapted treatments are still appropriate to be used if CF is not identified as a major focus of treatment, given the daily impact of the medical regimen and the physical limitations associated with disease progression.

Special adjustments should be made to established treatments addressing chronic pain, body image or nutrition, and substance misuse. The multisystemic effects of CF can cause pain in many different areas of the body. Depending on the location (e.g., chest wall, joints) and cause of pain (e.g., chronic cough, CF-related joint disease), treatments should be modified and the root cause addressed. The unique nutritional demands of CF impact growth and body images for both men and women, with difficulty achieving a healthy weight and having a shorter stature compared to peers. Individuals with CF may manipulate nutritional intake or GI medications to achieve a certain body type or exert control over their disease. Finally, substance misuse is an emerging area of clinical and research interest in CF. Individuals with CF commonly report pain due to things like cracked ribs, malabsorption, chronic constipation, or medications (Masson, Kirszenbaum, & Sermet-Gaudelus, 2017). If they have been prescribed pain medications and there is a concern for misuse, psychologists should work closely with the individual and their medical team to coordinate further assessment and determination for a treatment plan to be developed, which may include a plan for safe cessation of use.

Treatment can also be adapted to include and educate CF team members. Overall, members of the medical team benefit from education about the impact of mental health concerns on self-management. This information can also be used to modify team expectations. For example, pulmonary function testing can cue significant anxiety for patients, which subsequently negatively impacts the validity of this test. The medical team may choose to discontinue regular PFTs and instead use other markers (e.g., subjective symptoms, nutritional data) to regularly assess disease status.

CL clinicians should consider the unique ethnic and racial distribution of CF. As CF affects mostly Caucasian individuals, ethnic or racial minorities may feel underrepresented in patient materials, research studies, or the CF community. The CF Foundation and accredited CF centers are making efforts to diversify programming and increase the inclusion of minority groups. Health care preferences of cultural minorities may also differ from the larger population of individuals with CF. Mental health providers should carefully assess the impact of individual and familial racial, ethnic, and cultural identity status on disease beliefs and behaviors.

All therapy resources must be sanitized according to CF Foundation infection control guidelines (Saiman et al., 2014). Clinicians will need to plan ahead in making specific copies of materials that they may reuse with other patients. Objects like writing or drawing utensils, games, or toys should only be used for one individual with CF. If providers anticipate working with multiple people with CF, they may consider laminating commonly used materials or using resources that can be sanitized according to guidelines. Notably, there is a growing telehealth movement among mental health providers working with individuals with CF to circumvent some of the challenges associated with infection control.

Resources/Support

Having access to and collaborative relationships established with services such as child life, social work, psychiatry, and palliative care can aid in building a strong and comprehensive team that can address the individual needs of patients with CF and their families across the developmental lifespan proactively and more effectively. Including the CL provider in all team-based rounds is also critically important to ensure that emotional and behavioral health and needs are elevated alongside physical health outcomes and targets, to provide important context why individuals with CF are behaving and making decisions, and to provide recommendations for how to enhance patient–provider interactions when there are difficulties. The CL psychologist can also collaborate with the bedside teacher to promote academic success.

In-Hospital Consultation

One characteristic unique to the CF population is the close bond forged between patients, families, and CF care team members. Children and families have frequent, close interaction with care team members during hospitalizations. Additionally, frequent admissions over the child's lifetime can further deepen the familiarity between families and providers. With this context in mind, there are several aspects for CL providers to consider.

First, bedside staff (i.e., nurses, nurse practitioners, patient care assistants, respiratory therapists) typically have rich knowledge of the child and family's health history, cultural background, and current medical and psychosocial concerns. If the referral source is a nonbedside provider (e.g., attending, fellow, or resident), clinicians should make sure to additionally discuss the referral with the primary nurse or another provider familiar with the individual. Second, the close relationships between providers and families can make it challenging for providers to maintain appropriate boundaries or enforce expectations. This is a prime area for intervention based on the referral concern and identified treatment plan. Psychologists should emphasize the value of supporting children and families in meeting challenging, but developmentally appropriate, expectations.

Structural and systemic aspects of CF hospitalizations exist that inherently challenge mental health and adaptive functioning. First and foremost are the infection control procedures associated with CF care. During hospital admissions, individuals with CF are primarily confined to their hospital room. They are not allowed in public patient areas (e.g., therapeutic recreation rooms, hospital school settings), and they are prohibited from spending time with other CF patients. Understandably, these restrictions lead to feelings of isolation, frustration, and boredom.

Many CF admissions are also lacking in daily structure. Due to infection control guidelines, the "menu of inpatient activities" offered to an individual with CF is much smaller than other populations. The daily routine typically consists of four to five airway clearance treatments per day, frequent administration of oral and IV medications, physical exams and consultations by different medical subspecialties, physical therapy, and educational services. Besides airway clearance, these activities are not explicitly scheduled, and providers will approach patients at their convenience. This unpredictability can cause children and families to feel out of control, exacerbating underlying emotional concerns and impairing their ability to appropriately anticipate and participate in therapies.

When pertinent to the referral concern, mental health providers can creatively address lack of structure from different directions. Sleep hygiene is a common concern of families and medical providers. Psychologists should assess the patient's and their family's sleep patterns at home and determine differences present during inpatient stays. Often, environmental factors can be identified and adjusted. Common inpatient factors disrupting sleep during the night include administration of fluids, frequent medical care tasks, additional airway clearance treatments, and noisy staff activities in the hallway outside of hospital rooms. These possibilities should be investigated and addressed collaboratively with the bedside staff. Psychologists can also model and provide direct instruction to the bedside staff regarding interventions to promote daytime wakefulness.

While hospitalizations are considered a "routine" aspect of CF care, they are still disruptive and distressing to children and families. Significant demands can be placed on the person with CF to engage in medical care without appropriate support. The hospital can be a triggering environment for individuals with previous medical trauma, as they may be expected to cooperate with anxiety provoking medical events repeatedly during admissions (e.g., PICC line placement). Medical providers benefit from psychoeducation around medical trauma and phobias, observation of in vivo interventions delivered by mental health professionals, and subsequent instructions or guidelines for minimizing retraumatization and preparing the child for difficult medical tasks.

CL providers can collaborate with all inpatient medical providers throughout the treatment. Bedside staff are expected to deliver complex care to children with CF during admissions; however, most providers lack any training or support in behavior management. Psychologists can deliver staff training around behavioral issues, providing background on the function of behavior and specific behavior management strategies. This information should be delivered in the context of thoughtfully responding to promote productive interactions and adaptive patient responses. Specific providers that would benefit from this include nurses, patient care assistants, respiratory therapists, and physical therapists.

CL providers can partner with pharmacists in adherence promotion planning. Pharmacists can compile comprehensive lists of medications, treatments, and therapies. These include information about frequency, method, and timing parameters for administration. With this data, psychologists can work with children and families to create schedules to improve self-management at home after discharge. Individuals may go home with additional medications that are slowly withdrawn as they complete additional treatments. This should be considered and noted when creating schedules.

A final consideration for in-hospital consultation and intervention is the family's home environment. Children and adolescents receive significant support of daily treatments during hospitalizations; while this optimizes their recovery, it is not geared toward the promotion of independent skill development and is often very different from the typical daily routine at home. CL providers should strive to understand a family's priorities, capabilities, and needs for support outside of the hospital. With this foundation, CL providers can engage bedside staff and families in discussion around shared goals and collaboratively generate an inpatient behavioral plan providing scaffolding for self-management.

Outpatient Consultation

In accredited CF centers, outpatient CF care teams are likely to have a consistent interdisciplinary team, including the pulmonologist, nurse, dietitian, respiratory therapist (or airway clearance specialist), and social worker. Some CF social workers function in the more traditional medical social worker model, which includes resource allocation and supportive counseling. Some social workers are trained as mental health therapists and provide psychological screening and treatment. Recently, the CF Foundation supported the inclusion of mental health coordinators (MHC) in CF centers though a two-year grant mechanism, and within the last 2 years, over 110 CF centers have hired their own MHC, increasing the number of psychologists working with CF teams.

Consultation with the outpatient CF care team is critical, especially at two key times: at the time of admission and at the time of discharge. The outpatient team can aid CL care provision by readying people for an admission, including expectations and goals, one being the ultimate shared goal to restore health. In order to optimize care during the admission, the outpatient care team can communicate clear goals for the admission, including physical, emotional, and behavioral health goals with the CL team. For example, a goal sheet can be entered into the medical record that can be accessed by all inpatient care team members in order to promote more consistent expectations for care during the admission and for discharge.

The outpatient team can also share observations about how the individual coped with the decision to pursue an inpatient admission and can prepare the CL team for specific targets. Occasionally, the outpatient care team may have "high" expectations for what can be accomplished psychologically on the inpatient side because of beliefs that because the patient is "a captive audience," they may be more ready or more willing to receive the recommended treatment. In fact, given most people do not feel well for the first few days of an admission and the family may not be able to be present during the admission because of work and family demands, the inpatient admission will not always be an optimal time for patients and families to receive more intensive psychological treatment. Moreover, considering and planning for generalizability to the home environment is important given the environmental setting events between home and the hospital are likely quite different. Conversely, disease-specific thoughts and feelings may be better able to be processed during the admission because the admission may function as an extended "exposure period" that does not allow for the avoidance of disease-related care and emotional processing in the same way as it can in the home environment.

At the end of the admission, the CL psychologist can contribute to the discharge planning process and documentation. Progress with treatment goals and recommended targets for follow-up with the CF outpatient team or community resources can promote continuity of care between inpatient and outpatient care.

Case Example

Katy is a 17-year-old female admitted for a pulmonary exacerbation, and an inpatient referral was placed. She had CF, along with other diagnosed conditions, including chronic migraines, attention deficit hyperactivity disorder, major depressive disorder, generalized anxiety and posttraumatic stress disorder. She also experienced the sudden death of one of her parents. Katy had received regular outpatient therapy from the psychologist embedded within the CF Center. At the beginning of Katy's admission, the outpatient psychologist met with her in her hospital room to introduce the concept of meeting with an inpatient psychologist for more regular and frequent sessions in the hospital. Katy was agreeable to this idea, and the outpatient and inpatient provider jointly met with her to identify behavioral health goals for this admission. These included ongoing CBT and acceptance-based strategies to manage and treat her psychiatric conditions. Sleep hygiene was identified as an additional area for intervention. The inpatient psychologist facilitated a daily treatment schedule for Katy, also identifying periods of time that should be relatively free from interruptions to facilitate privacy and emotional "recharging." This schedule was reviewed with bedside providers, and the inpatient psychologist attended rounds to liaise with the medical team and stay aware of concerns or challenges throughout her admission. The inpatient psychologist met every other day with Katy to make progress on outpatient goals and facilitate patient-centered care in the hospital. An acute issue arose when a medical resident, unaware of her complex psychiatric history, performed a physical examination while she was asleep, inadvertently triggering symptoms of her PTSD. The inpatient psychologist was able to process this experience with Katy and facilitate her recovery from this trigger. The inpatient psychologist also provided psychoeducation to medical providers around general mental health concerns, PTSD, and the importance of consent and awareness with individuals with psychiatrically complex comorbidities.

References

Barker, D. H., & Quittner, A. L. (2016). Parental depression and pancreatic enzymes adherence in children with cystic fibrosis. *Pediatrics, 137*(2), 1–9. https://doi.org/10.1542/peds.2015-2296

Blackwell, L. S., & Quittner, A. L. (2015). Daily pain in adolescents with CF: Effects on adherence, psychological symptoms, and health-related quality of life. *Pediatric Pulmonology, 50*(3), 244–251. https://doi.org/10.1002/ppul.23091

Boat, T. F., Filigno, S., & Amin, R. S. (2017). Wellness for families of children with chronic health disorders. *Journal of the American Medical Association Pediatrics, 171*(9), 825–826. https://doi.org/10.1001/jamapediatrics.2017.1682

Borschuk, A. P., Everhart, R. S., Eakin, M. N., Rand-Giovannetti, D., Borrelli, B., & Riekert, K. A. (2016). Disease disclosure in individuals with cystic fibrosis: Association with psychosocial and health outcomes. *Journal of Cystic Fibrosis, 15*(5), 696–702. https://doi.org/10.1016/j.jcf.2016.02.011

Comeau, A. M., Accurso, F. J., White, T. B., Campbell, P. W., 3rd, Hoffman, G., Parad, R. B., … Cystic Fibrosis, F. (2007). Guidelines for implementation of cystic fibrosis newborn screening programs: Cystic Fibrosis Foundation workshop report. *Pediatrics, 119*(2), e495–e518. https://doi.org/10.1542/peds.2006-1993

Cystic Fibrosis Foundation. (2018a, December 2). *Bronchodilators*. Retrieved from https://www.cff.org/Life-With-CF/Treatments-and-Therapies/Medications/Bronchodilators/

Cystic Fibrosis Foundation. (2018b, December 2). *What is cystic fibrosis*. Retrieved from https://www.cff.org/What-is-CF/About-Cystic-Fibrosis/

Ernst, M. M., Johnson, M. C., & Stark, L. J. (2010). Developmental and psychosocial issues in cystic fibrosis. *Child and Adolescent Psychiatric Clinics of North America, 19*(2), 263–283. https://doi.org/10.1016/j.chc.2010.01.004

Filigno, S., Strong, S., Hente, E., Elam, M., Mara, C., & Boat, T. (2017). Promoting school success for students with cystic fibrosis: A novel empirically-based program. *Pediatric Pulmonology, 52*, S484–S484.

Filigno, S., Strong, S., Hente, E., Murphy, C., Elam, M., Mara, C., … Boat, T. (2018). We have a lot to learn: School needs and school absences for student with cystic fibrosis. *Pediatric Pulmonology, 53*, 407–407.

Friedman, D., Pinsky, H., Quittner, A., Salathe, M., Smith, B., & Georgiopoulos, A. (2018). Development of a CF-specific CBT intervention to prevent depression and anxiety in adults with CF. *Pediatric Pulmonology, 53*, 409–409.

Gravelle, A. M., Paone, M., Davidson, A. G., & Chilvers, M. A. (2015). Evaluation of a multidimensional cystic fibrosis transition program: A quality improvement initiative. *Journal of Pediatric Nursing, 30*(1), 236–243. https://doi.org/10.1016/j.pedn.2014.06.011

Grossoehme, D. H., Filigno, S. S., & Bishop, M. (2014). Parent routines for managing cystic fibrosis in children. *Journal of Clinical Psychology in Medical Settings, 21*(2), 125–135. https://doi.org/10.1007/s10880-014-9396-1

Jamieson, N., Fitzgerald, D., Singh-Grewal, D., Hanson, C. S., Craig, J. C., & Tong, A. (2014). Children's experiences of cystic fibrosis: A systematic review of qualitative studies. *Pediatrics, 133*(6), e1683–e1697. https://doi.org/10.1542/peds.2014-0009

Kazak, A. E., Brier, M., Alderfer, M. A., Reilly, A., Fooks Parker, S., Rogerwick, S., ... Barakat, L. P. (2012). Screening for psychosocial risk in pediatric cancer. *Pediatric Blood & Cancer, 59*(5), 822–827. https://doi.org/10.1002/pbc.24166

Li, S. S., Tumin, D., Krone, K. A., Boyer, D., Kirkby, S. E., Mansour, H. M., & Hayes, D., Jr. (2018). Risks associated with lung transplantation in cystic fibrosis patients. *Expert Review of Respiratory Medicine, 12*(11), 893–904. https://doi.org/10.1080/17476348.2018.1522254

Madan, A. S., Alpern, A. N., & Quittner, A. L. (2014). Transition from pediatric to adult cystic fibrosis care: A developmental framework. *European Respiratory Society Monograph, 64*, 272–285.

Masson, A., Kirszenbaum, M., & Sermet-Gaudelus, I. (2017). Pain is an underestimated symptom in cystic fibrosis. *Current Opinion in Pulmonary Medicine, 23*(6), 570–573. https://doi.org/10.1097/MCP.0000000000000427

Modi, A. C., Lim, C. S., Yu, N., Geller, D., Wagner, M. H., & Quittner, A. L. (2006). A multi-method assessment of treatment adherence for children with cystic fibrosis. *Journal of Cystic Fibrosis, 5*(3), 177–185. https://doi.org/10.1016/j.jcf.2006.03.002

Modi, A. C., Pai, A. L., Hommel, K. A., Hood, K. K., Cortina, S., Hilliard, M. E., ... Drotar, D. (2012). Pediatric self-management: A framework for research, practice, and policy. *Pediatrics, 129*(2), e473–e485. https://doi.org/10.1542/peds.2011-1635

O'Hayer, C., Aikens, R., O'Loughlin, C., Bennett, D., Lee, H., Hendry, M., & Stephen, M. (2018). ACT with CF: Promising conclusions of a telehealth pilot study of acceptance and commitment therapy for anxiety and depression. *Pediatric Pulmonology, 53*, 408–S2. Abstract 677.

Powers, S. W., Stark, L. J., Chamberlin, L. A., Filigno, S. S., Sullivan, S. M., Lemanek, K. L., ... Clancy, J. P. (2015). Behavioral and nutritional treatment for preschool-aged children with cystic fibrosis: A randomized clinical trial. *Journal of the American Medical Association Pediatrics, 169*(5), e150636. https://doi.org/10.1001/jamapediatrics.2015.0636

Quittner, A. L., Goldbeck, L., Abbott, J., Duff, A., Lambrecht, P., Sole, A., ... Barker, D. (2014). Prevalence of depression and anxiety in patients with cystic fibrosis and parent caregivers: Results of the international depression epidemiological study across nine countries. *Thorax, 69*(12), 1090–1097. https://doi.org/10.1136/thoraxjnl-2014-205983

Saiman, L., Siegel, J. D., LiPuma, J. J., Brown, R. F., Bryson, E. A., Chambers, M. J., ... Society for Healthcare Epidemiology of America. (2014). Infection prevention and control guideline for cystic fibrosis: 2013 update. *Infection Control and Hospital Epidemiology, 35*(Suppl 1), S1–S67. https://doi.org/10.1086/676882

Sanders, D. B., Zhang, Z., Farrell, P. M., Lai, H. J., & Wisconsin, C. F. N. S. G. (2018). Early life growth patterns persist for 12 years and impact pulmonary outcomes in cystic fibrosis. *Journal of Cystic Fibrosis, 17*(4), 528–535. https://doi.org/10.1016/j.jcf.2018.01.006

Smith, B. A., Modi, A. C., Quittner, A. L., & Wood, B. L. (2010). Depressive symptoms in children with cystic fibrosis and parents and its effects on adherence to airway clearance. *Pediatric Pulmonology, 45*(8), 756–763. https://doi.org/10.1002/ppul.21238

Stark, L. J., Quittner, A. L., Powers, S. W., Opipari-Arrigan, L., Bean, J. A., Duggan, C., & Stallings, V. A. (2009). Randomized clinical trial of behavioral intervention and nutrition education to improve caloric intake and weight in children with cystic fibrosis. *Archives of Pediatrics and Adolescent Medicine, 163*(10), 915–921. https://doi.org/10.1001/archpediatrics.2009.165

Talwalkar, J. S., Koff, J. L., Lee, H. B., Britto, C. J., Mulenos, A. M., & Georgiopoulos, A. M. (2017). Cystic fibrosis transmembrane regulator modulators: Implications for the management of depression and anxiety in cystic fibrosis. *Psychosomatics, 58*(4), 343–354. https://doi.org/10.1016/j.psym.2017.04.001

Tluczek, A., Orland, K. M., & Cavanagh, L. (2011). Psychosocial consequences of false-positive newborn screens for cystic fibrosis. *Qualitative Health Research, 21*(2), 174–186. https://doi.org/10.1177/1049732310382919

VanDevanter, D. R., Kahle, J. S., O'Sullivan, A. K., Sikirica, S., & Hodgkins, P. S. (2016). Cystic fibrosis in young children: A review of disease manifestation, progression, and response to early treatment. *Journal of Cystic Fibrosis, 15*(2), 147–157. https://doi.org/10.1016/j.jcf.2015.09.008

Sickle Cell Disease

Anna M. Hood, Emily A. McTate, Naomi E. Joffe, and Lori E. Crosby

Medical Basics

Sickle cell disease (SCD) is a life-threatening inherited red blood cell disorder affecting millions worldwide and is primarily seen in individuals of African ancestry. A minority of individuals in this population are of Hispanic, Asian Indian, or Middle Eastern descent (Hassell, 2010). There are approximately 100,000 individuals in the United States with SCD, of whom 40% are children and 90% are African American/Black (Brousseau, Panepinto, Nimmer, & Hoffmann, 2010).

Diagnosis of SCD most often occurs as part of newborn screening; however, screening was not universal in all states until 2006 (Ware, Montalembert, Tshilolo, & Abboud, 2017). SCD is a genetic mutation of the beta-globin gene that is inherited from each parent, resulting in the production of abnormal hemoglobin S that affects the shape (i.e., crescent versus round) and behavior of red blood cells. Sickle cells adhere to and obstruct blood vessels, limiting the ability of healthy red blood cells to carry oxygen-rich blood throughout the body (Rees, Williams, & Gladwin, 2010). SCD is an umbrella term for several genetic mutations of the beta-globin gene with varying clinical presentations. Sickle cell anemia (HbSS) represents 70% of cases, and along with hemoglobin S, beta thalassemia zero ($HbS\beta^0$) has the most severe clinical course (Piel, Hay, Gupta, Weatherall, & Williams, 2013). Hemoglobin SC and hemoglobin S beta thalassemia plus ($HbS\beta^+$) are other types of SCD with milder disease severity. Those who inherit only one abnormal gene (sickle cell trait) tend not to experience any symptoms but can pass SCD on to their children if their partner also has the trait or SCD (Frenette & Atweh, 2007).

Major medical complications of SCD are caused by hemolytic anemia (low red blood cell count), tissue damage (organ/tissue death due to lack of oxygen), and vaso-occlusion (sickling that results in lack of blood flow or pooling of blood) (Stuart & Nagel, 2004). Sickled red blood cells have an average lifespan of 8–40 days compared with healthy red blood cells, with a lifespan of 120 days. This causes the body to work harder to make new blood cells, resulting in fatigue, a common but underrecognized symptom of SCD. Acute pain from vaso-occulsion is the hallmark of SCD, often referred to as "pain

A. M. Hood (✉)
Developmental Neurosciences, UCL Great Ormond Street Institute of Child Health, London, UK
e-mail: ahood@ucl.ac.uk

E. A. McTate · N. E. Joffe · L. E. Crosby
Cincinnati Children's Hospital and Medical Center, Cincinnati, OH, USA

Department of Pediatrics, University of Cincinnati College of Medicine, Cincinnati, OH, USA

B. D. Carter, K. A. Kullgren (eds.), *Clinical Handbook of Psychological Consultation in Pediatric Medical Settings*, Issues in Clinical Child Psychology, https://doi.org/10.1007/978-3-030-35598-2_26

episodes." Acute pain is often unpredictable but can also be triggered by physiological and environmental factors such as temperature changes, stress, dehydration, and overexertion (Stuart & Nagel, 2004). Youth with SCD are also at risk for chronic pain related to repeated injury to the tissue, joints, or bones. Chronic pain can interfere with sleep and quality of life and result in functional disability (Ojelabi, Graham, & Ling, 2017). As acute and chronic pain experiences can co-occur, differentiation can be difficult for patients and healthcare providers (Williams & Tanabe, 2016).

Since red blood cells flow throughout the entire body, SCD can impact multiple systems through vaso-occlusion and by reducing oxygen supply when the red blood cell count is low. Damage can occur in the organs (e.g., heart, lungs, kidneys, spleen), the bones (e.g., death of bone tissue), the vascular system (e.g., narrowing of blood vessels in the eyes), and the brain (e.g., stroke), and patients are at an increased risk of infection. A common complication for children with SCD is acute chest syndrome, a pneumonia-like illness accompanied by pain caused by sickling in the lungs. Children with SCD are also at an increased risk of developing renal complications due to sickling in the capillaries of the kidneys. Acute splenic sequestration occurs when the spleen enlarges (splenomegaly) after rapidly pooling with blood due to blocked/narrowed arteries caused by sickled cells. Priapism affects young men and is a prolonged, typically painful erection of the penis, which ejaculation cannot relieve (Redding-Lallinger & Knoll, 2006). Death of bone tissue, known as avascular necrosis (AVN), can cause damage to the hip bones or shoulder joints due to repeated loss of blood supply. In the vascular system, blockage of the small blood vessels can cause damage to the eyes, known as retinopathy (Stuart & Nagel, 2004).

SCD also affects brain function, and children with SCD are at 200 to 400 times increased risk of overt stroke. Silent strokes/infarcts (i.e., infarcts not observable through neurologic examination) occur in 14–40% of children with SCD (DeBaun et al., 2012). Youths with SCD are at high risk for neurological or executive functioning deficits (Prussien, Jordan, DeBaun, & Compas, 2019). Annual eye exams, transcranial Doppler imaging (TCD), magnetic resonance imaging (MRI), and neuropsychological assessments are used to evaluate neurological impact and guide treatment.

Treatment for SCD and its complications are varied, with some interventions being more chronic in nature and others requiring acute emergency intervention and inpatient admission. Medical therapies remain limited, however, and there is no universal cure. Penicillin has been effective in reducing the rate of infections and mortality in young children with SCD and is typically prescribed as a preventative measure. Blood transfusion is a mainstay of treatment as it reduces the incidence of pain, acute chest syndrome, and stroke. Patients on regular transfusions require additional intervention to prevent chronic and life-threatening organ damage due to the buildup of excess iron. In 2017, Endari© became the first new treatment in 20 years as previously only Hydroxyurea© (HU) was available. These drugs improve oxygen delivery to tissue throughout the body, decrease acute and chronic aspects of SCD (e.g., pain, fatigue), and reduce hospitalizations (Ware et al., 2017).

Stem cell transplantation holds a promise as a curative therapy for SCD but is only available for the 14% of patients in the US who have a matched sibling donor. Further, there are significant associated risks, including infection and graft reactions (Bernaudin et al., 2007). Gene therapy (i.e., inserting genes to make normal red blood cells) and gene editing (genetic engineering in which DNA is inserted, deleted, modified, or replaced) are emerging as potentially curative therapies for SCD but remain in the early stages of evaluation.

Patient and Family Engagement

Stereotypical beliefs about mental health providers may lead patients/families to believe that their medical provider thinks that they are "faking," their symptoms are "all in their head," or they are "crazy." These beliefs can be exacerbated because

SCD patients' pain complaints, which are inherently subjective in nature, are often treated as false or exaggerated (Jenerette & Brewer, 2010). Therefore, it is important to understand that a referral to psychological services may inadvertently reinforce feelings of mistrust for patients with SCD.

Accordingly, rapport building is essential. Initially, the focus should be on developing a reciprocal relationship. Listening to and acknowledging the barriers faced by families will work to allay potential mistrust of mental health services (Cook et al., 2014). The CL psychologist can acknowledge the challenges of living with SCD (i.e., medical complications, perceived and actual discrimination, healthcare disparities related to minority status) while focusing on identifying strengths (e.g., problem-solving skills, active coping strategies) as many youths with SCD demonstrate optimal functioning, adaptation, and resilience.

Thoughtful presentation of the reason for referral is critical during initial interactions. Understanding the medical team's referral concerns is important but may or may not match the family's concerns. While balancing these competing demands can be difficult, prioritizing concerns identified by the patient and family will increase engagement and thus facilitate subsequent opportunities for intervention. Acceptance of psychological interventions can improve when presented as an *additional,* rather than *alternate,* treatment.

Maximizing the cultural competency of the CL psychologist is an important path to engagement (Whaley & Davis, 2007). Cultural sensitivity and exposure to African American/Black patients and families improve alliance building and rapport. Schwartz, Radcliffe, and Barakat (2007) developed a culturally sensitive roadmap for conducting clinical research with African American/Black families (Schwartz et al., 2007). Table 1 describes strategies for engaging in culturally sensitive practice with SCD patients and families to help with "buy-in" to psychosocial interventions and assessment while providing the groundwork for effective interventions.

Formulation

Along with clearly identifying and defining the presenting problem, both individual and cultural factors should be assessed (Kazdin, 2017). The patient's understanding of factors impacting their pain (e.g., differentiating between acute vs. chronic pain), as well as problematic patterns when responding to pain (e.g., not engaging in activity when experiencing pain), should be evaluated. Treatment adherence, quality of life, and patterns of coping are also important aspects of assessment for SCD patients. Since prevalence rates of mood and anxiety symptoms are disproportionately high for youths with SCD (Barakat, Lash, Lutz, & Nicolaou, 2006), assessment for mood and anxiety symptomology is essential, regardless of referral questions.

Some families experience *socioeconomic challenges* that impact disease management; they may have fewer economic and/or social resources acting as protective factors (Smith, Oyeku, Homer, & Zuckerman, 2006). Case conceptualization should include current family stressors and sources of support for the family (e.g., community, organizations). The Psychosocial Assessment Tool (PAT 3.0) (Kazak et al., 2018) is a brief, parent-report screener using a socioecological framework to assess family risk and resiliency factors. African American/Black families may have strong networks of extended family and friends (McAuliffe, 2008), so identifying and including these "key players" (e.g., friends, family, teachers, clergy) is an important component of assessment and intervention (Table 1).

Cognitive functioning is another area to be assessed in youths with SCD due to their increased risk for deficits in executive function (i.e., the ability to plan, organize, and shift easily from one task to another) (Hood et al., 2019) and information processing (Berkelhammer et al., 2007). One should assess whether the patient has challenges when completing tasks independently that require executive function skills (e.g., taking medication regularly) to determine if they need additional intervention. This may involve targeted questions during the clinical interview to identify deficits and impact on functioning (e.g., challenges with

Table 1 Cultural considerations in consultation-liaison psychology for children and adolescents with sickle cell disease

Factors	Key considerations	Applications
1. Family/ community	African American/Black families often have strong networks of family and friends (McAuliffe, 2008) Empowerment of the family system is a key factor in response to therapy (Barakat et al., 2006) There must be openness to engage key players in the management of their disease	• Multiple family members may be present and considered in the assessment and intervention stages • Patients can designate a support person (family member or friend) who may attend sessions and work with the patient to implement strategies (Schwartz et al., 2007) • Support patient in identifying people in their community who can support self-management (e.g., a coach, an extended family member, a trusted neighbor)
2. Minority status	Minority status represents a chronic stressor for patients due to issues of prejudice/discrimination Health disparities exist for minorities independent of other contextual and cultural factor Medical providers are likely part of the majority in the hospital/clinic setting—They may inadvertently reinforce racial dynamics that impact the patient–provider relationship	• Acknowledge and validate stressors related to minority status both within and outside the medical system (Schwartz et al., 2007) • Consider cultural and contextual factors that may influence patient and family decisions when communicating with medical providers. Some behaviors may signal to providers that patients and families are not engaged in care—To facilitate increased understanding, utilize the lens of the patient to understand why they may be engaging in a particular behavior
3. Culturally responsive approaches	Assessment and interventions should consider demands of African American/black parents to prepare their children with the skills to effectively navigate prejudice and discrimination Use culturally sensitive assessment materials, supportive materials (handouts, books, pamphlets), and language (i.e., understandable, not offensive, and at appropriate cognitive/reading level) (Schwartz et al., 2007)	• Recommendations should be respectful of nonmajority parenting styles – Join with parents around parenting challenges (e.g., managing behavior, adherence) – Work to understand their perspective and ask permission to use other techniques • Language of self-statements is flexible, broad, and chosen by the patient • Patients should be allowed to choose imagery to promote cultural consonance, including active events like sports or those taking place in familiar settings.Music may be incorporated into guided imagery (Schwartz et al., 2007) • Self-statements may be from the patient's cultural perspective and may include ethnic/racial pride and/ or be related to beliefs/faith
4. Stigma/ mistrust	The understanding of historical mistrust of the healthcare system may be related to a history of exploitation Microaggressions and provider bias impact health outcomes There may be stigma related to utilizing psychological services for patients with SCD	• Take necessary time to build rapport and trust. Do not pathologize problems (Schwartz et al., 2007) • Frame psychology as a way to manage their disease and facilitate positive interactions with the medical team • Clearly define goals and roles with the family/ patient. Respond quickly to patient and family comfort with a discussion of more sensitive information • Involve patients' trusted providers to support engaging in treatment • Support and reinforce openness, disclosure, and help-seeking behavior

(continued)

Table 1 (continued)

Factors	Key considerations	Applications
5. SES/ limited resources or barriers	Many African Americans/Blacks in the United States experience lower SES—a chronic stressor (Schwartz et al., 2007) Low SES contributes to disparities in health and creates barriers to access to healthcare Managing chronic illness may not be a family's most critical priority, but that does not indicate lack of concern about the illness	• Acknowledge/validate stressors related to limited resources • Steps toward achieving treatment goals should be manageable and realistic; provide guidance in identifying manageable steps to achieve goals when goals may conflict with basic survival • Highlight to medical providers that when a family prioritizes SES-related demands, it is necessary and does not equate to a lack of concern about health • Address and solve related stressors as they arise (e.g. utilizing social workers as needed) • Be flexible and accommodating with regard to scheduling and/or work schedules (jobs may have nontraditional hours), limited child care, and transportation issues • Provide guidance in identifying manageable steps to achieving goals related to managing the disease when such goals may compete with goals related to basic survival

Notes: *SCD* sickle cell disease, *SES* socioeconomic status

organization, impulsive behaviors, etc.) or formal neuropsychological evaluation referral for more serious concerns (e.g., academic concerns, nonadherence). Discussion about the reason for the referral must happen *before* it is suggested to other providers in order to minimize families' concerns and address any questions. Previous research has demonstrated that families are accepting of neuropsychological services when they are introduced respectfully and are family centered (Wills et al., 2010).

Interventions

Psychoeducation Increasing patient and family SCD knowledge has been shown to improve the use of active coping strategies for managing SCD (Kaslow et al., 2000). Ensuring accurate SCD-related disease knowledge is crucial as youths with SCD may have received disease education as a young child that may no longer be consistent with their developmental level and disease progression as a teen. Education about SCD should include basic medical knowledge (as presented earlier in this chapter and adapted to patient developmental and cognitive level), recognition and management of SCD-related complications, medication management, and when and how to access medical services. Recommendations for SCD psychoeducation are provided in the Appendix.

Psychoeducation on the physiological basis of pain, particularly the gate control theory of pain (Melzack & Wall, 1965), can serve as a framework for pain management interventions. The theory posits that pain signals travel along nerves in the spinal cord containing pain gates that can be open, partially opened, or closed. With open gates, all signals reach the brain, resulting in strong pain; if the gates are closed or partially open, then the pain experience may be lessened. Specific interventions such as distraction, imagery, relaxation, mindfulness techniques, etc. can be taught to patients to "close" gates to lessen the experience of pain. Parents should also receive education about the gate control theory as their response to their child's pain can contribute to whether pain nerve gates are open or closed.

Cognitive Behavioral Therapy Cognitive behavioral therapy (CBT) is the most often used intervention modality for patients with SCD and has the most empirical support for the treatment of pain and mood concerns. In fact, even one session of CBT for youths with SCD has been shown to reduce pain sensitivity, decrease negative thinking, increase active coping, and decrease school absences and hospital contacts (Gil et al., 1997, 2001). Specific to SCD, the CL psychologist should highlight variations in response strategies or interventions for acute-versus-chronic pain. For example, a heating pad and a warm bath may be more effective for acute pain than for chronic pain. Patients can be taught to close nerve gates through cognitive (e.g., teaching ways to decrease pain catastrophizing), behavioral (e.g., activity pacing, problem-solving), physical (e.g., diaphragmatic breathing), and emotional (e.g., mood management) pain-management strategies. Clinical biofeedback is an appropriate and engaging intervention and has been proven effective in reducing painful episodes, pain medication days, and anxiety (Cozzi, Tryon, & Sedlacek, 1987) and in improving quality of life (Myrvik, Campbell, & Butcher, 2012).

Targeted Adherence Interventions Some patients with SCD may be referred to the CL psychologist due to treatment nonadherence. For these patients, the Pediatric Self-Management Model can guide interventions (Modi et al., 2012). This model helps to identify modifiable influences at the individual, family, community, and healthcare system level that impact adherence and self-management (engagement in health-promoting behaviors). After assessing barriers at each level, the CL psychologist can identify intervention targets. For example, the assessment may reveal that a patient's family does not understand the benefits of medications (e.g., HU) and, as a result, has not been diligent about making sure that the child takes the medication. In these cases, the psychologist can focus on educating the family about the benefits of HU (e.g., pain, reducing long-term organ damage) and support them in using behavioral support strategies such as a pill box or a reminder system to ensure that the child takes the medication daily.

Motivational interviewing (MI) strategies are often appropriate and effective in the context of self-management (Lozano & Houtrow, 2018). Even one session of MI can have a lasting impact on improving self-management in chronic illness populations (Jensen et al., 2011). These interventions are guided by the patient's assessment and motivation for changes in their life. The Self-Management Personal Action Plan (Appendix) offers a guide for clinicians to effectively communicate with patients around self-management goals while respecting the patients' autonomy. By focusing on something that is important to patients (e.g., drinking more water) and then supporting them in setting achievable goals (i.e., a confidence level of 7 or higher), providers are meeting them at their level of readiness to change, giving them the skills they need to be effective in setting goals independently and eliciting conversation around forward movement.

Targeting Social Concerns Other patients with SCD may be referred because of psychosocial factors (e.g., financial concerns, social support, acute stressors) affecting the child or family's ability to manage the disease. Interventions will require the CL psychologist to collaborate with the multidisciplinary team, understand the impact of social determinants on health, and then apply interventions. Tools such as PAT (Kazak et al., 2018) identify levels of risk, thereby ensuring that intervention is directed toward the psychosocial factors having the greatest impact. For example, if a family's financial status is significantly impacting their ability to pay for the child's medication or attend clinic appointments, the CL psychologist can recommend social work involvement to connect the family to resources while helping the family improve problem-solving skills and strategies to advocate for their child's needs.

Alternative Therapies As a part of a comprehensive intervention, the CL psychologist should also consider referral to adjunctive or integrative services (e.g., therapeutic massage, yoga, aromatherapy, martial arts, etc.), which have demonstrated a positive impact on pain, mood, and anxiety symptoms for children with SCD (Lemanek, Ranalli, & Lukens, 2009; Moody et al., 2017).

Similarly, smart apps can also be a useful supplement to traditional therapeutic approaches. Mobile health (mHealth) tools have been shown to increase pain coping attempts and pain controllability (McClellan et al., 2008). The CL psychologist should keep in mind, when using mHealth tools in patients with SCD, that these tools are an adjunct to but not a replacement for psychology interventions (Schatz et al., 2015).

Adaptation

Inpatient Consultation For some patients with SCD, their first contact with a psychologist occurs during an inpatient admission. This gives CL psychologists an opportunity to help decrease potential stigma by contextualizing their role for families. Providers can begin by informing families that their services are focused on supporting individuals with chronic *physical* illness. It can be helpful to normalize challenges that are common when dealing with a chronic condition (e.g., missing out on things that their peers are doing, having to manage treatments, feeling frustrated). Additionally, it provides a potential opportunity to outline some of the areas that patients often work on with CL psychologists (e.g., coping with ongoing demands of treatment as they impact mood or behavior, finding ways to meet patient's treatment goals, learning ways to manage pain when pain impacts functioning, etc.). Then it is helpful to assess the patient's perception of how those things might be relevant to their goals (e.g., the patient may want to be able to keep a job or participate in cheerleading, etc.). Recurrent inpatient admissions, which are common for some patients with SCD, provide an opportunity for CL psychologists to develop relationships with the patient and family over time, particularly with patients who are unlikely to be seen by psychology in a SCD clinic. When possible, consistency of providers is recommended in order to form long-term bonds with the patient and family.

The majority of hospitalizations for SCD are for acute pain episodes or when symptoms suggest serious complications (Panepinto, Pajewski, Foerster, Sabnis, & Hoffmann, 2009). A CL psychologist consulted for pain during an inpatient admission may have a somewhat different focus in their assessment and intervention than in the outpatient setting as they may have only a few opportunities to intervene. An inpatient provider may focus more on the current pain episode and the impact of this episode on functioning and the reduction of suffering. CL psychologists can conduct a brief pain assessment (see Table 2), introduce the gate control theory of pain as a way to discuss the biopsychosocial model, and employ MI techniques to support the patient in engaging in behaviors consistent with effective pain management (e.g., getting up and out of bed, engaging in behavioral activation). With respect to pain management, the CL psychologist will need to acknowledge any distress that the patient experiences when they are asked to change responses to pain (e.g., continuing activity during acute pain episodes), particularly when patients and families are comfortable with existing interventions and are anxious about change. Additionally, the CL psychologist can support the medical team in their approach to pain management by educating and reinforcing the use of consistent terminology about pain by team members. If the medical team fails to recognize and acknowledge pain descriptions from the patient, the patient's pain experience may be invalidated, which can further alienate the patient in their confidence with the medical team.

It is important to asses for depression and anxiety as these symptoms have been found to be predictive of medical hospitalizations (Myrvik, Burks, Hoffman, Dasgupta, & Panepinto, 2013). Interventions for mood and anxiety may begin in the inpatient setting; however, they will likely require additional outpatient therapy sessions as response to treatment is typically longer than the duration of an inpatient admission. Interventions should target areas that are directly related to the current admission or potentially aimed at increasing likelihood that the patient would be engaged in services as an outpatient, if a referral seems appropriate.

Another significant adaptation involves the team-based nature of interventions. In addition to attending to culturally competent practices in

Table 2 Clinical considerations for the treatment of pain and medication adherence in children and adolescents with sickle cell disease

Referral concern	Formulation of assessment areas	Treatment goals/potential interventions
Pain	• Global assessment of pain experience to include current and historical experiences (pain experiences over lifetime, recent changes in pain experience, specifics of location, intensity, quality) • Functional analysis of pain experience (triggers: Weather, sleep, activity level, stressors, responses, consequences) • Assessment of the impact of pain on current functioning • Identification of what helps the pain (medications, rest, distraction, etc.) • Assessment of mood/anxiety symptoms (may or may not be directly related to pain) • Assessment of the patient's and family's goals for intervention (focus on pain control vs. increased functioning)	*Goals*: Increase in functioning and sense of control over the symptoms, developing both proactive and reactive skills *Interventions may include the following*: • Introduction of the gate control theory of pain, with goals being to (1) explain how pain works in the body, (2) increase internal locus of control around pain management, (3) gain buy-in for biobehavioral pain management strategies • Introduction of relaxation strategies (deep breathing, guided imagery, progressive muscle relaxation) • Use of motivational interviewing strategies to discuss areas within the patient's control (e.g., spending time up and out of bed, practicing strategies taught, engaging in healthy coping to manage current stressors) • Sleep hygiene • Activity pacing • Stress management • Hydration • Cognitive restructuring
Medication/ Treatment adherence	• Assessment of the impact of the illness on the patient's current functioning (e.g. impairs ability to engage in pleasant activities, school, etc.) • Assessment of the family's/ patient's current level of concern and motivation to make changes • Assessment of the family's/ patient's understanding of their role in managing the patient's SCD • Assessment of the current barriers to adherence, including system-level barriers • Attention to the patient's/family's values and goals	*Goals*: Match intervention type and target of intervention to the patient's/family's motivation to change area of concern. Support families in the communication of their goals/concerns to the medical team. Empower the patient/family to drive goal setting, not the psychologist or medical team *Interventions may include the following*: • Motivational interviewing (clarifying patient values, increasing awareness of the impact of various behaviors on values, encouraging change talk, increasing commitment to behaviors that are consistent with values (Crosby, Joffe, Peugh, Ware, & Britto, 2017) – Self-management training (supporting patients in developing skills to manage treatment demands) – Action planning (supporting patients in setting realistic goals that are consistent with what they want to work on) • Communication skill training • Introduction of tracking apps/calendars to identify barriers and monitor success • Exploring social support that the patient/family could use to share the burden of management *System interventions*: • Encouraging a regular assessment of barriers to adherence in clinics (every 2–3 months) • Considering implementing joint treatment approach, with a psychologist, medical provider/s, and social or community health worker (if needed) seeing the patient together for part of the session

their own work with patients, CL psychologists are in a unique position to facilitate improved cultural sensitivity (e.g., understanding of microaggressions and their impact on health) in the medical team. In the U.S., SCD has been historically conceptualized as a "Black disease" (Wakefield et al., 2018). Psychosocial providers must attend to multiple patient, family, and system-level aspects of patient care. Many patients with SCD have reported that interacting with medical providers has been experienced as a "battle" and that this may lead to their avoiding going to the ED when experiencing pain for fear of being perceived as malingering or opioid dependent, i.e., "drug seeking" (Haywood Jr et al., 2009). The inpatient setting often has providers (e.g., residents and fellows) with less exposure to the SCD population. Education with providers around avoiding pejorative language (e.g., "sicklers," "frequent flyers") can help decrease the negative impact of health-related stigma. Modeling respectful ways to talk about the relationship between psychosocial stressors and pain (e.g., "their pain experience is likely being exacerbated by…") can also be helpful in supporting patient-team communication (Conroy & Logan, 2014).

During an admission, problem-focused interventions may be more effective than preventative or general self-management strategies. MI can be effective for treatment adherence and pain in this setting, whether to increase engagement in behavioral strategies or to increase awareness of areas within a patient's control and then increasing participation in those activities. Additional targets may include establishing a consistent sleep schedule, behavioral activation (e.g., engaging with physical therapy, developing and adhering to a daily schedule), and beginning to address medication adherence challenges.

Outpatient Consultation

Patients with SCD may receive outpatient treatment in primary care settings or in an integrated sickle cell center. A method for reducing stigma and barriers to care in these settings is to integrate care, with physical and behavioral health services housed in the same facility (e.g., interdisciplinary teams, colocation of services, warm handoffs, etc.) (Kazdin, 2017). In the outpatient setting, a CL psychologist would ideally be embedded within the medical clinic as part of the hematology care team (Raphael & Oyeku, 2013). Other approaches are the continuity of care model, where patients are able to see the same psychologist when inpatient and outpatient, and/or holding integrated psychosocial/medical rounds, increasing the team's awareness of ongoing interventions and patient needs across domains (Hamann & Kendall, 2013). These care models allow providers to collaborate to address complex care needs and convey to the family the importance of equally addressing physical, psychological, and social factors (Crosby, Quinn, & Kalinyak, 2015). Other models of extending clinical care delivery include the use of telephonic, two-way video, email, and text-messaging modalities. These methods can increase access and convenience and can provide more real-time management of symptoms (Raphael & Oyeku, 2013).

Pain and adherence are the most common referral concerns in the outpatient setting, followed by referrals related to mood, developmental concerns (e.g., academic issues, behavioral challenges), and transition into adult care. Mortality risk is high for young adults with SCD (Quinn, Rogers, McCavit, & Buchanan, 2010), thus initiating behavioral interventions that target improving self-management and assertiveness/communication skills with a graduated approach when patients are in their early teenage years is highly recommended.

Other referral types in the outpatient setting may include treatment for pica, a psychological disorder common in SCD characterized by an appetite for nonnutritive substances. Using habit reversal therapy as a framework, providers intervene by helping patients in (1) increasing their awareness of the behavior (why/when am I eating paper?), (2) generating a competing response (e.g., eating a mint), (3) building motivation (what does pica get in the way of?), and (4) generalizing skills (e.g., from home to school) (Stiegler, 2005).

Preventative interventions targeting chronic pain management (e.g., stress management, sleep, nutrition, hydration, and activity pacing) may be more effectively implemented in an outpatient setting. Notably, while psychologists may actually have less frequent contact with patients during outpatient consultations within a clinic setting, they may have more opportunities for follow-up over time, which can provide increased continuity and reinforcement of patient skill development. In situations when referral concerns identified by the medical team are not shared by the family/patient, intervention should be collaborative, focus on building rapport, and include thorough assessment of the family's experience and values in order to improve willingness to return for future visits. Sessions may utilize MI techniques to highlight values and over time move toward change consistent with these values.

Outpatient consultation allows for a collaboration and should include regular interactions with the entire psychosocial team (e.g., social work, care manager, school liaison), as well as medical providers. This population has high "no show" rates for psychology and medical visits. The entire care team can reinforce the utility of psychological services to patients and families and provide practical help such as arranging for transportation, providing meal vouchers, allowing access to sibling play areas, and coordinating psychological and medical appointments. Another example of collaboration might be to ask the team to increase the frequency of medical visits in order to target adherence.

As SCD is most often diagnosed at birth, families tend to have strong ties with their medical team. As a consequence, there may be longstanding communication patterns, both adaptive and maladaptive, with medical providers. Research has demonstrated that children with SCD may engage passively during hematology visits when their parents are present, and patients respond less to physicians' efforts to build a relationship during the visit than do children with asthma or diabetes (Cox et al., 2017). This research suggests that engaging children with SCD during medical appointments can prove challenging, but shifting patterns of interactions may have positive impact. Strategies such as developmentally targeted self-management interventions to enhance patient independent communications with medical providers should ideally involve joint sessions with the patient, family, and medical team.

It is important that the CL psychologist keep the medical team informed regarding the interventions utilized in outpatient consultation so that they can support engagement and reinforce progress. Providing other providers on the team with the rationale and purpose of behavioral interventions is critical for increasing their knowledge and acceptance of integrated psychological consultation services. For example, MI techniques may not appear obviously efficacious to the referring provider. To support a consistent approach between psychological and medical services, it can be helpful to talk to the medical team about how change happens (i.e., change is not linear, change often happens slowly, changes in motivation are often precursors to observable behavior change) (Miller & Rollnick, 2002). These explanations can strengthen the medical teams' support of the intervention. Psychologists can then provide medical providers with specific strategies that are consistent with the treatment approach, e.g., the consulting psychologists can work with the team to ensure that discussions are consistent with evidence-based approaches to improving treatment adherence. Coordination will improve the patient experience by decreasing redundancy of discussions about adherence barriers and strategies (i.e., discussions about nonadherence primarily with the psychologist).

Case Example

Sean is a 13-year-old African American male with HbSS, who was admitted due to a pain episode. Sean has been prescribed HU since age five, and he regularly attends the sickle cell clinic. Historically, Sean has had very few pain episodes and only one hospitalization. However, over the past 4 months, he has had three admissions for pain. During his current admission, an initial psychology referral was placed due to concerns about medication adherence and pain. Per the medical team, the family was hesitant about the referral. Sean and his mother initially presented as guarded but became more engaged as the consultation progressed. The pediatric psychologist identified her role within the team. She acknowledged to the family that she was new to their care, acknowledging that they had spent years building rapport with other providers. Next, she asked the family's permission to learn more about the patient, treatment successes, and current challenges. Sean and his mother expressed worry and frustration about the recent change in Sean's pain. Sean shared that he was frustrated with the medical team's recommendation to "move around" when it "hurts to move." As the session proceeded, the family shared that Sean's mother had begun a new job, increasing Sean's responsibilities at home, and Sean was attending a new school. The family identified that their biggest concern was managing the current pain episode, which became the focus of the intervention. Employing CBT strategies and acknowledging Sean's early adolescent age, the intervention consisted of providing updated psychoeducation about SCD and pain processes, introducing behavioral strategies such as activity pacing and diaphragmatic breathing, and developing more adaptive cognitions regarding treatment demands (i.e., "moving is an important part of helping me recover from a pain crisis"). The CL psychologist contacted the school liaison specialist to address needed accommodations given his recent school change. The family was initially hesitant to try the new recommendations but was appreciative that the medical team was taking their concerns about addressing this pain crisis seriously. The psychologist advocated with the outpatient team for more frequent outpatient follow-up to monitor progress and reassure the family that their concerns were being taken seriously. After discharge, the family agreed to see the psychologist at Sean's next clinic visit.

At follow-up, the family was relieved that Sean had been readmitted for pain. Given their growing trust with the psychologist, Sean's mother for the first time expressed frustration that Sean "doesn't take his medicine like he is supposed to." Given these new concerns, the psychologist conducted a further assessment of the family's motivation, barriers, and expectations. Intervention shifted to adherence challenges. In the context of Sean's increased responsibilities, the psychologist worked with the family to identify common goals and expectations of independence, worked with Sean to better understand what he viewed as important and the value he found in taking his HU, and provided psychoeducation to his mother around developmentally sensitive ways to support Sean in making this transition to increased independence. Collaboration with the outpatient medical team included supporting manageable treatment goals for adherence and identifying roles of each team member to avoid potential dilution of the psychosocial interventions by multiple team members asking about adherence. The psychologist and Sean's family agreed to continue services and agreed that they would meet again during Sean's next outpatient medical appointment.

Conclusions

Patients with SCD face serious medical complications, and difficulties related to pain and/or medication adherence are often the primary reason for psychological consultation. Additionally, patients with SCD have increased risk for challenges with mood, anxiety, and developmental concerns, which should be areas of assessment and intervention for the CL psychologist. For some patients with SCD, their first contact with psychology occurs during an inpatient admission or clinic visit. In both settings, engagement and adaptation using culturally competent clinical practice can help to improve buy-in with this majority African American/Black population. Given the potential benefit of psychological interventions on pain management, mood/anxiety, quality of life, and functional outcomes, the next step for clinical research is to evaluate with more specificity how interventions can best be adapted to meet the needs of patients with SCD and their families.

Appendix: SCD Psychoeducation Resources

Patient and Family-Friendly Resources

Books

- Hope and Destiny: A Patient's and Parent's Guide to Sickle Cell Disease and Sickle Cell Trait (Platt, Eckman, & Hsu, 2016)
- Hope & Destiny Jr.: The Adolescent's Guide to Sickle Cell Disease (Hsu, Rodrigues, & Brandalise, 2013)

Websites

Sicklecellkids.org
Redbananasmovie.com

Self-Management
Personal Action Plan

My Personal Action Plan ________________________________
(Name)

1. Something I want to improve or change (a health goal or other personal goal):
____

2. How important is it to me to make this change? (circle a number)

0	1	2	3	4	5	6	7	8	9	10
Not at all Important									**Extremely Important**	

3. What might make it difficult for me to achieve my goal (what are the barriers)?
____

4. Steps I will take to make this change (for example, what, when, how, & with whom):
   A. ________________________________
   B. ________________________________
   C. ________________________________
   D. ________________________________

5. How certain am I that I can carry out this plan? (circle a number)

0	1	2	3	4	5	6	7	8	9	10
Very uncertain					**Moderately uncertain**					**Very certain**

6. Information or support I might need in accomplishing my goal:
____

7. I will know my plan is working when ________________________________

8. I will celebrate my success by ________________________________

I agree to this plan of action and will review my plan and progress on __________ with ______________ by:
(Date) (Name)

- ☐ email ________________________
- ☐ phone ________________________
- ☐ text message ________________________
- ☐ returning to clinic or other contact ________________________

Signature ________________________________ Date __________

Reviewed By ________________________________ Date __________

D1115
HIC 07/09

DTD1115

Cincinnati Children's
changing the outcome together

References

Barakat, L. P., Lash, L. A., Lutz, M. J., & Nicolaou, D. C. (2006). Psychosocial adaptation of children and adolescents with sickle cell disease. In R. T. Brown (Ed.), *Comprehensive handbook of childhood cancer and sickle cell disease: A biopsychosocial approach* (pp. 471–495). Oxford: Oxford University Press.

Berkelhammer, L. D., Williamson, A. L., Sanford, S. D., Dirksen, C. L., Sharp, W. G., Margulies, A. S., & Prengler, R. A. (2007). Neurocognitive sequelae of pediatric sickle cell disease: A review of the literature. *Child Neuropsychology, 13*(2), 120–131.

Bernaudin, F., Socie, G., Kuentz, M., Chevret, S., Duval, M., Bertrand, Y., … Bordigoni, P. (2007). Long-term results of related myeloablative stem-cell transplantation to cure sickle cell disease. *Blood, 110*(7), 2749–2756.

Brousseau, D. C., Panepinto, J., Nimmer, M., & Hoffmann, R. G. (2010). The number of people with sickle-cell disease in the United States: National and state estimates. *American Journal of Hematology, 85*(1), 77–78.

Conroy, C., & Logan, D. D. E. (2014). Pediatric multidisciplinary and interdisciplinary teams and interventions. In M. C. Roberts, B. S. Aylward, & Y. P. Wu (Eds.), *Clinical practice of pediatric psychology*. New York, NY: Guilford Press. pp. 93–108, 471–495.

Cook, B. L., Zuvekas, S. H., Carson, N., Wayne, G. F., Vesper, A., & McGuire, T. G. (2014). Assessing racial/ethnic disparities in treatment across episodes of mental health care. *Health Services Research, 49*(1), 206–229.

Cox, E. D., Swedlund, M. P., Young, H. N., Moreno, M. A., Schopp, J. M., Rajamanickam, V., & Panepinto, J. A. (2017). Family engagement in pediatric sickle cell disease visits. *Health Communication, 32*(1), 51–59.

Cozzi, L., Tryon, W. W., & Sedlacek, K. (1987). The effectiveness of biofeedback-assisted relaxation in modifying sickle cell crises. *Biofeedback and Self-Regulation, 12*(1), 51–61.

Crosby, L. E., Quinn, C. T., & Kalinyak, K. A. (2015). A biopsychosocial model for the management of patients with sickle-cell disease transitioning to adult medical care. *Advances in Therapy, 32*(4), 293–305.

Crosby, L. E., Joffe, N. E., Peugh, J., Ware, R. E., & Britto, M. T. (2017). Pilot of the chronic disease self-management program for adolescents and young adults with sickle cell disease. *Journal of Adolescent Health, 60*(1), 120–123.

DeBaun, M. R., Sarnaik, S. A., Rodeghier, M. J., Minniti, C. P., Howard, T. H., Iyer, R. V., … Quinn, C. T. (2012). Associated risk factors for silent cerebral infarcts in sickle cell anemia: Low baseline hemoglobin, sex, and relative high systolic blood pressure. *Blood, 119*(16), 3684–3690.

Frenette, P. S., & Atweh, G. F. (2007). Sickle cell disease: Old discoveries, new concepts, and future promise. *Journal of Clinical Investigation, 117*(4), 850.

Gil, K. M., Anthony, K. K., Carson, J. W., Redding-Lallinger, R., Daeschner, C. W., & Ware, R. E. (2001). Daily coping practice predicts treatment effects in children with sickle cell disease. *Journal of Pediatric Psychology, 26*(3), 163–173.

Gil, K. M., Wilson, J. J., Edens, J. L., Workman, E., Ready, J., Sedway, J., … Daeschner, C. W. (1997). Cognitive coping skills training in children with sickle cell disease pain. *International Journal of Behavioral Medicine, 4*(4), 364–377.

Hamann, H. A., & Kendall, J. (2013). Growing a psychosocial oncology program within a cancer center. *Oncology Issues, 28*(4), 32–39.

Hassell, K. L. (2010). Population estimates of sickle cell disease in the U.S. *American Journal of Preventive Medicine, 38*(4, Suppl), S512–S521. https://doi.org/10.1016/j.amepre.2009.12.022

Haywood, C., Jr., Beach, M. C., Lanzkron, S., Strouse, J. J., Wilson, R., Park, H., … Segal, J. B. (2009). A systematic review of barriers and interventions to improve appropriate use of therapies for sickle cell disease. *Journal of the National Medical Association, 101*(10), 1022–1033.

Hood, A. M., King, A. A., Fields, M. E., Ford, A. L., Guilliams, K. P., Hulbert, M. L., ... & White, D. A. (2019). Higher executive abilities following a blood transfusion in children and young adults with sickle cell disease. *Pediatric Blood & Cancer, 66*(10), e27899.

Hsu, L. L., Rodrigues, C. M., & Brandalise, S. R. (2013). *Hope and destiny: The patient and parent's guide to sickle cell disease and sickle cell trait revised* (4th ed.). Munster, IN: Hilton Publishing.

Jenerette, C. M., & Brewer, C. (2010). Health-related stigma in young adults with sickle cell disease. *Journal of the National Medical Association, 102*(11), 1050.

Jensen, C. D., Cushing, C. C., Aylward, B. S., Craig, J. T., Sorell, D. M., & Steele, R. G. (2011). Effectiveness of motivational interviewing interventions for adolescent substance use behavior change: A meta-analytic review. *Journal of Consulting and Clinical Psychology, 79*(4), 433.

Kaslow, N. J., Collins, M. H., Rashid, F. L., Baskin, M. L., Griffith, J. R., Hollins, L., & Eckman, J. E. (2000). The efficacy of a pilot family psychoeducational intervention for pediatric sickle cell disease (SCD). *Families, Systems, & Health, 18*(4), 381.

Kazak, A. E., Hwang, W.-T., Chen, F. F., Askins, M. A., Carlson, O., Argueta-Ortiz, F., & Barakat, L. P. (2018). Screening for family psychosocial risk in pediatric cancer: Validation of the Psychosocial Assessment Tool (PAT) Version 3. *Journal of Pediatric Psychology, 43*(7), 737–748.

Kazdin, A. E. (2017). Addressing the treatment gap: A key challenge for extending evidence-based psychosocial interventions. *Behaviour Research and Therapy, 88*, 7–18.

Lemanek, K. L., Ranalli, M., & Lukens, C. (2009). A randomized controlled trial of massage therapy in children with sickle cell disease. *Journal of Pediatric Psychology, 34*(10), 1091–1096.

Lozano, P., & Houtrow, A. (2018). Supporting self-management in children and adolescents with com-

plex chronic conditions. *Pediatrics, 141*(Suppl 3), S233–S241.
McAuliffe, G. (2008). *Culturally alert counseling: A comprehensive introduction* (Vol. 2). Thousand Oaks: Sage.
McClellan, C. B., Schatz, J. C., Puffer, E., Sanchez, C. E., Stancil, M. T., & Roberts, C. W. (2008). Use of handheld wireless technology for a home-based sickle cell pain management protocol. *Journal of Pediatric Psychology, 34*(5), 564–573.
Melzack, R., & Wall, P. D. (1965). Pain mechanisms: a new theory. *Science*, 150(3699), 971–979.
Miller, W. R., & Rollnick, S. (2002). *Motivational interviewing: Preparing people for change*. New York: The Guilford Press.
Modi, A. C., Pai, A. L., Hommel, K. A., Hood, K. K., Cortina, S., Hilliard, M. E., ... Drotar, D. (2012). Pediatric self-management: A framework for research, practice, and policy. *Pediatrics, 129*(2), e473–e485.
Moody, K., Abrahams, B., Baker, R., Santizo, R., Manwani, D., Carullo, V., ... Carroll, A. (2017). A randomized trial of yoga for children hospitalized with sickle cell vaso-occlusive crisis. *Journal of Pain and Symptom Management, 53*(6), 1026–1034.
Myrvik, M. P., Burks, L. M., Hoffman, R. G., Dasgupta, M., & Panepinto, J. A. (2013). Mental health disorders influence admission rates for pain in children with sickle cell disease. *Pediatric Blood & Cancer, 60*(7), 1211–1214.
Myrvik, M. P., Campbell, A. D., & Butcher, J. L. (2012). Single-session biofeedback-assisted relaxation training in children with sickle cell disease. *Journal of Pediatric Hematology/Oncology, 34*(5), 340–343.
Ojelabi, A., Graham, Y., & Ling, J. (2017). Health-related quality of life predictors in children and adolescents with sickle cell disease: A systematic review. *International Journal of Tropical Disease & Health, 22*(2), 1–14. https://doi.org/10.9734/IJTDH/2017/31954
Panepinto, J. A., Pajewski, N. M., Foerster, L. M., Sabnis, S., & Hoffmann, R. G. (2009). Impact of family income and sickle cell disease on the health-related quality of life of children. *Quality of Life Research, 18*(1), 5–13.
Piel, F. B., Hay, S. I., Gupta, S., Weatherall, D. J., & Williams, T. N. (2013). Global burden of sickle cell anaemia in children under five, 2010–2050: Modelling based on demographics, excess mortality, and interventions. *PLoS Medicine, 10*(7), e1001484.
Platt, A. F., Eckman, J., & Hsu, L. L. (2016). *Hope and destiny: The patient and parent's guide to sickle cell disease and sickle cell trait revised* (4th ed.). Munster, IN: Hilton Publishing.
Prussien, K. V., Jordan, L. C., DeBaun, M. R., & Compas, B. E. (2019). Cognitive function in sickle cell disease across domains, cerebral infarct status, and the lifespan: a meta-analysis. *Journal of Pediatric Psychology, 44*(8), 948–958.
Quinn, C. T., Rogers, Z. R., McCavit, T. L., & Buchanan, G. R. (2010). Improved survival of children and adolescents with sickle cell disease. *Blood, 115*(17), 3447–3452.
Raphael, J. L., & Oyeku, S. O. (2013). Sickle cell disease pain management and the medical home. *ASH Education Program Book, 2013*(1), 433–438.
Redding-Lallinger, R., & Knoll, C. (2006). Sickle cell disease—Pathophysiology and treatment. *Current Problems in Pediatric and Adolescent Health Care, 36*(10), 346–376.
Rees, D. C., Williams, T. N., & Gladwin, M. T. (2010). Sickle-cell disease. *The Lancet, 376*(9757), 2018–2031.
Schatz, J., Schlenz, A., McClellan, C. B., Puffer, E. S., Hardy, S., Pfeiffer, M., & Roberts, C. W. (2015). Changes in coping, pain and activity following cognitive-behavioral training: A randomized clinical trial for pediatric sickle cell disease using smartphones. *The Clinical Journal of Pain, 31*(6), 536.
Schwartz, L. A., Radcliffe, J., & Barakat, L. P. (2007). The development of a culturally sensitive pediatric pain management intervention for African American adolescents with sickle cell disease. *Children's Healthcare, 36*(3), 267–283.
Smith, L. A., Oyeku, S. O., Homer, C., & Zuckerman, B. (2006). Sickle cell disease: A question of equity and quality. *Pediatrics, 117*(5), 1763–1770.
Stiegler, L. N. (2005). Understanding pica behavior: A review for clinical and education professionals. *Focus Autism Other Dev Disabil, 20*(1), 27–38.
Stuart, M. J., & Nagel, R. L. (2004). Sickle-cell disease. *The Lancet, 364*(9442), 1343–1360.
Wakefield, E. O., Pantaleao, A., Popp, J. M., Dale, L. P., Santanelli, J. P., Litt, M. D., & Zempsky, W. T. (2018). Describing perceived racial bias among youth with sickle cell disease. *Journal of Pediatric Psychology, 43*(7), 779–788.
Ware, R. E., de Montalembert, M., Tshilolo, L., & Abboud, M. R. (2017). Sickle cell disease. *The Lancet, 390*, 311.
Whaley, A. L., & Davis, K. E. (2007). Cultural competence and evidence-based practice in mental health services: A complementary perspective. *American Psychologist, 62*(6), 563.
Williams, H., & Tanabe, P. (2016). Sickle cell disease: A review of nonpharmacological approaches for pain. *Journal of Pain and Symptom Management, 51*(2), 163–177.
Wills, K. E., Nelson, S. C., Hennessy, J., Nwaneri, M. O., Miskowiec, J., McDonough, E., & Moquist, K. (2010). Transition planning for youth with sickle cell disease: Embedding neuropsychological assessment into comprehensive care. *Pediatrics, 126*(Suppl 3), S151–S159.

Psychological Consultation in Pediatric Solid Organ Transplantation

Melissa K. Cousino, Kelly E. Rea, and Emily M. Fredericks

Medical Overview

Due to advancements in treatment and survival, solid organ transplantation (SOT) is a common intervention for pediatric patients with end-stage organ disease. Per the Organ Procurement and Transplantation Network (OPTN), nearly 2000 children (0–17 years) underwent SOT in 2017. On average, an additional 2000 pediatric patients remain on the national waitlist. Approximately half of pediatric patients receive a donor organ within a year of listing (based on OPTN data as of September 2018).

Pediatric Abdominal Transplantation Kidney transplantation is most common, with 746 pediatric kidney transplants performed in the US in 2017 (based on OPTN data as of September 2018). For patients under 6 years old, congenital anomalies of the kidney and urinary tract are the most common causes for end-stage kidney disease leading to kidney transplantation. Older children are more likely to require kidney transplantation due to focal segmental glomerulosclerosis and glomerulonephritis. Five-year kidney graft survival ranges from 91% (living donor recipient under 11 years old) to 75% (deceased donor recipient over 11 years old), with overall 5-year patient survival rates of 98% (Hart et al., 2018). In 2017, 599 US children underwent liver transplantation (based on OPTN data as of September 2018). Primary diseases resulting in need for pediatric liver transplantation most commonly include cholestatic biliary atresia or metabolic disease. Five-year graft survival of pediatric liver transplants exceeds 80%, with 5-year patient survival rates of 86% (Kim et al., 2018).

Pediatric Thoracic Transplantation Incidence of pediatric heart transplantation has increased in the past decade with 431 US transplants performed in 2017 (based on OPTN data as of

M. K. Cousino (✉)
C.S. Mott Children's Hospital, Ann Arbor, MI, USA

University of Michigan Transplant Center, Ann Arbor, MI, USA

Department of Pediatrics, University of Michigan Medical School, Ann Arbor, MI, USA
e-mail: melcousi@med.umich.edu

K. E. Rea
Department of Psychology, University of Georgia, Athens, GA, USA

E. M. Fredericks
C.S. Mott Children's Hospital, Ann Arbor, MI, USA

University of Michigan Transplant Center, Ann Arbor, MI, USA

Department of Pediatrics, University of Michigan Medical School, Ann Arbor, MI, USA

Susan B. Meister Child Health Evaluation and Research (CHEAR) Center, Ann Arbor, MI, USA

B. D. Carter, K. A. Kullgren (eds.), *Clinical Handbook of Psychological Consultation in Pediatric Medical Settings*, Issues in Clinical Child Psychology, https://doi.org/10.1007/978-3-030-35598-2_27

September 2018). The most common causes for pediatric heart transplantation are congenital heart disease, dilated cardiomyopathy, and myocarditis. Overall, 5-year patient survival following pediatric heart transplantation is 79%; however, one in ten recipients will die within a year of transplant (Colvin et al., 2018). Most commonly offered for patients with cystic fibrosis or pulmonary hypertension, pediatric lung transplantation occurs less frequently, with 44 pediatric lung transplants performed in the US in 2017 (based on OPTN data as of September 2018). Five-year survival following pediatric lung transplantation is 58% (Valapour et al., 2018).

Treatment Regimen and Complications Other types of pediatric SOTs include intestinal, pancreas, and multiorgan transplants. Regardless of transplant type, post-SOT care requires daily medication administration, regular blood draws, frequent follow-up visits, and occasional procedures, such as biopsies. SOT recipients will take immunosuppressant medications daily for the remainder of their lives to prevent the body from rejecting the transplanted organ. These medications are accompanied by potential sides effects, including high blood pressure, weight gain, increased rates of infection, and increased risk for some types of cancer, as well as new-onset diabetes (Magee, Krishnan, Benfield, Hsu, & Shneider, 2008).

Psychosocial Overview

Psychological Functioning SOT is associated with increased psychosocial stressors for patients and families. Although some research suggests that patient psychological functioning improves following SOT, increased risk for long-term internalizing and externalizing problems exists for a subset of pediatric SOT recipients (Fredericks, Zelikovsky, Aujoulat, Hames, & Wray, 2014; Shellmer, Brosig, & Wray, 2014). For example, among 64 pediatric kidney and liver SOT recipients, child-reported scores of psychosocial functioning were significantly better than average; however, parent-reported scores indicated higher rates of internalizing problems when compared to controls (Wu, Aylward, Steele, Maikranz, & Dreyer, 2008). Others have supported these parent-reported findings. Of 23 kidney SOT recipients, 17% endorsed significant depressive symptoms (Dobbels, Decorte, Roskams, & Van Damme-Lombaerts, 2010). Similarly, in a study of 38 liver SOT recipients (≤16 years), 22% and 19% exceeded clinical cutoffs for internalizing and externalizing problems, respectively (Fredericks, Lopez, Magee, Shieck, & Opipari-Arrigan, 2007). Approximately 20–50% of pediatric heart or heart-lung SOT recipients have been found to have impaired psychological functioning (e.g., Cousino et al., 2018; DeMaso, Kelley, Bastardi, O'Brien, & Blume, 2004). Posttraumatic stress symptoms are also higher in pediatric SOT populations when compared with national averages, with reported rates of approximately 15% (Mintzer et al., 2005) to 30% (Shemesh et al., 2000).

Health-related quality of life (QOL) in pediatric SOT populations is well researched. Improvements in QOL have been observed post-SOT; however, pediatric SOT recipients continue to have lower QOL than healthy controls (Anthony, BarZiv, & Ng, 2010; Fredericks et al., 2012; Uzark et al., 2012). Factors associated with poorer long-term QOL in SOT recipients include lower family income, higher family conflict, sleep-related problems, history of a rejection episode, and poorer adherence behaviors (Devine et al., 2011; Fredericks et al., 2012).

Adherence and Self-management Adherence to immunosuppressant medications is critical for SOT recipients. Medication nonadherence is associated with morbidity and mortality, including acute rejection, graft loss, and death (Dobbels et al., 2010). Medication nonadherence is common in pediatric SOT populations, with prevalence rates up to 50–70% (Shemesh et al., 2004). Adolescents are at four times higher risk of medication nonadherence than adults are (Dobbels, Van Damme-Lombaert, Vanhaecke, & Geest, 2005; Shemesh et al., 2004). Researchers have identified a number of correlates associated with nonadherence in pediatric SOT populations, including older child age, poorer child psychosocial functioning, limited medication knowledge, adolescent-reported medication barriers, executive functioning deficits, greater parental distress, and lower family cohesion (Dew et al., 2009; Dobbels et al., 2005; Gutiérrez-Colina et al., 2015; Simons, McCormick, Devine, & Blount, 2010).

Academic and Neuropsychological Outcomes End-stage disease can impact intellectual, academic, and neurocognitive functions (Alonso & Sorensen, 2009). In a sample of pediatric thoracic SOT recipients, 40% had clinically significant cognitive delays (Brosig, Hintermeyer, Zlotocha, Behrens, & Mao, 2006). In a multicenter study of pediatric liver SOT recipients, 26% had mild-to-moderate cognitive delays (Sorensen et al., 2011). Deficits in the areas of academic functioning, executive functioning, memory, language, visual-spatial skills, and attention have also been documented among pediatric SOT populations (Haavisto, Korkman, Holmberg, Jalanko, & Qvist, 2011; Kaller, Langguth, Ganschow, Nashan, & Schulz, 2010; Sorensen et al., 2011). Common risk factors associated with poor neurocognitive outcomes include earlier age of disease onset and longer disease duration, poor growth prior to SOT, and longer hospitalizations during the first year post SOT (Wayman, Cox, & Esquivel, 1997).

Parent and Family Functioning A recent systematic review of 37 studies concluded that parents of pediatric SOT patients experience significant stress and mental health problems throughout the course of SOT (Cousino, Rea, Schumacher, Magee, & Fredericks, 2017). Researchers have reported rates of clinically significant psychological symptoms (Douglas, Hulson, & Trompeter, 1998; Tarbell & Kosmach, 1998) and posttraumatic stress symptoms (Farley et al., 2007; Young et al., 2003) in greater than 50% of parents of pediatric SOT recipients. Factors associated with poorer parent and family functioning in SOT populations include greater family conflict, increased parenting stress, patient emotional and behavioral problems, increased medication barriers, and poorer adherence outcomes (Cousino, Rea, Schumacher, et al., 2017).

Role of Psychology Consultant and Models of Service

Given the myriad of patient and family psychosocial stressors, psychologists are valuable members of pediatric SOT teams. Multidisciplinary SOT teams include physicians, surgeons, transplant coordinators, nurses, social workers, dieticians, child life specialists, and psychologists, among others. The Center for Medicaid and Medicare Services (CMS) mandates that a pretransplant psychosocial evaluation be completed by a social worker for each SOT candidate. Professional societies have recommended that a psychologist also be included in SOT teams; however, the role and level of integration of the psychologist varies from center to center. At some centers, psychologists are integrated members of SOT teams, providing assessment and treatment throughout the transplant process in its entirety and regularly attending selection meetings. At other centers, psychology services are accessed through hospital-based consultation-liaison programs (Skillings & Lewandowski, 2015).

Among pediatric inpatient consultation-liaison (CL) services, 37% report a medium-to-high number of referrals for pretransplant psychology/psychiatry evaluations (Shaw, Wamboldt, Bursch, & Stuber, 2006). In addition to pretransplant evaluations, inpatient psychology/psychiatry services may be requested for adjustment to illness, nonadherence to treatment, procedural anxiety, and disposition and referral. Some inpatient SOT populations may also require more traditional, longer term psychotherapy services due to prolonged hospital stays while waiting for a donor organ. Some centers offer dedicated transplant psychology services within outpatient transplant specialty clinics. Pre- and post-SOT patients are seen by an array of multidisciplinary providers while attending these comprehensive clinics. Psychologists working within outpatient specialty clinics tend to provide brief psychosocial assessment with emphasis on identifying patients in need of additional intervention services (Cousino et al., 2018). Psychology consultation in outpatient clinics is also likely to focus on issues related to nonadherence (e.g., mood, sleep issues, lack of parental monitoring), learning and school-based concerns (Da Cruz et al., 2019), risk assessments and safety planning, and promoting readiness for transition to adult-based SOT care (Fredericks et al., 2015).

Evidence-Based Assessment and Intervention for Common Referrals

Pretransplant Psychosocial Evaluation All SOT candidates must undergo a psychosocial assessment prior to SOT listing. At some centers, pre-SOT psychology evaluations are standard practice. At other centers, pre-SOT psychology evaluations may only be requested following a social work evaluation or as needed for more concerning psychiatric or behavioral issues (Skillings & Lewandowski, 2015). The primary aims of the psychosocial assessment is to identify patient and family strengths and weaknesses, particularly as they may relate to adherence to medication management, early identification of signs of serious complications, and close medical follow-up. Additionally, the assessment should help to target potential needs for additional psychosocial interventions and/or resources critical to addressing pre-, in-hospital-, and posttransplant adjustment and adherence (Lefkowitz, Fitzgerald, Zelikovsky, Barlow, & Wray, 2014). Primary domains of the pre-SOT psychosocial evaluation should minimally include patient and family history of adherence to treatment (e.g., medications, appointments, diet), barriers to medical management (e.g., pill swallowing, procedural distress), disease and SOT-related knowledge, illness-related self-management skills, allocation of treatment responsibility, cognitive and/or neurodevelopmental functioning, patient and parent/extended family mental health history, including treatments, patient and parent coping skills, social support, family functioning, and abuse and legal history (Fung & Shaw, 2008; Lefkowitz et al., 2014). Patient healthcare communication and medical decision-making preferences may also be assessed via interview or clinical tools, such as *My CHATT* (Cousino, Rea, & Mednick, 2017).

Unlike adult SOT, where a number of established standardized psychosocial assessment tools exists, the only comprehensive pre-SOT screening tool specific to pediatrics is the 17-item Pediatric Transplant Rating Instrument (P-TRI) (Fung & Shaw, 2008). This semi-structured interview was designed to identify developmental, psychosocial, and family risks for poor post-SOT adherence; however, associations between the P-TRI and post-SOT outcomes have yet to be well established, and additional revisions to improve interrater reliability are needed (Fisher et al., 2011; Lefkowitz et al., 2014). Thus, some psychologists include a variety of other domain-specific assessment measures as part of the pre-SOT evaluation (see Appendix 2).

While considerable clinical effort often goes into conducting the required pre-SOT psychosocial evaluation, the research fails to show that pre-SOT psychosocial risk factors are predictive of poorer post-SOT outcomes (e.g., Lefkowitz et al., 2014). Particularly in the case of pediatric patients, it is rare for a child to be denied listing for a transplant due to psychosocial concerns alone. Rather, the efforts of the psychologist and other social support services are directed toward developing interventions and resources to address mitigating risk factors in order to promote a favorable long term posttransplant outcome. Clinically, the pre-SOT psychosocial evaluation experience often serves the important process of the psychosocial transplant team members joining with the patient and family in the longer term posttransplant coping and adjustment process.

Tips and tools: a sampling of assessment measures used in pediatric SOT, along with a sample pretransplant psychology evaluation template, are provided in Appendices 1 and 2.

Psychological Functioning Due to the high incidence of emotional and behavioral concerns in children and adolescents whose medical conditions require SOT, mental health interventions are frequently needed. Cognitive behavioral therapy (CBT) remains the most documented and empirically supported treatment approach for child anxiety and depressive disorders (Compton et al., 2004); however, few have examined CBT interventions specific to pediatric SOT. In adults pre-SOT, CBT interventions (e.g., cognitive restructuring, problem-solving) have been shown to improve QOL, mood stability, and social relations (Rodrigue, Baz, Widows, & Ehlers, 2005).

Tips and tools: worksheets and CBT-based activities used in general child clinical settings can be easily adapted to meet the emotional and behavioral needs of SOT patients. For example, positive self-statement generation can be especially helpful for children struggling with self-esteem and body-image issues triggered by scars, infusion therapy, or devices. Thought challenging and relaxation training are particularly useful for anxiety related to procedures, return to school, and medical visits. To bolster mood and improve QOL, especially for inpatients, positive event scheduling can be incorporated via the implementation of daily schedules (including child life therapies), hospital scavenger hunts, and "special events" (movie nights, outdoor picnic).

Adherence and Self-management Adherence to treatment, particularly lifesaving immunosuppressant medications, is one of the most challenging factors to predict and address with pediatric SOT patients, especially adolescents and young adults. For the busy clinician, it is frustrating to note that, to date, there remains a lack of an accepted "gold standard" method for assessing adherence in pediatric SOT recipients. Measures of adherence among SOT populations include patient- and caregiver-reported questionnaires or interviews, objective measures (e.g., electronic medication monitoring technology, pill counts, prescription refill rates), and drug assays. Electronic medication monitoring tends to be the standard measure of adherence, yet there are barriers associated with this method, such as cost and the possibility that these devices may interfere with established adherence routines (Shellmer & Zelikovsky, 2007). Adherence behavior has the potential to be modified, yet available pediatric adherence promotion interventions generally demonstrate heterogeneous and relatively small-effect sizes (Kahana, Drotar, & Frazier, 2008; Pai & McGrady, 2014). In a recent review of adherence-promoting interventions among SOT recipients, few intervention studies led to improvements in SOT-related medical outcomes. Adherence interventions tend to show greater improvements in secondary outcomes, such as improved QOL and decreased healthcare utilization (Duncan et al., 2017).

Established self-management skills are also critically important when SOT recipients transfer to adult-based care. Assessment of transition-related skills should include measures of self-management skills, health-related knowledge, adherence, and psychosocial functioning. Transition readiness interventions demonstrating some improvements in transfer outcomes among SOT patients include promotion of regimen and health-related knowledge (Fredericks et al., 2015; Pahl et al., 2018).

Tips and tools: due to the lack of a "gold standard" adherence assessment that can be easily implemented by busy clinicians, one may simply rely on asking patients, "In the past 2 weeks, how many doses of (medication) have you missed? How many doses have you taken more than two hours late?" Promoting active problem-solving with patients and families to address contributors to nonadherence is one of the more clinically useful interventions. Strategies that families may agree upon (with the guidance and approval of their medical team) include changing the timing of medication so that it is more amenable with school/social/sleep schedule, setting phone or home device alarms, using video chat with parents when away from home to increase monitoring, using a keychain pill holder with a spare dose of medications, etc. Using behavioral rewards to enhance treatment adherence may also be helpful. Table 1 includes medication reminder

Table 1 SOT and related apps

App		Cost	Platform	Brief description
Medication adherence				
	TransplantHero	Free	iOS, Android	Alerts users when it is time to take their medications, allows users to share medication schedules with others, and can send them notifications of missed dosages
	Teen Pocket Path (TPP)	Free	Android	Helps track medication taking with reminders and history of adherence, as well as providing general organ information
	MediSafe	Free, in-app purchases	iOS, Android	Gives medication reminders, prescription refill reminders, drug interaction warnings, and caregiver alerts when doses are missed and tracks adherence progress over time
Transplant specific information				
	Care After Kidney Transplant	Free	iOS, Android	Provides learning on how to stay healthy post-kidney transplant and answers frequently asked questions about how and why it is important to follow medical recommendations
	Organ Transplant—Terms	Free	iOS	Allows searching for and bookmarking common transplant-related terms and phrases for learning and discussing with medical providers
	Our Journey with Heart Transplant	Free	iOS	Helps families identify what they need to know before taking their child home from the hospital following a heart transplant
	Our Journey with Liver Transplant	Free	iOS	Helps families identify what they need to know before taking their child home from the hospital following a liver transplant
Medical/hospital resources				

App		Cost	Platform	Brief description
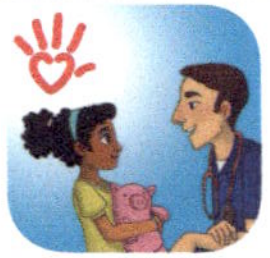	Simply Sayin'—Medical Jargon for Families	Free	iOS	Provides a mobile resource of pictures, sounds, and a family-friendly glossary of terms to facilitate clear conversations between the healthcare provider, child, and family
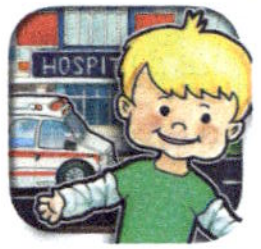	My PlayHome Hospital	$2.99	iOS, Android	Is an open-ended play game to introduce kids to a hospital/medical setting and allow them to explore or role-play in a variety of hospital settings
Fluid intake				
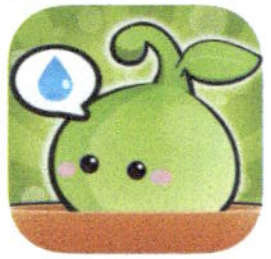	Plant Nanny	Free, in-app purchases	iOS, Android	Provides kid-friendly reminder to meet daily fluid goals, keeps your plant alive by meeting water goals throughout the day and drinking water regularly
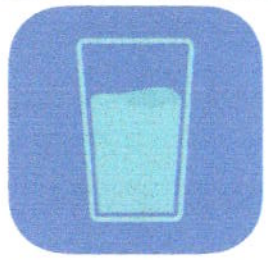	Daily Water	Free	iOS	Sets daily water goals, gives alerts when it is time to hydrate, tracks progress, emails graphs and tracking information to family members, friends, or doctors
	Hydro Coach	Free, in-app purchases	Android	Sets daily water goals, gives alerts when it is time to hydrate, tracks weekly and monthly progress, shares water intake with family members, friends, or doctors

Table 2 Resources for patients and families

Resource	Brief description
Information about transplant: Websites/handouts	
What Every Parent Needs to Know UNOS Parent Guide	A comprehensive guide for parents who have children facing an organ transplant, guiding parents through the transplant process and post-transplant management
Transplant Families http://transplantfamilies.org/	An online and in-person community of families facing transplantation
Boston Children's Hospital Experience Journals: Transplant Journal https://experiencejournal.com/journals/transplant/	A collection of stories and personal experiences from patients and families about what it has been like to have a solid organ transplant
UNOS: Transplant Living https://transplantliving.org/	A patient-oriented website providing information on what happens before and after transplantation
Books for parents	
My Child Needs a Transplant, Now What? By Tandy & James Owen	A book written by parents of a child who received a liver transplant to help answer other parents' questions and help parents going through a similar process realize they are not alone
Your Child in the Hospital: A Practical Guide for Parents By Nancy Keene	A guide for parents of children with a variety of illnesses, tips for visiting the hospital, woven together with inspiring stories of parents who have been through similar experiences
When Pigs Fly By Gretchen Cooke and Jennifer Cooke Rinehart	The story of a young woman's liver transplant, written by a mother and daughter to serve as an inspiration to organ transplant patients, their families, and friends
Books for kids	
Brave Just Like Me By Kimberly Ruff	A book inspired by the true story of a young girl facing organ transplants, hospitalizations, and medical procedures, encouraging children going through similar situations to "be brave and know that you are not alone"
Medikidz Explain Organ Transplant By Kim Chilman-Blair	A story of five superheroes, each specializing in a different organ, explaining organ transplants in a kid-friendly way, geared toward children ages 10–13
Your Transplant Adventure By Matt Butler and Tanya Smith	A picture book created for young patients and/or siblings to depict the solid organ transplant process; common questions young children have are asked with simple, honest answers to follow
What Every Kid Needs to Know About Organ Transplants By UNOS	A free PDF download from UNOS to help children and their families feel more at ease with the organ transplantation process in an understandable format
Organizations, foundations, and support groups	
Donate Life https://www.donatelife.net	National and state organizations committed to increased organ, eye, and tissue donation
Children's Organ Transplant Association	An association that helps children and young adults who need lifesaving organ transplants by providing fundraising assistance
Local support groups by state	https://transplantliving.org/community/support-groups/
Summer camps by state	https://transplantliving.org/children/camps

apps and fluid-tracking apps to assist patients in adhering to their medical regimen. Increased check-ins with psychosocial and/or medical teams may also be needed. A table of transition-readiness assessments used in pediatric SOT is provided in Appendix 2. Some resources for patients and families to improve regimen and health-related knowledge can be found in Table 2.

Academic Support It is common for SOT psychosocial team members, particularly psychologists with psychoeducational expertise, to recommend interventions specifically addressing educational needs. Da Cruz et al., 2019 found that this occurred in almost a third of clinical encounters. Psychology interventions in this area are likely to include psychoeducation (e.g., education about 504/IEP services), advocacy efforts (e.g., writing letters), and liaising directly with schools. 504/IEP services that are specifically pertinent to SOT patients include access to water/use of water bottles, unlimited restroom breaks, access to handwashing, and breaks for medication administration. In addition, SOT patients will require homebound school services in the weeks to months following surgery. A subset of patients may need these services while awaiting SOT. Intellectual and academic assessments will inform additional 504/IEP needs. These assessments may be completed by SOT psychologists; however, it is more common that referrals are made for comprehensive neuropsychological testing.

Tips and tools: Da Cruz et al., 2019 have made available an educational need assessment for SOT patients that can be used to determine current academic supports and potential areas for additional intervention.

Procedural Distress and Pill Swallowing In addition to the surgery itself, pediatric SOT patients undergo many procedures, ranging from frequent blood draws to dialysis port placements and cardiac catheterizations. In the most extreme forms, when a child in need of a transplant engages in behaviors that make conducting even basic clinical procedures difficult or impossible, it can serve as a barrier to being listed for transplant. In these instances, cognitive-behavioral interventions, distraction, and clinical hypnosis have been shown to be effective (Uman, Chambers, McGrath, & Kisely, 2008). Given the significance of posttransplant medication adherence on patient survival, psychologists are often called upon to provide interventions to address pill-swallowing difficulties. Behavioral approaches, including modeling, shaping, and positive reinforcement, have been effective in teaching children to swallow pills (Blount, Dahlquist, Baer, & Wuori, 1984; Patel, Jacobsen, Jhaveri, & Bradford, 2015).

Tips and tools: "Poke plans" (e.g., where a child will sit, what he/she will do during a procedure), medical play (i.e., desensitization), relaxation strategies, and active distraction (e.g., "I spy") are useful interventions. A sample dressing change plan is provided in Appendix 3.

Palliative and End-of-Life Care Although survival following SOT has improved in recent decades, SOT is accompanied by risks of morbidity and shortened life expectancy. Psychological interventions specific to end-of-life care may be needed for some patients. Interventions may include symptom management (e.g., nonpharmacological interventions for pain and nausea), treatment of emotional or behavioral problems, grief and bereavement, and communication and decision-making support. A recent survey of pediatric SOT providers indicated that less than 20% engage their pediatric transplant patients (<18 years) in advance care planning discussions and only ~30% discuss advance care planning with their young adult patients (Cousino, Schumacher, Magee, et al., 2019). However, pilot research indicated that young patients pre-heart SOT want to engage in these discussions (Cousino, Miller, Smith, et al., 2019).

Tips and tools: resources such as a *Voicing My Choices* and *VitalTALK* are helpful tools for navigating such discussions. *My CHATT* (Cousino, Rea, & Mednick, 2017) can serve as a starting point for gauging patient preferences for discussing end-of-life care.

Case Example

As this chapter illustrates, psychological consultation in pediatric SOT covers a range of presenting problems and may occur across a variety of clinical settings with practices varying from center to center. This case example highlights the important role of pediatric psychological consultation in SOT.

Case "Lily" was born with complex single ventricle congenital heart disease. She underwent Fontan surgery at age four. She subsequently developed protein-losing enteropathy (PLE) and was hospitalized with symptoms of worsening heart failure at age eight. A transplant (SOT) psychology consultation was requested to assess current psychological functioning, risks, and protective factors as part of a standard multidisciplinary pretransplant evaluation for consideration to be listed for heart transplantation. Due to Lily's age, SOT psychology met with her parents first. Parent interview included clinical interview in the following domains (see Appendix 1 for sample pretransplant evaluation template): patient/family regimen knowledge/adherence/transplant knowledge, allocation of responsibility for health management tasks, patient coping with the illness/procedures/hospitalizations and a potential need for transplant, patient/family health-related communication and decision-making preferences, patient developmental history, patient/family mental health, abuse, and trauma history, patient current psychological functioning, patient/family academic/vocational history, and patient/family social history. Parent interview revealed intact family functioning with strong social support, history of untreated maternal anxiety, and excellent parental understanding of the disease, regimen, and transplant process with no adherence concerns. Her parents endorsed notable concerns about Lily's functioning, primarily in the areas of anxiety, sleep, and coping with medical procedures. While symptoms of anxiety had been present for greater than 6 months, they had worsened over the past month in the setting of Lily's decompensating health.

One-to-one interview with Lily followed, along with administration of a child anxiety self- and parent-report scale. Similar to parent report, Lily endorsed excessive and intrusive worry thoughts about transplant, hospitalizations, new people/activities, school performance, and separation from parents. Symptoms of anxiety interfered with daily functioning with notable impact on sleep (e.g., delayed sleep onset of >2 h most nights), sibling relations (e.g., increased irritability and conflict), and medical care (e.g., withdrawing and hiding from clinicians while hospitalized). Although Lily recognized that a heart transplant was needed, she was unable to speak about it without becoming highly distressed. She demonstrated above developmental level knowledge of her disease and treatment regimen. She was able to name most of her medications and their functions. She swallowed pills without issue but required significant parent/clinician intervention to complete procedures, such as blood draws. Based on parent and patient interviews, along with clinically elevated scores on anxiety measurements, a diagnosis of generalized anxiety disorder was made, and a recommendation was shared with the family and transplant team that Lily participate in bi-weekly cognitive behavioral therapy throughout the transplant listing/waiting process. In addition, the mother was referred to a clinical psychologist treatment for her anxiety. No major psychological contraindications to transplant listing were noted.

Lily began bi-weekly psychotherapy with the SOT psychologist as her evaluation continued. Cognitive behavioral interventions were provided to target anxiety and sleep, including emotion identification, relaxation skill training (utilizing heart rate variability and electrodermograph biofeedback, Wild Divine®), identification of distressing automatic thoughts, thought challenging, positive statement generation, and behavioral reinforcement. In addition, desensitization, clinical hypnosis (e.g., relaxation was induced via guided imagery of Lily swimming in a pool, and suggestions were given to turn pain and burn controls down), and procedural coping plans were provided to target procedural distress specific to blood draws. After eight outpatient sessions, Lily demonstrated excellent progress. She was able to speak more comfortably about transplant, conflict with siblings had significantly decreased, and sleep onset was occurring within 30 min without need for parental intervention.

Unfortunately, though, Lily had not yet been listed for transplant due to various medical concerns (e.g., PLE flare-ups, worsening liver disease). The evaluation was put on hold until her PLE was better controlled. This caused understandable stress and burden on Lily and her family. Lily noted she had "worked so hard to be ready for this, but it may not happen." At age nine, Lily began to have more questions about her life expectancy, but she was uninterested in discussing her concerns further. She made comments to parents about school, stating "what's the point?" SOT psychology continued to provide supportive interventions for Lily, now primarily in the inpatient setting, with diagnosis of adjustment disorder with depressed mood. In light of her depression, Lily began to exhibit medication refusal behaviors, stating that she did not like the side-effects associated with many of her PLE-related medications. In response, psychology consultation also began to include adherence-focused interventions. Behavioral plans with rewards were implemented, along with team/family meetings to review medication schedule/burden. Helpful changes were made, such as adjusting the timing of her diuretics to decrease impact on sleep. In addition, a dopamine infusion was started, requiring PICC line placement. Psychology sessions engaged Lily in thought challenging and problem-solving interventions specific to home-going with the PICC. Of greatest concern to Lily was her inability to swim over the summer. Prior to discharge, the psychologist held a session with her family, younger siblings included, to assist them in generating a list of nonaquatic summer activities. Lily and her sisters decided to enroll in Lego and theater camps. Her mood was bolstered with improvements in medical adherence and health. After 3 months without a PLE flare-up, Lily underwent reevaluation to be listed for transplant. Psychosocial reevaluation was conducted and, due to improvements in anxiety, mood, sleep, and adherence, no additional therapy needs were identified and Lily/her family were encouraged to contact a psychologist as needed. Continued check-ins would be provided in the transplant clinic.

Lily received her heart transplant at age ten. Her surgery was successful, but psychology was consulted while she was inpatient to address labile and aggressive mood, triggered by pain and steroid induction. Supportive and environmental interventions were applied, including the establishment of "quiet times," decreasing the number of providers in the room, and scheduling times for preferred activities (art, games). She was discharged 3 weeks post transplant in both great health and spirits. She continues to be seen by transplant psychology for check-ins in heart transplant follow-up clinics.

Summary and Conclusions

In the last few decades, SOT has become almost a routine in children's hospital settings, with significant improvement in survival and quality of life for the young recipients. However, favorable outcome is highly dependent on a host of individual, family, and healthcare team factors. Pediatric psychologists and other psychosocial service providers are playing an increasingly important role in facilitating these improvements. As such, even more efforts have to be made to identify and refine effective assessment and intervention strategies to inform our consultation to the SOT process.

Appendix 1: Sample Pretransplant Psychology Evaluation Template

PRE-TRANSPLANT PSYCHOLOGY EVALUATION

MEDICAL HISTORY:

MEDICAL COPING, ADHERENCE, KNOWLEDGE.

Patient Regimen Knowledge/Adherence:

Name Medical Condition:

Name Medications, Dosing, Timing, Function:

System for Remembering Medications:

Adherence Rating (Self):

Adherence Rating (Parent):

Diet:

Appointments:

Patient Transplant-Specific Knowledge:

Why transplant?

Process?

Post-transplant treatment demands?

Risks?

Not cure?

Allocation of Responsibility for Health Management Tasks:

Remembering medications?

Filling/organizing pillbox?

Refilling prescriptions?

Noticing health changes?

Contacting medical team, making appointments?

Providing medical updates during medical visits?

Patient Coping with Illness, Procedures, Hospitalizations and Transplant:

Patient Motivation For/Desire to be Listed:

Problems Taking Medications:

Patient Communication/Decision-Making Preferences:

Patient Coping Strategies that are Helpful:

DEVELOPMENTAL HISTORY:

Complications of pregnancy or delivery:

Developmental milestones:

PATIENT AND FAMILY MENTAL HEALTH HISTORY:

Patient Mental Health History (Previous Diagnoses, Treatment, Hospitalizations):

Family Mental Health Diagnoses:

PATIENT CURRENT PSYCHOLOGICAL FUNCTIONING:

MOOD: Mood (___/10), Concentration, Energy, Anhedonia, Worthlessness, Hopelessness, Fatigue, Appetite, Sleep, Mania, SI

ANXIETY: Worries (___/10), Phobias, Habits/Tics, Panic Attack, O/C, Separation.

PSYCHOSIS: A/V H, Delusions, Paranoia

SUBSTANCE: Alcohol, Cigarettes, Drugs, OTC, Rx, Etoh, Marijuana, Crack/Cocaine, Sedatives, Inhalents – Abuse/Depend

BEHAVIOR/ATTENTION: ADHD, PICA, Behavior Problems, Developmental Disabilities

TRAUMA: Physical, sexual, neglect, PTSD, CPS involvement

SI/RISK BEHAVIORS: SI Thoughts, SIB, Sexually Active (Y/N), Dangerous Behaviors, Aggression, Stealing, Truancy

RISK ASSESSMENT:

ACADEMIC FUNCTIONING:

Current Grade:

School:

School grades:

School concerns/support:

Special education services:

School support specific to transplant:

FAMILY AND SOCIAL FUNCTIONING:

Lives with:

Family relations/stressors:

Hobbies/activities:

Peers:

Peers aware of/response to transplant:

MENTAL STATUS EXAM.

SUMMARY/IMPRESSIONS.

DSM-5 DIAGNOSES (IF APPLICABLE).

RECOMMENDATIONS.

Online Appendix 2: Sample of Assessment Measures Commonly Used in Pediatric SOT

Abbreviation	Measure name	Reference	Construct	# of items	Who completes?	Validated SOT?	Brief description
Screening measures							
PAT2.0	Psychosocial Assessment Tool	Pai et al. (2008)	Psychosocial functioning	57 items, 7 subscales	Parent	Yes	Screener for psychosocial risk for families of children with a variety of chronic illnesses
PedsQL 3.0 Transplant Module	Pediatric Quality of Life Inventory	Weissberg-Benchell et al. (2010)	Health-related QoL	46 items, 8 subscales,	Child and parent	Yes	Child self-report and/or parent-proxy report of children's SOT specific health-related QoL
CHQ-PF-50/ CF-87	Child Health Questionnaire Parent/ Child Form	Landgraf, Abetz, and Ware (1996) and Landgraf and Abetz (1997)	Health-related QoL	50 items/87 items	Child & parent	Yes	Child self-report and/or parent-proxy report of children's health-related QoL
CBCL	Child behavior checklist	Achenbach and Edlebrock (1993)	Psychological functioning	8 subscales, 118 items	Parent		Standardized parent report of behavioral problems and social competencies in children
PIP	Pediatric inventory for parents	Streisand, Braniecki, Tercyak, and Kazak (2001)	Psychological functioning	42 items, 4 subscales	Parent	Yes	Parent report of parenting stress related to caring for a child with a chronic illness
FAD	Family assessment device	Miller, Epstein, Bishop, and Keitner (1985)	Family functioning	60 items, 6 subscales	Parent		Parent report regarding the organization of the family, communication, and problem-solving
Adherence/barriers							
AMBS	Adolescent Medication Barriers Scale	Simons and Blount (2007)	Barriers to adherence	17 items, 3 subscales	Child	Yes	Child self-report of perceived barriers to medication adherence
PMBS	Parent Medication Barriers Scale	Simons and Blount (2007)	Barriers to adherence	16 items, 4 subscales	Parent	Yes	Parent-proxy reported of child's barriers to medication adherence
MAM	Medical Adherence Measure	Zelikovsky and Schast (2008)	Medication adherence	Interview, 4 domains	Child and parent	Yes	Semi-structured interview assessing medication knowledge and regimen adherence
Transition readiness							
RTQ	Readiness for Transition Questionnaire	Gilleland, Amaral, Mee, and Blount (2012)	Readiness for transition	22 items, 3 subscales	Child and parent	Yes	Child and parent-reported transition readiness, responsibility/involvement in healthcare tasks
TRAQ	Transition Readiness Assessment Questionnaire	Sawicki et al. (2011)	Readiness for transition	29 items, 2 subscales	Child		Skill-focused tool to assess readiness for transition to adult healthcare
TRS:A/YA	Transition Readiness Scale	Fredericks et al. (2010)	Readiness for transition	38 items, 4 subscales	Child	Yes	Adolescent perceived and demonstrated self-management skills and transition readiness
TRS:P	Transition Readiness Scale	Fredericks et al. (2010)	Readiness for transition	36 items, 5 subscales	Parent	Yes	Parent perception of their adolescent's skills and transition readiness
ATR-PF/CF	Allocation of Treatment Responsibility Scale	Pai et al. (2010)	Allocation of responsibility	18 items, 3 subscales	Child and parent	Yes	Child and parent-reported distribution of treatment tasks across family members

Online Appendix 3: Sample Procedural Plan (PICC Dressing Change)

JOEY'S STICKER SWITCHEROO PLAN

Quiet time is best for Joey! Please try to limit discussion/noise during sticker change.

Sit on bed with mom

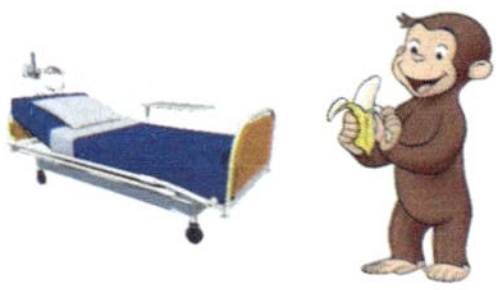

Movie turned on quietly

Masks on

Nurse to hold arm gently as sticker edges are peeled back

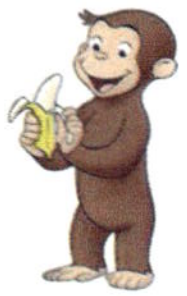

Joey to count to 10 before each cleaning swab is started

1, 2, 3 … 10!

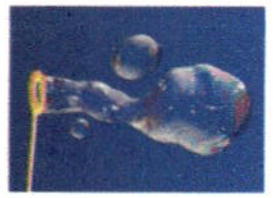

Deep breaths during cleaning

Mask party after!

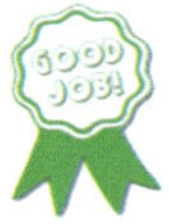

References

Achenbach, T. M., & Edlebrock, C. (1993). *Manual for the child behavior checklist and revised child behavior profile*. Burlington: University of Vermont, Department of Psychiatry.

Alonso, E. M., & Sorensen, L. G. (2009). Cognitive development following pediatric solid organ transplantation. *Current Opinion in Organ Transplantation, 14*(5), 522–525.

Anthony, S. J., BarZiv, S. P., & Ng, V. L. (2010). Quality of life after pediatric solid organ transplantation. *Pediatric Clinics of North America, 57*(2), 559–574.

Blount, R. L., Dahlquist, L. M., Baer, R. A., & Wuori, D. F. (1984). A brief, effective method for teaching children to swallow pills. *Behavior Therapy, 15*, 381.

Brosig, C., Hintermeyer, M., Zlotocha, J., Behrens, D., & Mao, J. (2006). An exploratory study of the cognitive, academic, and behavioral functioning of pediatric cardiothoracic transplant recipients. *Progress in Transplantation, 16*(1), 38–45.

Colvin, M., Smith, J. M., Hadley, N., Skeans, M. A., Carrico, R., Uccellini, K., … Kasiske, B. L. (2018). OPTN/SRTR 2016 annual data report: Heart. *American Journal of Transplantation, 18*(S1), 291–362.

Compton, S. N., March, J. S., Brent, D., Albano, A. M., Weersing, V. R., & Curry, J. (2004). Cognitive-behavioral psychotherapy for anxiety and depressive disorders in children and adolescents: An evidence-based medicine review. *Journal of the American Academy of Child & Adolescent Psychiatry, 43*(8), 930–959.

Cousino, M. K., Miller, V. A., Smith, C., Uzark, K., Lowery, R., Rottach, N., ... & Schumacher, K. R. (2019). Medical and end-of-life decision making in adolescents' pre-heart transplant: A descriptive pilot study. *Palliative Medicine*, doi: 10.1177/0269216319874689.

Cousino, M. K., Rea, K. E., & Mednick, L. M. (2017). Understanding the healthcare communication needs of pediatric patients through the My CHATT tool: A pilot study. *Journal of Communication in Healthcare, 10*(1), 16–21.

Cousino, M. K., Rea, K. E., Schumacher, K. R., Magee, J. C., & Fredericks, E. M. (2017). A systematic review of parent and family functioning in pediatric solid organ transplant populations. *Pediatric Transplantation, 21*(3), 1–13.

Cousino, M. K., Schumacher, K. R., Magee, J. C., Wolfe, J., Yu, S., Eder, S. J., & Fredericks, E. M. (2019). Communication about prognosis and end-of-life in pediatric organ failure and transplantation. *Pediatric Transplantation, 23*(3), e13373.

Cousino, M. K., Schumacher, K. R., Rea, K. E., Eder, S., Zamberlan, M., Jordan, J., & Fredericks, E. M. (2018). Psychosocial functioning in pediatric heart transplant recipients and their families. *Pediatric Transplantation, 22*(2).

da Cruz, K., Cousino, M. K., Smith, T., … Fredericks, E. M. (2019). Educational needs in families of pediatric liver and kidney transplant recipients: a quality improvement project. *Pediatric Transplantation, 23*(4), e13412.

DeMaso, D. R., Kelley, S. D., Bastardi, H., O'Brien, P., & Blume, E. D. (2004). The longitudinal impact of psychological functioning, medical severity, and family functioning in pediatric heart transplantation. *The Journal of Heart and Lung Transplantation, 23*(4), 473–480.

Devine, K. A., Reed-Knight, B., Loiselle, K. A., Simons, L. E., Mee, L. L., & Blount, R. L. (2011). Predictors of long-term health-related quality of life in adolescent solid organ transplant recipients. *Journal of Pediatric Psychology, 36*(8), 891–901.

Dew, M. A., Dabbs, A. D., Myaskovsky, L., Shyu, S., Shellmer, D. A., DiMartini, A. F., … Shapiro, R. (2009). Meta-analysis of medical regimen adherence outcomes in pediatric solid organ transplantation. *Transplantation, 88*(5), 736.

Dobbels, F., Decorte, A., Roskams, A., & Van Damme-Lombaerts, R. (2010). Health-related quality of life, treatment adherence, symptom experience and depression in adolescent renal transplant patients. *Pediatric Transplantation, 14*(2), 216–223.

Dobbels, F., Ruppar, T., De Geest, S., Decorte, A., Van Damme-Lombaerts, R., & Fine, R. N. (2010). Adherence to the immunosuppressive regimen in pediatric kidney transplant recipients: A systematic review. *Pediatric Transplantation, 14*(5), 603–613.

Dobbels, F., Van Damme-Lombaert, R., Vanhaecke, J., & Geest, S. D. (2005). Growing pains: Non-adherence with the immunosuppressive regimen in adolescent transplant recipients. *Pediatric Transplantation, 9*(3), 381–390.

Douglas, J. E., Hulson, B., & Trompeter, R. S. (1998). Psycho-social outcome of parents and young children after renal transplantation. *Child: Care, Health and Development, 24*(1), 73–83.

Duncan, S., Annunziato, R. A., Dunphy, C., LaPointe Rudow, D., Shneider, B. L., & Shemesh, E. (2017). A systematic review of immunosuppressant adherence interventions in transplant recipients: Decoding the streetlight effect. *Pediatric Transplantation, 22*(1), e13086.

Farley, L. M., DeMaso, D. R., D'Angelo, E., Kinnamon, C., Bastardi, H., Hill, C. E., … Logan, D. E. (2007). Parenting stress and parental post-traumatic stress disorder in families after pediatric heart transplantation. *The Journal of Heart and Lung Transplantation, 26*(2), 120–126.

Fisher, M., Storfer-Isser, A., Shaw, R. J., Bernard, R. S., Drury, S., Ularntinon, S., & Horwitz, S. M. (2011). Inter-rater reliability of the Pediatric Transplant Rating Instrument (P-TRI): Challenges to reliably identifying adherence risk factors during pediatric pre-transplant evaluations. *Pediatric Transplantation, 15*(2), 142–147.

Fredericks, E. M., Dore-Stites, D., Calderon, S. Y., Well, A., Eder, S. J., Magee, J. C., & Lopez, M. J. (2012). Relationship between sleep problems and health-related quality of life among pediatric liver transplant recipients. *Liver Transplantation, 18*(6), 707–715.

Fredericks, E. M., Dore-Stites, D., Well, A., Magee, J. C., Freed, G. L., Shieck, V., & James Lopez, M. (2010). Assessment of transition readiness skills and adherence in pediatric liver transplant recipients. *Pediatric Transplantation, 14*, 944. https://doi.org/10.1111/j.1399

Fredericks, E. M., Lopez, M. J., Magee, J. C., Shieck, V., & Opipari-Arrigan, L. (2007). Psychological functioning, nonadherence and health outcomes after pediatric liver transplantation. *American Journal of Transplantation, 7*(8), 1974–1983.

Fredericks, E. M., Magee, J. C., Eder, S. J., Sevecke, J. R., Dore-Stites, D., Shieck, V., & Lopez, M. J. (2015). Quality improvement targeting adherence during the transition from a pediatric to adult liver transplant clinic. *Journal of Clinical Psychology in Medical Settings, 22*(2–3), 150–159.

Fredericks, E. M., Zelikovsky, N., Aujoulat, I., Hames, A., & Wray, J. (2014). Post-transplant adjustment—the later years. *Pediatric Transplantation, 18*(7), 675–688.

Fung, E., & Shaw, R. J. (2008). Pediatric Transplant Rating Instrument–a scale for the pretransplant psychiatric evaluation of pediatric organ transplant recipients. *Pediatric Transplantation, 12*(1), 57–66.

Gilleland, J., Amaral, S., Mee, L., & Blount, R. (2012). Getting ready to leave: Transition readiness in adolescent kidney transplant recipients. *Journal of Pediatric Psychology, 37*, 85.

Gutiérrez-Colina, A. M., Eaton, C. K., Lee, J. L., Reed-Knight, B., Loiselle, K., Mee, L. L., ... Blount, R. L. (2015). Executive functioning, barriers to adherence, and nonadherence in adolescent and young adult transplant recipients. *Journal of Pediatric Psychology, 41*(7), 759–767.

Haavisto, A., Korkman, M., Holmberg, C., Jalanko, H., & Qvist, E. (2011). Neuropsychological profile of children with kidney transplants. *Nephrology Dialysis Transplantation, 27*(6), 2594–2601.

Hart, A., Smith, J. M., Skeans, M. A., Gustafson, S. K., Wilk, A. R., Robinson, A., ... Israni, A. K. (2018). OPTN/SRTR 2016 annual data report: Kidney. *American Journal of Transplantation, 18*(S1), 18–113.

Kahana, S., Drotar, D., & Frazier, T. (2008). Meta-analysis of psychological interventions to promote adherence to treatment in pediatric chronic health conditions. *Journal of Pediatric Psychology, 33*(6), 590–611.

Kaller, T., Langguth, N., Ganschow, R., Nashan, B., & Schulz, K.-H. (2010). Attention and executive functioning deficits in liver-transplanted children. *Transplantation, 90*(12), 1567–1573.

Kim, W. R., Lake, J. R., Smith, J. M., Schladt, D. P., Skeans, M. A., Harper, A. M., ... Kasiske, B. L. (2018). OPTN/SRTR 2016 annual data report: Liver. *American Journal of Transplantation, 18*(S1), 172–253.

Landgraf, J. M., Abetz, L., & Ware, J. E. (1996). *The CHQ user's manual*. Boston: The Health Institute, New England Medical Center.

Landgraf, J. M., & Abetz, L. N. (1997). Functional status and well-being of children representing three cultural groups: Initial self-reports using the chq-cf87. *Psychology & Health, 12*, 839–854.

Lefkowitz, D. S., Fitzgerald, C. J., Zelikovsky, N., Barlow, K., & Wray, J. (2014). Best practices in the pediatric pretransplant psychosocial evaluation. *Pediatric Transplantation, 18*(4), 327–335.

Magee, J. C., Krishnan, S. M., Benfield, M. R., Hsu, D. T., & Shneider, B. L. (2008). Pediatric transplantation in the United States, 1997–2006. *American Journal of Transplantation, 8*(4p2), 935–945.

Miller, I. W., Epstein, N. B., Bishop, D. S., & Keitner, G. I. (1985). The McMaster family assessment device: Validity and reliability. *Journal of Marital and Family Therapy, 11*, 345.

Mintzer, L. L., Stuber, M. L., Seacord, D., Castaneda, M., Mesrkhani, V., & Glover, D. (2005). Traumatic stress symptoms in adolescent organ transplant recipients. *Pediatrics, 115*(6), 1640–1644.

Pahl, E., Andrei, A., Hof, K. V., Liu, M., Shankel, T., Chinnock, R., ... Addonizio, L. J. (2018). Pediatric heart transplantation: Transitioning to adult care TRANSIT. *The Journal of Heart and Lung Transplantation, 37*(4), S392–S393.

Pai, A. L. H., Gray, E., Kurivial, K., Ross, J., Schoborg, D., & Goebel, J. (2010). The allocation of treatment responsibility scale: A novel tool for assessing patient and caregiver management of pediatric medical treatment regimens. *Pediatric Transplantation, 14*, 993.

Pai, A. L. H., & McGrady, M. (2014). Systematic review and meta-analysis of psychological interventions to promote treatment adherence in children, adolescents, and young adults with chronic illness. *Journal of Pediatric Psychology, 39*(8), 918–931.

Pai, A. L. H., Patiño-Fernández, A. M., McSherry, M., Beele, D., Alderfer, M. A., Reilly, A. T., ... Kazak, A. E. (2008). The Psychosocial Assessment Tool (PAT2.0): Psychometric properties of a screener for psychosocial distress in families of children newly diagnosed with cancer. *Journal of Pediatric Psychology, 33*(1), 50–62.

Patel, A., Jacobsen, L., Jhaveri, R., & Bradford, K. K. (2015). Effectiveness of pediatric pill swallowing interventions: A systematic review. *Pediatrics, 135*(5), 883–889.

Rodrigue, J. R., Baz, M. A., Widows, M. R., & Ehlers, S. L. (2005). A randomized evaluation of quality-of-life therapy with patients awaiting lung transplantation. *American Journal of Transplantation, 5*(10), 2425–2432.

Sawicki, G. S., Lukens-Bull, K., Yin, X., Demars, N., Huang, I. C., Livingood, W., ... Wood, D. (2011). Measuring the transition readiness of youth with special healthcare needs: Validation of the TRAQ—Transition readiness assessment questionnaire. *Journal of Pediatric Psychology, 36*, 160.

Shaw, R. J., Wamboldt, M., Bursch, B., & Stuber, M. (2006). Practice patterns in pediatric consultation–liaison psychiatry: A national survey. *Psychosomatics, 47*(1), 43–49.

Shellmer, D., Brosig, C., & Wray, J. (2014). The start of the transplant journey: Referral for pediatric solid organ transplantation. *Pediatric Transplantation, 18*(2), 125–133.

Shellmer, D. A., & Zelikovsky, N. (2007). The challenges of using medication event monitoring technology with pediatric transplant patients. *Pediatric Transplantation, 11*(4), 422–428.

Shemesh, E., Lurie, S., Stuber, M. L., Emre, S., Patel, Y., Vohra, P., … Shneider, B. L. (2000). A pilot study of posttraumatic stress and nonadherence in pediatric liver transplant recipients. *Pediatrics, 105*(2), e29–e29.

Shemesh, E., Shneider, B. L., Savitzky, J. K., Arnott, L., Gondolesi, G. E., Krieger, N. R., … Schmeidler, J. (2004). Medication adherence in pediatric and adolescent liver transplant recipients. *Pediatrics, 113*(4), 825–832.

Simons, L. E., & Blount, R. L. (2007). Identifying barriers to medication adherence in adolescent transplant recipients. *Journal of Pediatric Psychology, 32*, 831.

Simons, L. E., McCormick, M. L., Devine, K., & Blount, R. L. (2010). Medication barriers predict adolescent transplant recipients' adherence and clinical outcomes at 18-month follow-up. *Journal of Pediatric Psychology, 35*(9), 1038–1048.

Skillings, J. L., & Lewandowski, A. N. (2015). Team-based biopsychosocial care in solid organ transplantation. *Journal of Clinical Psychology in Medical Settings, 22*(2–3), 113–121.

Sorensen, L. G., Neighbors, K., Martz, K., Zelko, F., Bucuvalas, J. C., Alonso, E. M., & Studies of Pediatric Liver Transplantation (SPLIT), and Functional Outcomes Group (FOG). (2011). Cognitive and academic outcomes after pediatric liver transplantation: Functional Outcomes Group (FOG) results. *American Journal of Transplantation, 11*(2), 303–311.

Streisand, R., Braniecki, S., Tercyak, K. P., & Kazak, A. E. (2001). Childhood illness-related parenting stress: The pediatric inventory for parents. *Journal of Pediatric Psychology, 26*, 155.

Tarbell, S. E., & Kosmach, B. (1998). Parental psychosocial outcomes in pediatric liver and/or intestinal transplantation: Pretransplantation and the early postoperative period. *Liver Transplantation and Surgery, 4*(5), 378–387.

Uman, L. S., Chambers, C. T., McGrath, P. J., & Kisely, S. (2008). A systematic review of randomized controlled trials examining psychological interventions for needle-related procedural pain and distress in children and adolescents: An abbreviated Cochrane review. *Journal of Pediatric Psychology, 33*(8), 842–854.

Uzark, K., Griffin, L., Rodriguez, R., Zamberlan, M., Murphy, P., Nasman, C., … Varni, J. W. (2012). Quality of life in pediatric heart transplant recipients: A comparison with children with and without heart disease. *The Journal of Heart and Lung Transplantation, 31*(6), 571–578.

Valapour, M., Lehr, C. J., Skeans, M. A., Smith, J. M., Carrico, R., Uccellini, K., … Kasiske, B. L. (2018). OPTN/SRTR 2016 annual data report: Lung. *American Journal of Transplantation, 18*(S1), 363–433.

Wayman, K. I., Cox, K. L., & Esquivel, C. O. (1997). Neurodevelopmental outcome of young children with extrahepatic biliary atresia 1 year after liver transplantation. *The Journal of Pediatrics, 131*(6), 894–898.

Weissberg-Benchell, J., Zielinski, T. E., Rodgers, S., Greenley, R. N., Askenazi, D., Goldstein, S. L., … Varni, J. W. (2010). Pediatric health-related quality of life: Feasibility, reliability and validity of the PedsQL™ transplant module. *American Journal of Transplantation, 10*, 1677.

Wu, Y. P., Aylward, B. S., Steele, R. G., Maikranz, J. M., & Dreyer, M. L. (2008). Psychosocial functioning of pediatric renal and liver transplant recipients. *Pediatric Transplantation, 12*(5), 582–587.

Young, G. S., Mintzer, L. L., Seacord, D., Castaneda, M., Mesrkhani, V., & Stuber, M. L. (2003). Symptoms of posttraumatic stress disorder in parents of transplant recipients: Incidence, severity, and related factors. *Pediatrics, 111*(6), e725–e731.

Zelikovsky, N., & Schast, A. P. (2008). Eliciting accurate reports of adherence in a clinical interview: Development of the medical adherence measure. *Pediatric Nursing, 34*(2), 141–146.

Part III

Cross-Cutting Issues in Consultation-Liaison Practice

Developmental Considerations in Consultation-Liaison Psychology

Maia M. Noeder and Allyson L. Davis

Developmental Considerations in Consultation-Liaison Psychology

Developmental disabilities (DDs) are a varied group of impairments in motor, cognitive, linguistic, or behavioral functioning that arise before adulthood and persist throughout the lifespan of an individual (CDC, 2018). These conditions affect approximately 15 percent of children between the ages of 3 and 17 years currently living in the United States. Learning disabilities are the most common DD, followed by attention-deficit/hyperactivity disorder (ADHD), "other" developmental delay (i.e., cerebral palsy, down syndrome and other congenital abnormalities, vision and hearing impairments, and intellectual disabilities), and autism spectrum disorder (ASD, Boyle et al., 2011). Males are twice as likely to be diagnosed with any DD compared with females, as are children insured by Medicaid compared to those with private insurance (Boyle et al., 2011).

Children with DD have increased hospital usage compared with their typically developing peers (Nageswaran, Parish, Rose, & Grady, 2011), making this an important topic for consultation-liaison (CL) psychologists. Assessment of children under the age of 3 years who had been hospitalized more than 30 days in a tertiary care hospital found that 54% were eligible for early intervention services with an additional 36% eligible for screening and monitoring (Feldman, Ploof, Hofkosh, & Goehring, 1993). An investigation by Petersen, Kube, Whitaker, Graff, and Palmer (2009) in an acute care hospital setting determined that 33.5% of children met the criteria for DD. A retrospective evaluation revealed that approximately one third of these children may not have a formal diagnosis of DD upon admission, indicating that providers are frequently unaware that they are caring for children with DD. Medically, children with DD have a higher prevalence of medical conditions than the general pediatric population with particularly high rates of asthma, allergies (food, skin, respiratory), gastrointestinal complaints, and neurological conditions such as seizures (Schieve et al., 2012).

Pediatric patients with DD can require additional support and planning in the hospital setting due to lack of cooperation with instructions, as

M. M. Noeder (✉)
Division of Behavioral Health, Nemours/Alfred I. duPont Hospital for Children, Wilmington, DE, USA

Pediatrics, Sidney Kimmel Medical College - Thomas Jefferson University, Philadelphia, PA, USA
e-mail: Maia.Noeder@nemours.org

A. L. Davis
Division of Behavioral Health, Nemours/Alfred I. duPont Hospital for Children, Wilmington, DE, USA

B. D. Carter, K. A. Kullgren (eds.), *Clinical Handbook of Psychological Consultation in Pediatric Medical Settings*, Issues in Clinical Child Psychology, https://doi.org/10.1007/978-3-030-35598-2_28

well as internalizing and externalizing behaviors (Bruininks, Woodcock, Weatherman, & Hill, 1997). Youths with intellectual disabilities (IDs) are three to four times as likely to exhibit psychopathology symptoms compared with typically developing children (Einfeld & Tonge, 1996; Emerson, Einfeld, & Stancliffe, 2010; Wallander, Dekker, & Koot, 2003). Although prevalence rates vary across sample and DD classification, a large-scale investigation of children with ID found that 41% met the criteria for a psychiatric condition, with only 10% of those children receiving mental health interventions during the course of the investigation (Einfeld et al., 2006). Lakhan (2013) found that common comorbid psychiatric conditions in a sample of children with ID included behavioral problems (80.9%), enuresis (10.3%), ADHD (6.5%), ASD (4.2%), anxiety (2.7%), and depression (2.3%).

Children with DD in the hospital setting frequently have increased need for developmentally informed, evidenced-based assessment and intervention, and pediatric psychologists are uniquely qualified to provide research-informed support and expertise. Furthermore, patient characteristics have the potential to create significant barriers to the team during procedures and medical care. Thus, pediatric psychologists are poised to lend knowledge to multidisciplinary teams and implement skilled interventions, potentially increasing the likelihood of successful medical care.

Formulation

While information gathering is always a critical component of the inpatient CL process, a thorough initial assessment guides psychological treatment while also providing valuable information for the entire care team. Given the variable nature of impairments among children with DD, assessments that gather information from the entire family are imperative. As a result, a family-centered care approach, characterized by a collaborative partnership between caregivers and the medical team (Kuo et al., 2012), has long been considered the gold standard when working with youths with DD (Hockenberry & Wilson, 2018; Shelton & Stepanek, 1994). Viewing caregivers as valuable experts also encourages "buy in" and commitment to psychological interventions. In addition, contacting special educators, nurses, early intervention specialists, and other outside providers can yield valuable information regarding the child's functioning, effective interventions, and behavior management techniques. Ideally, family-centered care begins before the family arrives at the hospital so that personalized care can be initiated at the first point of contact (Blake, 2010). A plan for the patient's care may be established by obtaining information prior to admission, during either ongoing outpatient care or a preadmission interview (Van der Walt & Moran, 2001). If a plan cannot be established in advance, assessment may be completed as part of the CL service.

During the formulation phase of CL, assessing the following areas (in addition to a standard diagnostic interview) is a way to aspire toward family-centered, developmentally appropriate care (Scarpinato et al., 2010; Van der Walt & Moran, 2001).

- **Developmental level**: discussing and identifying a child's developmental level guides intervention planning and helps other care team members provide patients with developmentally appropriate information and directions. Caregivers can be encouraged to describe a child's developmental level using age, grade, or skill (e.g., adaptive, academic, verbal, etc.) as a developmental marker.
- **Communication**: caregivers of children with DD frequently identify communication as the primary barrier that their children face while inpatient (Davignon, Friedlaender, Cronholm, Paciotti, & Levy, 2014). DDs can result in a wide range of abilities and preferences for both expressive and receptive communication. How does the child express needs? How does the child communicate "yes" and "no?" Does the child use a picture exchange communication system (PECS) to communicate nonverbally? Receptively, does the child process information better when it is presented

verbally or visually? Does the child experience difficulties recognizing nonverbal communication, gestures, or facial expressions? How does the family communicate an upcoming transition to the child? How would the family prefer that the medical team communicate with their child about medical procedures and care?
- **Preferences**: identifying preferred rewards, objects, and interests can be helpful when creating positive reinforcement plans to encourage compliance with medical care. Preferred items can also be used to provide comfort during an extended hospitalization. Identifying dislikes and sensitivities is equally important and helps providers avoid potential emotional or behavioral triggers.
- **Behavioral/emotional functioning**: given the increased prevalence of internalizing and externalizing behaviors in the DD population, special attention should be paid to a child's present and past behavioral and emotional functioning. What are the child's typical warning signs for dysregulation? What does it look like when the child is dysregulated? What interventions have been most helpful to deescalate challenging behavior? Which coping strategies have been most successful?

Intervention

Evidence-based practices for children with DD in the inpatient setting have three common themes (Koski, Gabriels, & Beresford, 2016):

1. Patient care is guided by collaboration and information gathering with the child's primary caregivers during the formulation phase.
2. A process to communicate caregiver information to the patient's care team is established. While the implementation of this process is outside the scope of this chapter, a positive relationship between the pediatric psychologist and the rest of the multidisciplinary team can allow psychology to act as a conduit between caregivers and the care team.
3. The patient environment is modified, when possible, based on information gathered via caregiver interview. This could include alterations to the number of providers allowed to enter the room at one time, lighting, sounds, one-on-one support and monitoring, arrangement of furniture, decorations, and etcetera.

Taken as a whole, these practices support the creation of caregiver-driven, proactive, multidisciplinary care plans that serve as frameworks for intervention. Proactive care plans that document information about the child's developmental level, communication skills, preferences, and behavioral/emotional functioning, as well as intervention recommendations, have been shown to provide an effective way to manage distress and agitation for children with DD (Nicholas et al., 2016). Care plans are most successful when they are flexible and prioritize caregiver knowledge and expertise over one-size-fits-all recommendations (Muskat et al., 2015). Pediatric psychologists can facilitate and/or direct the creation of these care plans in conjunction with the medical care team given their specialized training in developmental differences, psychopathology, and hospital-based intervention strategies.

There are a number of evidence-based practices that can enhance the care plan of a child with DD and manage challenging situations that arise while inpatient. Transitions and procedures are frequent triggers of behavioral dysregulation while inpatient, but dysregulation can be managed with developmentally informed preparation. Providing patients with step-by-step instructions, delivered in a multimodal approach that includes verbal, pictorial, video, and kinesthetic sources of information, gives children with DD multiple opportunities to overcome possible communication limitations (Browne, 2006; Giarelli, Souders, Pinto-Martin, Bloch, & Levy, 2005; Scarpinato et al., 2010). Social stories, developed by Carol Gray (1994), are a research-supported method of describing an event step by step using an illustrated story format and allow for rehearsal and desensitization prior to procedures and transitions (Kokina & Kern, 2010). These stories are readily available without cost online and also come in a blank template format that can be personalized for a particular child's medical experience (see Appendix 1 for resources). During the procedure or transition itself, sensory-based toys that have been carefully selected based on children's preferences and sensory needs can be useful distractions. Positive reinforcement plans for specific targeted behaviors in the inpatient setting can encourage compliance with medical provider requests, procedures, and medication use (Koontz, Slifer, Cataldo, & Marcus, 2003; Scarpinato et al., 2010). Picture schedules are an effective way for many children with delayed verbal skills to prepare for upcoming transitions and treatments and have been found to reduce both parent anxiety and parent perceptions of their child's anxiety (Chebuhar, McCarthy, Bosch, & Baker, 2013).

If a patient with DD would benefit from a course of psychotherapy while inpatient, traditional evidence-based practices can be utilized but often require modifications. Cognitive behavioral therapy (CBT) has shown particular effectiveness when modified for use with ASD (Attwood, 2003; Vasa et al., 2014; Walters, Loades, & Russell, 2016). Attwood (2003) describes a CBT treatment plan for mood challenges (e.g., anxiety, depression, and anger) that includes emotion education (emotion labeling and exploration, as well as the use of an intensity thermometer), cognitive restructuring (encouraging flexible thinking and perspective taking, often enhanced by social stories), stress relief (relaxation strategies accompanied by modification of the patient environment), self-reflection, and practice. Key differences from the traditional CBT model include a heavier focus on visual aids and activities over verbal techniques. This variation helps overcome possible language barriers. Similarly, purely behavioral interventions are more efficacious for children with low-functioning ASD than interventions that are more cognitively driven (i.e., verbally mediated strategies; Rosen, Connell, & Kerns, 2016; Walters et al., 2016). Relaxation strategies are generally delivered in a more structured and directive way than standard practice (Walters et al., 2016), while supplemental treatment modules can be added to the treatment plan to address special/restricted interests and social challenges (Vasa et al., 2014).

Solution-focused brief therapy (SFBT) appears to be a promising family-based approach for children with profound IDs (Lloyd & Dallos, 2006) and could likely be implemented in a hospital consult setting given that it is intended to be brief and targeted. Overall, this modified SFBT approach emphasizes empowerment, integration of patient goals into the family's narrative, and acceptance of a child's abilities while also identifying the family's vision of a preferred future. Treatment steps include (1) identifying strengths and challenges; (2) assessing past improvements, discussing prior coping strategies, and prioritizing parents as experts; (3) clarifying the family's end goal state using De Shazer's (1988) miracle question:

> Suppose that one night when you were asleep there was a miracle and this problem was solved. The miracle occurs while you are sleeping, so you do not immediately know that it has happened. When you wake up what is the first thing you will notice that will let you know there has been a miracle? (Lloyd & Dallos, 2006, p. 374).

Additional steps include (4) scaling, (5) identifying concrete goals, and (6) eliciting family-driven problem-solving.

Special Considerations for Autism Spectrum Disorder

ASD is a chronic, neurodevelopmental disability that affects 1 in 59 individuals in the United States (Baio et al., 2018; CDC, 2018). ASD is characterized by impairments in social communication and interaction, as well as restricted and repetitive interests and behaviors (American Psychiatric Association, 2013). Children with ASD have been found to be represented in hospital admissions at a rate of 65.6 per 100,000 admissions, have a significantly higher length of service (6.5 days vs. 4.2 days), and a higher total charge ($24,862 vs. $23,225) compared with non-ASD peers (Lokhandwala, Khanna, & West-Strum, 2012). Adolescents with ASD have been noted to access emergency department services at four times the rate of non-ASD adolescents (Liu, Pearl, Kong, Leslie, & Murray, 2017). The most common hospital admission medical diagnoses for children with ASD include epilepsy and seizures (36%), gastrointestinal disturbances (16%), and respiratory disturbances (10%; Scarpinato et al., 2010). Additional presenting concerns include orthopedic, mood/behavioral difficulties, sleep issues, and food/skin allergies (Kopecky, Broder-Fingert, Iannuzzi, & Connors, 2013; Muskens, Velders, & Staal, 2017; Scarpinato et al., 2010).

In conjunction with higher rates of utilization, parents of children with ASD report greater dissatisfaction with care teams and concerns about receiving suboptimal and less timely care when compared to parents of children with ADHD (Zablotsky, Kalb, Freedman, Vasa, & Stuart, 2014). Parent qualitative interview results reveal a number of care concerns for children with ASD in the hospital setting (Muskat et al., 2015). Parents of children with ASD noted communication challenges related to receptive and expressive language, which are exacerbated by the high-stress hospital environment. Communication of physical state, pain levels, and pain location can be particularly difficult. The sensory sensitivities commonly exhibited by children with ASD were also noted as a particular challenge in the hospital setting. The need for physical contact during medical examinations, the high frequency of noises in hospital rooms, olfactory triggers such as new soaps, tissues, and cleaning supplies, and new food exposures can all present problems. Parents reported that the number of care providers entering the room of a child with ASD can be an additional challenge and can result in negative behaviors. Asking children with ASD to wait for care or procedures in waiting rooms and lack of flexibility in hospitals were also highlighted as negative experiences.

Children with ASD frequently present with increased rates of behavior challenges compared to non-ASD peers, as well as other children with DD (Johnson & Rodriguez, 2013; Kozlowski & Matson, 2012). Challenging behaviors can include aggression, noncompliance, self-injurious behaviors, and hyperactivity (Browne, 2006; Johnson & Rodriguez, 2013; Lowe et al., 2007; Scarpinato et al., 2010; Skinner, Ng, McDonald, & Walters, 2005). However, medical teams are often ill-prepared to manage the high levels of dysregulation observed in this population (Inglese, 2009; Johnson & Rodriguez, 2013; Muskat et al., 2015). Furthermore, hospitalization is likely to exacerbate negative behaviors in children with ASD, thus increasing stress for parents and caregivers, as well as medical teams (Inglese, 2009; Johnson & Rodriguez, 2013; Muskat et al., 2015).

Given the increased behavior challenges of children with ASD, modifications to improve the hospital experience and better prepare teams for managing behaviors are necessary (Table 1). In order to address noncompliance, as well as decrease tantrums or meltdowns that may include aggression, strategies that are likely beneficial

Table 1 Inpatient modifications for children with ASD

Difficulty	Recommendations
Challenging behavior	• Implement positive reinforcement systems • Allow children to engage in distracting activities • Modify the environment to decrease triggers for negative behaviors • Provide opportunities for physical activity • Allow time for children to process instructions and procedures • Limit disruptions to calming behaviors • Consult with psychiatry regarding medication management
Behavioral rigidity	• Establish structure and routines for each day in the hospital • Allow children to choose activities when possible • Limit changes to medical teams • Use visual schedules that children can follow
Sensory sensitivity	• Limit unnecessary sensory input (e.g., keep the door closed, dim lights as needed, etc.) • Plan ahead for sensory needs • Prepare children for necessary sensory stimulation • Limit the number of providers in the room

include utilizing visual schedules (Appendix 2) to prepare children for medical procedures, reducing sensory stimulation, implementing positive reinforcement systems, and allowing children to engage in distracting activities (Chebuhar et al., 2013; Inglese, 2009; Johnson & Rodriguez, 2013; Souders, DePaul, Freeman, & Levy, 2002). Additionally, children may engage in disruptive behaviors due to pain, which should be monitored using pain scales tailored to the child's developmental level and treated accordingly (Inglese, 2009; Johnson & Rodriguez, 2013). Children with ASD may also engage in negative behaviors due to the disruption of rituals or self-stimulatory behaviors, which may be comforting and often should not be interrupted or prevented in hospital settings (Johnson & Rodriguez, 2013; Scarpinato et al., 2010). Increased rates of hyperactivity and comorbid ADHD are observed in children diagnosed with ASD (Leyfer et al., 2006). These symptoms are best addressed through increased opportunities for physical activity and appropriate management of psychiatric medications (Golnik & Nadia Maccabee-Ryaboy, 2010; Johnson & Rodriguez, 2013). Self-injurious behaviors may also be observed in children with ASD, particularly in response to increased frustration or pain. Possible strategies for decreasing self-injury include improved communication methods and frequent pauses in order to allow children to calm and process information (Browne, 2006; Inglese, 2009; Johnson & Rodriguez, 2013). In addition to disruptive behaviors, children with ASD can display behavioral rigidity and inflexibility, which pose challenges in the hospital setting (Muskat et al., 2015; Scarpinato et al., 2010). To address these challenges, it is important to implement as much structure as possible by using visual schedules (Appendix 2), establishing daily routines, allowing children to choose activities, and limiting changes in medical teams (Davignon et al., 2014; Kopecky et al., 2013; Scarpinato et al., 2010).

Sensory sensitivities are commonly observed in children with ASD and may lead to anxiety or disruptive behaviors (Johnson & Rodriguez, 2013; Kopecky et al., 2013; Lowe et al., 2007; Muskat et al., 2015). In hospital settings, sensory challenges include difficulty tolerating touch, as well as sensitivity to sounds, smells, and lights (Muskat et al., 2015; Scarpinato et al., 2010). These sensitivities are likely to have a negative impact on both medical treatment and patients' overall hospital stay. In order to address these challenges and improve care and experiences for children with ASD, strategies that appear to be beneficial include limiting unnecessary sounds (e.g., silencing machines, keeping doors closed, strategically assigning a child's room) whenever possible (Scarpinato et al., 2010). Additionally, it is important to plan ahead for sensory challenges and ensure that distraction methods, positive reinforcement, and visual cues or schedules for necessary sensory stimulation are readily available (Johnson & Rodriguez, 2013; Muskat et al., 2015; Scarpinato et al., 2010). It is also beneficial to limit the number of health care professionals who are in the room with a child who is diagnosed with ASD in order to avoid overstimulation or confusion (Muskat et al., 2015).

Similar to children with other DD diagnoses, best practices for children with ASD include thorough assessment of each patient's needs across developmental level, communication, preferences, and behavioral/emotional functioning (Kopecky et al., 2013; Muskat et al., 2015; Scarpinato et al., 2010). Consistent with recommendations above for establishing care plans across categories of DD, it is crucial for parents and caregivers to inform both assessment and care for children with ASD (Inglese, 2009; Muskat et al., 2015). Furthermore, care plans specific to children with ASD may need to be expanded to include social considerations (e.g., social demands in the hospital setting, need for social supports) and safety concerns (e.g., eloping behaviors) in order to tailor care to needs of children with ASD and their families (Broder-Fingert et al., 2016). Autism-specific care plans have been shown to improve experiences for patients, parents, and health care providers (Broder-Fingert et al., 2016). Psychologists within CL services may play an important role by developing autism care plans with parents and caregivers, as well as training medical teams in the use of these plans. Additionally, it is important for psychologists with knowledge related to ASD to provide training and consultation for physicians and nurses who may have less experience with this population (McGonigle et al., 2014).

Applications to Outpatient Medical Settings

While the previously described practices can be applied across settings, there are additional opportunities and factors to consider when serving children with DD in an outpatient consultative environment. Children with ASD in particular are overrepresented in the outpatient setting with an average of 41.5 annual outpatient visits (compared with 3.3 in the general pediatric population; Liptak, Stuart, & Auinger, 2006). At the same time, a large-scale investigation by Kogan et al. (2008) found that 25% of parents of children with emotional, developmental, or behavioral problems and 31% of parents of children diagnosed with ASD reported at least one unmet outpatient health care need. A significant barrier when seeking appropriate services is provider inexperience with a child's diagnosis (Chiri & Warfield, 2012).

Given this high level of utilization combined with observed barriers to diagnostically informed care, pediatric psychologists can be significant resources for children with DD presenting in primary care and outpatient settings. Psychologists can improve access to informed care by utilizing and encouraging other providers to utilize available training. Autism Case Training (ACT) (Division of Birth Defects, National Center on Birth Defects and Developmental Disabilities (NCBDDD), Centers for Disease Control and Prevention (CDC), 2018), is an effective teaching tool (Major, Peacock, Ruben, Thomas, & Weitzman, 2013) and is freely available online (www.cdc.gov/ncbddd/actearly/act.html). Warm handoffs, in which a psychologist is available for liaison during medical appointments, are an additional opportunity to support patient families and medical providers while disseminating developmentally and diagnostically appropriate information (Hoffses et al., 2016).

Primary care is an ideal setting for brief, targeted interventions given the high frequency of pediatrician visits for children with DD. Primary Care Stepping Stones Triple P (PCSSTP) is a research supported parent-training intervention for children with developmental disabilities, specifically within the primary care setting (Tellegen & Sanders, 2014). Derived from Stepping Stones Triple P (SSTP) (Tellegen & Sanders, 2013), which emphasizes positive parenting strategies that improve child behavior, parenting styles, and parent satisfaction (Whittingham, Sofronoff, Sheffield, & Sanders, 2009), PCSSTP consists of four brief sessions (15–30 min) and targets one to two specific child behaviors, such as noncompliance or aggression. Treatment includes behavior tracking, discussion of parent perceptions of the targeted behavior(s), and psychoeducation regarding parent-implemented behavior management strategies (Tellegen & Sanders, 2012). This brief, targeted, and effective protocol is an ideal tool for CL work in the outpatient setting as it can be used during both warm handoffs and scheduled outpatient visits.

Case Study

A 10-year-old male who was nonverbal and diagnosed with comorbid ASD and ID, as well as co-occurring medical conditions that included epilepsy, was admitted to the hospital due to compulsive picking of a wound that prevented it from healing following surgery. When the medical team attempted to restrain him in order to prevent picking, he became agitated and began to demonstrate disruptive behaviors. A psychology consult was placed in order to implement a behavior plan for managing both skin picking and disruptive behaviors. During the consultation, his mother reported that his understanding of the need to stop picking his wound, as well as the need to keep his hands covered or restrained, was limited. She also noted that he consistently engages in self-stimulatory behaviors with his hands, which he could not do when they were covered. The combination of limited understanding and restriction of self-stimulatory behaviors that often soothe him appeared to be exacerbating his frustration and escalating negative behaviors.

Given this information, the psychologist worked with his mother to establish a reinforcement system paired with visuals for leaving his hands covered and keeping them away from his wound (e.g., "hands down" or "nice hands") based on reward systems and motivators, which his mother described as successful during ABA therapy. Additionally, the psychologist provided education to the medical team regarding the importance of taking a behavioral approach and using the reward system, rather than attempting to explain the reasons for leaving his wound alone or trying to restrain him.

Conclusion

Patients with DD are overrepresented in inpatient and outpatient medical settings and require additional attention given barriers to care and internalizing and externalizing behaviors. Viewing family caregivers as patient experts and focusing on developmental level, communication, preferences, and behavioral/emotional functioning during the formulation phase of CL allows for the development of care plans that can help patients overcome challenging situations. CL psychologists are uniquely trained and positioned to develop care plans for children with DD, educate members of the multidisciplinary team, and provide developmentally appropriate evidence-based interventions.

Appendix 1: Resources for Social Stories

Books:

Gray, C. (2010). *The new social story book.* Arlington, TX: Future Horizons.

Timmins, S. (2016). *Successful Social Stories for young children with autism.* London: Jessica Kingsley Publishers.

Timmins, S. (2017). *Successful Social Stories for school and college students with autism.* London, UK: Jessica Kingsley Publishers.

Websites:

http://www.pbisworld.com/tier-2/social-stories
https://www.autism.org.uk/about/strategies/social-stories-comic-strips.aspx

Appendix 2: Sample Visual Schedule

7:00 a.m.	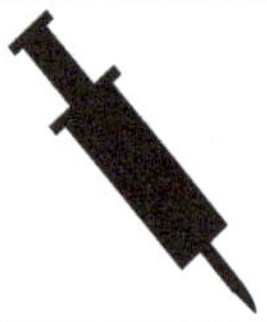	Labs/blood draw
8:00 a.m.		Breakfast
10:00 a.m.	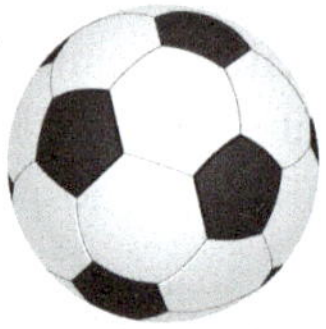	Physical therapy
11:00 a.m.	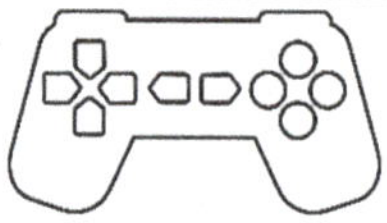	Child life
12:00 p.m.	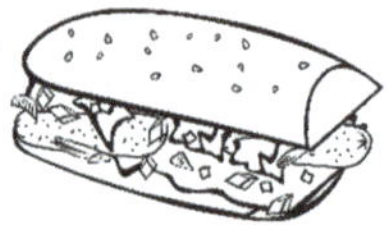	Lunch
2:00 p.m.	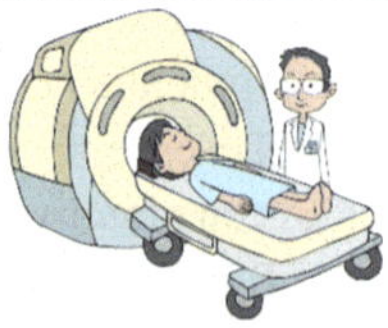	MRI
5:00 p.m.	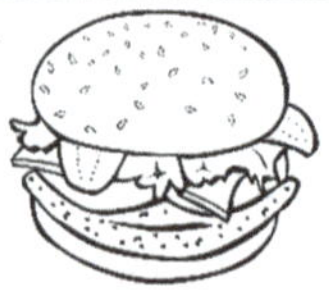	Dinner
9:00 p.m.	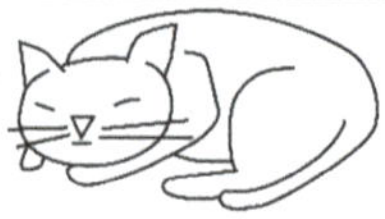	Bedtime

References

American Psychiatric Association. (2013). *Diagnostic and statistical manual of mental disorders (DSM-5)*. Washington, DC: American Psychiatry Association.

Attwood, T. (2003). Framework for behavioral interventions. *Child and Adolescent Psychiatric Clinics of North America, 12*, 65–86.

Baio, J., Wiggins, L., Christensen, D. L., Maenner, M. J., Daniels, J., Warren, Z., … Durkin, M. S. (2018). Prevalence of autism spectrum disorder among children aged 8 years—Autism and developmental disabilities monitoring network, 11 sites, United States, 2014. *MMWR Surveillance Summaries, 67*(6), 1.

Blake, K. (2010). Spectrum disorders a new generation of complex patients. *Pennsylvania Nurse, 65*(4), 9–11. 15.

Boyle, C. A., Boulet, S., Schieve, L. A., Cohen, R. A., Blumberg, S. J., Yeargin-Allsopp, M., … Kogan, M. D. (2011). Trends in the prevalence of developmental disabilities in US children, 1997–2008. *Pediatrics, 127*(6), 1034–1042.

Broder-Fingert, S., Shui, A., Ferrone, C., Iannuzzi, D., Cheng, E. R., Giauque, A., … Kuhlthau, K. (2016). A pilot study of autism-specific care plans during hospital admission. *Pediatrics, 137*(Suppl 2), S196–S204.

Browne, M. (2006). Communication with the child who has autism spectrum disorder: A practical introduction. *Paediatric Nursing, 18*(1), 14–17.

Bruininks, R., Woodcock, R., Weatherman, R., & Hill, H. (1997). *Scales of independent behavior—Revised*. Rolling Meadows, IL: Riverside Publishing.

Centers for Disease Control and Prevention (CDC). (2018). *Developmental disabilities*. Retrieved from April 19, 2018, from https://www.cdc.gov/ncbddd/developmentaldisabilities/facts.html

Chebuhar, A., McCarthy, A. M., Bosch, J., & Baker, S. (2013). Using picture schedules in medical settings for patients with an autism spectrum disorder. *Journal of Pediatric Nursing, 28*(2), 125–134.

Chiri, G., & Warfield, M. E. (2012). Unmet need and problems accessing core health care services for children with autism spectrum disorder. *Maternal and Child Health Journal, 16*(5), 1081–1091.

Davignon, M. N., Friedlaender, E., Cronholm, P. F., Paciotti, B., & Levy, S. E. (2014). Parent and provider perspectives on procedural care for children with autism spectrum disorders. *Journal of Developmental & Behavioral Pediatrics, 35*(3), 207–215.

De Shazer, S. (1988). Utilization: The foundation of solutions. In *Developing Ericksonian therapy: State of the art* (pp. 112–124).

Division of Birth Defects, National Center on Birth Defects and Developmental Disabilities (NCBDDD), Centers for Disease Control and Prevention (CDC). (2018). *Autism care landing page*. Retrieved from February 2, 2019, from https://www.cdc.gov/ncbddd/actearly/act.html

Einfeld, S. L., Piccinin, A. M., Mackinnon, A., Hofer, S. M., Taffe, J., Gray, K. M., … Tonge, B. J. (2006). Psychopathology in young people with intellectual disability. *JAMA, 296*(16), 1981–1989.

Einfeld, S. L., & Tonge, B. J. (1996). Population prevalence of psychopathology in children and adolescents with intellectual disability: II epidemiological findings. *Journal of Intellectual Disability Research, 40*(2), 99–109.

Emerson, E., Einfeld, S., & Stancliffe, R. J. (2010). The mental health of young children with intellectual disabilities or borderline intellectual functioning. *Social Psychiatry and Psychiatric Epidemiology, 45*(5), 579–587.

Feldman, H. M., Ploof, D. L., Hofkosh, D., & Goehring, E. L. (1993). Developmental needs of infants and toddlers who require lengthy hospitalization. *American Journal of Diseases of Children, 147*(2), 211–215.

Giarelli, E., Souders, M., Pinto-Martin, J., Bloch, J., & Levy, S. E. (2005). Intervention pilot for parents of children with autistic spectrum disorder. *Pediatric Nursing, 31*(5), 389.

Golnik, A., & Nadia Maccabee-Ryaboy, B. A. (2010). Autism: Clinical pearls for primary care. *Contemporary Pediatrics, November*, 42–59.

Gray, C. (1994). *The new social story book*. Arlington, TX: Future Horizons.

Hockenberry, M. J., & Wilson, D. (2018). *Wong's nursing care of infants and children-E-book*. Philadelphia: Elsevier Health Sciences.

Hoffses, K. W., Ramirez, L. Y., Berdan, L., Tunick, R., Honaker, S. M., Meadows, T. J., … Stancin, T. (2016). Topical review: Building competency: Professional skills for pediatric psychologists in integrated primary care settings. *Journal of Pediatric Psychology, 41*(10), 1144–1160.

Inglese, M. D. (2009). Caring for children with autism spectrum disorder, Part II: Screening, diagnosis, and management. *Journal of Pediatric Nursing, 24*(1), 49–59.

Johnson, N. L., & Rodriguez, D. (2013). Children with autism spectrum disorder at a pediatric hospital: A systematic review of the literature. *Pediatric Nursing, 39*, 131–141.

Kogan, M. D., Strickland, B. B., Blumberg, S. J., Singh, G. K., Perrin, J. M., & van Dyck, P. C. (2008). A national profile of the health care experiences and family impact of autism spectrum disorder among children in the United States, 2005–2006. *Pediatrics, 122*(6), e1149–e1158.

Kokina, A., & Kern, L. (2010). Social Story™ interventions for students with autism spectrum disorders: A meta-analysis. *Journal of Autism and Developmental Disorders, 40*(7), 812–826.

Koontz, K. L., Slifer, K. J., Cataldo, M. D., & Marcus, C. L. (2003). Improving pediatric compliance with positive airway pressure therapy: The impact of behavioral intervention. *Sleep, 26*(8), 1010–1015.

Kopecky, K., Broder-Fingert, S., Iannuzzi, D., & Connors, S. (2013). The needs of hospitalized patients with autism spectrum disorders: A parent survey. *Clinical Pediatrics, 52*(7), 652–660.

Koski, S., Gabriels, R. L., & Beresford, C. (2016). Interventions for paediatric surgery patients with comorbid autism spectrum disorder: A systematic literature review. *Archives of Disease in Childhood, 101*, 1090–1094.

Kozlowski, A. M., & Matson, J. L. (2012). An examination of challenging behaviors in autistic disorder versus pervasive developmental disorder not otherwise specified: Significant differences and gender effects. *Research in Autism Spectrum Disorders, 6*(1), 319–325.

Kuo, D. Z., Houtrow, A. J., Arango, P., Kuhlthau, K. A., Simmons, J. M., & Neff, J. M. (2012). Family-centered care: Current applications and future directions in pediatric health care. *Maternal and Child Health Journal, 16*(2), 297–305.

Lakhan, R. (2013). The coexistence of psychiatric disorders and intellectual disability in children aged 3–18 years in the Barwani District, India. *ISRN Psychiatry, 2013*, 875873.

Leyfer, O. T., Folstein, S. E., Bacalman, S., Davis, N. O., Dinh, E., Morgan, J., … Lainhart, J. E. (2006). Comorbid psychiatric disorders in children with autism: Interview development and rates of disorders. *Journal of Autism and Developmental Disorders, 36*(7), 849–861.

Liptak, G. S., Stuart, T., & Auinger, P. (2006). Health care utilization and expenditures for children with autism: Data from US national samples. *Journal of Autism and Developmental Disorders, 36*(7), 871–879.

Liu, G., Pearl, A. M., Kong, L., Leslie, D. L., & Murray, M. J. (2017). A profile on emergency department utilization in adolescents and young adults with autism spectrum disorders. *Journal of Autism and Developmental Disorders, 47*(2), 347–358.

Lloyd, H., & Dallos, R. (2006). Solution-focused brief therapy with families who have a child with intellectual disabilities: A description of the content of initial sessions and the processes. *Clinical Child Psychology and Psychiatry, 11*(3), 367–386.

Lokhandwala, T., Khanna, R., & West-Strum, D. (2012). Hospitalization burden among individuals with autism. *Journal of Autism and Developmental Disorders, 42*(1), 95–104.

Lowe, K., Allen, D., Jones, E., Brophy, S., Moore, K., & James, W. (2007). Challenging behaviours: Prevalence and topographies. *Journal of Intellectual Disability Research, 51*(8), 625–636.

Major, N. E., Peacock, G., Ruben, W., Thomas, J., & Weitzman, C. C. (2013). Autism training in pediatric residency: Evaluation of a case-based curriculum. *Journal of Autism and Developmental Disorders, 43*(5), 1171–1177.

McGonigle, J. J., Migyanka, J. M., Glor-Scheib, S. J., Cramer, R., Fratangeli, J. J., Hegde, G. G., … Venkat, A. (2014). Development and evaluation of educational materials for pre-hospital and emergency department personnel on the care of patients with autism spectrum disorder. *Journal of Autism and Developmental Disorders, 44*(5), 1252–1259.

Muskat, B., Burnham Riosa, P., Nicholas, D. B., Roberts, W., Stoddart, K. P., & Zwaigenbaum, L. (2015). Autism comes to the hospital: The experiences of patients with autism spectrum disorder, their parents and health-care providers at two Canadian paediatric hospitals. *Autism, 19*(4), 482–490.

Muskens, J. B., Velders, F. P., & Staal, W. G. (2017). Medical comorbidities in children and adolescents with autism spectrum disorders and attention deficit hyperactivity disorders: A systematic review. *European Child & Adolescent Psychiatry, 26*(9), 1093–1103.

Nageswaran, S., Parish, S. L., Rose, R. A., & Grady, M. D. (2011). Do children with developmental disabilities and mental health conditions have greater difficulty using health services than children with physical disorders? *Maternal and Child Health Journal, 15*(5), 634–641.

Nicholas, D. B., Zwaigenbaum, L., Muskat, B., Craig, W. R., Newton, A. S., Cohen-Silver, J., … Kilmer, C. (2016). Toward practice advancement in emergency care for children with autism spectrum disorder. *Pediatrics, 137*(Suppl 2), S205–S211.

Petersen, M. C., Kube, D. A., Whitaker, T. M., Graff, J. C., & Palmer, F. B. (2009). Prevalence of developmental and behavioral disorders in a pediatric hospital. *Pediatrics, 123*(3), e490–e495.

Rosen, T. E., Connell, J. E., & Kerns, C. M. (2016). A review of behavioral interventions for anxiety-related behaviors in lower-functioning individuals with autism. *Behavioral Interventions, 31*(2), 120–143.

Scarpinato, N., Bradley, J., Kurbjun, K., Bateman, X., Holtzer, B., & Ely, B. (2010). Caring for the child with an autism spectrum disorder in the acute care setting. *Journal for Specialists in Pediatric Nursing, 15*(3), 244–254.

Schieve, L. A., Gonzalez, V., Boulet, S. L., Visser, S. N., Rice, C. E., Braun, K. V. N., & Boyle, C. A. (2012). Concurrent medical conditions and health care use and needs among children with learning and behavioral developmental disabilities, National Health Interview Survey, 2006–2010. *Research in Developmental Disabilities, 33*(2), 467–476.

Shelton, T. L., & Stepanek, J. S. (1994). *Family-centered care for children needing specialized health and developmental services*. Bethesda, MD: Association for the Care of Children's Health.

Skinner, S. R., Ng, C., McDonald, A., & Walters, T. (2005). A patient with autism and severe depression: Medical and ethical challenges for an adolescent medicine unit. *Medical Journal of Australia, 183*(8), 422–424.

Souders, M. C., DePaul, D., Freeman, K. G., & Levy, S. E. (2002). Caring for children and adolescents with autism who require challenging procedures. *Pediatric Nursing, 28*(6), 555–562.

Tellegen, C. L., & Sanders, M. R. (2012). Using primary care parenting interventions to improve outcomes in children with developmental disabilities: A case report. *Case Reports in Pediatrics, 2012*, 150261.

Tellegen, C. L., & Sanders, M. R. (2013). Stepping stones triple P-positive parenting program for children with disability: A systematic review and meta-analysis. *Research in Developmental Disabilities, 34*(5), 1556–1571.

Tellegen, C. L., & Sanders, M. R. (2014). A randomized controlled trial evaluating a brief parenting program with children with autism spectrum disorders. *Journal of Consulting and Clinical Psychology, 82*(6), 1193.

Van der Walt, J. H., & Moran, C. (2001). An audit of perioperative management of autistic children. *Pediatric Anesthesia, 11*(4), 401–408.

Vasa, R. A., Carroll, L. M., Nozzolillo, A. A., Mahajan, R., Mazurek, M. O., Bennett, A. E., … Bernal, M. P. (2014). A systematic review of treatments for anxiety in youth with autism spectrum disorders. *Journal of Autism and Developmental Disorders, 44*(12), 3215–3229.

Wallander, J. L., Dekker, M. C., & Koot, H. M. (2003). Psychopathology in children and adolescents with intellectual disability: Measurement, prevalence, course, and risk. In L. Glidden (Ed.), *International review of research in mental retardation* (pp. 93–134).

Walters, S., Loades, M., & Russell, A. (2016). A systematic review of effective modifications to cognitive behavioural therapy for young people with autism spectrum disorders. *Review Journal of Autism and Developmental Disorders, 3*(2), 137–153.

Whittingham, K., Sofronoff, K., Sheffield, J., & Sanders, M. R. (2009). Stepping Stones Triple P: An RCT of a parenting program with parents of a child diagnosed with an autism spectrum disorder. *Journal of Abnormal Child Psychology, 37*(4), 469.

Zablotsky, B., Kalb, L. G., Freedman, B., Vasa, R., & Stuart, E. A. (2014). Health care experiences and perceived financial impact among families of children with an autism spectrum disorder. *Psychiatric Services, 65*(3), 395–398.

Disruptive Behavior and Noncompliance

Anne Reagan, Emily Mudd, and Courtney Landau Fleisher

Disruptive Behavior in the Medical Setting

Pediatric psychologists are frequently consulted by our pediatrician and subspecialist colleagues to address the problem of patient externalizing behaviors in consultation-liaison (CL) work. Research has identified disruptive behaviors as the most common reason for referral for mental health services (Loeber, Burke, Lahey, Winters, & Zera, 2000), and studies have found that children with disruptive behavior are referred more for psychology consults while hospitalized than are children without externalizing behaviors (Carter et al., 2003). The impact of the child's disruptive behavior and noncompliance on their own welfare, the family, the medical staff, and the overall quality of care can be severe, including impairing important relationships with healthcare providers, increasing the possibility of unintentional injury, and increasing the length of stay and cost of hospitalization (Doupnik et al., 2016; Modi & Quittner, 2006).

Related to disruptive patient behaviors that can adversely impact patient care and welfare are problems with patient and family adherence and compliance (or nonadherence and noncompliance; see Chap. 32), which are often used interchangeably when discussing disruptive behaviors of pediatric patients. Adherence refers to behaviors associated with medical advice such as taking medications or making lifestyle changes. Previous investigations have defined the term "compliance" as fact driven, i.e., a child either did or did not follow a regimen as prescribed (McDonald, Garg, & Haynes, 2002). In the current chapter, however, we are referring to disruptive behaviors as those characterized by explosive behavior, interpersonal aggression, defiance, and enduring impairment.

Regardless of etiology, disruptive behavior in pediatric patients can result in significant negative health outcomes, and in terms of the adverse effects of these behaviors on the provision of effective medical care, consulting pediatric psy-

A. Reagan (✉)
Golisano Children's Hospital, Syracuse, NY, USA

Department of Pediatrics, SUNY Upstate Medical University, Syracuse, NY, USA
e-mail: ReaganA@upstate.edu

E. Mudd
Cleveland Clinic, Cleveland, OH, USA

Cleveland Clinic Lerner College of Medicine of Case Western Reserve University, Cleveland, OH, USA

C. L. Fleisher
University of Vermont Medical Center, Burlington, VT, USA

Departments of Psychiatry and Pediatrics, Robert Larner MD College of Medicine, Burlington, VT, USA

B. D. Carter, K. A. Kullgren (eds.), *Clinical Handbook of Psychological Consultation in Pediatric Medical Settings*, Issues in Clinical Child Psychology, https://doi.org/10.1007/978-3-030-35598-2_29

chologists can provide invaluable resources for assessing and identifying the function of the behavior and implementing appropriate interventions needed to improve health outcomes. As specialists in the delivery of child and adolescent mental health services, pediatric psychologist consultation is particularly crucial when the patient has specific behavioral conditions (e.g., ADHD, trauma, depression, anxiety) requiring psychotherapeutic expertise.

Assessment of Disruptive Behavior

There have been few assessments designed and validated to evaluate patient behavioral dysregulation on a medical inpatient unit (see Chap. 11). One assessment measure that has been validated for use in the inpatient medical setting is the Pediatric Inpatient Behavior Scale (PIBS) (Kornenberger, Carter, & Thomas, 1997), which has been shown to be sensitive to identifying both internalizing and externalizing behaviors that may impair response to treatment and be disruptive to the optimal provision of nursing and medical care in the hospitalized child. Clinicians may also choose to adapt scales designed for the prediction of externalizing and violent behaviors in inpatient pediatric psychiatric settings (Brief Rating of Aggression for Children and Adolescents; Almvik, Woods, & Rasmussen, 2000) and with older adolescents and young adults (Brøset Violence Checklist; Barzman, Mossman, Sonnier, & Sorter, 2012). Other standardized behavioral rating scales, such as the Behavioral Assessment System for Children (BASC-3) (Reynolds & Kamphaus, 2009) and Child Behavior Checklist (CBCL) (Achenbach, 2009) are useful for identifying longer term problems with externalizing behaviors, which may be exacerbated by the demands of medical treatment and hospitalization.

Once the potential for aggressive or disruptive behavior has been identified, via formal assessment or observation, an assessment of any externalizing behavior should begin with both parent and patient interviews. In order to create an effective behavior plan to be carried out in the inpatient medical setting, a functional analysis of the behavior should be completed in order to identify the antecedents to the action, in addition to the potential consequences that may serve to reinforce these behavioral responses. In developing a behavioral plan, the consulting psychologist must identify and objectively define the problem behavior and antecedent/consequent conditions, help formulate demonstrable outcome goals, design and implement an intervention plan, monitor plan implementation, evaluate the effectiveness of the plan, and put in place mechanisms for the maintenance of the intervention.

Functional Analysis Case Example Felix is a 12-year-old male admitted for the management of his type 1 diabetes. He becomes irritable and engages in verbal aggression with the nursing staff when his evening dose of long-acting insulin is scheduled, resulting in a delay of medication administration and meal times. In this scenario, the antecedent is the presentation of the insulin for administration, the externalizing behavior is verbal agitation and nonadherence, and the reinforcement is delaying appropriate medication administration, likely a major contributor to his poor diabetes management. In the context of this assessment, the targeted intervention would be to determine the source and function of his verbal aggression and to address or change the reinforcing contingencies (e.g., reinforce the fact that the patient is communicating while ignoring the content of what he is saying and continuing with the insulin administration) to a positive contingency (e.g., explaining that when the patient can communicate in a constructive manner, it will be possible to discuss the situation and address his negative mood state and subsequently reinforce his compliance with insulin administration with a walk around the unit, a trip to the playroom, television time, video games, etc.). This behavioral plan gradually results in timely insulin administration with more appropriate communication between Felix and the staff. Longer term interventions are applied to transferring these skills to parents/caregivers to address these behaviors beyond the hospital admission.

Addressing Disruptive Behavior in the Inpatient Medical Setting

On an inpatient pediatric consultation-liaison (CL) service, assessment and treatment of disruptive behavior and nonadherence is paramount for patient, family, and healthcare team functioning and safety. The accepted standard-of-care treatment for oppositional behavior in outpatient settings is parent training intervention (parent psychoeducation, parent–child interaction therapy, individual and family behavioral therapy). However, such extensive parenting intervention is not always practical, or even feasible, in the environment of the medical unit. Additionally, even though parent behavioral management training has significant empirical support, it has yet to be validated with all populations of children and families (Lundahl, Riser, & Lovejoy, 2006), including hospitalized medically ill children. With pharmacotherapy being minimally effective for oppositional behavior (particularly in the shorter term of many pediatric hospital stays), despite evidence that medication is increasingly being chosen over psychosocial intervention to address disruptive behavior (Epstein, Fonnesbeck, Potter, Rizzone, & McPheeters, 2015), the prevention of behavioral dysregulation and behavioral modification remain the treatments of choice for managing disruptive behaviors in the hospital setting.

General Behavioral Management Procedures

The inpatient psychology CL team plays a valuable role in assessing the patient/family and teaching frontline staff how to assess for increasing patient irritability and escalating oppositional behavior that, if neglected, may result in aggression and sometimes even violent behavior. As externalizing behaviors escalate, optimally there should be a corresponding intervention to mitigate the situation. For all patients considered to be at risk of behavioral escalation, particularly at a time when they are relatively calm and well behaved, the team should ideally plan for addressing those conditions likely to provoke patient distress, assess child and family coping skills and preferences, and create a behavioral contingency plan with the patient and family. When there is an escalation in disruptive behaviors (e.g., the patient engages in disrespectful or threatening verbalizations, increased anxiety, and agitation), the initial clinical response should focus on deescalation via engaging in empathic listening with calm supportive statements, coaching the patient and their family in the use of more effective coping strategies, and actively modeling and reinforcing more adaptive behaviors.

Ideally, these are skills that many pediatric providers may engage in naturally. However, if the patient's behavior escalates to increased agitation, aggressive actions toward objects (e.g., kicking a chair, throwing things), and physical refusal to comply with medical procedures, then these behaviors are best addressed via the setting of clear limits and consequences, self-soothing and grounding techniques (clinical biofeedback, mindfulness exercises, diaphragmatic breathing), and deescalation techniques (utilize empathy, be nonjudgmental, allow silence for reflection, try to focus on the emotional response rather than on the content of the speech). If the patient continues to escalate and becomes verbally threatening (e.g., directing anger and threats at a specific person, intimidation, yelling) it is important to give the child reasonable physical space while remaining present (at a distance) to maintain supervision and providing brief, concise, and concrete directives.

Finally, if despite these efforts to defuse the situation the patient continues to engage in oppositionality and becomes physically threatening or violent (e.g., pulls out their IV, attempts to run from the room or medical unit, makes threatening posturing toward the staff, is physically assaultive toward others), safety is the first priority, and physical restraint may be indicated as a last resort. In order to minimize the child's and their family's experience of the restraint as traumatic, the restrainer should calmly narrate their behavior, including why they are using this intervention ("I can't let you hurt yourself or anyone else; we have to keep you safe"), allowing the restrainer to maintain a safety framework while reassuring the patient and their family that the restraint is not intended as a punishment. Most pediatric hospitals have established very specific procedures for the use of restraint by their staff and security, and the pediatric psychologist should be thoroughly informed of these procedures. Following an efficacious treatment application of a parent training intervention, safe and appropriate restraint skills should be communicated and taught to the parents of the patient as well, as needed.

Skill Building Cognitive Behavioral Interventions

Once the behaviors of concern and treatment goals have been clearly operationally defined via functional analysis, it is important to consider the most efficacious intervention strategies for the specific behavior change. Behavioral interventions have been shown to be effective for pediatric adherence with varied medical conditions and procedures related to oncology, neuroimaging, neurodevelopmental disabilities, and insertion of intravenous catheters (Slifer et al., 2002; Slifer, Babbitt, & Cataldo, 1995; Slifer, Cataldo, Cataldo, Llorente, & Gerson, 1993). Interventions typically fall into three categories: operant techniques/contingency management, cognitive behavioral skill-building techniques, and schedule management.

Behavioral Interventions Operant interventions target changing aversive behaviors through reinforcement schedules (Skinner, 1937). Using positive reinforcement within the context of a consult service to increase prosocial behaviors can be effective in reducing disruptive behavior. Anderson and Collier (1999) demonstrated the effectiveness of behavioral interventions using contingent reinforcement on an inpatient service in increasing adherence to medication. As with all behavioral intervention, resorting to negative reinforcement/punitive techniques should only be made in the context of having established reinforcing procedures previously. Given the short and/or uncertain duration of most hospitalizations, it is likely to be most efficacious to focus on positive reinforcement strategies.

Cognitive Therapies Cognitive behavioral therapy (CBT) strategies can be effective in helping hospitalized children increase their knowledge of their medical condition and treatments, which can decrease anxiety and improve behavioral regulation. Utilization of CBT techniques, such as exposure therapy for needle phobia or processing emotions that accompany a new chronic illness diagnosis, are relevant and an appropriate application. Such exposures can be in vivo or employ observations of peer models via video from a social learning perspective (Ernst, 2011).

Children often exhibit disruptive behavior (e.g., aggression, poor self-control, and noncompliance) when having difficulties with emotion identification and regulation. A child may feel his heart beating fast or see his fists clenched, but he may not realize that this is an indication that he is becoming fearful and angry. Having the child track his rapid heartbeat and the tension in his fists and simultaneously drawing attention to the connection between the behavior and the emotion can build emotional awareness. Pediatric psychologists can introduce the cognitive triangle to elucidate the connection between the mind (thoughts, feelings) and the body (actions), a chief concept to treatment success in reducing behavioral dysregulation. Once a child is able to identify his emotional state, the implementation of positive coping skills can assist with the regulation of the autonomic nervous system. In teaching a child that once he feels his heart beating faster he can engage in strategies such as diaphragmatic breathing to reduce his heart rate (which can be enhanced with clinical biofeedback technology; see Chap. 37), this decreases his anxiety/fear, allowing him to engage in more adaptive coping skills (e.g., distraction), further improving his emotional state and reducing behavioral dysregulation in turn.

Scheduling Though schedules are often unpredictable in the inpatient medical setting, for youths who experience lengthy admissions, implementing a daily schedule can be an effective intervention to increasing predictability and a sense of security in an otherwise uncontrollable environment. For example, a child who has difficulty with emotional regulation during rehabilitation therapies may benefit from having physical therapy and occupational therapy at the same times each day to increase predictability and decrease ambiguity. Scheduling wake and sleep times daily can also be very beneficial in regulating the child's circadian rhythm, which can have lasting effects on emotional and behavioral regulation the next day.

Regardless of the intervention chosen to manage behavior, each intervention must match the targeted behavior and be individualized for each child, in addition to including frontline medical staff (nurses, child life, patient care assistants, etc.).

Addressing Disruptive Behavior in the Outpatient Medical Setting

Pediatric psychologists play an integral role in improving treatment outcomes in the outpatient medical setting. Having access to a psychologist during a routine clinic appointment or as part of follow-up after hospital discharge is valuable for both the prevention of new disruptive behaviors and continuing intervention for a problematic behavior identified in the hospital. In conjunction with an outpatient medical appointment, the psychologist may meet with patients and families to identify and address challenging/disruptive behaviors or behavior patterns that interfere with adherence to treatment requirements and disease management.

Coordination Between Inpatient and Outpatient Services When disruptive behaviors are identified during an inpatient admission, outpatient psychology follow-up is one of the many recommendations frequently resulting from an inpatient psychology consultation. An important consideration is how information flows between inpatient and outpatient services. For the outpatient clinician, it is important to obtain inpatient psychology or psychiatry consult notes, as well as details about any assessment, diagnosis, or clinical interventions that were started in order to achieve optimal continuity of care.

Functional Case Example In the case example earlier of Felix, the coordination of services initiated in the inpatient setting is crucial for a follow-up in an outpatient medical setting, ideally accessing psychology follow-up soon after discharge. The behavioral plan can be further developed and expanded upon with a continued use of positive reinforcement, if it has been successful, or by adding other techniques such as negative reinforcement (e.g., restricting technology use around the time when medication is due and until care is completed) or with the use of negative contingencies (e.g., loss of allowance or access to preferred activity when medication administration time is missed). The family system element can be expanded upon by educating caregivers on how to implement interventions with consistency (especially if the patient lives in more than one home), as well as recognizing and changing maladaptive caregiver responses (one caregiver may display a stronger response or be identified as the disciplinarian while the other caregiver is more passive, resulting in caregiver conflict, which disrupts medication administration). Avoiding power struggles would also be an important focus as disruptive behavior can be elicited when a patient feels threatened or forced to complete a task. Highlighting where there are opportunities for the patient to have a choice and independence in their care (based on what is developmentally appropriate) can be the longer term focus of outpatient services. These interventions are able to be developed in more detail over time with follow-up in the outpatient setting.

Prevention/Early Intervention Pediatric psychologists provide interventions for health promotion and disease prevention in the outpatient medical setting. Programs that focus on the prevention of child abuse and drug use have shown positive outcomes in efforts aimed at reducing the rates of social, behavioral and academic problems (Weisz, Sandler, Durlak, & Anton, 2005). Clinical work in the outpatient medical setting can focus on the promotion of healthy child development while managing the psychological stressors of acute or chronic medical conditions. In addition to the universal intervention of screening for anxiety and depression, a practice increasingly common in pediatric primary and subspecialty care, psychologists can work with medical providers in outpatient clinics to identify patients at high risk for challenging behaviors. A targeted intervention of teaching parents the value of attending to positive behaviors and how to give developmentally appropriate direct commands can prevent or address disruptive and noncompliant behavior early on, and these efforts can be generalized to impact healthcare adherence regimens, which may improve health outcomes.

When fully integrated in an outpatient medical setting, psychologists often serve as interventionists when acute problematic behavior presents in clinic and interferes with medically necessary treatments. For example, a pediatric psychologist may be integrated into an outpatient pediatric pulmonology center where a teenage patient with cystic fibrosis presents for a clinic appointment and the caregiver mentions that the patient has been more resistant and oppositional regarding the completion of daily vest treatments for pulmonary respiratory therapy, to the point of verbal aggression toward family members and refusal. By employing a combination of frameworks and techniques, including functional assessment of behavior, individual and family clinical interview, motivational interviewing, and setting treatment goals around a successful completion of medically necessary treatment, the psychologist may be able to help the patient and their family process and better understand the underlying cause of the behavior. This hopefully would result in a decrease of oppositional behavior and decreased conflict at home, with an underlying goal of avoiding hospitalization due to not following the prescribed medical treatment (i.e., worsening pulmonary function and respiratory infection).

Behavioral Interventions Austin, Dunn, Johnson, and Perkins (2004) identified challenging behaviors common in pediatric patients with epilepsy, with several unique aspects of seizure disorders contributing to the development and maintenance of behavior problems in this population, including neurodevelopmental and family dynamic factors. As mentioned earlier, emotional dysregulation can manifest in physical ways (rapid heart rate, tension in fists), but patients can also externalize disruptive behavior with symptoms that mirror medical symptoms. For example, a teenage patient presents to an outpatient neurology clinic for concern of increase in seizure activity at home. The neurologist determined that the described episodes are inconsistent with an expected seizure presentation. Upon further questioning, the neurologist suspects that the episodes are behavioral in nature and conducts a warm hand-off to the psychologist in the clinic. Following a brief clinical interview, the psychologist determines that these episodes occur after a demand or a limitation is placed on the patient. The demands historically have been ones that the patient identifies as difficult to complete (i.e., cleaning a bedroom, completing school work), or the limitation is in contrast to what the patient desires (e.g., staying out past curfew, participating in a social activity), often resulting in the escalation of behaviors at home. A few minutes later, the teen starts to shake or become limp, and they fall to the floor. The psychologist can use this as an opportunity to work with the family and identify the appropriate responses and management of this behavior, with the treatment goal of reducing the frequency and intensity of the behavior. Often these presentations are connected to avoidant or attention-seeking behaviors, in addition to maladaptive coping in response to stressors associated with their chronic illness. Interventions should focus on parent training (e.g., redirection when behaviors start to escalate, planned ignoring), psychoeducation, and behavioral interventions such as contingency planning or setting up positive reinforcement when demands are met. Psychologists working with these patients would also want to address family dynamics and identify if there are elements (e.g., caregiver's tone of voice or general delivery of the demand, chaotic schedule where the child feels rushed to complete demands, dyads within the family system) that may elicit certain behaviors. Other useful interventions include CBT techniques that prime the patient to more accurately identify their emotional state and choose a more adaptive behavioral response (e.g., use of visual cues to slow down thought processes, worksheets such as emotion faces, thermometer, or volcano activity worksheets).

Behavioral interventions should reflect the clinic environment and be sensitive to the resources available to the patient and family system. All team members play a role in helping to support clinical interventions. The medical team, nurses, and other clinical staff can also provide additional observations of the patient and family, and share insight or concern about particular interactions and behaviors. The medical team can provide valuable data regarding compliance (or noncompliance) with medical regimen. When there is a behavioral plan in place, various members of the medical team may ask the patient about his or her progress and express interest in the plan and the patient's success as reinforcement. If the patient and family know the entire treatment team is engaged and in support of the goals and process, it provides a more consistent and clear message of the significance of the behavioral plan.

Clinical Assessment Pediatric psychologists can recommend assessments or complete screeners to identify variables that may contribute to disruptive behavior. For example, some children with neurodevelopmental disorders may struggle in an academic setting, and this can cause frustration, school avoidance, or acting out. There may be significant benefit from academic accommodations based on performance on neuropsychological assessments, and psychologists in an outpatient medical setting are uniquely positioned to communicate information to schools while advocating for patients' medical, academic, and behavioral needs. Social skills groups provided in an outpatient setting can be implemented to address ongoing social needs that are common with children who have chronic medical needs. Parent skills training can also be utilized in this setting, with a focus on containing and managing difficult behaviors when parents and patients present with behavioral concerns. Outpatient psychotherapy can also help normalize certain behaviors that are common with acute and chronic medical conditions (e.g., tic disorders), as well as address the anxiety (experienced by both patients and parents) that accompanies associated behaviors.

Adaptations

Involving Caregivers as Treatment Team Members in Intervention

Importance of Parent Involvement Research evaluating effective treatments for decreasing disruptive and noncompliant behavior highlights the importance of caregiver involvement in mitigating problematic behavior across interventions (Epstein et al., 2015; Gleason, Goldson, Yogman, & AAP Council on Early Childhood, 2016; Lundahl et al., 2006), although the effect size of the results and the population with whom they are most effective is less clear. Comparing the effectiveness of three treatment modalities to waitlist control or treatment as usual, interventions that included a parenting component had a higher probability of being the most efficacious treatment (86%) compared with those intervening exclusively with the child (14%) (Epstein et al., 2015). Interventions focused on strengthening parent–child interactions and attachment, reducing harsh discipline, and fostering parents' ability to promote children's social, emotional, and language development were most effective. Additional aspects of parent intervention include teaching positive methods for increasing desired behavior and, in turn, reducing undesired behavior.

The Broader Treatment Team Children and families often develop enduring relationships with nurses, physicians, and other medical caregivers of the team that they see repeatedly at clinic visits. This continuity offers opportunities to establish routines and develop trusting relationships (Njoroge, Hostutler, Schwartz, & Mautone, 2016), which allows for additional familiar adults who may assist in managing challenging behaviors. The balance of achieving clear and consistent communication in the inpatient setting can be difficult, however, due to the multitude of caregivers who must align their message over the course of days or weeks. Pediatrically trained nurses and physicians are often facile with incorporating developmentally appropriate language into their practice, but applying these skills with disruptive or noncompliant behavior that interferes with medical care adds a layer of complexity. Child life specialists may be brought in to alleviate providers serving in dual roles when medical procedures are anticipated to be or become difficult for a child or family member.

Family/Teamwork in the Inpatient Setting Disruptive behavior patterns that existed within family systems prior to a child's hospital admission can become amplified in periods of stress or even lead to hospitalization. Change may need to happen in the family system and the environment in order to reduce disruptive behavior and increase the likelihood for compliance. In the case of Felix, described earlier, a family session could be scheduled to ascertain what challenges interfere with Felix receiving his insulin at home. Being in the hospital where appropriate administration of insulin is ensured while Felix undergoes a workup for additional medical contributors to his poorly managed type 1 diabetes, a pediatric psychologist could simultaneously work with the family to improve communication, establish developmentally appropriate roles, set reasonable expectations for Felix in managing his condition, or set the groundwork for addressing other problems amenable to behavioral health intervention after discharge. Such an admission could be highly efficient in diagnosing and beginning to modify a serious situation.

Family/Teamwork in the Outpatient Setting Parents and guardians are invaluable partners in collaborative problem-solving around the manifestations of disruptive behavior and noncompliance that arises during a visit or procedure. When pediatric psychologists engage in such collaborative problem-solving, developmentally appropriate family-centered care is optimized (Walsh, 2004). Flexibility and creativity on the part of the clinician engaging with the family is important as space and time constraints in the outpatient setting may require a dedicated outpatient psychological visit to develop a plan to address situations that arise repeatedly (Guilfoyle, Follansbee-Junger, & Modi, 2013; Njoroge et al., 2016). A warm handoff between the physician and psychologist increases the likelihood that the child and their family will comply with follow-ups (Njoroge et al., 2016).

Cultural Factors in Involving Caregivers in Intervention Studies have investigated incorporating ethnoculturally specific concepts into evidence-based practices (EBP) for disruptive and noncompliant behavior (e.g., Calzada, 2010; Gross, Belcher, Budhathoki, Ofonedu, & Uveges, 2018; Lau, Fung, & Yung, 2010). Evidence has not found treatment by ethnicity interactions across White, Latino, and African American families in reducing abusive parenting practices (e.g., Parent–Child Interaction Therapy; Chaffin et al., 2004), and few ethnic differences were found across White, Latino, African American, and Asian American families with regard to child conduct outcomes and attrition in completing the Incredible Years (IY) intervention (Reid, Webster-Stratton, & Beauchaine, 2001). Identified central concepts inherent in successful parent training programs for children include educating parents about the benefits of positive reinforcement to promote desired behaviors, the importance of ignoring irritating as opposed to unsafe behaviors, and how to respond to unacceptable behaviors in a clear, consistent, and safe manner (Gleason et al., 2016). Aside from keeping the core concepts needed for achieving behavior change in mind, approaching treatment from a culturally humble stance (Hook, Davis, Owen, Worthington Jr., & Utsey, 2013) is essential to achieve desired outcomes while maintaining therapeutic rapport with the patient and family.

Medical Trauma: Contributions to Disruptive Behavior

A medical setting that embeds trauma-informed care into its culture offers the opportunity to prevent cycles of disruptive behavior through clinician education and changes in practice behavior (see Chap. 19). A meta-analysis of studies investigating pediatric medical traumatic stress (PMTS) reported rates of 30% (Price, Kassam-Adams, Alderfer, Christofferson, & Kazak, 2016). Subjectively traumatic experiences can activate the sympathetic nervous system, thus signaling the body to respond with a fight or flight response. When faced with trauma reminders, patients may become emotionally or behaviorally dysregulated and, thus, disruptive during the clinical encounter (Lieberman, Ghosh Ippen, & Van, 2015; Saxe, Ellis, & Brown, 2015). Pediatric psychologists can help educate providers about the concepts of trauma-informed care as they relate to their specific professions (Healthcaretoolbox.org; Kassam-Adams, Schneider, & Kazak, 2018) and aid clinicians in employing changes in their practice to reduce distress and increase a sense of trust in the situation for children and family members. Supporting primary care pediatricians in accessing resources developed by their own guild (aap.org/traumaguide; American Academy of Pediatrics, 2014) can be a useful approach to affecting systemic change that positively impacts disruptive behavior in the busy outpatient medical setting.

When a child comes into the acute care medical setting having experienced a traumatic injury or illness, the opportunity is ripe for pediatric psychologists to assess for traumatic stress responses. Given that prior history of trauma puts the youth at increased risk of traumatic stress reactions, gathering information about historical experiences of trauma exposure is also indicated and can lead to a discussion that yields important information about triggers and responses. When triggers have a tendency to lead to disruptive behavior, the pediatric psychologist can pass along information about things to avoid, if possible, and if triggers are inevitable given the setting, the psychologist can work with the patient and their family to identify various coping strategies to manage in those situations. Sharing information about trauma triggers and likely responses often results in greater empathy for the child and a willingness on the part of the provider to problem-solve about ways to manage the situation.

Collaborative Consultation to Address Disruptive Behaviors

Collaborating with others within a multidisciplinary team is one of the most important skills that a pediatric psychologist must hone. When reduction of disruptive behaviors and noncompliance have been identified as a goal, getting "buy-in" to the process is crucial to successfully implement behavioral interventions across a system. The ability to effectively educate our medical colleagues by conveying knowledge of clinical interventions and helping them to understand conceptualizations has been identified as a core competency for pediatric psychologists (Palermo et al., 2014). Intentions and concepts of clinical skills and interventions must be made accessible to medical colleagues so opportunities for reinforcement and modeling are not missed. Collaborating with medical colleagues and other hospital or clinic staff is critical as well, in part because their interactions and observations of the patient's disruptive behavior can be important when determining antecedents and functions of oppositional behavior. With proper collaboration and training, a patient's interactions with physicians, nurses, physical therapists, occupational therapists, social workers, and child life specialists can be opportunities for intervention and progress.

In an effort to manage disruptive behavior in the inpatient setting, pediatric psychologists can champion efforts for the implementation of institution-wide training that focuses on verbal deescalation and behavior management. Some institutions have found it helpful to supplement broader trainings to meet the needs of their institution or specific population of patients. Trainings related to behavior management and program implementation are skills that pediatric psychologists can demonstrate and spread knowledge to medical providers and other staff.

Pediatric psychologists should also be viewed as valuable resources for child life when tasked with safely managing difficult patients, as well as physical, occupational, and speech therapists when working with disruptive or noncompliant patients to achieve specific functionality goals. Whether in the inpatient or outpatient setting, these additional ancillary services should be encouraged to collaborate with CL psychology services to aid in their clinical work. Cotreatment sessions with physical therapy provide an example of an opportunity to work collaboratively on reinforcing desired behaviors and increasing compliance with treatment goals. This type of collaboration is best served when psychology is fully integrated into a system and when the environment supports integration and fluidity in the engagement of psychology services.

The field of medicine has turned toward order sets (OS) and care pathways to improve reliable and consistent access to evidence-based care for a range of interventions and processes. Research in the pediatric setting has demonstrated that the use of these methods has yielded improvements in efficiency and quality of care (Ballard et al., 2008; Bartlett, Parente, Morales, Hauser, & McLean, 2017; Bekmezian, Chung, & Yazdani, 2009; Dayal & Alvarez, 2015) and resource utilization (Guttmann et al., 2007) across a variety of illness conditions. To date there only appears to be one published study of the use of OS in a behavioral health setting (Strauss, Olbrycht, & Woo, 2013), and this research described the process of establishing standards for psychiatric admissions into various programs and the implementation of electroconvulsive therapy (ECT). Patients with psychiatric conditions are increasingly being served on inpatient medical floors and in hospital emergency departments while awaiting appropriate psychiatric placement. The process of establishing and implementing OS is generally a multidisciplinary one that identifies best practices to address a specific patient population or problem followed by an iterative process of determining how those practices can be put into place on a given floor or in a specific unit, taking tasks, responsibilities, and workflow of providers into account. Without sufficient staffing for psychologists to carry out behavioral management plans on medical floors, pediatric psychologists can participate with medical teams to standardize and operationalize the care we provide into OS that nurses, patient observers, child life specialists, physicians, and other providers can carry out to reinforce positive behavioral change on medical floors.

Case Example

Angel was a 2.5-year-old previously healthy female who lived at home with her mother and father. Angel was admitted with severe lead toxicity following her primary care provider (PCP) visit because the level of lead in her blood had more than doubled in the 6 months. Additionally, the PCP recently referred Angel to be evaluated for autism spectrum disorder (ASD). The psychology CL service was consulted to provide support to the patient and family, along with identifying services that would be needed at discharge.

Upon initial evaluation, Angel was observed to be a highly active toddler who engaged with several objects around the room while the CL team interviewed her mother. Shortly after the interview began, Angel became emotionally dysregulated as she cried and verbally expressed agitation, though words were not discernible. Angel's parents were unable to attend to Angel due to their own distress about the situation. Angel began hitting her head with her hands and eventually began to hit her head on the wall. The CL team observed that a likely function of Angel's behavior in the moment was to get adult attention and assistance with regulating her emotions. The parents were felt to be emotionally unavailable to soothe Angel in the moment, so the CL team engaged the child life specialist to assist with the regulation of Angel while they met individually with her parents.

Angel's mother acknowledged concerns about language development and noted that the idea of an autism evaluation had been raised in the past. With the increase in lead levels, Angel's PCP posited lead toxicity as the possible etiology of Angel's delay. Additional concerns about behavior included Angel's "extreme anger" during periods of dysregulation where she would "plant herself on the floor" and "space out" while engaging in verbal agitation. She had also been physically aggressive toward herself and property, at times ending in self-inflicted injury. The parents expressed that they did not have the knowledge or expertise to manage these behaviors and felt helpless as to how to go about making changes to their parenting approach for fear of "spoiling her." Additionally, the parents were often unable to be present at the hospital due to several competing demands, including caring for their other young child, searching for housing, and completing the lead testing requested by the medical team. Recognizing the importance of early intervention for children with autism, along with the significant wait times for evaluations by the State Department of Health Child Development Clinic in the area, the CL team assisted Angel's mother in completing the paperwork necessary for Angel to be placed on the waitlist for an autism evaluation.

Behavioral strategies developed for Angel and her family over their 15-day hospital admission included individual, family system/parenting, medical team/hospital, and social system level interventions. With the assistance of child life specialist colleagues, sensory toys that helped Angel calm down when she was distressed were identified and kept in her room to help soothe her when caregivers were absent and during necessary medical evaluations and procedures. Concepts that had previously been presented in a series of lectures to pediatric trainees and nurses in highlighting the effectiveness of behavioral interventions, such as redirection with young children and positive reinforcement for modifying behavior, were referenced (Gleason et al., 2016) when putting together a behavior plan for Angel. Having prepared the hospital staff with these resources, they felt comfortable applying them directly with Angel and modeling them for Angel's parents when they came in during evening hours and on weekends. Angel's parents were particularly accepting of feedback from the nursing staff. Though significant concerns about parental supervision remained (e.g., insufficient monitoring of Angel's behavior while she was in the hospital, at times posing risks to her safety), the parents' improvements in confidence in using such strategies as redirection and positive reinforcement were noted, along with increases in Angel's use of language and more appropriate behavior and self-regulation. Angel was seen by her PCP three days following hospital discharge. The CL service contacted the PCP social worker to ensure that all of the recommendations were communicated, including ASD assessment and home-based early intervention. Furthermore, given the traumatic nature of this situation for the family, the CL team recommended child-parent psychotherapy (CPP), a dyadic, relationally based EBP treatment model, to help the family in returning Angel to a normal developmental trajectory.

References

Achenbach, T. M. (2009). *The Achenbach System of Empirically Based Assessment (ASEBA): development, findings, theory, and applications*. Burlington, VT: University of Vermont Research Center for Children, Youth, & Families.

Almvik, R., Woods, P., & Rasmussen, K. (2000). The Broset violence checklist: Sensitivity, specificity, and interrater reliability. *Journal of Interpersonal Violence, 15*(12), 1284–1296.

American Academy of Pediatrics. (2014). *Trauma toolbox for primary care*. Retrieved from https://www.aap.org/en-us/advocacy-and-policy/aap-health-initiatives/healthy-foster-care-america/Pages/Trauma-Guide.aspx

Anderson, C. A., & Collier, J. A. (1999). Managing very poor adherence to medication in children and adolescents: An inpatient intervention. *Clinical Child*

Psychology and Psychiatry, 4, 393–402. https://doi.org/10.1177/1359104599004003009

Austin, J. K., Dunn, D. W., Johnson, C. S., & Perkins, S. M. (2004). Behavioral issues involving children and adolescents with epilepsy and the impact of their families: Recent research data. *Epilepsy & Behavior, 5*(3), 33–41. https://doi.org/10.1016/j.yebeh.2004.06.014

Ballard, D. J., Ogola, G., Fleming, N. S., Heck, D., Gunderson, J., Mehta, R., … Kerr, J. D. (2008). The impact of standardized order sets on quality and financial outcomes. In K. Henriksen, J. B. Battles, M. A. Keyes, et al. (Eds.), *Advances in patient safety: New directions and alternative approaches* (Culture and redesign) (Vol. Vol. 2). Rockville, MD: Agency for Healthcare Research and Quality (US). https://www.ncbi.nlm.nih.gov/books/NBK43723/?report=reader

Bartlett, K. W., Parente, V. M., Morales, V., Hauser, J., & McLean, H. S. (2017). Improving the efficiency of care for pediatric patients hospitalized with asthma. *Hospital Pediatrics, 7*(1), 31–38. https://doi.org/10.1542/hpeds.2016-0108

Barzman, D., Mossman, D., Sonnier, L., & Sorter, M. (2012). Brief Rating of Aggression by Children and Adolescents (BRACHA): A reliability study. *The Journal of the American Academy of Psychiatry and the Law, 40*(3), 374–382.

Bekmezian, A., Chung, P. J., & Yazdani, S. (2009). Standardized admission order set improves perceived quality of pediatric inpatient care. *Journal of Hospital Medicine, 4*(2), 90–96.

Calzada, E. (2010). Bringing culture into parent training with latinos. *Cognitive and Behavioral Practice, 17*, 167–175.

Carter, B. D., Kronenberger, W. G., Baker, J., Grimes, L. M., Crabtree, V. M., Smith, C., & McGraw, K. (2003). Inpatient pediatric consultation-liaison: A case-controlled study. *Journal of Pediatric Psychology, 28*(6), 423–432. https://doi.org/10.1093/jpepsy/jsg032

Chaffin, M., Silovsky, J. F., Funderburk, B., Valle, L. A., Brestan, E. V., Balachova, T., … Bonner, B. L. (2004). Parent-child interaction therapy with physically abusive parents: Efficacy for reducing future abuse reports. *Journal of Consulting and Clinical Psychology, 72*(3), 500–510. https://doi.org/10.1037/0022-006X.72.3.500

Dayal, A., & Alvarez, F. (2015). The effect of implementation of standardized, evidence-based order sets on efficiency and quality measures for pediatric respiratory illnesses in a community hospital. *Hospital Pediatrics, 5*(12), 624–629. https://doi.org/10.1542/hpeds.2015-0140

Doupnik, S. K., Lawlor, J., Zima, B. T., Coker, T. R., Bardach, N. S., Hall, M., & Berry, J. G. (2016). Mental health conditions and medical and surgical hospital utilization. *Pediatrics, 138*(6), e20162416. https://doi.org/10.1542/peds.2016-2416

Epstein, R. A., Fonnesbeck, R., Potter, S., Rizzone, K. H., & McPheeters, M. (2015). Psychosocial interventions for child disruptive behaviors: A meta-analysis. *Pediatrics, 136*(5), 947–960.

Ernst, M. M. (2011). The coping club: a new user-generated resource for children with pain and other medical condition. *Pediatric Pain Letter, 13*(2), 20–23.

Gleason, M. M., Goldson, E., Yogman, M. W., & AAP Council on Early Childhood. (2016). Addressing early childhood emotional and behavioral problems. *Pediatrics, 138*(6), e20163025.

Guilfoyle, S. M., Follansbee-Junger, K., & Modi, A. C. (2013). Development and preliminary implementation of a psychosocial service into standard medical care for pediatric epilepsy. *Clinical Practice in Pediatric Psychology, 1*(3), 276–288.

Guttmann, A., Zagorski, B., Austin, P. C., Schull, M., Razzaq, A., To, T., & Anderson, G. (2007). Effectiveness of emergency department asthma management strategies on return visits in children: a population-based study. *Pediatrics, 120*(6), e1402–e1410.

Hook, J. N., Davis, D. E., Owen, J., Worthington, E. L., Jr., & Utsey, S. O. (2013). Cultural humility: Measuring openness to culturally diverse clients. *Journal of Counseling Psychology, 60*(3), 353–366. https://doi.org/10.1037/a0032595

Kassam-Adams, N., Schneider, S., & Kazak, A. (2018). *Health Care Toolbox*. Retrieved from http://www.Healthcaretoolbox.org

Kornenberger, W. G., Carter, B. D., & Thomas, D. (1997). Assessment of behavior problems in pediatric inpatient settings: Development of the pediatric inpatient behavior scale. *Children's Health Care, 26*, 211–232.

Lau, A. S., Fung, J. J., & Yung, V. (2010). Group parent training with immigrant Chinese families: Enhancing engagement and augmenting skills training. *Journal of Clinical Psychology, 66*, 880–894.

Lieberman, A. F., Ghosh Ippen, C., & Van Horn, P. (2015). *Don't hit my mommy! A manual for child-parent psychotherapy with young children exposed to violence and other trauma* (2nd ed.). Washington, DC: Zero to Three.

Loeber, R., Burke, J. D., Lahey, B. B., Winters, A., & Zera, M. (2000). Oppositional defiant and conduct disorder: A review of the past 10 years, part I. *Journal of the American Academy of Child and Adolescent Psychiatry, 39*(12), 1468–1484.

Lundahl, B., Riser, H. J., & Lovejoy, M. C. (2006). A meta-analysis of parent training: Moderators and follow-up effects. *Clinical Psychology Review, 26*, 86–104.

McDonald, H. P., Garg, A. X., & Haynes, R. B. (2002). Interventions to enhance patient adherence to medication prescriptions. *Scientific Review. Journal of the American Medical Association, 288*(22), 2868–2879. https://doi.org/10.1001/jama.288.22.2868

Modi, A. C., & Quittner, A. L. (2006). Barriers to treatment adherence for children with cystic fibrosis and asthma: What gets in the way? *Journal of Pediatric Psychology, 31*(8), 846–858. https://www.nctsn.org/what-is-child-trauma/about-child-trauma

Njoroge, W. F. M., Hostutler, C. A., Schwartz, B. S., & Mautone, J. A. (2016). Integrated behavioral health in primary care. *Current Psychiatry Reports, 18*, 106. https://doi.org/10.1007/s11920-016-0745-7

Palermo, T. M., Janicke, D. M., McQuaid, E. L., Mullins, L. L., Robins, P. M., & Wu, Y. P. (2014). Recommendations for training in pediatric psychology: Defining core competencies across training levels. *Journal of Pediatric Psychology, 39*(9), 965–984. https://doi.org/10.1093/jpepsy/jsu015

Price, J., Kassam-Adams, N., Alderfer, M. A., Christofferson, J., & Kazak, A. E. (2016). Systematic review: A reevaluation and update of the integrative (trajectory) model of pediatric medical traumatic stress. *Journal of Pediatric Psychology, 41*(1), 86–97.

Reid, M. J., Webster-Stratton, C., & Beauchaine, T. P. (2001). Parent training in head start: a comparison of program response among African American, Asian American, Caucasian, and Hispanic mothers. *Prevention Science, 2*(4), 209–227.

Reynolds, C. R., & Kamphaus, R. W. (2009). *Behavior Assessment System for Children—Second Edition (BASC-2): Progress Monitor (PM)*. Bloomington, MN: Pearson.

Saxe, G. N., Ellis, B. H., & Brown, A. D. (2015). The social environment and the service system: Traumatic stress responses are embedded in a social context. In *Trauma system therapy for children and teens* (2nd ed., pp. 64–81). New York, NY: The Guilford Press.

Skinner, B. F. (1937). Two types of conditioned reflex: a reply to Konorski and Miller. *Journal of General Psychology, 16*, 272–279.

Slifer, K. J., Babbitt, R. L., & Cataldo, M. D. (1995). Simulation and counterconditioning as adjuncts to pharmacotherapy for invasive pediatric procedures. *Journal of Development and Behavioral Pediatrics, 16*(3), 133–141. https://doi.org/10.1097/00004703-199506000-00001

Slifer, K. J., Cataldo, M. F., Cataldo, M. D., Llorente, A. M., & Gerson, A. C. (1993). Behavior analysis of motion control for pediatric neuroimaging. *Journal of Applied Behavior Analysis, 26*(4), 469–470.

Slifer, K. J., Eischen, S. E., Tucker, C. L., Dahlquist, L. M., Busby, S., Sulc, W., & Hilley, L. (2002). Behavioral treatment for child distress during repeated needle sticks. *Behavioural and Cognitive Psychotherapy, 30*(1), 57–68. https://doi.org/10.1017/S1352465802001066

Strauss, J., Olbrycht, P., & Woo, V. (2013). Behavioral health order sets in a hybrid information environment. *The Open Medical Informatics Journal, 7*, 30–33. https://doi.org/10.2174/1874431120130607002

Walsh, F. (2004). Family resilience: A framework for clinical practice. *Family Process, 42*, 1–18. https://doi.org/10.1111/j.1545-5300.2003.00001.x

Weisz, J. R., Sandler, I. N., Durlak, J. A., & Anton, B. S. (2005). Promoting and protecting youth mental health through evidence-based prevention and treatment. *American Psychologist, 60*(6), 628–648. https://doi.org/10.1037/0003-066X.60.6.628

Distressed Parents and Family Issues

Laura Judd-Glossy and Eileen Twohy

It is well established that caring for a child or adolescent with an acute or chronic illness is taxing for parents and family members. Medical hospitalization, particularly when it is prolonged, challenges even the most resilient of caregivers. The majority of families are able to manage this distress and maintain respectful and collaborative relationships with medical providers and staff. Occasionally, however, caregivers behave in a negative manner that interferes directly or indirectly with the relationship with the medical team, which can result in adverse outcomes. This chapter will review disruptive family behaviors that occur in pediatric medical settings, factors that contribute to these problematic behaviors, and strategies to address and prevent these behaviors, using the Strengthening Alliances with Families Team (SAFTeam) as a model (Judd-Glossy, Twohy, Penner, & Carubia, 2017).

L. Judd-Glossy (✉)
Departments of Psychiatry and Pediatric Surgery, University of Colorado School of Medicine, Aurora, CO, USA

Children's Hospital Colorado, Aurora, CO, USA
e-mail: Laura.Judd-Glossy@childrenscolorado.org

E. Twohy
Department of Psychiatry and Behavioral Medicine, University of Washington School of Medicine, Seattle, WA, USA

Seattle Children's Hospital, Seattle, WA, USA

Difficult Encounters with Family Members

There is a substantial literature describing "difficult patients," particularly in adult medicine (Hinchey & Jackson, 2011; Meadow, 1992). This literature tends to focus on the perceptions of physicians or other providers, without accounting for systemic factors that may help to explain "difficult" behavior. In this chapter, we choose to describe "disruptive behavior" or "difficult patient encounters," in the interest of taking a less pejorative stance toward patients and families (Fiester, 2012). However, the "difficult patient" literature does provide valuable information about the factors that may lead to disruption in relationships between families and healthcare providers.

"Difficult patients" are commonly defined as those who display relatively mild, but bothersome behavior (e.g., an expression of dissatisfaction or disagreement with a provider; Robiner & Petrik, 2017). Other mildly difficult behaviors include patients who require a greater than average amount of time with providers (Mack, Ilowite, & Taddei, 2017), who are frequently late to appointments (Breuner & Moreno, 2011), who have poor adherence to their medical regimen (Meltzer et al., 2009), or who are generally inflexible (Meadow, 1992). While these behaviors are not necessarily disrespectful or unsafe,

B. D. Carter, K. A. Kullgren (eds.), *Clinical Handbook of Psychological Consultation in Pediatric Medical Settings*, Issues in Clinical Child Psychology, https://doi.org/10.1007/978-3-030-35598-2_30

they can have a negative impact on patient care. For example, in a study of NICU providers in a medical simulation, a mildly rude comment made by a parent led to decreased performance by the medical team in regard to diagnosis and intervention and also hindered team communication and collaboration (Riskin et al., 2017).

At times, family behavior can rise to another level of disruption, including overt aggression toward staff and providers (Robiner & Petrik, 2017). This may be evidenced as verbal aggression (disrespectful language, name-calling, cursing, threats), stalking, or physical violence. It may also include unsafe behaviors that show a "blatant disregard for medical recommendations" (Robiner & Petrik, 2017, p. 29) such as making unauthorized changes to medical equipment. Phillips (2016) reported multiple incidents of extreme violence in the healthcare setting, with several providers being killed by current or former patients. While physical assault is relatively uncommon, aggressive behavior of any kind can have a detrimental effect on medical care. Providers who experience high levels of disruptive behavior in their patients may be at elevated risk for burnout, job dissatisfaction, decreased productivity, and decreased feelings of safety as compared to providers who have fewer disruptive patients (Phillips, 2016).

Studies have also examined short-term outcomes for "difficult" patients. Adult patients who were rated by medical providers as "difficult" were more likely to describe how their expectations for their medical visit were *not* met compared to patients who were not described as difficult (Hinchey & Jackson, 2011). The so-called "difficult" group also reported lower levels of trust and satisfaction in their providers and higher levels of stress in the previous week. Finally, these patients also noted worsening physical symptoms over the 2 weeks following their medical visit and had increased healthcare utilization over the next 6 months. In sum, the perception of being "difficult" is related to a negative healthcare experience for both patients and providers.

Identification

While it can be virtually impossible to consistently predict which patients and families may exhibit disruptive behavior, it is worth considering the risk factors that may relate to these behaviors. The Pediatric Psychosocial Preventative Health Model (PPPHM) presents a framework for evaluating the psychosocial needs of families in the setting of acute or chronic illnesses (Kazak, 2006). The PPPHM uses a social ecological framework to consider areas of both risk and resilience for pediatric patients and their families, dividing them into three categories based on these factors and corresponding psychosocial needs.

The universal category, which includes the majority of patients and their families, is comprised of families who are generally functioning in a healthy way and experiencing a normative level of stress regarding their child's acute or chronic illness (Kazak, 2006). Families in the universal category are considered to be resilient with satisfactory to excellent coping skills and do not typically require high levels of psychosocial support (Kazak, Schneider, Didonato, & Pai, 2015). The next category is the targeted group, which includes patients and families who may have psychosocial difficulties outside of their child's medical illness that increase their risk for maladaptive coping. Targeted families may display acute distress and often benefit from evidenced-based treatment (e.g., cognitive-behavioral therapy; Kazak et al., 2015). Finally, the families at highest risk are considered the clinical/treatment group. This group has the most significant risk factors and may display increasing levels of distress across illness or hospitalization. The clinical/treatment group is often comprised of the smallest number of families, and also typically requires the highest level of resources and supports (Kazak, 2006). When considering families across these three levels of psychosocial risk and need, families in the clinical/treatment group are expected to be at the highest risk for displaying challenging and disruptive behavior.

Risk Factors

Risk factors for high levels of distress and disruptive behavior can be broken down into three subsets: patient and family factors, provider factors, and larger systemic factors.

Patient and Family Factors Parenting a child with an acute or chronic illness impacts the psychosocial functioning of caregivers. In their systemic review of parenting stress across many pediatric chronic illnesses, Cousino and Hazen (2013) found that parents of children with chronic illness experienced more parenting stress than parents of healthy children. A patient's functional status constitutes another important risk factor. In a study of parents with babies in the NICU, mothers of young children who had lower functioning, as evidenced by fewer age-appropriate behaviors, experienced poorer family adjustment in comparison to mothers of children with higher functioning (Rodrigues & Patterson, 2007). Similarly, patients who were medically complex, had little chance of recovery, and had experienced multiple failures in treatment were at elevated risk for being part of "difficult patient encounters" as defined by their medical providers (Robiner & Petrik, 2017). In addition, patients who presented with more than five somatic concerns were more commonly described as challenging than those who had no or fewer somatic symptoms (Breuner & Moreno, 2011).

From a psychosocial standpoint, parents with mental health disorders, including anxiety, were more often labeled as difficult or challenging by their child's pediatric provider (Meadow, 1992). This is consistent with the adult literature, which has found that mental health concerns, including depression and anxiety, were a strong contributor to being identified as difficult (Hinchey & Jackson, 2011). Family disagreement, including parental criticism of children, also increased the perception of a family being difficult (Meadow, 1992). Other family factors that may contribute to increased risk for psychosocial problems include households headed by single or minor parents, families with limited social or financial supports, or siblings with behavioral concerns (Kazak, 2006).

Provider Factors Medical providers and staff play an important role in supporting a family's ability to cope with challenging situations and, conversely, provider characteristics and practices can also play a role in family's disruptive behavior. Within pediatric medicine, few studies have examined the role of pediatric providers in difficult patient or family encounters. Meltzer et al. (2009) found that nurses and physicians who perceived pediatric patients and families to be "difficult" were more likely to engage in "distancing behaviors," including referring patients to psychosocial professionals. Similarly, in a study of pediatric oncologists and parents in which both groups rated the level of difficulty in the provider/family relationship, difficulties with "communication and understanding" were identified as a primary concern in difficult relationships (Mack et al., 2017, p. 677). Parents in the study noted that their trust in their child's provider was negatively impacted when they did not feel that the provider understood their concerns or communicated with them well (Mack et al., 2017).

The adult treatment literature has also examined physician-related factors that contribute to the description of patients as "difficult." Physicians who scored lower on the Physician Beliefs Scale, a measure of attitudes about the psychosocial aspects of patient care that has been associated with communication skills and time spent discussing psychosocial concerns, were more likely to experience patient encounters as "difficult" (Jackson & Kroenke, 1999). Other factors include physicians who own mental health and experience of stress (Krebs, Garrett, & Konrad, 2006), the quantity of hours that they worked (Krebs et al., 2006), and the percentage of patients with psychiatric or substance abuse concerns (Krebs et al., 2006). The level of experience also had an effect, as doctors with fewer than 10 years of experience rated 23% of their patient encounters as difficult, whereas providers with more than 20 years of experience rated only 2% of encounters as difficult (Hinchey & Jackson,

2011). Finally, patients who present with greater diagnostic uncertainty are more likely to be identified by their providers as difficult, which may be a reflection of the provider's decreased confidence in treating certain diagnoses (Breuner & Moreno, 2011).

System Factors Hospitals and medical clinics have their own unique culture that may contribute to a family's level of distress and difficulty. For example, families may experience frequent changes in the leadership of their child's medical team and feel that they have limited time to speak with their providers, given weekly rotations for many attendings, increasing expectations for productivity and billing, as well as overall high staffing levels (Breuner & Moreno, 2011; Meltzer et al., 2009). This lack of continuity of care was identified as a factor in difficult provider/parent relationships, as described by both pediatric oncology providers and parents (Mack et al., 2017). In addition, the more specialists there are involved with a patient and family, the more opportunities there are for miscommunication and confusion (Steinmiller & Ely, 2015). Thus, for families of pediatric patients with chronic illnesses requiring lengthy hospital stays, many opportunities for miscommunication and lack of continuity exist, which can contribute to the family's level of distress and maladaptive coping.

The SAFTeam

One model for addressing disruptive family behavior in the medical setting is the SAFTeam (Strengthening Alliances with Families Team), a multidisciplinary approach to providing evaluation and support in response to challenging interactions among healthcare providers, patients, and families. The SAFTeam model was developed in 2009 as an innovative service implemented by the consultation-liaison (CL) psychiatry team in a large pediatric hospital. It is built on a commitment to professionalism, sensitivity, interdisciplinary respect, and effective communication. The model assumes that (1) effective communication between providers and families is essential for quality care, (2) communication becomes more challenging when families are perceived to be "difficult," and, therefore, (3) interventions that improve communication, support the medical team and family, and address complex patient/family dynamics are necessary in order to optimize family-centered care. The SAFTeam is intended not only to improve care to patients and families but also to support team members and prevent burnout.

SAFTeam consultation requests are made by the primary medical or surgical team and are managed and implemented by the CL team. In the electronic health record (EHR) consultation request, teams identify the reason for their concern. Commonly selected reasons for the consultation include "disrespectful interpersonal behavior," "unreasonable demands," and "obstructions to care." During the first call from the requesting team, it is determined whether a SAFTeam meeting is needed immediately or if the team should first undertake recommended preliminary steps. These first steps include direct communication to the family by the primary medical attending, social worker, and/or the charge nurse to address the concern, with an emphasis on empathy and validation. Often, direct and caring communication is enough to diffuse the need for any further action. If these steps have already been taken and disruptive family behavior continues or escalates, a SAFTeam meeting is scheduled by an administrative assistant assigned to the consulting medical team as soon as possible, typically within 24–48 h of the consult request. While it can be challenging for all team members to attend on such short notice, we have had success with rapidly gathering core members of the team. This likely reflects the value placed on the SAFTeam process.

The SAFTeam meeting is facilitated by a member of the CL team and comprised of a multidisciplinary group of team members. Other attendees include members of the risk management team (hospital body tasked with identifying and mitigating risk), social work, physician members of the primary medical or surgery teams including the attending and treating interns or residents, the nursing unit manager, primary care team members including charge and/or bedside nurses, patient representative, and any other team members involved in the issue to be discussed. Depending on the concern, a member of the ethics team may be invited to attend. Patients and family members are not present during SAFTeam meetings, which are intended to serve a different function than care conferences, where family members are included. Our experience is that the absence of family members during SAFTeam meetings allows for team members to be open, receive support, and develop consensus around a unified plan.

SAFTeam meetings are typically 60 min in duration. The patient's medical presentation, treatment course, and current clinical status are briefly introduced by a member of the medical team (often a resident), followed by a discussion of any concerning family behavior and/or obstructions to care. The SAFTeam representative facilitates the development of recommendations for how to respond to this behavior and a clear plan for how to proceed. This plan typically includes identification of both care team responsibilities and family responsibilities. If needed, a behavior contract for family member behavior is drafted, often with the assistance of the risk management team. Perhaps most importantly, decisions are made during the SAFTeam meeting about which team members will communicate with the family about the plan for behavioral expectations and when this communication will occur. This conversation is often facilitated by the primary attending physician and the team social worker, sometimes with the assistance of a member of the risk management team. However, other team members may be identified as more appropriate, particularly if they have developed a therapeutic relationship with the family.

The SAFTeam consultant who facilitates the meeting is typically not involved in meeting directly with family members, taking only a "behind the scenes" role. If a member of our team is already involved with the case, an alternate member takes on the SAFTeam role. She or he documents the SAFTeam meeting in the EHR, with emphasis on the specific recommendations generated during the meeting. In the days and weeks following the meeting, the SAFTeam consultant follows up with the primary team about implementation of recommendations and any need for follow-up meetings. More than half of SAFTeam consult requests are resolved after one meeting, with the vast majority requiring two or fewer meetings.

SAFTeam Case Example

Jon is a three-month-old ex-32-week biracial male with a complex medical history, including congenital heart disease, who was transferred to the NICU shortly after birth. Maternal history was notable for limited prenatal care and use of marijuana during pregnancy. Jon initially benefitted from respiratory support, but was weaned to room air after several weeks. He also experienced difficulties with oral feeds and benefitted from nasogastric supplementation.

Social Background Jon was born to unmarried partners who had been together for several years. The couple had several previous pregnancies that all ended in miscarriages. The NICU social worker noted concerns for parents' mental health and substance abuse in her initial psychosocial assessment, including postpartum depression. Parents also indicated concerns that their home environment was unstable and unsafe for a medically complex child.

Hospital Course During Jon's hospitalization, his parents were able to secure a room at a local Ronald McDonald House. However, it was challenging for them to come to the bedside regularly due to the mother's recovery from labor and depressed mood. Given concerns about perinatal substance use, a report was made to child protective services. Within 2 weeks of Jon's birth and hospitalization, staff reported concerns about the mother's behavior, as she was reportedly labile and verbally aggressive toward staff. In addition, both parents were observed to be frequently sleeping and inattentive to the patient's needs during the brief periods that they were at bedside.

Shortly after Jon's birth, his parents were out of state for nearly 8 weeks and had little communication with the medical team during this time. Jon was reportedly improving and nearing readiness for discharge.

Reason for Consult The SAFTeam consult was called due to concerns about multiple incidents of parental verbal aggression observed on hospital grounds. During the initial consult call, the medical team described their concerns (Jon's parents had been overheard yelling at one another in a hospital sleep room). The mother reportedly also yelled at a bedside nurse and made negative comments about the quality of care that her child was receiving, stating, "he would be better off at another hospital where people care about kids," and physically posturing in a way that made the nurse feel threatened. NICU staff provided parents with the hospital's written behavioral expectations and notified them that they could be asked to leave if behavioral expectations were violated. Two days later, hospital security observed parents again yelling at one another on hospital grounds. Given multiple incidents of disruptive behavior, they were asked to leave by staff and security and were informed that they could not return to bedside until they participated in a meeting to review behavioral expectations with hospital personnel. The medical team stated that they were unsure how to proceed. While they did not feel it was fair to keep Jon and his parents separated, they were also worried about staff and safety. Several primary nurses had already asked not to work with Jon due to the stress they experienced when interacting with his parents.

SAFTeam Meeting The SAFTeam meeting was held to address these concerns. Participants included the NICU floor leadership, medical attending, charge nurse, bedside nurse, social worker, risk management representative, patient advocate, and psychologist (acting in the SAFTeam facilitator role). NICU providers and staff presented Jon's medical and psychosocial history. They reviewed concerns regarding parents' disruptive behavior as well as their limited and inconsistent engagement with the patient. Nursing shared concerns about caring for Jon, given yelling and negative comments made by his mother. The group discussed concerns about the parents' level of stress, mother's possible untreated postpartum depression, and the family's apparent lack of social support. Psychosocial team members provided options for connecting the family to resources, including potential psychotherapeutic support for Jon's mother.

The decision was made by the group for NICU leadership, social worker, and hospital security to meet with parents to discuss a behavioral contract. This contract specified that parents could only be at bedside certain days of the week for a designed period of time, to ensure that there would be adequate providers and staff on the floor to address any concerning behavior. In addition, it specified that any inappropriate or aggressive behavior could result in further restrictions to visitation. Other recommendations to the team included reemphasizing that the hospital has zero tolerance for disrespectful or aggressive behavior, recommending that nursing staff enter the room in pairs to increase comfort, and instructing staff to immediately speak with their supervisor if they felt threatened by parents. Finally, staff members were encouraged to document concerning behavior in an objective manner in the EHR.

Following the SAFTeam meeting, a meeting was held with parents, NICU social worker, and floor manager to review the behavioral contract. Security was notified of the meeting and was available nearby in preparation for any behavioral escalation. Parents were respectful in the meeting and voiced their understanding of the current limitations to their visits. The social worker facilitated a conversation about the parents' understandable stress and the recommendation that they may benefit from additional sources of support. The SAFTeam consultant (CL psychologist) followed up with the NICU social worker several times in the week following the meeting to discuss progress and determine if additional SAFTeam meetings needed to be held. In this case, given that parents were respectful during the meeting and were observed by nursing to be appropriate at bedside, the decision was made by NICU social worker to discontinue formal SAFTeam supports. However, the NICU team was aware that they could follow up with the SAFTeam at any time with additional concerns.

General Recommendations

Implementation of the SAFTeam over nearly a decade has revealed a number of effective strategies for responding to challenging family member behavior. While a formal SAFTeam does not exist in all settings, these strategies can be applied broadly to consulting psychologists and multidisciplinary teams in various settings.

1. **Engage a multidisciplinary team.** One of the most effective elements of this approach to responding to challenging family behavior is likely its engagement of multiple disciplines. It is not uncommon for the team to extend beyond those providing patient care. Risk management is regularly involved, and additional participants can include partners from disciplines such as security, patient relations, and ethics. These varied perspectives enrich the creative problem-solving process, and meeting together allows for the establishment of consistent messaging to the family.
2. **Maintain safety.** It should go without saying that employees have the right to feel safe at work. Healthcare workers are, however, at increased risk for workplace violence compared to workers in other settings (Phillips, 2016). Frontline staff members should often be reminded by leaders of their right to feel safe and of the hospital's commitment to zero tolerance for violence in the workplace. Thus, team members are "given permission" to address concerns about their personal safety and teams are guided in taking practical steps to maintain a safe environment. For example, a security guard may be placed nearby during a meeting in which there is any expectation that family member behavior might escalate. These interventions are especially recommended in light of evidence that support from supervisors protects against harassment and violence in the workplace (Phillips, 2016).
3. **Hold families accountable.** A common theme in this approach is a discussion about behavioral expectations for family members. Although written behavioral expectation documents are generally available in healthcare organizations, providers and staff do not necessarily receive instruction in how to respond to behavior that departs from these expectations. Further, individuals working in pediatric healthcare settings may be more likely to tolerate misbehavior. This may result from compassion for the patient who is not responsible for family behavior, empathy for the plight of distressed families, and/or a tendency to overfocus on families' rights as compared to families' responsibilities (Robiner & Petrik, 2017). Ethics experts note that both providers and patients/families are obligated to cooperate in the interest of carrying out an agreed-upon treatment plan (Center for Practical Bioethics Ethics Committee Consortium, 2000). Although repairing blocks to the therapeutic relationship is prioritized, it is also considered appropriate for providers to transfer care if a therapeutic relationship cannot be reestablished (Center for Practical Bioethics Ethics Committee Consortium, 2000).
4. **Maintain the standard of care.** Risk management professionals participating in these multidisciplinary meetings can regularly remind the team of the importance of maintaining a consistent standard of care. Adjusting this standard to accommodate a family member's disruptive behavior (e.g., changing a medication schedule to decrease staff interaction with an aggressive parent) or tolerating behavior that impedes team members' ability to provide care (e.g., a family member whose yelling negatively affects a nurse's concentration) is inappropriate patient care and increases legal risk.
5. **Objectively document**. Team members should *objectively* document any concerning

family member behavior, including direct quotes of inappropriate language. Clear, objective documentation of behavior can be used to justify needed interventions, such as establishment of a behavioral contract or removal of family members from the hospital.

6. **Emphasize family strengths and protective factors.** It is natural for team members who are dealing with disruptive family behavior to lose sight of the strengths and protective factors that are present in all families. Meeting as a team to discuss and implement solutions can allow for a shift in perspective that includes recognition of the family's strengths. Even simply reestablishing that the healthcare team and the family "are here for the same reason" (i.e., the well-being of the child) can be enough to redirect team members who find themselves in a deficit-focused perspective.
7. **Increase psychosocial support.** The calling together of a multidisciplinary team can serve to increase psychosocial support for families, both by identifying resources that may be beneficial and by assisting providers in learning how to have challenging conversations about disruptive behavior. Psychosocial team members may recommend phrases or approaches drawn from their specialized behavioral training that attending physicians, residents, and other team members can utilize when communicating with parents.
8. **Empower team members.** A current that runs under many, if not all, of the recommendations listed above is the empowerment of team members. Rather than directly addressing problematic family behavior, facilitators can assist the team in developing a clear plan of action that the *team* implements. Individual team members are empowered to take action as needed in order to ensure workplace safety and maintain the standard of care. These actions include having a low threshold for asking family members to step out of the room and/or calling security if family member behavior interferes with staff safety or patient care. While setting these limits may feel inconsistent with our role as caring professionals, it is at times necessary in order to keep patients, team members, and families safe.

A Proactive Approach

In addition to developing and implementing effective strategies for responding to disruptive behavior by family members, teams are encouraged to also consider prevention. While it is not expected that all disruptive family behavior can be prevented, the incidence of such behavior—and the extent to which it disrupts—may be reduced in systems that take a proactive approach. Psychologists and other psychosocial providers play a critical role in developing a hospital culture that promotes healthy family involvement in pediatric care. The following sections provide specific, proactive recommendations that can be expected to reduce the likelihood of disruptive family behavior and/or assist teams in managing such behavior.

Normalize the Experience A first step in the proactive approach to working with distressed family members is to normalize this experience, both for clinicians and for families. As reviewed in the first section of the chapter, pediatric hospitalization is, in itself, a distressing event. Fiester (2012) warns against pathologizing the "difficult" patient, noting that some of the behaviors often attributed to the presence of a psychiatric disorder in the "difficult" patient encounter (e.g., hostility, anger, depression, anxiety, noncompliance) can also be considered normative responses to stress. Educational programs for medical providers and other team members ought to prepare clinicians for the inevitability of working with patients and families who demonstrate challenging behaviors and/or with whom the clinician feels ineffective (Robiner & Petrik, 2017). While psychologists, social workers, and other psychosocial professionals play a crucial role, "psychosocial concerns" should not be relegated to these professionals alone. Psychologists and other psychosocial providers may assist where there are educational gaps, both via formal teaching opportunities and as members of integrated medical teams.

Focus on the relationship(s) Also crucial to the proactive approach is to frame any disruption that may arise as a symptom of the relationship, rather than a problem that is rooted in the family. As reviewed earlier, a fairly robust literature delineates the characteristics and management of the "difficult" patient or parent (e.g., Hinchey & Jackson, 2011). Teams are encouraged to shift from focusing on the "difficult patient" to recognizing the challenges that exist within the relationship (Blackall & Green, 2012). The term "relationship-centered care" describes a framework for recognizing the value and importance of relationships across all areas of healthcare, including between clinician and patient, among clinicians, and between the clinician and the community at large (Beach, Inui, and Relationship-Centered Care Research Network, 2006). In pediatric medicine, the relationship is almost always more complex than the patient-physician dyad, necessarily including parents and other family members.

Reframe the Behavior "Difficult" behavior can be reframed as a skills deficit or a coping strategy, rather than as noncompliance (Dudzinski & Alvarez, 2017). For example, a family member who is yelling may lack the skill to communicate during stressful events, and a caregiver who is absent from the bedside of a sick child may be attempting to cope with distressing emotions through avoidance. Recognizing skills deficits and/or misguided attempts to cope can increase team member empathy (Dudzinski & Alvarez, 2017). Likewise, communicating awareness of a patient's or family's strengths or competencies can aid in relationship building (Blackall & Green, 2012). Kazak articulates an approach in which "behaviors of family members are viewed as well-intentioned efforts to solve problems, and interventions are directed toward channeling the energy of the system toward new solutions to challenging situations" (Kazak, Simms, & Rourke, 2002; p. 140).

Challenge the Traditional Medical Model Clinicians working in a pediatric hospital environment are encouraged to consider the ways in which the traditional medical model may lend itself to relationship challenges with parents. Adult patients have described discomfort participating in shared decision-making with their physicians for multiple reasons, including fear of being considered "difficult" and hesitation about challenging the authority of the physician (Frosch, May, Rendle, Tietbohl, & Elwyn, 2012). This power dynamic is further complicated in pediatric decision-making, where team members provide medical expertise, but the parent or caregiver should generally be considered the unequivocal authority on her or his individual child (Kazak et al., 2002). Traditional biomedical, physician-centered interviewing strategies have been challenged in the rise of patient-centered and family-centered care, with a shift toward less interrupting and more open-ended collection of information (Barrier, Li, & Jensen, 2003). Robiner and Petrik (2017) describe how psychologists, who utilize a biopsychosocial rather than a biomedical approach to conceptualization and intervention, can play an important role in assisting traditional medical systems to become more family-centered and relationship-focused.

Build Regular Opportunities for Consultation Built-in opportunities for consultation and team debriefing may also reduce the need for a reactive response such as the SAFTeam. Two observations from SAFTeam facilitators support this hypothesis. First, the SAFTeam seems to work very effectively when it is requested early, before behavior has escalated to the point that a reactive response is necessary. A second observation is that one of the key elements of the SAFTeam process seems to be the opportunity for team members to express grievances and concerns and to receive support. Clinicians who experience challenging encounters with family members benefit from support and consultation by colleagues, and regular opportunities for debriefing may allow for behavior concerns to be proactively addressed before they escalate.

Diversity and Healthcare Disparities

Culture and diversity must be considered in discussions about how to care for and communicate with families in the healthcare setting. Racial and ethnic disparities exist in healthcare and affect treatment decisions (e.g., Nelson, 2002). Children with special healthcare needs who are Latino, African American, or live in households with a non-English primary language were found to have lower odds of receiving family-centered care (e.g., providers spending enough time, listening carefully, being sensitive to family's values and customs) as compared to nonminority peers (Coker et al., 2010). Compared with white parents, black and Hispanic parents of children with special healthcare needs are more likely to be dissatisfied with healthcare and to experience difficulties related to ease of service use (Ngui & Flores, 2006).

Members of care teams must carefully attend to ways in which bias may impact clinician behavior and perceptions of family member behavior. In a 1992 English study of physicians' views on "difficult and unlikable parents," being from the Indian subcontinent was endorsed by two thirds of physicians as a difficult or unlikeable characteristic, reportedly due to the lack of availability of interpreters (Meadow, 1992). One of 31 factors identified as challenging or complicating pediatric medical care in a tertiary hospital setting was "language/cultural differences that impede discharge and/or plan of care" (Steinmiller & Ely, 2015). Valenzuela and Smith (2016) found that families experience multiple disparities during interactions with healthcare providers, including feeling less understood, spending less time, receiving less information, hearing fewer partnership-building statements, and hearing more about certain topics (e.g., violence, smoking, drug use) as compared to nonminority youth.

It is not known what role diversity factors play in the incidence of disruptive family behavior nor in what ways family behavior in the pediatric medical setting may vary across groups. However, it is crucial to understand that minority families experience disparities in healthcare outcomes. Consistent with our general recommendations related to focusing on relationships and understanding the function of family member behavior, teams are encouraged to learn about families' health beliefs and practices (Flores, 2000). This is a recommended practice with *all* families, and it is especially critical when working with families whose culture differs from the majority group and/or the treating clinicians. The Cultural Formulation Interview from the *Diagnostic and Statistical Manual of Mental Disorders* (American Psychiatric Association, 2013) includes open-ended questions that can help to elicit information about family members' understandings of illness, health, and treatment. Practical steps toward reducing racial and ethnic disparities in healthcare include diversifying the workforce of medical professionals, improvement of interpreter services, availability of language-appropriate health education materials, and cross-cultural education for team members (Betancourt, Green, Carrillo, & Owusu Ananeh-Firempong, 2016).

Conclusion

While the majority of patients and families coping with pediatric hospitalization manage their distress in an adaptive manner and maintain respectful relationships with their medical teams, situations do arise in which family members interfere with care or exhibit disruptive behavior. These behaviors clearly impact patient care as well as the relationship between the family and the medical providers. Few models for addressing disruptive family member behavior are described in the literature. The SAFTeam is an example of a collaborative approach to provide evaluation and support in response to challenging and disruptive behaviors in one large pediatric hospital. It is recommended that clinicians discuss and document strategies that may have been developed in other pediatric settings, in order to improve currently available tools. In addition, formal investigation into both preventive and reactive models for addressing challenging family behavior in the pediatric setting is needed.

Acknowledgments We would like to acknowledge Jenny Reese, MD, and Harrison Levine, MD, who first developed the SAFTeam model at Children's Hospital Colorado in 2009.

References

American Psychiatric Association. (2013). *Diagnostic and statistical manual of mental disorders* (5th ed.). Washington, DC: American Psychiatric Association.

Barrier, P. A., Li, J. T. C., & Jensen, N. M. (2003). Two words to improve physician-patient communication: What else? *Mayo Clinic Proceedings, 78*(2), 211–214.

Beach, M. C., Inui, T., & Relationship-Centered Care Research Network. (2006). Relationship-centered care: A constructive reframing. *Journal of General Internal Medicine, 21*(1), S3–S8.

Betancourt, J. R., Green, A. R., Carrillo, J. E., & Owusu Ananeh-Firempong, I. I. (2016). Defining cultural competence: A practical framework for addressing racial/ethnic disparities in health and healthcare. *Public Health Reports, 118*(4), 293–302.

Blackall, G. F., & Green, M. J. (2012). "Difficult" patients or difficult relationships? *The American Journal of Bioethics, 12*(5), 8–9.

Breuner, C. C., & Moreno, M. A. (2011). Approaches to the difficult patient/parent encounter. *Pediatrics, 127*(1), 163–169.

Center for Practical Bioethics Ethics Committee Consortium. (2000). *Guidelines for providing ethical care in difficult provider-patient relationships*. Kansas City: Kansas City Area Ethics Committee Consortium.

Coker, T. R., Rodriquez, M. A., & Flores, G. (2010). Family-centered care for US children with special health care needs: Who gets it and why? *Pediatrics, 125*(6), 1159–1167.

Cousino, M. K., & Hazen, R. A. (2013). Parenting stress among caregivers of children with chronic illness: A systematic review. *Journal of Pediatric Psychology, 38*(8), 809–828.

Dudzinski, D. M., & Alvarez, C. (2017). Repairing "difficult" patient-clinician relationships. *AMA Journal of Ethics, 19*(4), 364–368.

Fiester, A. (2012). The "difficult" patient reconceived: An expanded moral mandate for clinical ethics. *The American Journal of Bioethics, 12*(5), 2–7.

Flores, G. (2000). Culture and the patient-physician relationship: Achieving cultural competency in health care. *Pediatrics, 136*(1), 14–23.

Frosch, D. L., May, S. G., Rendle, K. A., Tietbohl, C., & Elwyn, G. (2012). Authoritarian physicians and patients' fear of being labeled 'difficult' among key obstacles to shared decision making. *Health Affairs, 31*(5), 1030–1038.

Hinchey, S. A., & Jackson, J. L. (2011). A cohort study assessing difficult patient encounters in a walk-in primary care clinic, predictors and outcomes. *Journal of General Internal Medicine, 26*(6), 588–594.

Jackson, J. L., & Kroenke, K. (1999). Difficult patient encounters in the ambulatory clinic: Clinical predictors and outcomes. *Archives of Internal Medicine, 159*(10), 1069–1075.

Judd-Glossy, L., Twohy, E., Penner, A., & Carubia, B. (2017, April). SAFTeam*: An innovative consultation model to support family-centered care in challenging patient/provider relationships*. Poster presented at the annual conference of the Society of Pediatric Psychology.

Kazak, A. E. (2006). Pediatric Psychosocial Preventative Health Model (PPPHM): Research, practice, and collaboration in pediatric family systems medicine. *Families, Systems & Health, 24*(4), 381.

Kazak, A. E., Schneider, S., Didonato, S., & Pai, A. L. H. (2015). Family psychosocial risk screening guided by the Pediatric Psychosocial Preventative Health Model (PPPHM) using the Psychosocial Assessment Tool (PAT). *Acta Oncologica, 54*(5), 574–580.

Kazak, A. E., Simms, S., & Rourke, M. T. (2002). Family systems practice in pediatric psychology. *Journal of Pediatric Psychology, 27*(2), 133–143.

Krebs, E. E., Garrett, J. M., & Konrad, T. R. (2006). The difficult doctor? Characteristics of physicians who report frustration with patients: An analysis of survey data. *BMC Health Services Research, 6*, 128.

Mack, J. W., Ilowite, M., & Taddei, S. (2017). Difficult relationships between parents and physicians of children with cancer: A qualitative study of parent and physician perspectives. *Cancer, 123*(4), 675–681.

Meadow, R. (1992). Difficult and unlikeable parents. *Archives of Disease in Childhood, 67*(6), 697–702.

Meltzer, L. J., Steinmiller, E., Simms, S., Grossman, M., Li, Y., & Team, T. C. C. C. (2009). Staff engagement during complex pediatric medical care: The role of patient, family, and treatment variables. *Patient Education and Counseling, 74*(1), 77–83.

Nelson, A. (2002). Unequal treatment: Confronting racial and ethnic disparities in health care. *Journal of the National Medical Association, 94*(8), 666.

Ngui, E. M. & Flores, G. (2006). Satisfaction with care and ease of using health care services among parents of children with special health care needs: The roles of race/ethnicity, insurance, language, and adequacy of family-centered care. *Pediatrics, 117*(4), 1184–1196.

Phillips, J. P. (2016). Workplace violence against health care workers in the United States. *The New England Journal of Medicine, 374*(17), 1661–1669.

Riskin, A., Erez, A., Foulk, T. A., Riskin-Geuz, K. S., Ziv, A., Sela, R., … Bamberger, P. A. (2017). Rudeness and medical team performance. *Pediatrics, 139*(2), 1–11.

Robiner, W. N., & Petrik, M. L. (2017). Managing difficult patients: Roles of psychologists in the age of interdisciplinary care. *Journal of Clinical Psychology in Medical Settings, 24*(1), 27–36.

Rodrigues, N., & Patterson, J. M. (2007). Impact of severity of a child's chronic condition on the functioning of two-parent families. *Journal of Pediatric Psychology, 32*(4), 417–426.

Steinmiller, E. A., & Ely, E. (2015). Patient, family, and provider complex care situations in pediatric acute medical care: Creation of the Red Flags Situation Assessment Tool. *Journal for Specialists in Pediatric Nursing, 20*(4), 290–297.

Valenzuela, J. M., & Smith, L. (2016). Topical review: Provider–patient interactions: An important consideration for racial/ethnic health disparities in youth. *Journal of Pediatric Psychology, 41*(4), 473–480.

Psychiatric Emergencies: Self-Harm, Suicidal, Homicidal Behavior, Addiction, and Substance use

Simona Bujoreanu, Sara Golden Pell, and Monique Ribeiro

Psychiatric Emergencies

An emergency involves an immediate danger of harm to one or more people (self-induced or based on a threat to the person's life or development) for which an acute intervention is required. Defining psychiatric emergency depends on whose perspective is taken into consideration. For example, one outpatient medical provider might perceive treatment nonadherence as a psychiatric emergency (passive suicidality), while another provider might see the same behavior as developmentally within the realm of adolescent poor decision-making. As psychologists in medical settings, it is very likely that medical providers will turn to our expertise to assess, intervene, and manage acute or perceived psychiatric emergencies. In receiving a request for consultation, it is important that psychologists differentiate right away between the "urgency" and "emergency" of the consultation question, by considering the continuum of psychiatric acuity. At one end, a youth reporting fleeting thoughts of death, a nurse noticing healed scars on the forearm, a teenager reporting smoking marijuana, etc., constitute urgent psychiatric concerns, while at the other end of the spectrum, behaviors such as an agitated youth throwing things in the clinic waiting room, a youth reporting suicidal ideation and plan during medical admission, or a noticeable altered mental status due to substance ingestion, all constitute psychiatric emergencies. This chapter will address cross-cutting issues of diagnostic assessment and management of acute safety concerns and other psychiatric emergencies, as well as intervention and treatment recommendations across outpatient (specialty and primary care clinics) and inpatient medical settings.

Diagnosis and Medical Basis

Pursuing a detailed diagnostic evaluation, as the acute situation affords, can allow psychologists to reach a conclusion about the current psychiatric diagnoses. Ensuring diagnostic clarity allows the psychologist to put forth a hypothesis about the reasons for the presentation, creates a basis for intervention and alliance building with the youth and family, and can lead to the appropriate treatments and disposition planning.

Differential diagnosis is the process by which clinicians consider the given symptom presentation across the spectrum of competing, although not mutually exclusive psychiatric systems before choosing a single diagnosis that best explains the given presentation (First, 2017). For example, a symptom such as acute decline in

S. Bujoreanu (✉) · S. G. Pell · M. Ribeiro
Boston Children's Hospital, Boston, MA, USA

Department of Psychiatry, Harvard Medical School, Boston, MA, USA
e-mail: Simona.Bujoreanu@childrens.harvard.edu

B. D. Carter, K. A. Kullgren (eds.), *Clinical Handbook of Psychological Consultation in Pediatric Medical Settings*, Issues in Clinical Child Psychology, https://doi.org/10.1007/978-3-030-35598-2_31

mood and associated irritability can be due to depression, social anxiety, trauma, psychosis, or substance use.

Several aspects are important to consider in the process of diagnostic interview such as the availability of information from the youth/family/collateral sources. Clinicians rely on a collaborative, honest communication about the nature or severity of the symptoms with the youth/family/collateral sources. In addition, the ability to observe the youth in the acute situation and understand the context leading to or perpetuating the psychiatric emergency can provide equally valuable information. Finally, it is important to integrate developmental factors and cultural perspectives in establishing the presence or absence of a mental disorder. Especially for psychologists working with youth with medical conditions, it is important to be alert in the differential diagnosis process to the potential that what might appear to be at face value a psychiatric emergency (e.g., agitation or behavioral dysregulation) can be better explained at times by physiological conditions (the presence of a medication impacting the central nervous system or direct effects of a general medical condition). In the context of working with medically involved youth, it is important to think of a psychiatric emergency both as a "casual comorbidity" in which the psychiatric presentation is a direct result of physical illness and can have impact on the course or severity of the physical illness and as a "coincidental comorbidity" in instances in which psychiatric presentations are not related with physiological conditions (Shaw & DeMaso, 2010). Therefore, close collaboration with medical colleagues and clear communication about psychiatric impressions, diagnoses, and formulation can guide the best next clinical steps and management of an emergency in the medical setting.

Agitation

Agitation is an acute behavioral emergency (heightened state of anxiety, emotional arousal, and/or increased motor and/or verbal activity) requiring immediate intervention to control symptoms and decrease the risk of injury to self or others. Actual causes for agitation are hard to identify especially in the crisis moment; hence the differential diagnoses for agitated behaviors should be broad and should include several factors, more often than not in combination: preexisting psychiatric disorders (e.g., attention deficit/hyperactivity symptoms, oppositional and defiant behaviors, conduct concerns, autism-related struggles, intellectual disabilities, etc.), new psychiatric developments (e.g., mania, anxiety, psychosis, trauma), psychosocial concerns (e.g., child protective concerns, acute on chronic lack of access to mental health treatment, academic stressors, etc.), and medical issues (e.g., intoxication, substance withdrawal, delirium, organic brain syndromes, pain, sensory concerns, infectious or metabolic processes, etc.). Attempts to determine the underlying cause of the agitation should be made, nevertheless, as they often guide treatment choices (Chun et al., 2016). The sheer fact of being in a medical setting (clinic, emergency room, hospital room, procedure unit) could be the trigger for agitation even in youth without any identifiable risk factors, as these environments are stimulating, unpredictable, and taxing to psychological and physiological resources of youth and their caregivers (e.g., fear, pain, fatigue, discomfort, novelty, hunger, etc.).

Psychologists should collaborate with physicians to ensure that an appropriate examination has taken place as it can provide important information with regard to potential triggers for the agitation especially for youth who do not have a history of agitation at baseline and/or have intellectual disabilities or autism spectrum disorder diagnoses. For instance, an assessment of the gait, pupil size, general appearance, and a review of recent vital signs can provide important clues regarding the presence of physical or genetic disease, intoxication, and developmental/functional disability (Gerson, Malas, & Mroczkowski, 2018). Having basic knowledge of the existence of such conditions and related presentations will empower the psychologist to work together with the medical teams and advocate for the appropriate medical investigation at the same time as psychological factors are explored.

Suicidality

Suicide is a particular concern for youth as the second leading cause of death among young individuals (19.2 deaths in every 100,000 males aged 15–24 years). As important as it is to assess for risk factors (prior engagement in self-harm or suicide attempts; being a 15–19-year-old female adolescent; history of depression, ADHD, anxiety, alcohol and substance abuse; school failure; family relational struggles; childhood sexual abuse), it is equally important to not assume that the absence of risk factors is evidence of absence of suicidal ideation or plans (Hawton, Saunders, & O'Connor, 2012). Suicide screening procedures have been implemented in medical settings in the last decades, and there are many screening tools available to clinicians across many disciplines (Ambrose & Prager, 2018).

Self-Harm

Nonsuicidal self-injury (NSSI), or self-harm, is a direct and deliberate action (cutting, burning, biting, poisoning) with the intent of destructing bodily tissue and with an undetermined intent to die (Cha et al., 2016). Self-harm is thought of as a maladaptive way to regulate and cope with emotions triggered by stressors, low self-esteem, bullying, and negative body image (O'Reilly, Kiyimba, & Karim, 2016). Assessing for a history of self-harm, quantifying the frequency and triggers, qualifying the means, and assessing for signs and symptoms concerning for additional psychological and psychiatric disorders should be part of the psychologist's routine assessment during a consultation. The presence of major depressive disorder and hopelessness, anxiety disorders, disruptive behavior disorders, or substance use, particularly alcohol and cigarettes, increases the risk for self-harm; hence, the psychologist should be alert to the fact that the NSSI might be a signal for deeper, potentially unrecognized psychiatric struggles, especially as there is mounting evidence in the field that the presence of NSSI is a predictor of future suicide attempt (Cha et al., 2016; Hawton et al., 2012). Repetition of self-harm is also common in adolescents, especially ones presenting with risk factors as outlined above, so safety planning for discharge is an appropriate intervention. Additionally, there are many other known risk factors for NSSI that psychologists should assess for and address in treatment, such as onset of sexual activity, history of sexual abuse, sexual orientation concerns, exposure to others' self-harm/suicide attempts, family adversity (e.g., poor parenting styles and parental divorce), interpersonal difficulties both with peers and adults, social isolation, and bullying. The literature also highlights associations between self-harm and personality styles from perfectionism and low self-esteem to borderline personality traits/disorders and learned behaviors (Cha et al., 2016; Hawton et al., 2012).

Homicidal/Violent Behavior

A broad look at violent behavior in adolescents between 2004 and 2008 showed that about a third of youths engaged in at least one violent behavior (e.g., a serious fight at school or work, group-against-group fight, or an attack on others with the intent to seriously hurt them) (SAMHSA, 2010). The differential diagnosis for NSSI and violent behaviors should move beyond pure psychiatric explanations, especially when encountering youth in medical settings, as the potential of harm to others and agitation can also present in youth with developmental disabilities, physiological/medical causes, or both. Youth with developmental disabilities are likely to exhibit tantrums, aggression, or self-injury as part of the regular repertoire of behaviors (estimated prevalence of aggression in youth with autism is about 35%) or when triggered by being in the hospital/clinic (Carroll et al., 2014). While behavioral treatment of aggression can be challenging in the acute setting, preemptive planning before the clinic visit or hospital admission with families and medical teams can reduce the impact of lack of structure, loss of routine, novelty of staff and medical cares, pain reactions, and sensory overload. In addition, via collaboration with parents and providers who know the child (e.g., teachers, applied behavior analysis specialists), context can be provided for the "function" of an aggressive behavior and its triggers. Collaboration with psychiatry colleagues in their expertise for psychiatric medication management is also highly recommended (Gerson et al., 2018).

In assessing the risk for violence, psychologists should focus on exploring possible risk factors which can include both static (i.e., age, sex, and history of abuse) and dynamic/modifiable factors that can be altered and, therefore, can be targets for intervention (e.g., substance abuse, lack of psychiatric treatment). While the presence of substance abuse and psychosis has been reported to increase the risk of violence, mental illness is estimated to be a very small contributor to the overall violence in the United States (Saxton, Resnick, & Noffsinger, 2018). Determination about whether there is duty to warn and protect as evidenced by the Tarasoff ruling (Adi & Mathbout, 2018), thoughtful documentation of a risk assessment (with or without use of instruments) guiding decision-making, and the elaboration of a discharge plan that addresses clinical presentation aiming at treatment and risk reduction are also within the scope of the consulting psychologist (Copelan, 2006; Saxton et al., 2018).

Substance Abuse and Addiction

Substance use is among the most common psychiatric disorders of adolescence and is associated with substantial morbidity and mortality. Heavy use, abuse, and dependence are the strongest predictors of continued substance use disorders in adulthood and of psychosocial impairment such as school failure, early parenthood, high-risk sexual behavior, and legal problems (Hicks et al., 2014). Mental illness comorbidity both precedes and develops as a consequence of substance use, with disruptive behavior and mood disorders (depression and bipolar disorders) as the most frequent psychiatric diagnoses (Hersh, Curry, & Kaminer, 2014). Medically ill youth, while at similar risk for using substances compared to their healthy counterparts (Snyder, Truong, & Law, 2016), are likely to experience more adverse effects from substances by the impact on their medical condition via organ dysfunction, medication interactions, invalidation of lab tests, and associated risky behaviors that can adversely affect their health, such as nonadherence.

Obtaining an adequate history of substance use, qualifying and quantifying substances of choice, and assessing for signs and symptoms concerning for psychological and physiological dependence with or without the use of well-established tools should be part of the psychologist's routine assessment during a consultation (Knight, Sherritt, Shrier, Harris, & Chang, 2002; Sterling et al., 2015). A negative urine drug screen in the presence of a suspicious history is not particularly meaningful as many recreational drugs such as hallucinogens and synthetic cannabinoids are not detected on a standard toxicology screen (Rocker & Oestreicher, 2018).

Formulation

A developmental biopsychosocial formulation gives a multidimensional picture of the youth and family that goes beyond diagnostic labels and beyond a simple medical-model explanation. The formulation allows the psychologist to put forward hypotheses about underlying causes and precipitants of the psychiatric emergency, about factors leading to the continuation of the crisis, while at the same time allowing for reflection on strengths and ameliorating factors that could be used in developing a comprehensive and supportive treatment plan (Winters, Hanson, & Stoyanova, 2007). In the process of responding to psychiatric emergencies, psychologists can use case formulation to succinctly highlight the major issues in a manner that is useful for the multidisciplinary approach, via clear and simple terminology, by answering the questions "what is this case about?," "why is this happening for this youth?," "what can be done (immediately and in the long run)?," and "how?" Creating a youth-/family-centered formulation can be a powerful intervention in itself in building alliance with youth and caregivers and by increasing empathy, understanding, and effective communication with medical and nursing staff. Painting a developmental, cultural, biopsychosocial multifaceted picture of the youth in crisis can reduce stigma and increase understanding, which in turn can decrease negative affect in staff toward the youth/family and positively impact collaboration with medical providers in managing and avoiding future psychiatric crises (Jellinek & McDermott, 2004).

One of the major approaches to case formulation is the biopsychosocial model (Winters et al., 2007). As relevant, it is important to also include developmental and cultural factors in the formulation, as many times developmental stages and milestones and cultural values and practices are informing the clinical presentation, especially in the context of working with medically complex youth. Another model for case formulation is the "four Ps" which puts forward hypotheses about underlying *predisposing* aspects (e.g., genetics, life events, temperament), *precipitants* of the current problems (e.g., specific triggers), factors leading to the *perpetuation* of the presenting problem, and the individual and systems strengths conceptualized as *protective* factors that could be used in developing a treatment plan (Winters et al., 2007).

Engagement

Never has the statement "treat others how you want to be treated" rang more true than in times of emergency/crisis. To engage youth and families, it is important to think about the entire interaction from the beginning to the end. In a medical setting, youth and families are meeting many new providers, so it is important to introduce yourself and explain your role when engaging in the care of the young patient. This will, in turn, invite the opportunity to clarify the relationship and names of caregivers, as well as how they prefer to be addressed. Never assume the adults accompanying the youth are the parents. Also, asking the youth for the preferred way to be addressed is important for the beginning stages of engagement, especially with respect and awareness toward gender identity.

Another early starting point for alliance building and engaging the youth/family is asking about families' expectations and their understanding about what the reason for the psychologist's presence is in the management and treatment of the youth. In addition, another basic strategy to engage caregivers and older adolescents is to acknowledge the areas in which they are more knowledgeable than the clinicians. Starting from a place of empowerment rather than coming in as the expert can begin to create the alliance. Because youth and families meet various providers, are answering many questions, and have to retell the event several times, it is helpful to ask the youth/caregiver where they want to start. It is best to offer the youth/caregiver a choice of how/where/when we start: "I understand you have talked to a lot of different people. I want to make good use of your time. Do you want to start by telling me what is important to know or would it be helpful if I tell you what I understand from reading your chart and talking to the members of your team; you can correct anything I have wrong and/or fill in information I might be missing."

At times, the psychiatric crisis has started well before the youth arrives in the medical setting, and hence, caregivers are blindsided by the emergency. As a psychologist in the medical setting, it is important to recognize that youth/families might not want mental health involvement in their treatment; therefore, close collaboration with the medical team for integrating recommendations in the overall treatment plan of the youth and for delivering the recommendations to the families can reduce resistance and increase participation in the psychiatric treatment. In contrast, there might be times when the psychologist may need to advocate for the youth/family's needs and educate the medical providers and the rest of the multidisciplinary treatment team. Difficult conversations and interactions can be productive in the midst of a psychiatric emergency if engagement and alliances are part of the framework. At times, the psychologists' best intervention is building the therapeutic relationship that allows an opportunity to "plant a seed" via support and psychoeducation with the knowledge that other providers are going on to "nurture and water" that seed toward behavior change. This intervention is not only relevant in the work with the youth/family but also in collaborating with providers as part of systemic changes. Psychologists in medical settings can make the difference in engaging both the youth/family and the medical team in the management, reduction, and treatment of psychiatric emergencies.

In psychiatric emergencies, clinicians can override the parent/guardian/young adult's consent for psychiatric evaluation and treatment. Ideally, when assessing and managing psychiatric emergencies, psychologists should maintain the delicate balance between respecting youth/family's confidentiality and engaging external supports (e.g., family, mental health systems), as collaboration will lead to a more positive and productive experience for all involved, including providers. Having transparent open conversations that invite youth and caregivers to ask questions and offer potentially opposing perspectives allows for the youth and family to join the providers in the decision-making process. Families are often scared, feel out of control, and may even be blaming themselves for their child being in the midst of a psychiatric crisis. Understanding caregivers' experience allows providers to remain compassionate partners with them through the process, one moment at a time. Engaging families and youth will also allow for more collaboration with other providers outside the hospital, via consented collateral contacts, as understanding how the youth and/or family present in other settings gives more context to the psychiatric emergency. Talking with collaterals is best practice for managing the psychiatric crisis and planning for next steps.

In summary, when considering engaging the family in assessing and managing psychiatric emergencies, it is important that the psychologist acts in authentic, transparent, knowledgeable, yet humble, and flexible ways. Even in the most challenging situations, a relationship can be initiated and an alliance formed to help the youth through the psychiatric emergency and moving toward next steps.

Intervention

In the medical setting, providing youth in psychiatric emergencies with a safe environment is paramount for everybody, no matter what causes it (e.g., NSSI, agitation, suicidality, altered mental status, etc.). A first general intervention in any psychiatric emergency ensures a safe environment by providing the youth with a separate room/removed space from which unnecessary and potentially unsafe objects have been removed: cords, sharp objects (e.g., glass, aluminum cans), medications (either that the youth/families have with them or left in the room by the medical staff), objects that can be thrown, and, in extreme emergency cases, even pieces of furniture. Additionally, it is important that the youth is constantly observed for safety. Determining the most appropriate person to observe the patient largely depends on the resources available in the setting (clinical assistant, care companion). Careful thought should be given before a family member is asked to fulfill this role, especially for the most high-risk cases of suicide attempts, self-harm, and violence to others in the context of interpersonal/family dynamics. For the patient who is at risk of hurting others by becoming aggressive and/or attempts to elope, consider collaboration with hospital security (Lelonek et al., 2018). Guidelines for working with agitated patients in medical settings have been developed with focus on the safety of the individual and the treating staff, managing emotions and regaining control of behavior, utilizing age-appropriate and the least-restrictive methods possible, and recognizing that coercive interventions may exacerbate the agitation. Some of the principles of de-escalation are respect for personal space, not being provocative, establishing verbal contact, being concise, identifying desires and feelings, listening closely to what the patient is saying, agreeing or agreeing to disagree, setting clear limits, offering choices and optimism, and debriefing the patient, family, and staff (Chun et al., 2016; Marzullo, 2014; Richmond et al., 2012).

At an interpersonal level, psychologists should facilitate safety planning for the youth in collaboration with the youth and caregivers, with focus on the trigger for the psychiatric emergency (NSSI, substance intoxication, suicidal thoughts, etc.) and as informed by a biopsychosocial case formulation that was agreed upon by the youth and caregivers. The core of safety planning involves identifying (1) triggers and warning signs both internally for the individual and externally for the family/caregivers, (2) concrete/spelled out coping skills, (3) natural supports and (4) additional professional resources and agencies in the community that are already in place and can be contacted for help, and (5) ways to make the environment safe at home and on the way from the hospital to home (Suicide Prevention Resource Center, 2018). Creating a visual (pictorial/nonverbal) safety plan with the youth/family can address unique communication and learning styles in a developmentally sensitive manner (e.g., Likert scale, traffic light, the "Zones of Regulation") (Kuypers, 2018). Finally, behavior management plans and daily schedules should be utilized for youth who are boarding for psychiatric placement or who are hospitalized on the medical units. Close collaboration with other hospital specialists and tapping into additional resources in the medical setting (child life specialists, augmentative communication specialists, social workers, etc.) is crucial. Two very important additional steps are to inform the youth's medical team (physicians, nurses) about the behavioral interventions and plans as a means to provide consistency and predictability and reduce behavioral escalations, and to document useful interventions in the medical records for future admissions/clinic visits.

For suicidal youth, the family-based crisis intervention (FBCI) has been used successfully in the emergency room and outpatient settings and has been shown to prevent the need for psychiatric hospitalization (Wharff et al., 2017). The FBCI is a single visit structured intervention that utilizes elements of cognitive-behavioral, narrative, and family systems therapy along with safety planning. The visit is broken into three meetings: one with the youth separately, another with the family/caregivers separately, and the final meeting with youth and family/caregivers together. The goal of the three meetings is to operationalize a "joint crisis narrative" that allows improvement in intrafamilial communication, collaborative safety planning, and effecting changes that enable the youth to feel and remain safe at home.

When working with youth presenting with substance abuse, motivational interviewing is a well-established empirically based treatment. Over the years, motivational interviewing has evolved to be an intervention that can be used for a variety of psychiatric presentations in which the focus is on behavior change, such as nonadherence to medical treatments, reducing NNSI, etc. Motivational interviewing allows clinicians to build an alliance with the youth and work with their resistance to behavior change by creating an opportunity to observe the discrepancy between youth's behavior and their wishes/self-image while supporting youth's belief that successful behavior changes can take place (SAMHSA, 2018). The screening, brief intervention, and referral to treatment (Sterling et al., 2015) is another evidence-based practice that can be used to prevent the development of a substance use disorder and/or prevent the progression of substance-related disorders with adolescents across settings such as schools or primary cares (D'Amico et al., 2018).

Finally, when addressing psychiatric emergencies, psychologists should be knowledgeable about levels of psychiatric care and how to access such supports for youth in need, in collaboration with case managers and health insurances. The levels of care in the mental health-care system range from the most intensive services (inpatient psychiatric units and residential treatment programs) to less intensive services (outpatient partial hospitalization/day programs, intensive evening programs), to outpatient therapy. Based on the psychiatric emergency, the diagnostic evaluation, case formulation, and the youth/family needs and input, the youth might need to be connected with various behavioral health treatments once the crisis is stabilized and treatment planning starts. For youth who require safety and stabilization at an inpatient psychiatric unit, the ideal situation is that the youth and the guardian are in agreement with this plan. When the legal guardian does not agree with the psychiatric admission despite the assessment of acute safety concerns, the clinician can invoke the state's laws defining the standards for involuntary treatment. Each practicing psychologist should be knowledgeable about the legal coordinates of practicing in their state with regard to age of consent for psychiatric treatment and involuntary psychiatric treatment (Testa & West, 2010). Ideally, it is best to collaborate with family and understand their hesitation with the plan (e.g., stigma of mental health, cultural and/or religious beliefs). Empathic listening and validation of guardians' concerns/questions/hesitancies, yet a transparent and collaborative approach, as well as some extra time for processing the information, are helpful in gaining buy-in from the guardians.

Adaptation

Engaging families and youth in the process of evaluating and managing psychiatric emergencies as much as possible allows for opportunity to continue with intervention once the crisis has stabilized. Working in clinics, pediatricians' offices, or on the medical floors creates challenges for psychologists with regard to youth/family's time availability, access to private space, ability to respect privacy, individual/family stage of readiness for change and their availability (emotional and cognitive) for psychiatric treatment, developmental needs, cultural and contextual needs and values, etc. Therefore, psychologists have to work within the flexibility and fidelity framework (Kendall & Beidas, 2007) and combine empirically supported treatment principles, clinical expertise, and individual client characteristics in their treatment interventions. Psychological treatment in the medical setting should be pragmatic and preventative, with focus on immediate impact and concrete opportunities for behavior change and alignment with youth/family's needs. In contrast with the outpatient psychotherapeutic work, for psychologists working in medical settings, less is more: in the context of the inherent time limitations, providing a few interventions with observable/measurable positive outcome can lead to further behavior change through attitude change, strengthening of working alliance, knowledge about the benefit of behavioral health, and empowerment for further access of treatment in the community, outside of the hospital setting.

Resources/Support

Detailed knowledge about available resources, both clinical expertise and environmental resources that can facilitate and enhance the psychological interventions in psychiatric emergencies, is key. Utilizing clinical expertise to assess and intervene during a psychiatric emergency can be enhanced by utilizing standardized assessment and intervention tools many of which are readily available online. While other chapters of this book address collaborating with psychosocial teams and psychiatry colleagues in medical settings, it is important to highlight other providers like nursing, behavior response teams, care companions, physical and occupational therapists, etc., that can enhance the care of the patient through collaboration on environmental interventions (e.g., reducing sensory overload in the room, room safety proofing, maintenance of daily schedule and behavioral plans). Additional resources and interventions should focus on ensuring the ability to communicate in one's own language and fostering communication by collaborating with language interpreters and augmentative communication specialists; supporting families and ensuring family-centered care through partnering with chaplaincy, cultural brokers, and social work; ensuring safety (e.g., consulting with child protection teams, security, legal counsel); and devising appropriate and realistic disposition planning through work with resource specialists and case managers.

Along with understanding the resources available within the work setting, it is important to understand resources available in the psychologist's geographic area of practice, especially when addressing psychiatric emergencies, as it is important that psychologists understand how/when youth can be hospitalized involuntarily for psychiatric or substance-related treatment.

In-Hospital Consultation and Outpatient Consultation

The role of a psychologist in the medical setting might vary based on the actual setting of the work. Providing consultation in an inpatient medical setting vs. in an outpatient specialty or primary care clinic presents unique advantages and challenges for the psychologist to navigate in order to best address the needs of youth, caregivers, and medical providers. Independent on the setting, the psychologists' role is likely to involve effective collaboration, communication, and coordination of care. Other common goals in working with medically involved youth in outpatient settings include promoting emotional wellness, providing early identification of mental health problems and interventions, integrating culturally sensitive and evidence-based mental health services, and increasing comfort, knowledge, and abilities in diagnosing and responding to mental health problems (DeMaso et al., 2009).

Case Example

Dan is a 13-year-old white male with autism spectrum disorder, anxiety, and a medical history of seizure disorder. He is a freshman in high school in a regular classroom and has an individualized educational plan to assist him with social pragmatics and speech therapy. Dan has had a difficult time transitioning to high school and has been increasingly anxious. He presented to a previously scheduled neurology clinic after he had a behavioral outburst at school and a challenging morning during which his parents had a difficult time getting him to school. He had an anxiety attack during class and was escorted to a quiet room where he engaged in light head banging. He was redirected with support from the school nurse. In the clinic, he was given a screening instrument to assess for depression which revealed moderately/severe range for depression. An emergency consultation was arranged by Dan's neurologist with the clinic's psychologist for a safety assessment. While being assessed by the psychologist, Dan reported worsening mood and anxiety symptoms over the past month. He described difficulties with sleep and appetite due to constant anxious thoughts about having to attend school every day. He feels he "does not fit" and, therefore, does not see a future for himself. Dan disclosed cutting the past 2 weeks and feeling increasingly hopeless. When asked about suicide, he was vague, "I wish I was not around sometimes." When asked about whether he had a plan to end his life, he reported "I don't know, but one can always find ideas online." He stated he did not feel comfortable telling his parents how he felt because "they don't get it." Due to significant concerns for worsening depression and safety, after the psychologist discussed with Dan and his parents the clinical impressions and recommendations, a plan was made to transfer him to the emergency department (ED) for psychiatric assessment, management, and disposition. The psychologist called the ED to alert the staff of the arrival of a youth in psychiatric crisis. The clinic nurse, psychologist, security, and the family all escorted Dan to the ED.

In the ED, Dan was assessed briefly by nursing in the triage area and moved to an ED bedspace. After appropriate safety measures were taken (e.g., removing unnecessary objects and cables from the room, belonging search for safety, a one-to-one constant observer, etc.), he was evaluated by an emergency psychiatry clinician. During the evaluation, Dan became agitated requiring a brief physical hold by security staff and requiring administration of medication (lorazepam), which he took orally. As a result, it was deemed that Dan could not be safely discharged to the community and required higher level of psychiatric care. Due to the lack of available psychiatric beds, and since Dan waited in the ED for 48 hours, the medical team decided to transfer Dan to a medical unit to continue boarding for an inpatient psychiatry unit placement. Dan transferred to the medical unit in good behavioral control. Again, similar safety measures were taken for the room. Over the next few days that Dan remained in the hospital, he was seen daily by the consultation-liaison (CL) psychologist for ongoing assessment, brief interventions, and continued work for a safe disposition plan. Since the one time in the ED, Dan did not have any further episodes of acute agitation, did not require any restraints, and did not need emergent psychiatric medications. He expressed remorse for his behavior in the ED and was able to process with the CL psychologist and his parents the precipitant to both his acute agitation and to his presentation to the hospital. CL psychologist, Dan, and his parents created a safety scale which was utilized daily to assess his psychiatric acuity and safety. In addition, the psychologist worked with Dan on concrete cognitive and behavioral skill building (e.g., understanding the connection between thoughts, actions, body reactions, and feelings, learning relaxation strategies and cognitive techniques to identify and challenge automatic/irrational thoughts). Finally, the psychologist provided brief family work to help clear communication and guide some of the interactions between the parents and Dan, to reduce stress in the home. The CL psychologist communicated with Dan's school, primary care physician (PCP), and neurologist throughout his boarding process and also collaborated with the unit's child life specialist to create structure and routine during his days with the goal of appropriate behavioral activation and emotion regulation.

After 5 days boarding on the medical unit, Dan stabilized psychiatrically. Dan continued to experience significant anxiety and depressive symptoms, mainly related to school stressors. A plan was made with Dan and his parents to attend a partial hospitalization program where he could get intense psychological therapy together with a psychotropic medication evaluation. Prior to discharge, the CL psychologist engaged parents, Dan, school, and PCP in safety planning which included coping tools and signs and symptoms that Dan should return to the nearest ED for psychiatric re-evaluation.

Appendix: Attachments: Resources

https://www.samhsa.gov/

"The Substance Abuse and Mental Health Services Administration is the agency within the U.S. Department of Health and Human Services that leads public health efforts to advance the behavioral health of the nation."

https://www.integration.samhsa.gov/about-us/about-cihs

"The SAMHSA Center for Integrated Health Solutions (CIHS) promotes the development of integrated primary and behavioral health services to better address the needs of individuals with mental health and substance use conditions, whether seen in specialty behavioral health or primary care provider settings."

Alcohol and substance abuse screening tools

https://www.integration.samhsa.gov/clinical-practice/sbirt/CRAFFT_Screening_interview.pdf

https://www.samhsa.gov/sbirt

Motivational interviewing tools

https://www.integration.samhsa.gov/clinical-practice/motivational-interviewing

Depression screening tools

http://www.cqaimh.org/pdf/tool_phq9.pdf

https://www.nimh.nih.gov/labs-at-nimh/asq-toolkit-materials/index.shtml

Safety planning tools

www.sprc.org

https://www.zonesofregulation.com/index.html

References

Adi, A., & Mathbout, M. (2018). The duty to protect: Four decades after tarasoff. *The American Journal of Psychiatry Residents' Journal, 13*, 6. https://doi.org/10.1176/appi.ajp-rj.2018.130402

Ambrose, A. J. H., & Prager, L. M. (2018). Suicide evaluation in the pediatric emergency setting. *Child and Adolescent Psychiatric Clinics of North America, 27*(3), 387–397. https://doi.org/10.1016/j.chc.2018.03.003

Carroll, D., Hallett, V., McDougle, C. J., Aman, M. G., McCracken, J. T., Tierney, E., … Scahill, L. (2014). Examination of aggression and self-injury in children with autism spectrum disorders and serious behavioral problems. *Child and Adolescent Psychiatric Clinics of North America, 23*(1), 57–72. https://doi.org/10.1016/j.chc.2013.08.002

Cha, C. B., Augenstein, T. M., Frost, K. H., Gallagher, K., D'Angelo, E. J., & Nock, M. K. (2016). Using implicit and explicit measures to predict nonsuicidal self-injury among adolescent inpatients. *Journal of the American Academy of Child and Adolescent Psychiatry, 55*(1), 62–68. https://doi.org/10.1016/j.jaac.2015.10.008

Chun, T. H., Mace, S. E., Katz, E. R., & American Academy of Pediatrics; Committee on Pediatric Emergency Medicine; American College of Emergency Physicians; Pediatric Emergency Medicine Committee. (2016). Executive summary: Evaluation and management of children and adolescents with acute mental health or behavioral problems. Part I: Common clinical challenges of patients with mental health and/or behavioral emergencies. *Pediatrics, 138*(3), e20161571. https://doi.org/10.1542/peds.2016-1571

Copelan, R. (2006). Assessing the potential for violent behavior in children and adolescents. *Pediatrics in Review, 27*(5), e36–e41.

D'Amico, E. J., Parast, L., Shadel, W. G., Meredith, L. S., Seelam, R., & Stein, B. D. (2018). Brief motivational interviewing intervention to reduce alcohol and marijuana use for at-risk adolescents in primary care. *Journal of Consulting and Clinical Psychology, 86*(9), 775–786. https://doi.org/10.1037/ccp0000332

DeMaso, D. R., Martini, D. R., Cahen, L. A., Bukstein, O., Walter, H. J., Benson, S., … Medicus, J. (2009). Practice parameter for the psychiatric assessment and management of physically ill children and adolescents. *Journal of the American Academy of Child and Adolescent Psychiatry, 48*(2), 213–233. https://doi.org/10.1097/CHI.0b013e3181908bf4

First, M. B. (2017). *The DSM-TM handbook of differential diagnosis*. Washington, DC: American Psychiatric Association Publishing.

Gerson, R., Malas, N., & Mroczkowski, M. M. (2018). Crisis in the Emergency Department: The evaluation and management of acute agitation in children and adolescents. *Child and Adolescent Psychiatric Clinics of North America, 27*(3), 367–386. https://doi.org/10.1016/j.chc.2018.02.002

Hawton, K., Saunders, K. E., & O'Connor, R. C. (2012). Self-harm and suicide in adolescents. *Lancet, 379*(9834), 2373–2382. https://doi.org/10.1016/S0140-6736(12)60322-5

Hersh, J., Curry, J. F., & Kaminer, Y. (2014). What is the impact of comorbid depression on adolescent substance abuse treatment? *Substance Abuse, 35*(4), 364–375. https://doi.org/10.1080/08897077.2014.956164

Hicks, B. M., Johnson, W., Durbin, C. E., Blonigen, D. M., Iacono, W. G., & McGue, M. (2014). Delineating selection and mediation effects among childhood personality and environmental risk factors in the development of adolescent substance abuse. *Journal of Abnormal Child Psychology, 42*(5), 845–859. https://doi.org/10.1007/s10802-013-9831-z

Jellinek, M. S., & McDermott, J. F. (2004). Formulation: Putting the diagnosis into a therapeutic context and treatment plan. *Journal of the American Academy of Child and Adolescent Psychiatry, 43*(7), 913–916. https://doi.org/10.1097/01.chi.0000125090.35109.57

Kendall, P., & Beidas, R. S. (2007). Smoothing the trail for dissemination of evidence-based practices for youth: Flexibility within fidelity. *Professional Psychology: Research and Practice, 38*(1), 13–20.

Knight, J., Sherritt, L., Shrier, L., Harris, S. H., & Chang, G. (2002). Validity of the CRAFFT substance abuse screening test among adolescent clinic patients. *The Archives of Pediatrics & Adolescent Medicine, 156*, 607–614.

Kuypers, L. (2018). Retrieved September 19, 2018, from http://www.zonesofregulation.com/index.html

Lelonek, G., Crook, D., Tully, M., Trufelli, K., Blitz, L., & Rogers, S. C. (2018). Multidisciplinary approach to enhancing safety and care for pediatric behavioral health patients in acute medical settings. *Child Adolesc Psychiatric Clin N Am, 27*, 491–500.

Marzullo, L. R. (2014). Pharmacologic management of the agitated child. *Pediatric Emergency Care, 30*(4), 269–275;. ; quiz 276–268. https://doi.org/10.1097/PEC.0000000000000112

O'Reilly, M., Kiyimba, N., & Karim, K. (2016). "This is a question we have to ask everyone": Asking young people about self-harm and suicide. *Journal of Psychiatric and Mental Health Nursing, 23*(8), 479–488. https://doi.org/10.1111/jpm.12323

Richmond, J. S., Berlin, J. S., Fishkind, A. B., Holloman, G. H., Jr., Zeller, S. L., Wilson, M. P., … Ng, A. T. (2012). Verbal de-escalation of the agitated patient: Consensus statement of the American Association for Emergency Psychiatry Project BETA De-escalation Workgroup. *The Western Journal of Emergency Medicine, 13*(1), 17–25. https://doi.org/10.5811/westjem.2011.9.6864

Rocker, J. A., & Oestreicher, J. (2018). Focused medical assessment of pediatric behavioral emergencies. *Child and Adolescent Psychiatric Clinics of North America, 27*(3), 399–411. https://doi.org/10.1016/j.chc.2018.02.003

Saxton, A., Resnick, P., & Noffsinger, S. (2018). Chief complaint: Homicidal. Assessing violence risk. Current Psychiatry, 17(5):26–35.

Shaw, R. J., & DeMaso, D. R. (2010). *Textbook of pediatric psychosomatic medicine*. Arlington, VA: American Psychiatric Publishing.

Snyder, L. L., Truong, Y. K., & Law, J. R. (2016). Evaluating substance use and insulin misuse in adolescents with type 1 diabetes. *The Diabetes Educator, 42*(5), 529–537. https://doi.org/10.1177/0145721716659149

Sterling, S., Kline-Simon, A. H., Satre, D. D., Jones, A., Mertens, J., Wong, A., & Weisner, C. (2015). Implementation of screening, brief intervention, and referral to treatment for adolescents in pediatric primary care: A cluster randomized trial. *JAMA Pediatrics, 169*(11), e153145. https://doi.org/10.1001/jamapediatrics.2015.3145

Substance Abuse and Mental Health Services Administration. (2018). *Motivational interviewing*. Retrieved from https://www.integration.samhsa.gov/clinical-practice/motivational-interviewing

Substance Abuse and Mental Health Services Administration, Office of Applied Studies. (2010). The National Survey on Drug Use and Health report: Violent behaviors and family income among adolescents. Rockville, MD.

Suicide Prevention Resource Center. (2018). *Suicide prevention resource center*. Retrieved September 19, 2018, from http://www.sprc.org/

Testa, M., & West, S. G. (2010). Civil commitment in the United States. *Psychiatry (Edgmont), 7*(10), 30–40.

Wharff, E. A., Ginnis, K. B., Ross, A. M., White, E. M., White, M. T., & Forbes, P. W. (2017). Family-based crisis intervention with suicidal. Adolescents: A randomized clinical trial. *Pediatric Emergency Care, 35*, 170. https://doi.org/10.1097/PEC.0000000000001076

Winters, N. C., Hanson, G., & Stoyanova, V. (2007). The case formulation in child and adolescent psychiatry. *Child and Adolescent Psychiatric Clinics of North America, 16*(1), 111–132. , ix. https://doi.org/10.1016/j.chc.2006.07.010

Treatment Adherence Within Consultation-Liaison Services

Rachelle R. Ramsey and Christina E. Holbein

Treatment Adherence Within Consultation-Liaison Services

Treatment adherence is defined as the extent to which a person's behavior matches medical advice from a health-care professional (Modi et al., 2012). Although often associated with a patient's accuracy in taking medications as prescribed, adherence can refer to a range of other behaviors, including healthy lifestyle habits (e.g., dietary choices, physical activity regimens, fluid intake, sleep), physical therapy programs, supplemental feeds, blood glucose checks, and airway clearance procedures. Patient nonadherence is a major public health concern with approximately 50% of pediatric patients being nonadherent to their prescribed medications (Rapoff, 2010) and even higher rates of nonadherence (i.e., 65–90%) in adolescents (Hommel & Baldassano, 2010; Logan, Zelikovsky, Labay, & Spergel, 2003). Treatment adherence is critical for the maintenance of optimal health outcomes; nonadherence has been associated with poorer health outcomes, drug resistance, poorer health-related quality of life, and increased morbidity and mortality (DiMatteo, 2004; Rapoff, 2010). Further, nonadherent patients significantly influence the health-care system, with higher rates of health-care utilization and resulting health-care costs in excess of $300 billion annually (DiMatteo, 2004; McGrady & Hommel, 2013).

It is quite common for a consultation-liaison (CL) service provider to encounter issues related to treatment adherence challenges. In fact, emergency department visits or hospital admissions may serve as opportunities to reinforce the importance of treatment adherence and implement tailored strategies for improving adherence (Drotar, 2013). Consultations may be directly related to adherence, as in the case of a child admitted for an asthma exacerbation who has not taken his preventative and rescue medications as prescribed. Alternatively, a CL psychologist may determine that treatment adherence is one of multiple concerns (e.g., a patient with postsurgical pain management concerns who admits she forgets to take her medication at the appropriate times and often

R. R. Ramsey (✉)
Cincinnati Children's Hospital Medical Center, Cincinnati, OH, USA

Division of Behavioral Medicine and Clinical Psychology, Department of Pediatrics, University of Cincinnati College of Medicine, Cincinnati, OH, USA
e-mail: Rachelle.Ramsey@cchmc.org

C. E. Holbein
Children's Hospital of Philadelphia, Philadelphia, PA, USA

Department of Child and Adolescent Psychiatry and Behavioral Sciences, Children's Hospital of Philadelphia, Philadelphia, PA, USA

B. D. Carter, K. A. Kullgren (eds.), *Clinical Handbook of Psychological Consultation in Pediatric Medical Settings*, Issues in Clinical Child Psychology, https://doi.org/10.1007/978-3-030-35598-2_32

does not stay ahead of the pain). In both of these cases, it is important to have a clear conceptualization of treatment adherence, a thorough process for assessing adherence, and knowledge of evidence-based adherence interventions.

The aims of this chapter are to (1) provide a solid foundation regarding conceptualization of treatment adherence within a contextual framework, (2) offer guidance for comprehensive assessment of treatment adherence and related barriers, (3) describe evidence-based adherence interventions and recommendations in the context of CL service, and (4) guide efforts at communicating adherence-related issues with physicians, nurses, and other medical providers. A case example is provided at the conclusion of this chapter to demonstrate the application of assessment, intervention, and interdisciplinary collaboration related to nonadherence.

The Pediatric Self-Management Model

Use of a conceptual framework is essential for a full understanding of the dynamic interplay of factors and processes that affect treatment adherence and potential targets for intervention. Areas for consideration include factors across patient, family, provider, and larger systems (e.g., communities, schools, health-care settings). Several theoretical models, including the health belief model (Strecher & Rosenstock, 1997), common sense model of self-regulation (Leventhal & Ian, 2012), theory of planned behavior (Conner & Armitage, 1998), and the transtheoretical model of change (Prochaska & DiClemente, 1982), have been proposed to describe the complex associations between treatment adherence and other contextual factors.

While the aforementioned theoretical health self-management models have associated strengths and weaknesses (Hommel, Ramsey, Rich, & Ryan, 2017), the pediatric self-management model (PSMM) (Modi et al., 2012) is ideal for conceptualizing pediatric treatment adherence because it accounts for multiple contextual and developmental factors and processes associated with treatment adherence. Within the PSMM (Fig. 1), contextual factors and processes are organized across four domains (i.e., individual, family, community, and health-care system), which are further divided into modifiable and nonmodifiable influences. In clinical practice, modifiable influences are factors that may be targeted by intervention strategies. For example, a caregiver's knowledge about his or her child's medical condition and treatment plan (i.e., modifiable family influence) can be increased as a result of educational interventions. Alternatively, nonmodifiable influences are the factors that must be considered when developing or adapting adherence interventions. For example, a patient's cultural background is a nonmodifiable individual influence that may affect treatment adherence and must be considered in treatment planning and intervention implementation. Altogether, contextual influences interact with social (e.g., communication), emotional (e.g., stress management), and cognitive (e.g., attention) processes to determine whether a patient will be successful in performing adherence behaviors consistent with the treatment plan.

Evidence-Based Assessment of Adherence

A comprehensive assessment of adherence requires the integration of data from multiple sources: (1) a review of the medical chart, (2) input from the medical team, and (3) an adherence assessment with the patient and family (Hommel, Greenley, Maddux, Gray, & Mackner, 2013; Quittner, Modi, Lemanek, Ievers-Landis, & Rapoff, 2008). Integrating information from all sources allows for the development of a thorough, informed conceptualization of treatment adherence and associated treatment recommendations.

Medical Chart Review

First, gather information about the patient's presenting concern(s) and any past or present adherence concerns through a careful review of the

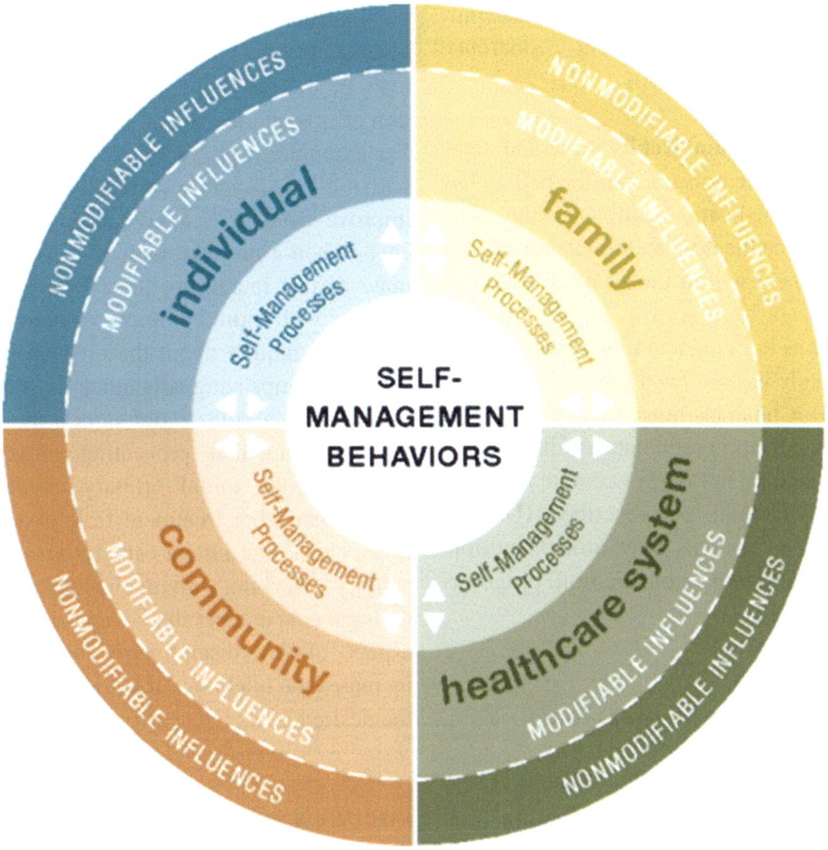

Fig. 1 Pediatric Self-Management Model (Modi et al., 2012), Reproduced with permission from Pediatrics, 129, e473–85, ©2012 by the AAP

medical chart. When reviewing the patient's chart, recent clinic notes or documentation by medical providers, social workers, or behavioral medicine specialists may mention concerns related to nonadherence or potential barriers. Additional material to review includes bioassay data and frequency of medication refills. Finally, a review of a clearly documented treatment plan is critical when determining whether the patient is appropriately following their regimen and should always be confirmed with the medical team.

Bioassays For some medical conditions, bioassays (i.e., metabolites present in the blood, urine, or saliva, viral loads, drug trough levels) may provide valuable information about medication adherence (Drotar, 2013; Hommel et al., 2017). Although some bioassays (e.g., HbA1c, coagulation international normalized ration [INR], HIV antiviral loads) may commonly be assessed for the current admission or visit, others may be included in previous encounters within the chart. Of note, bioassays are often influenced by many other factors (e.g., puberty, drug metabolism, pharmacokinetics, tendency to adhere to treatment shortly before a clinic visit ["white coat adherence"]) (Driscoll et al., 2016; Duncan, Mentrikoski, Wu, & Fredericks, 2014; Hommel et al., 2017). It should also be noted that bioassays provide little insight into patterns of adherence, may not be sensitive enough to detect mild nonadherence, and typically only represent recent adherence due to short half-lives of many medications (Lehmann et al., 2014). Therefore, bioassay data is often best used as a preliminary screener for nonadherence and should be used in conjunction with other information gleaned from the medical chart and discussions with patients, families, and medical providers when conceptualizing the patient's treatment adherence (Hommel & Baldassano, 2010).

Pharmacy/Prescription Refills Potential nonadherence may be demonstrated if the patient has not requested medication refills at the time expected based on the dose and time elapsed. For example, a patient with a three-month prescription who has not been seen in clinic in over 6 months and has not contacted the medical team for a refill likely has not been taking medication as prescribed. Clinicians must be cautious when interpreting medication refill data as filling medications on time does not imply accurate administration of medication as prescribed (Duncan et al., 2014) and patients may utilize multiple pharmacies or enroll in automatic refill programs (Hommel et al., 2017).

Discussion with the Medical Team

When an adherence consultation is requested, it is important to gather more in-depth information from the medical team. Questions to ask include the team's evidence for nonadherence, the patient's history of adherence, the team's perceived understanding of the patient's adherence barriers, and their goals and recommendations for the patient. It may be helpful to inquire whether the medical team has previously addressed nonadherence with the patient and what strategies may have been recommended or implemented in the past. Despite the critical information gleaned from consultation with medical providers, this information should be interpreted in conjunction with other sources; in fact, it is important to note that physicians tend to overestimate their patients' treatment adherence, with their assessments often influenced by observable cues (e.g., gender, language skills, internalizing symptoms) (Miller et al., 2002; Pabst, Bertram, Zimmermann, Schiffer, & de Zwaan, 2015). Rapport and social desirability between the patient and providers can also influence the quality of information about treatment adherence that is communicated to the medical team (Lehmann et al., 2014).

Finally, ensuring that the CL psychologist understands the medical team's goals and how realistic the goals are will inform psychoeducation efforts and the selection of a treatment plan. For example, a physician may expect a patient with multiple psychosocial risk factors to quickly improve from 50% adherence to 100% adherence, when a more realistic goal for the patient may start at increasing to 65% adherence. For patients with more complex regimens, it can be helpful to inquire about the medical team's priorities for improving adherence. In the case of a patient with a spinal cord injury, the physician may indicate that preventing pressure sores should be the initial primary target behavior rather than other treatment tasks (e.g., medications, clean intermittent catheterization, physical activity). Working with medical providers to help their patients to meet shared goals is an important aspect of interdisciplinary collaboration and increases the likelihood that the patient will meet the desired goals (Nancarrow et al., 2013).

Interview with the Patient and Family

To accurately assess adherence, clinical interviews must be conducted as a collaborative effort by providers, patients, and families to improve health outcomes (Zelikovsky & Schast, 2008). Adherence can be a challenging and emotional topic to broach with patients and families, resulting in defensiveness, fear of disappointing medical providers, attempts to avoid consequences, or discouragement (Drotar, 2013; Duncan et al., 2014; Lehmann et al., 2014). As a result, patients tend to overestimate their actual rates of adherence when compared with more objective electronic monitoring methods (Hommel & Baldassano, 2010). When discussing medication adherence, a nonjudgmental interpersonal style with clear, simple language and normalization of any difficulties can increase the patient's comfort and the validity of information (Duncan et al., 2014; Hommel & Baldassano, 2010; Stiratt et al., 2015). It can be helpful to emphasize that the goal of the discussion is to improve the patient's health outcomes (Zelikovsky & Schast, 2008).

Table 1 How to talk to patients and families about treatment adherence

Strategy	Examples
Use simple language	"I would like to talk about what it's like for you to take your medication the way your doctor has prescribed" "One thing I do as a pediatric psychologist is to help patients follow the treatment plans that their medical team creates for them"
Normalize adherence challenges	"Most of us miss doses at times. What has been your experience?" "A lot of teens tell me they have a hard time remembering their inhalers. What things get in the way or make it hard for you?"
Be specific	"Please tell me the last time you took this medication" "How many doses do you think you missed this week?"
Ask about the treatment's effect on quality of life	"Tell me how you feel about taking these pills" "How do you feel about having to give up foods with gluten?"
Ask about side effects	"What kind of side effects have you experienced?"
Identify the problem	"What medications do you find the most difficult to take?" "When do you struggle most to take your medications?"
Use data to facilitate an open conversation about adherence	"It looks like the last time you requested a three-month refill for your child's medicine was 6 months ago. This information often shows me that families might be having some difficulty making sure their child is taking their medication when they're supposed to. This is a really common issue that we see with families in the hospital. I would like to talk more about this with you to see how we can best support you to manage your child's health"

Note. Table adapted from Medication Adherence-Promotion Resources (https://www.cincinnatichildrens.org/research/divisions/c/adherence/map)

When objective adherence information (e.g., pharmacy refills, bioassays) is available, it is best used to facilitate a collaborative discussion about the patient's treatment rather than as evidence that the patient and family have not truthfully reported any nonadherence (Duncan et al., 2014). See Table 1 for communication strategies and examples.

In addition to maintaining a collaborative nature, a comprehensive evaluation of adherence requires the provider to understand the frequency, timing, and magnitude of nonadherence. To improve the detail and accuracy of information, it is important to provide a specific, relatively brief time frame appropriate for the given medical condition (Duncan et al., 2014; Stiratt et al., 2015; Zelikovsky & Schast, 2008). A seven-day time frame may be appropriate for a patient taking twice daily medication, while a three- or six-month time frame better suits a patient receiving monthly injections. Further, more general terms (e.g., "sometimes," "often") and Likert-type ratings can be misinterpreted and result in imprecise information (Duncan et al., 2014; Williams, Amico, Bova, & Womack, 2013). It is essential for the CL psychologist to ask questions that allow for understanding of (1) the patient and family's knowledge of the prescribed treatment, (2) how often the patient accurately complies with the prescribed treatment plan, (3) how often the patient has missed or neglected treatment behaviors and/or has been late/early in completing a treatment for which timeliness is critical (e.g., taking a morning medication in the evening) (Zelikovsky & Schast, 2008), and (4) the barriers that impede the patient's adherence. The patient's knowledge of his/her medical condition(s) and associated treatment is critical because patients who are unsure of their treatment plan and why it is important for their health will likely struggle to follow through with their medical team's plan (Drotar, 2013; Zelikovsky & Schast, 2008). Each medication and/or treatment component should be individually assessed, as rates of adherence differ by treatment component (Duncan et al., 2014); however, the psychologist may want to prioritize obtaining information about the medical team's primary concern for nonadherence.

Use of a validated clinical interview can ensure that fundamental aspects of treatment adherence are systematically assessed. The medical adherence measure (MAM) (Zelikovsky

& Schast, 2008) is a semi-structured interview for assessing treatment adherence across three domains: medication, nutrition, and clinic appointments. There are also optional modules for specific patient populations (i.e., dialysis, cystic fibrosis, urologic conditions requiring catheterization, and weight management). For each type of treatment task, the MAM evaluates the patient's knowledge of the treatment, self-reported adherence behaviors, strategies that have been used to support adherence, and barriers. Although it may be impractical to implement the full 20-minute MAM during a consult, review of the measure may be helpful to inform the assessment process.

Self-Report Questionnaire Measures of Adherence

Self-report questionnaires allow for an inexpensive, comprehensive, and standardized evaluation of specific adherence behaviors, barriers, or related factors (e.g., beliefs about treatment, family involvement) (Lehmann et al., 2014; Quittner et al., 2008) that can complement the information acquired from the clinical interview. In an outpatient clinic setting, paper-and-pencil or electronic measures can be provided at the time of check-in, with scoring completed before the patient interview. Providers can review questionnaire results and interpretation with families when discussing adherence challenges, barriers, and potential therapeutic interventions. Disadvantages of self-report questionnaire measures include a tendency for overreporting adherence (e.g., social desirability bias), inaccurate recall, and challenges in using them with children 8 years and younger (Lehmann et al., 2014; Quittner et al., 2008). If the workflow allows, providers should choose the most appropriate self-report measures for their clinical use and medical populations. General adherence measures can be used with a wide array of medical populations with common treatment regimens (e.g., daily medication, attending clinic appointments). Although there is no "gold standard" self-report general adherence measure, several questionnaires have been used with multiple pediatric populations: Medication Adherence Self-Report Inventory (MASRI) (Walsh, Mandalia, & Gazzard, 2002), Medication Adherence Report Scale (MARS) (Thompson, Kulkarni, & Sergejew, 2000), and Brief Adherence Rating Scale (BARS) (Byerly, Nakonezny, & Rush, 2008). We refer readers to an excellent review of pediatric treatment adherence measures (Quittner et al., 2008) to aid in selecting condition-specific measures. Condition-specific measures may also provide rich information about condition-specific regimen tasks and barriers and can be identified through a search of the pediatric adherence literature. While some measures may be somewhat lengthy for use in a consultation, they may be successfully abbreviated while continuing to provide valuable clinical information (Varnell Jr. et al., 2017).

Other Adherence Assessment Tools

Although there are other well-validated methods of assessing treatment adherence, they may be somewhat less practical for a psychologist working within an inpatient CL service. Pill counts (i.e., comparing the number of pills to the amount expected to be available based on prescription dosage and time elapsed) can provide a cost-effective, objective measure of adherence, although many patients may not have their medication containers with them during a clinic visit or hospital admission (Duncan et al., 2014; Hommel et al., 2017; Hommel & Baldassano, 2010).

While electronic monitors (e.g., MEMS pill bottle cap, electronic pillboxes, electronic inhaler caps, CPAP machines, glucose monitor) can provide objective adherence data, identification of adherence patterns, and continuous "real-time" monitoring (Duncan et al., 2014; Lehmann et al., 2014; Quittner et al., 2008), they are only helpful in a consultation model if the patient has been using an electronic monitor prior to the consultation. This information is rare with the exception of patients using glucose meters and pumps for managing type 1 diabetes. In this case, the data within these monitors can be visually analyzed to determine patterns (e.g., the patient does not have blood glucose readings on their meter during weekends) and provide feedback; however, it is important to explore additional possibilities (e.g., the patient uses other glucose meters that they did not bring with them, their pump malfunctioned) other than nonadherence when examining such data.

Treatment Adherence Barriers and Interventions

After obtaining information about current treatment knowledge and adherence, an assessment of treatment barriers allows for a clearer understanding of each patient's unique challenges. Barriers to optimal treatment adherence can be found across the four domains of the PSMM (Modi et al., 2012). While some barriers may be condition specific (e.g., discomfort from a chest therapy vest is associated with reduced use in a child with cystic fibrosis, math learning disability interferes with insulin calculations), many others are observed across multiple conditions (e.g., forgetting, low parental involvement; see Table 2 for a comprehensive list).

It may be helpful to distinguish between *volitional* nonadherence (e.g., an adolescent patient chooses not to take a medication due to side effects and peer reactions) and *unintentional* nonadherence (e.g., a patient missed several doses of growth hormone at his father's home because the supplies were left at his mother's house) (Duncan et al., 2014). Family factors, including family stressors (e.g., lack of parental supervision, poor household organization and routines) (Modi et al., 2012; Zelikovsky & Schast, 2008) and family involvement (e.g., who is responsible for treatment behaviors) (Pai et al., 2010), are also critical to assess. Although patients may volunteer some barriers, it can also be helpful to ask about specific barriers (e.g., social pressures, financial challenges, motivation; see Table 2). If time allows, self-report questionnaires, including the Parent and Adolescent Medication Barriers Scales (Simons & Blount, 2007; Simons, McCormick, Devine, & Blount, 2010) and the Illness Management Survey (Logan et al., 2003), can be used to systematically assess adherence barriers. Assessment of barriers over time is key; although adherence barriers tend to remain stable over time without intervention (Ramsey, Zhang, & Modi, 2018), barriers may vary as the patient develops, treatment regimens are altered, or family circumstances change. Understanding these barriers are an integral component for implementing or adapting adherence-focused interventions.

Evidence-Based Adherence-Promotion Interventions

Upon gathering information form the medical team, patient, and family regarding the patient's treatment regimen, understanding of the regimen, current adherence behaviors, and barriers to adherence, the CL psychologist must efficiently compile this information to provide brief adherence-promotion interventions and recommendations for both the patient and the medical team. The goal of a CL psychologist is to select and deliver an intervention(s) to the patient to improve adherence to treatment recommendations and to provide the medical team with recommendations for aiding in the adherence success of the patient. It is important for all CL psychologists to consider that "perfect" adherence is often an unobtainable goal. In addition, the CL psychologist should understand the time frame of the consultation and whether they will have the opportunity to meet with the patient and family one time or several times, as this will also influence intervention selection. Finally, although adherence rates to various treatment components may vary, patients who struggle with nonadherence to their medical treatment may also struggle to adhere to adherence-promotion recommendations. This does not mean that the CL psychologist should not provide recommendations; rather, interventions and recommendations should be presented in a straightforward manner, feasible for the family to implement, and agreed upon by patient and/or caregivers. If outpatient behavioral medicine providers are available, referrals can be placed for short-term outpatient interventions to

Table 2 Common barriers and interventions for treatment adherence

	Barrier	Possible CL interventions
Individual	Forgetting	Setting reminders or alarms, pairing with common activity (e.g., meals, bedtime), change in location of treatment or supplies, self-monitoring (e.g., tracking on logs, calendars, and/or mobile apps)
	Lack of knowledge about disease or treatment	Education about disease and treatment
	Time management, busy schedule, interference with activities	Planning for the time and location of treatment, setting reminders or alarms
	Low motivation, disease burnout	Investigation of health beliefs, incentive/reward system
	Perceived benefits of treatment	Review benefits of treatment, connect benefits with patient values
	Wanting to feel "normal," not feeling "different"	Planning for the time and location of treatment, referral for outpatient treatment
	Internalizing symptoms (i.e., anxiety, depression)	Referral for outpatient treatment
	Fatigue, falling asleep	Setting reminders or alarms, altering treatment times (e.g., after dinner instead of at bedtime)
	Feeling unwell	Utilize help from caregivers
	Oppositional behaviors	Referral for outpatient treatment, behavioral family systems therapy, alter time of day or treatment delivery method to an optimal time of day
Family	Family conflict, chaos, and stress	Behavioral family systems therapy, referral to social work to assist with transportation, financial needs, etc.
	Caregiver's lack of knowledge about disease or treatment	Education about disease and treatment
	Lack of family support	Referral to social work
	Transfer of treatment responsibility from caregiver to child	Problem-solving related to sharing treatment responsibility
	Insufficient caregiver involvement and supervision	Education about developmentally appropriate responsibility, problem-solving related to sharing treatment responsibility, altering time or location of treatment (e.g., at end of school day instead of home)
Community	Community settings (e.g., school, shopping center, restaurant) not conducive to treatment	Problem-solving about alternative treatment locations, encourage education and problem-solving with community providers regarding disease and treatment needs
	Lack of social support	Referral for outpatient treatment
	Fear that peers will learn about child's disease, social stigma	Referral for outpatient treatment
	Embarrassment about taking medications in front of others	Problem-solving alternative locations to take medication
Health system	Patient-provider communication difficulties Patient-provider rapport	Education about treatment priorities, communicate with medical providers about patient's concerns, model asking questions to physician about treatment Provide support and reinforce importance of treatment, utilize other medical team members (e.g., nurse, occupational therapist) with whom patient has better rapport
	Health insurance difficulties, cost of supplies or medications	Referral to social work
Medication specific	Unpleasant side effects (e.g., weight gain, loss of appetite)	Encourage conversation with medical providers, motivational interviewing

(continued)

Table 2 (continued)

Barrier	Possible CL interventions
Taste of medication or supplemental feeds	Suggest pharmacy add flavors to liquid medications, taste preferred food/drink before and/or after taking medication
Difficulty swallowing pills	Behavioral pill swallowing intervention, referral for brief outpatient treatment
Availability of medicine (e.g., running out, left at home)	Setting reminders or alarms, collaborating with pharmacy for automatic refills or home delivery
Complex regimens (e.g., multiple medications, dosing schedules)	Discuss with medical team possibility of simplifying medical regimen
Needle phobia/fear of painful injections	Referral for brief outpatient treatment (graded exposure therapy)

Note. Barriers have been adapted from the modifiable factors of the Pediatric Self-Management Model (Modi et al., 2012)

improve adherence, although appointment attendance could also prove to be difficult. Given the characteristics of patients with suboptimal adherence, it is important for the CL provider to provide clear and direct recommendations during their consultation in case follow-up is suboptimal.

Evidence-based adherence-promotion interventions can be categorized as educational, behavioral, and organizational (Duncan et al., 2014). Intervention selection will be influenced by the information obtained from the medical team, the patient, and the family during the psychologist's assessment of adherence and barriers. In general, the family's barriers will heavily impact the selection of the adherence-promotion intervention. *Educational approaches* seek to provide patients and families with knowledge and skills by providing them with information regarding the illness, its prescribed medical regimen, and specific benefits of adherence (Rapoff, 2010). For patients with knowledge barriers, a CL psychologist can educate the family about the treatment regimen (e.g., dosing, timing), provide written instructions of treatment, allow the patient to ask questions about the regimen, and/or inform the patient of the medical team's treatment priorities. It can be helpful for CL psychologists to be present when the medical team reviews the treatment plan so that they can model and encourage patients and families to ask medical providers questions about their treatment regimen during future hospitalizations and follow-up appointments (Duncan et al., 2014). CL psychologists can also provide education or request that support staff from the medical team provide instruction and time to practice the use of treatment regimen behaviors (e.g., how to correctly use an inhaler, how to calculate an insulin-to-carbohydrate ratio). Treatment knowledge serves as the foundation upon which other adherence skills are built, and a patient cannot adherence to their treatment if they do not understand the purpose and requirements of their regimen. Educating the patient and family on any inconsistencies or uncertainties is an excellent and often necessary first step for a CL psychologist. However, it is important to remember that education alone has a much lower impact on improving sustained adherence than combined education and behavioral interventions (Graves, Roberts, Rapoff, & Boyer, 2010; Kahana, Frazier, & Drotar, 2008).

Behavioral interventions are provided to patients and families with modifiable barriers (e.g., forgetting, busy schedule, oppositional behaviors) by targeting the antecedents (e.g., forgetting) and/or consequences (e.g., rewards) of the adherence behaviors. When behavioral techniques are added to education, there is a significant increase in effect sizes compared to either educational or behavioral interventions alone (Graves et al., 2010). Behavioral approaches consistent with the goals and time frame of a CL psychologist may include techniques such as implementing patient self-monitoring, setting up reminders to take medications, problem-solving, goal setting, establishing reward or token systems, and increasing parental supervision (Duncan et al., 2014). During a brief or one-time consult, a CL psychologist may set small goals and prescriptively provide basic recommendations such as using visible or audible reminders (e.g., pill box, cell phone alarms) and pairing treatment with an already established daily activity (e.g., eating dinner, brushing teeth). Setting small, achievable goals that have a high likelihood of success may improve confidence in a patient's abilities to be adherent to their regimen (Harris et al., 2015). If time allows, it is often beneficial to engaging in a more in-depth problem-solving intervention with the family to increase patient and family buy-in.

For all consults, recommendations for self-monitoring through the use of monitoring logs, electronic monitoring devices (e.g., mobile applications), or parental supervision can also increase adherence. Although not always possible, studies have suggested that providing children and their families with graphs or feedback on how their adherence influences health outcomes may be reinforcing and improve adherence (Duncan et al., 2014). The use of mobile apps that allow for reminders, self-monitoring, and feedback to increase adherence has increased over the past several years. A recent review examined and analyzed the content of 420 free adherence-promotion apps (Ahmed et al., 2018); although the efficacy of most apps has not been scientifically examined, familiarity with the content and quality of several general adherence-promotion apps would allow for informed app recommendations.

Depending on the patient's age and the barriers the patient and family are experiencing, behavioral adherence-promotion approaches that target the whole family may be most effective. These interventions often require outpatient behavioral medicine visits and typically cannot be delivered within the context of a single consultative visit. However, it is important for the CL psychologist to be aware of possible outpatient adherence-promotion interventions in order to make appropriate, specific recommendations and to lay the groundwork for the importance of this type of intervention. For example, Behavioral Family Systems Therapy (BFST) for diabetes includes weekly sessions focused on problem-solving and communication training, along with cognitive modification and functional-structural family therapy (Wysocki et al., 2007). Two other studies demonstrated improved adherence with family-based behavioral interventions utilizing a combination of education, problem-solving, and communication techniques (Hommel et al., 2012; Modi, Guilfoyle, & Rausch, 2013). Contingency-based behavioral interventions that focus on providing rewards or consequences for completing treatment behaviors have also been shown to be effective (Rapoff, 2010). Although the basics of a token economy system can be taught to parents within a consultation, additional outpatient sessions may be needed to refine or modify the original plan. In addition, interventions aimed at decreasing parent-child conflict and increasing the sharing of adherence responsibility may be beneficial for families (Anderson, Brackett, Ho, & Laffel, 1999).

The third category of adherence-promotion interventions is *organizational approaches* that involve changing the environment or factors outside of the patient and/or family. Within the context of CL work, one strategy is to collaborate with the medical team to decrease regimen complexity (Greenley, Kunz, Walter, & Hommel, 2013). For example, switching a child to a medication that can be taken once per day vs. twice per day can increase adherence. If a simpler regimen is not an option (e.g., for an adolescent with spina bifida), working with the medical team to create a treatment priority hierarchy (e.g., "It is most important that you complete your bowel regimen daily. Swimming to reduce your weight is important, but less important than your bowel regimen") can serve as a guide for adherence areas to address first. In addition, another organizational approach is providing insight to the medical team pertaining to the patient and family's barriers to help inform their care. For instance, informing the medical team of a mother's low health literacy and recommending that the team provide succinct, written instructions for medical regimens could improve that child's adherence. Similarly, discussing a patient's move across town and the difficulties that exist with getting to medical appointments could lead to offering clinic appointments at a different location to improve clinic access. In line with the PSMM, coordinating efforts within the patient's community, including school, local therapists, or extracurricular coaches/leaders, may assist in improving adherence away from home.

When delivering CL consultations for children with nonadherence, it is important to remember that using a combination of several empirically based strategies increases the likelihood of improved adherence (Kahana et al., 2008; Pai & McGrady, 2014). For example, patients who do not know their treatment regimen and have little parental supervision for medication taking may require both an educational strategy and a behavioral strategy. Also, given the consultative and liaison nature of CL work, the psychologist would likely be most effective in improving adherence by providing interventions across several of the categories depicted in the pediatric self-management model (e.g., education, behavioral, organizational).

Case Study: Ethan

Patient Information

Ethan is a 9-year-old Caucasian male with spina bifida attending an outpatient clinic visit with his mother. He uses a wheelchair in most settings. His physician consults the pediatric psychologist because Ethan frequently experiences pressure sores and urinary tract infections thought to be related to poor adherence to treatment recommendations, including performing skin checks, periodic pressure relief exercises, and clean intermittent catheterization ("cathing"). The physician also expresses concern about obesity and Ethan's sedentary lifestyle. When asked to prioritize, the physician states that she is currently most concerned about adherence to cathing.

Assessment

A thorough chart review reveals that Ethan has visited the ED three times in the past 6 months for spina bifida complications. His BMI is listed at 32. The chart indicates that Ethan and his mother briefly worked with a psychologist when he was five for behavior management strategies, and he currently has a 504 Plan at school for ADHD.

During the clinical interview, Ethan's mother states that caregivers try to remind him to cath and perform pressure relief exercises in his wheelchair, but he often responds by becoming oppositional and saying "I'll do it later." It is particularly difficult in the evenings when Ethan is engaged in video games or other preferred activities. Ethan reports that he forgets these treatment tasks after he is reminded and feels like he is getting nagged. Ethan and his parents sometimes fight about his nonadherence, resulting in a loss of privileges. Ethan also indicates that he forgets pressure checks at school and skips cathing about 2 days each week because he does not want to miss important information in math class. Regarding exercise, Ethan and his mother are unsure of what exercises are safe for him and have not looked into adaptive sports in their area.

Relevant Barriers

Regimen complexity, executive function deficits (e.g., forgetting, planning ahead) associated with spina bifida and ADHD, oppositional behavior, family conflict, school-based obstacles.

Intervention

The psychologist and family make a plan to address cathing adherence at this visit. Education about positive behavior management strategies (e.g., praising desired behaviors, positive reinforcement) is provided. Ethan, his mother, and the psychologist develop a reward system in which he can earn points toward a reward each time he caths on his own or after one reminder. The psychologist also recommends that Ethan's mother work with his teacher to determine whether there may be a more appropriate time for him to cath (e.g., silent reading time instead of math). It is suggested that Ethan try using alarms on his tablet to provide reminders for cathing in the evenings, which the family feels may be less irritating or annoying for him.

Referrals

Ethan's mother agrees to schedule an outpatient treatment visit with the psychologist in 2 weeks to review and refine strategies and to follow up on addressing adherence to pressure relief exercises and skin checks. The clinic social worker is consulted to provide Ethan's mother with information about local adaptive sports organizations.

Conclusions

Treatment nonadherence is an issue commonly encountered by psychologists working within a pediatric CL setting. An informed conceptualization of treatment adherence includes assessing individual, family, community, and health system factors that may be modified when addressing adherence. A thorough assessment of adherence may include a medical chart review, interviews with the patient and family, and discussion with the medical team. Awareness of the patient's and family's unique adherence barriers is essential for the selection and implementation of appropriate interventions. Effective adherence interventions are derived from educational, behavioral, and organizational approaches, with a combination of strategies often being the most beneficial. Overall, sensitive and clear communication and collaboration with all patients, families, and medical providers is critical in the assessment and treatment of patient nonadherence.

References

Ahmed, I., Ahmad, N. S., Ali, S., Ali, S., George, A., Saleem Danish, H., … Darzi, A. (2018). Medication adherence apps: Review and content analysis. *JMIR mHealth and uHealth, 6*(3), e62. https://doi.org/10.2196/mhealth.6432

Anderson, B. J., Brackett, J., Ho, J., & Laffel, L. M. (1999). An office-based intervention to maintain parent-adolescent teamwork in diabetes management. Impact on parent involvement, family conflict, and subsequent glycemic control. *Diabetes Care, 22*(5), 713–721.

Byerly, M. J., Nakonezny, P. A., & Rush, A. J. (2008). The Brief Adherence Rating Scale (BARS) validated against electronic monitoring in assessing the antipsychotic medication adherence of outpatients with schizophrenia and schizoaffective disorder. *Schizophrenia Research, 100*(1–3), 60–69. https://doi.org/10.1016/j.schres.2007.12.470

Conner, M., & Armitage, C. J. (1998). Extending the theory of planned behavior: A review and avenues for further research. *Journal of Applied Social Psychology, 28*(15), 1429–1464.

DiMatteo, M. R. (2004). Variations in patients' adherence to medical recommendations: A quantitative review of 50 years of research. *Medical Care, 42*(3), 200–209.

Driscoll, K. A., Wang, Y., Bennett Johnson, S., Lynch, R., Stephens, H., Willbur, K., … Deeb, L. C. (2016). White coat adherence in pediatric patients with type 1 diabetes who use insulin pumps. *Journal of Diabetes Science and Technology, 10*(3), 724–729. https://doi.org/10.1177/1932296815623568

Drotar, D. (2013). Strategies of adherence promotion in the management of pediatric chronic conditions. *Journal of Developmental and Behavioral Pediatrics, 34*(9), 716–729. https://doi.org/10.1097/DBP.0b013e31829f6781

Duncan, C. L., Mentrikoski, J. M., Wu, Y. P., & Fredericks, E. M. (2014). Practice-based approach to assessing and treating non-adherence in pediatric regimens. *Clin Pract Pediatr Psychol, 2*(3), 322–336. https://doi.org/10.1037/cpp0000066

Graves, M. M., Roberts, M. C., Rapoff, M., & Boyer, A. (2010). The efficacy of adherence interventions for chronically ill children: A meta-analytic review. *Journal of Pediatric Psychology, 35*(4), 368–382. https://doi.org/10.1093/jpepsy/jsp072

Greenley, R. N., Kunzm J. H., Walter, J., & Hommel, K. A. (2013). Practical strategies for enhaning adherence to treatment regimen in infalmmatory bowel disease. *Inflammatory Bowel Disease 19*(7), 1534–45. https://doi.org/10.1097/MIB.0b013e3182813482.

Harris, M. A., Wagner, D. V., Wilson, A. C., Spiro, K., Heywood, M., & Hoehn, D. (2015). Novel interventions in children's healthcare for youth hospitalized for chronic pain. *Clin Pract Pediatr Psychol, 3*(1), 48–58.

Hommel, K. A., & Baldassano, R. N. (2010). Brief report: Barriers to treatment adherence in pediatric inflammatory bowel disease. *Journal of Pediatric Psychology, 35*(9), 1005–1010. https://doi.org/10.1093/jpepsy/jsp126

Hommel, K. A., Greenley, R. N., Maddux, M. H., Gray, W. N., & Mackner, L. M. (2013). Self-management in pediatric inflammatory bowel disease: A clinical report of the North American Society for Pediatric Gastroenterology, Hepatology, and Nutrition. *Journal of Pediatric Gastroenterology and Nutrition, 57*(2), 250–257. https://doi.org/10.1097/MPG.0b013e3182999b21

Hommel, K. A., Hente, E. A., Odell, S., Herzer, M., Ingerski, L. M., Guilfoyle, S. M., & Denson, L. A. (2012). Evaluation of a group-based behavioral intervention to promote adherence in adolescents with inflammatory bowel disease. *European Journal of Gastroenterology & Hepatology, 24*(1), 64–69. https://doi.org/10.1097/MEG.0b013e32834d09f1

Hommel, K. A., Ramsey, R. R., Rich, K. L., & Ryan, J. L. (2017). *Adherence to pediatric treatment regimens* (5th ed.). New York, NY: The Guilford Press.

Kahana, S. Y., Frazier, T. W., & Drotar, D. (2008). Preliminary quantitative investigation of predictors of treatment non-adherence in pediatric transplantation: A brief report. *Pediatric Transplantation, 12*(6), 656–660.

Lehmann, A., Aslani, P., Ahmed, R., Celio, J., Gauchet, A., Bedouch, P., … Schneider, M. P. (2014). Assessing medication adherence: Options to consider. *International Journal of Clinical Pharmacy, 36*(1), 55–69. https://doi.org/10.1007/s11096-013-9865-x

Leventhal, H., & Ian, B. (2012). *The common-sense model of self-regulation of health and illness* (1st ed.). London: Routledge.

Logan, D., Zelikovsky, N., Labay, L., & Spergel, J. (2003). The illness management survey: Identifying adolescents' perceptions of barriers to adherence. *Journal of Pediatric Psychology, 28*(6), 383–392.

McGrady, M. E., & Hommel, K. A. (2013). Medication adherence and health care utilization in pediatric chronic illness: A systematic review. *Pediatrics, 132*(4), 730–740. https://doi.org/10.1542/peds.2013-1451

Miller, L. G., Liu, H., Hays, R. D., Golin, C. E., Beck, C. K., Asch, S. M., … Wenger, N. S. (2002). How well do clinicians estimate patients' adherence to combination antiretroviral therapy? *Journal of General Internal Medicine, 17*(1), 1–11.

Modi, A. C., Guilfoyle, S. M., & Rausch, J. (2013). Preliminary feasibility, acceptability, and efficacy of an innovative adherence intervention for children with newly diagnosed epilepsy. *Journal of Pediatric Psychology, 38*(6), 605–616. https://doi.org/10.1093/jpepsy/jst021

Modi, A. C., Pai, A. L., Hommel, K. A., Hood, K. K., Cortina, S., Hilliard, M. E., … Drotar, D. (2012). Pediatric self-management: A framework for research, practice, and policy. *Pediatrics, 129*(2), e473–e485. https://doi.org/10.1542/peds.2011-1635

Nancarrow, S. A., Booth, A., Ariss, S., Smith, T., Enderby, P., & Roots, A. (2013). Ten principles of good interdisciplinary team work. *Human Resources for Health, 11*, 19. https://doi.org/10.1186/1478-4491-11-19

Pabst, S., Bertram, A., Zimmermann, T., Schiffer, M., & de Zwaan, M. (2015). Physician reported adherence to immunosuppressants in renal transplant patients: Prevalence, agreement, and correlates. *Journal of Psychosomatic Research, 79*(5), 364–371. https://doi.org/10.1016/j.jpsychores.2015.09.001

Pai, A. L., Gray, E., Kurivial, K., Ross, J., Schoborg, D., & Goebel, J. (2010). The Allocation of Treatment Responsibility scale: A novel tool for assessing patient and caregiver management of pediatric medical treatment regimens. *Pediatric Transplantation, 14*(8), 993–999. https://doi.org/10.1111/j.1399-3046.2010.01391.x

Pai, A. L., & McGrady, M. (2014). Systematic review and meta-analysis of psychological interventions to promote treatment adherence in children, adolescents, and young adults with chronic illness. *Journal of Pediatric Psychology, 39*(8), 918–931. https://doi.org/10.1093/jpepsy/jsu038

Prochaska, J. O., & DiClemente, C. C. (1982). Transtheoretical therapy: Toward a more integrative model of change. *Psychotherapy: Theory, Research & Practice, 19*(3), 276.

Quittner, A. L., Modi, A. C., Lemanek, K. L., Ievers-Landis, C. E., & Rapoff, M. A. (2008). Evidence-based assessment of adherence to medical treatments in pediatric psychology. *Journal of Pediatric Psychology, 33*(9), 916–936;. discussion 937-918. https://doi.org/10.1093/jpepsy/jsm064

Ramsey, R. R., Zhang, N., & Modi, A. C. (2018). The stability and influence of barriers to medication adherence on seizure outcomes and adherence in children with epilepsy over 2 years. *Journal of Pediatric Psychology, 43*(2), 122–132. https://doi.org/10.1093/jpepsy/jsx090

Rapoff, M. A. (2010). *Issues in clinical child psychology. Adherence to pediatric medical regimens* (2nd ed.). New York, NY: Springer Publishing.

Simons, L. E., & Blount, R. L. (2007). Identifying barriers to medication adherence in adolescent transplant recipients. *Journal of Pediatric Psychology, 32*(7), 831–844. https://doi.org/10.1093/jpepsy/jsm030

Simons, L. E., McCormick, M. L., Devine, K., & Blount, R. L. (2010). Medication barriers predict adolescent transplant recipients' adherence and clinical outcomes at 18-month follow-up. *Journal of Pediatric Psychology, 35*(9), 1038–1048. https://doi.org/10.1093/jpepsy/jsq025

Stiratt, M. J., Dunbar-Jacob, J., Crane, H. M., Simoni, J. M., Czajkowski, S., Hilliard, M. E., & Ogedegbe, G. (2015). Self-report measures of medication adherence behavior: Recommendations on optimal use. *Translational Behavioral Medicine, 5*(4), 470–482.

Strecher, V. J., & Rosenstock, I. M. (1997). *The health belief model*. Cambridge: Cambridge University Press.

Thompson, K., Kulkarni, J., & Sergejew, A. A. (2000). Reliability and validity of a new Medication Adherence Rating Scale (MARS) for the psychoses. *Schizophrenia Research, 42*(3), 241–247.

Varnell, C. D., Jr., Rich, K. L., Nichols, M., Dahale, D., Goebel, J. W., Pai, A. L. H., … Modi, A. C. (2017). Assessing barriers to adherence in routine clinical care for pediatric kidney transplant patients. *Pediatric Transplantation, 21*(7), e13027. https://doi.org/10.1111/petr.13027

Walsh, J. C., Mandalia, S., & Gazzard, B. G. (2002). Responses to a 1 month self-report on adherence to antiretroviral therapy are consistent with electronic data and virological treatment outcome. *AIDS, 16*(2), 269–277.

Williams, A. B., Amico, K. R., Bova, C., & Womack, J. A. (2013). A proposal for quality standards for measuring medication adherence in research. *AIDS and Behavior, 17*(1), 284–297. https://doi.org/10.1007/s10461-012-0172-7

Wysocki, T., Harris, M. A., Buckloh, L. M., Mertlich, D., Lochrie, A. S., Mauras, N., & White, N. H. (2007). Randomized trial of behavioral family systems therapy for diabetes: Maintenance of effects on diabetes outcomes in adolescents. *Diabetes Care, 30*(3), 555–560. https://doi.org/10.2337/dc06-1613

Zelikovsky, N., & Schast, A. P. (2008). Eliciting accurate reports of adherence in a clinical interview: Development of the Medical Adherence Measure. *Pediatric Nursing, 34*(2), 141–146.

Pediatric Gender Identity: Consultation on Matters of Identity, Transgender Concerns, and Disorders/Differences of Sex Development

Christine E. Brady and Michelle M. Ernst

Pediatric Gender Identity: Consultation on Matters of Identity, Transgender Concerns, and Disorders/Differences of Sex Development

Broadly, gender identity refers to a person's sense of self as a gendered (or not) individual. A person's "gender identity" is distinct from other constructs such as biological "sex" characteristics (e.g., chromosomes, internal/external anatomy, and hormonal activity), sexual orientation (the gender that a person is romantically or sexually attracted to), and gender assignment (the gender that parents and/or medical professional assigns to an infant at birth, typically based on the appearance of the genitals). Most people are *cisgender;* that is, they develop a gender identity consistent with their initial gender assignment. In most, but not all cultures, gender has typically been confined to the gender binary (i.e., the two primary categories of female/male), with transgender referring to a person assigned one of those categories at birth (e.g., male) who identifies as the other category (e.g., female). Recently, the dichotomy of the gender binary has been questioned by both research findings and sociocultural movements such as LGBTQ activism (Hyde, Bigler, Joel, Tate, & Anders, 2018), resulting in an expansion of categories recognized (by some individuals and groups) to include a number of other identities including bi-gender, gender nonconforming (GNC), and genderqueer (gender terminology quickly changes; a number of websites provide definitions, e.g., https://www.apa.org/pi/lgbt/programs/safe-supportive/lgbt/key-terms.pdf).

Indeed, there is a paradigm shift in expression of gender identity underway in the United States and other countries. At the time of writing this chapter, New York City and four states offer a gender X designation on birth certificates, and three states plus Washington, DC, offer gender-neutral driver licenses (Trotta, 2018). A recent large-scale study of US adults from 19 states analyzed 2014 data and found the prevalence of adults identifying as transgender (0.6% of the sample, 1,400,000 total persons) had doubled over the past 10 years, with 18–24-year-old adults (the youngest age group) more likely to identify as transgender (Flores, Herman, Gates, & Brown, 2016). A

C. E. Brady (✉)
Kaiser Permanente,
Santa Clara, California, United States

Child Psychiatry, Kaiser Permanente,
Santa Clara, California, United States
e-mail: Christine.X.Brady@kp.org

M. M. Ernst
Cincinnati Children's Hospital Medical Center,
Cincinnati, OH, USA

Division of Behavioral Medicine and Clinical Psychology, University of Cincinnati School of Medicine, Cincinnati, OH, USA

B. D. Carter, K. A. Kullgren (eds.), *Clinical Handbook of Psychological Consultation in Pediatric Medical Settings*, Issues in Clinical Child Psychology, https://doi.org/10.1007/978-3-030-35598-2_33

population-based study of high school students found that 2.7% identified as "transgender, genderqueer, genderfluid, or unsure about [your] gender identity"; those youth identifying as such reported compromised physical and mental health (Rider, McMorris, Gower, Coleman, & Eisenberg, 2018).

Pediatric psychologists consulting in inpatient and outpatient medical settings are likely to encounter youth who experience gender identity in a variety of ways. Given that youth may not easily disclose to others, providing appropriate and effective consultative services is critical. In this chapter we briefly review gender identity development, gender dysphoria, and current terminology relevant to gender. We then discuss assessment of gender concerns, as well as assessment of relevant psychosocial risk and resiliency factors, and highlight potential interventions, with a focus on transgender individuals and youth with a disorder/difference of sex development (DSD).

Gender Identity Development

Gender identity is most appropriately conceptualized as a multidimensional construct, including aspects such as *gender typicality* (whether behaviors/interests conform to gender stereotypes), *gender contentedness* (the degree to which a person feels glad to be their gender), and *pressure to conform* to gender stereotypes (Egan & Perry, 2001; Yunger, Carver, & Perry, 2004). Importantly, these dimensions can operate independently of each other. For example, a person can have interests that are atypical of their gender yet be content in their gender. Extensions of the multidimensional model now include the potential for determining the degree to which an individual feels similar or dissimilar to both genders (Martin, Andrews, England, Zosuls, & Ruble, 2017). Research investigating the multidimensional model of gender identity (Egan & Perry, 2001) suggests that different aspects of gender identity interact to pose different risks for adjustment. For example, preadolescents' perceived gender atypicality most strongly predicted later internalizing behaviors when youth also reported high pressure to conform to gender stereotypes (Yunger et al., 2004). Research has identified both psychosocial and biological influences on gender identity development. For example, the development of cognitive gender schemas is thought to influence gender identity, framing children as active participants in this identity development through information processing activities. Social influences include early socialization, modeling and reinforcement for gender-typical behaviors by family and peers, as well as the perceived and experienced costs/benefits of belonging to a "social category." Biological theories emphasize the influence of prenatal sex hormones on both gendered behavior and identity (de Vries, Kreukels, Steensma, & McGuire, 2014; Ruble, Martin, & Berenbaum, 2006).

Gender identity develops over time (de Vries et al., 2014; Ruble et al., 2006). Male versus female gender behavior differences are present at birth; newborn girls spend longer time looking at interpersonal features of stimuli than do boys. Infants as young as 3–4 months old distinguish between male and female features, and by 2 years of age children understand gender labels. Three-year-old children can usually identify their own gender and are more likely to play with gender-typical toys. The degree to which an individual engages in sex-typical behavior is relatively constant from toddlerhood through adolescence (de Vries et al., 2014). Gender variant behavior often is first noticed in early childhood and may range from children playing with gender-atypical toys and dressing in atypical clothing to children expressing a desire to be the other gender, intense anatomic dysphoria, or insisting that they are the other gender.

Gender dysphoria (GD) is diagnosed when there is (1) "marked incongruence between one's experienced/expressed gender and assigned gender, of at least 6 months' duration," and (2) this incongruence is associated with clinically significant distress (American Psychiatric Association, 2013, pp. 452–453). The majority of children with GD no longer meet criteria by the time they reach adolescence or adulthood (Ristori &

Steensma, 2016); childhood GD intensity, older age at GD diagnosis, female assignment at birth, and early cross-gender identification predict persistent GD into adolescence (Steensma, McGuire, Kreukels, Beekman, & Cohen-Kettenis, 2013). Childhood GD has a high association with a lesbian, gay, or bisexual orientation (Ristori & Steensma, 2016). Adolescents presenting with GD typically report significant gender variant behavior occurred earlier in childhood, although a more recent "late-onset" GD first presenting in adolescence has been reported (Cohen-Kettenis & Klink, 2015).

Transgender/GNC Youth and Psychosocial Functioning

There is a rapidly growing body of literature describing the mental health disparities experienced by transgender and GNC youth. The documented increased risk for mental health problems has been linked to the dysphoria/distress experienced when one's gender assignment does not match their gender identity as well as the stress experienced from societal discrimination and prejudice (e.g., Cass' Minority Stress Model; Hatzenbuehler & Pachankis, 2016).

ADHD and ASD Higher rates of externalizing disorders such as ADHD and ASD have been found in the transgender population. In a recent study of a large sample of transgender youth (588 transgirls and 745 transboys), Becerra-Culqui et al. (2018) observed increased rates of ADHD in transgender children (15%) and adolescents (19.5%) compared to epidemiological estimates ranging from 5 to 10% in the general population. Indeed, ADHD was the most common mental health diagnosis observed in the child sample; however, the reason for this phenomenon is unknown. ADHD is associated with increased risk taking and impulsive behavior; thus clinicians should be aware of the presence of ADHD and work with trans youth to manage symptoms as it could lead to health risks, e.g., sexually transmitted infections (STIs) or substance use.

In the same study, 7% of the transgirls and 3% of transboys met criteria for ASD (versus 1% of the general population). It is important to note that this study did not perform a full diagnostic assessment for ASD and solely utilized a standardized diagnostic interview; however, other studies have observed similar increased rates of ASD in transgender youth (e.g., de Vries, Noens, Cohen-Kettenis, van Berckelaer-Onnes, & Doreleijers, 2010). Theories posited to explain the co-occurrence of ASD and GD include the male brain theory, fetal testosterone exposure, lack of attention paid to social constructs and schemas like gender, or that the social impairment experienced by those with GD (e.g., social isolation) may mimic symptoms of high functioning ASD (Glidden, Bouman, Jones, & Arcelus, 2016). Although these individuals present as more complex, they should not be excluded from receiving transgender-related medical treatment if deemed appropriate and gender dysphoria should not be seen/treated as a symptom of ASD.

Anxiety and Depression The occurrence of internalizing disorders in transgender youth has been well established. Becerra-Culqui et al. (2018) found anxiety to be the second most common diagnosis in children and adolescents with GD (15% and 38%, respectively). Chodzen, Hidalgo, Chen, and Garofalo (2018) found that internalized transphobia (i.e., the shame one feels about their identity) positively predicted a diagnosis of generalized anxiety disorder in a sample of adolescent with GD. Indeed, many youths with GD describe having few friends and self-isolate due to shame and fear. Among adolescents with GD, depression is the most common mental health diagnosis, occurring in over half of the adolescent sample (Becerra-Culqui et al., 2018). Transgender and GNC youth are at increased risk for self-harm, suicide ideation, and suicide attempts. A recent large-scale study comparing rates of suicide attempts between transgender youth and cisgender youth found 50.8% of transmen and 29.9% of transwomen had attempted suicide compared to 17.6% for cisgender females and 9.8% for cisgender males (Toomey,

Syvertsen, & Shramko, 2018). Notably, risk for suicide attempts doubles if families moderately reject a trans family member and the risk triples if there is a high amount of rejection (Klein & Golub, 2016). Factors found to protect against poor mental health outcomes in this population include positive self-esteem, supportive family and peer relationships, and community connections (Johns, Beltran, Armstrong, Jayne, & Barrios, 2018). Other studies have noted the positive effects of social transition (e.g., allowing youth to wear what they choose) and other people using youth's preferred name (Durwood, McLaughlin, & Olson, 2017; Russell, Pollitt, Li, & Grossman, 2018). Supportive environments and especially parental support can reduce risk for internalizing symptoms to levels found in the general population (Ryan, Russell, Huebner, Diaz, & Sanchez, 2010).

The CL psychologist is unlikely to receive a consultation for gender identity specifically unless they are working within a clinic that serves this population. However, nonspecialized practitioners are likely to interface with these youth under a variety of circumstances. Psychologists should be aware that consultation requests received for such concerns as "behavioral problems," "family stress," "suicide attempt," etc., may include a gender identity component. Given the high rate of occurrence of mental health issues in these youth, it is important that psychological consultation services in medical settings establish sensitive assessment strategies to identify and competently address these issues.

Table 1 Categories of disorders/differences of sex development

DSD category	Examples
Sex chromosome DSD	
45,X	Turner syndrome
47,XXY	Klinefelter syndrome
45,X/46,XY	Mixed gonadal dysgenesis
46,XX/46,XY	Chimeric
46,XY DSD	
Disorders of gonadal (testicular) development	Complete/partial gonadal dysgenesis
Disorders in androgen synthesis or action	17-Hydoxysteroid dehydrogenase deficiency, 5α reductase deficiency
Others	Severe hypospadias
46,XX DSD	
Disorders of gonadal (ovarian) development	Gonadal dysgenesis
Androgen excess	21 hydroxylase deficiency
Others	Vaginal atresia

Note. Ovotesticular DSD can be classified in any category depending on karyotype

Table based on classification presented in Lee, P. A., Houk, C. P., Ahmed, S. F., & Hughes, I. A. (2006). Consensus statement on management of intersex disorders. *Pediatrics, 118,* e488–500. doi:https://doi.org/10.1542/peds.2006-0738

Disorder(s)/Differences of Sex Development (DSD)

DSD are defined as congenital conditions in which a person's sex chromosomes, internal or external reproductive anatomy, or gonads have developed atypically (Lee, Houk, Ahmed, & Hughes, 2006). Incidence of DSD is estimated to be 1:4500–5000 live births (Sax, 2002). DSD are classified into three categories based on karyotype (Table 1) and range in acuity from presenting as a medical emergency, e.g., salt-wasting Congenital Adrenal Hyperplasia (CAH), to conditions for which no medical or surgical care is required, e.g., mild hypospadias. DSD often co-occur with other congenital anomalies that may pose greater mortality risk (e.g., congenital heart disease). DSD are most commonly diagnosed during the neonatal period when the infant's genitalia are first clearly visualized, and gender assignment may be delayed while further diagnostic workup proceeds including karyotyping and other genetic testing, imaging studies of internal structures, and lab work detailing sex hormone levels. Assignment of infant gender in such cases takes into consideration a variety of factors: medical diagnosis, implications for hormone therapy, fertility potential, genital appearance, surgical options, predicted gender identity given diagnosis (when evidence is available), and caregiver preference (Lee et al., 2006). Other common diagnostic time points include surgical exploration of an inguinal hernia in girls, atypical or absent pubertal development, or fertility challenges; thus, psychologists may be supporting patients and families across the developmental span in coping with a new diagnosis.

Medical care related to DSD often involves hormone therapy to influence genital development or steroids (in the case of CAH). Surgical treatment may be indicated in some conditions, e.g., if atypical gonadal development or placement increases cancer risk, or when the formation of urogenital structures block urine or menstrual fluid flow. Surgery may also occur to change the appearance of atypical genitals. These procedures are commonly initiated by the parents of infants, but have become the focus of controversy of advocacy and human rights groups due to the inability of the infant to consent to these irreversible and "not medically urgent" procedures (Human Rights Watch, 2017). Of note, many persons/families affected by these conditions reject the term DSD, expressing concerns that the term medicalizes, pathologizes, or stigmatizes the condition. Some individuals prefer condition-specific terminology (e.g., CAH), or prefer the term "intersex," which has a stronger association with identity and the gender spectrum (Johnson et al., 2017). As with transgender pronouns, asking individuals and families what term they prefer is the recommended patient-centered approach.

DSD and Psychosocial Functioning Most individuals with DSD maintain their assigned gender throughout their lifetime, although higher rates of both gender change and nonbinary gender identification (compared to the general population) have been documented (e.g., 3% gender change, 4% nonbinary gender; Kreukels et al., 2018). Findings from studies on more general psychological functioning and quality of life are mixed, with some reporting overall good psychological adjustment, while others note significant psychiatric and social concerns (e.g., Engberg et al., 2017; Meyer-Bahlburg, Khuri, Reyes-Portillo, & New, 2016; Nordenström, 2015). The adjustment of caregivers has also been explored, particularly during infancy, with many caregivers of infants with a DSD reporting high levels of distress (e.g., Pasterski, Mastroyannopoulou, Wright, Zucker, & Hughes, 2014).

Gender Identity: Consultation and Assessment

Given the psychosocial risk associated with GD, it is recommended that evaluations of preadolescents and older patients should routinely include an assessment of gender identity. Normalizing approaches can decrease fear and stigma related to disclosure. For example, a question such as "some children see themselves as a girl, some see themselves as a boy, and some see themselves as both of those or something entirely different—how do you see yourself?" conveys that a range of responses are acceptable. If youth appear to be unclear or questioning their gender identity, their uncertainty and level of confusion and/or distress can be queried. It is important to remember that youth may be questioning, or identify as nonbinary or transgender, without notable distress. Assessing level of distress is important as dysphoria contributes to negative mental health outcomes such as suicide attempts. Questions assessing this include the following: "How do you feel about your body?" "What would you change about your body if anything?" "Are there specific times when you feel worse about your body or gender? What makes it worse?"

Assessment via clinical interview should include eliciting an individual/family's gender narrative or gender journey. Gender is a multifaceted, internal, social construct and every journey is unique; many youth are eager to share the details of their story, which can help in building rapport. One aspect of establishing a diagnosis of GD is establishing a developmental timeline in order to establish consistency, insistency, and persistency. Two particular factors have been shown to predict stability of transgender identity into adolescence and adulthood: intensity of GD and tendency to discuss gender cognitively rather than affectively ("I am a boy" versus "I feel like a boy"; Steensma et al., 2013). Both factors can be assessed through the gender narrative. If gender identity appears to be a large aspect of the case conceptualization or referral question, self-report rating scales of body image/dissatisfaction and gender identity can also be used, such as the body image scale (for older children/adolescents; Lindgren & Pauly, 1975), the transgender congruence scale (validated for 18 and older but appropriate for older adolescents; Jones, Bouman, Haycraft, & Arcelus, 2018), the multidimensional gender identity scale (for children/adolescents; Egan & Perry, 2001), and the gender identity interview (Zucker et al., 1993; for review see Zucker, 2005), all of which are brief enough for the medical consultation setting. Patients may be more forthcoming if these areas are explored without parental presence. Parental input will likely be required for younger patients, which can be facilitated via a parent-report measure assessing child gender identity (Johnson et al., 2004). Of note, these measures have limited evidence supporting psychometric validity and reliability (this research is ongoing), particularly when used within the DSD population.

Beyond gender, consultations with patients reporting gender concerns and/or DSD condition should include the areas of functioning typically assessed in behavioral health consultations, such as family, school and peer functioning, and overall emotional/behavioral functioning (see the Assessment chapter). Peer victimization has been shown to influence the relationship between gender atypicality and psychosocial adjustment (Smith & Juvonen, 2017). Thus, the quality of peer relationships should be carefully assessed. Finally, given the high rates of self-harm, suicidal ideation, and suicide attempts in these populations, particularly in transgender youth, a thorough risk-safety assessment should be performed. Risk factors that should be assessed include parental support, peer support, school support, degree of affirmation, co-occurring depression, substance use, previous self-harm or suicide attempts, and family history of suicide. Conversely, protective factors should also be assessed including level of acceptance and support (parental, peer, school, societal), as well as access to and utilization of mental health services. For transgender youth, initiating transition may also be protective.

Of note, a psychosocial evaluation of youth and families with DSD or GD should be conducted with the standard pediatric psychology focus on *resiliency* factors. Though these populations are at higher risk for mental health difficulties, they should not be treated as innately pathological. Especially with GD, mental health professionals have often been rightfully perceived as functioning as "gatekeepers" to patients' access to life-saving treatments (e.g., hormonal therapies). Assessment of individuals requesting transition is now conceptualized as an avenue to confirm diagnosis of GD, evaluate knowledge and informed consent capabilities, and ultimately lead to appropriate referrals for medical and mental health interventions. The pediatric psychologist consultant should play an active role in facilitating referral to appropriate and competent providers.

Psychosocial Interventions for Transgender/Gender Nonconforming Youth

Addressing Mental Health Concerns The American Psychological Association (APA) has produced competency guidelines for psychologists treating individuals who identify as transgender or gender nonconforming (American Psychological Association, 2015). Affirmative care is the current primary therapeutic framework with transgender/gender nonconforming youth, which supports variability in gender expression based on research suggesting that lack of acceptance poses significant psychosocial risk (Edwards-Leeper, Leibowitz, & Sangganjanavanich, 2016; but see Berenbaum, 2018, for cautions related to this approach). Though there are currently no specific evidence-based therapies for this population, there are numerous evidence-based therapies used in the treatment of depression and anxiety that are appropriate for their clinical concerns. For example, a transgender youth who is afraid to go out in public may benefit from exposure therapy. A transgender youth with depression and/or self-harm may benefit from cognitive-behavioral therapy or dialectical behavior therapy. Given that many transgender youths are in situations that cannot be changed (e.g., being misgendered in public), many may benefit from acceptance and commitment therapy which strives to acknowledge emotional situations while promoting value-based behavior.

Addressing Family Dynamic Issues In addition to treating mental health difficulties, there are other tasks therapists can help transgender patients complete that have been shown in the research to have positive effects on well-being. As stated earlier, there is an increased risk for depression and suicide if families reject their children after coming out. Pediatric psychologists embedded in medical settings are uniquely positioned to facilitate family sessions that foster healthy, positive communication in addressing barriers in accepting and supporting their transgender child, including informing them of the damaging effects of rejection and the positive effects of their understanding and acceptance. One study found that supportive parents, defined in this study as those providing help, advice, and confidant support, increased transgender individual's life satisfaction, lowered the burden of being transgender, and reduced depressive symptoms (Simons, Schrager, Clark, Belzer, & Olson, 2013).

Additionally, data has shown that using affirmed name and pronouns reduces depressive symptoms, suicidal ideation, and behaviors. Russell et al. (2018) found that by adding one additional setting where a youth's chosen name and pronouns were used reduced depressive symptoms by five points (0–60 scale), suicidal ideation by 29%, and suicide behaviors by 56%. Providers should review their institutional policies regarding names and pronouns and advocate for patients to be referred to by their preferred name and pronouns when in the medical setting. Some electronic medical records have included a nickname or AKA in addition to legal name as well as a gender marker in addition to sex. Of note, it is important to ask a patient's permission before changing the chart ("Would you like me to make a note in your chart of your preferred name and pronouns? This way other staff will know how to refer to you"). Not all patients and families will be ready to socially transition in the medical setting.

In line with this research, Durwood et al. (2017) observed that socially transitioned youth (e.g., out and asking to be affirmed in multiple settings) showed no significant differences in self-worth or depressive symptoms when compared to cisgender peers. A very individualized approach is critical when working with youth who experience GD and desire social transition (Edwards-Leeper et al., 2016). The psychologist provider role can include exploring motivations and expectations for transition, identifying the range of possibilities for initiating or progressing transition, bolstering peer and family support, and problem-solving to optimize a healthy and safe social transition. Transition ideally begins in the home with caregivers and immediate family and then extends to other settings such as school or work. Social transition requires that schools allow transgender patients to go by affirmed name and pronouns, use affirmed gender facilities (bathroom/locker rooms), participate on affirmed gender teams, and above all else have access to a safe environment conducive to learning. Psychological intervention can function as an initial liaison between the family and school, increasing effective communication and reducing stress.

Addressing Health and Wellness Behaviors Lastly, patient and family negative health behaviors should be addressed. For example, transgender youth are at higher risk for substance use (Day, Fish, Perez-Brumer, Hatzenbuehler, & Russell, 2017) and STIs (highest rates of HIV are observed in the transgender female population; Kellogg, Clements-Nolle, Dilley, Katz, & McFarland, 2001). Psychological interventions should promote positive health behaviors to reduce rates of substance use and STIs. Moreover, providers may have unique opportunities if a patient is seeking gender-affirming hormone therapy. In addition to writing letters of support to medical providers on behalf of their patients, providers can also address smoking and weight management. Patients seeking estrogen therapy will be at increased risk for stroke; those risks are increased with smoking. Similarly, patients seeking testosterone will be at increased risk for high cholesterol; being a healthy weight and maintaining a balanced diet can decrease this risk.

Diverting Families from Controversial Approaches With transgender youth, the approach commonly known as conversion therapy should be avoided due to its harmful effects. This highly questionable approach, sometimes referred to as reparative therapy, aims to change an individual's sexual orientation or gender identity to conform to societal norms (i.e., heterosexual and cisgender). A recent retrospective study exploring long-term outcomes of adults who were referred for conversion therapy in adolescence revealed higher rates of depression, suicidal thoughts, suicide attempts, lower educational attainment, and lower weekly income (Ryan, Toomey, Diaz, & Russell, 2018). The APA, American Academy of Child and Adolescent Psychiatry, and the American Academy of Pediatrics have all deemed this therapy unethical. Numerous states have outlawed the therapy (14 states and the District of Columbia when this chapter was written) and more have pending bills awaiting approval. Families interested in seeking this form of therapy should be given the above information and should be cautioned from participating in such an approach.

DSD Given the complexity of DSD, care consensus statements and clinical guidelines advise that affected individuals and their families receive care within the context of a multidisciplinary team, including the presence of a behavioral health specialist (Cools et al., 2018; Lee et al., 2006). Thus, working with teams to routinely consult psychology when DSD is known or suspected is recommended. While DSD-specific psychological interventions have not been developed or tested, evidence-based treatments from other chronic conditions may be of use (Eccleston, Palermo, Fisher, & Law, 2012). Therapeutic tasks are largely dependent on time of diagnosis, developmental level of the patient, specific DSD condition, and setting (Sandberg, Gardner, & Cohen-Kettenis, 2012). With neonatal diagnosis, psychologists consulting on inpatient units or at outpatient medical visits can target parental postpartum depression or anxiety, coping with differences in infant's physical appearance, receiving unexpected and unwelcomed news, and dealing with uncertainty (particularly if gender assignment is delayed). In addition, caregivers may have been given inaccurate information from medical providers who do not have expertise in the condition; thus, it is essential that behavioral health providers optimize family knowledge to enhance both coping and decision-making. In addition, consulting psychologists can facilitate effective and supportive physician-family communication, including emphasizing the healthy aspects of the infant (Liao & Simmonds, 2013). Coaching caregivers in self-care and using cognitive-behavioral strategies to enhance coping may be helpful, as has been demonstrated in studies of caregivers in the NICU (not specific to DSD; Mendelson, Cluxton-Keller, Vullo, Tandon, & Noazin, 2017). Problem-solving interventions (Sahler et al., 2005) may also be of use, particularly in working with families on information-sharing strategies related to their family, friends, and other people involved in the infant's care, with the goal of enhancing social support and decreasing shame-inducing secrecy. In addition, it is within the role of the psychologist consultant to insist that families are receiving a robust shared decision-making process related to all important decisions such as gender assignment and medical and surgical interventions (Tamar-Mattis, Baratz, Baratz Dalke, & Karkazis, 2014).

As children age, ongoing education for parents on gender identity is important, for example, that their child can be content with their gender assignment even as they display gender atypical behaviors and the risk of compromised child adjustment when a child perceives parental pressure to conform to gender stereotypes. Educating parents on the harms associated with withholding developmentally appropriate information from children about their anatomical differences, medical condition, or future fertility is essential, as is supporting hesitant parents in the act of information sharing with their child in a developmentally appropriate manner (Liao & Simmonds, 2013).

Providing psychological support to patients with a DSD depends on developmental stage and presenting concerns. With younger children, body acceptance and highlighting child strengths are a general good strategy, as is education related to gender identity/roles/behaviors ("You can be a boy who likes to dance!")—a number of children's books are available that celebrate differences (https://www.dsdfamilies.org/parents/childrens-books). As children age, assessing for gender concerns or stigma/shame related to karyotype or body image is important to facilitate positive self-image and adjustment; if these concerns are noted, psychoeducation and cognitive-behavioral strategies may be implemented (perhaps specifically targeting differences; Clarke, Thompson, Jenkinson, Rumsey, & Newell, 2013). In adolescence and young adulthood, providing support and problem-solving around interpersonal/sexual intimacy or experimentation, interpersonal communication with significant others, and fertility concerns may be targets of intervention. Behavioral health providers may also assist with the treatment burden associated with DSD, such as increasing adherence to hormone therapy, coping with medical exams (Tishelman, Shumer, & Nahata, 2017), or decreasing anxiety related to vaginal dilation.

Conclusion

Pediatric psychologists' systems orientation and competence in assessment, enhancing emotion/behavior regulation, and communication dovetail with the needs of youth with DSD and/or gender variance and their families. The current dynamic sociocultural zeitgeist of gender identity creates opportunities for consulting psychologists to positively influence the experience of individuals and families by facilitating comprehensive health care that is up-to-date, person-centered, and informed by scientific evidence.

References

American Psychiatric Association. (2013). *Diagnostic and statistical manual of mental disorders* (5th ed.). Washington, DC: American Psychiatric Press.

American Psychological Association. (2015). Guidelines for psychological practice with transgender and gender nonconforming people. *American Psychologist, 70*, 832–864.

Becerra-Culqui, T. A., Liu, Y., Nash, R., Cromwell, L., Flanders, W. D., Getahun, D., ... Millman, A. (2018). Mental health of transgender and gender nonconforming youth compared with their peers. *Pediatrics, 141*, e20173845. https://doi.org/10.1542/peds.2017-3845

Berenbaum, S. A. (2018). Evidence needed to understand gender identity: Commentary on Turban & Ehrensaft (2018). *Journal of Child Psychology and Psychiatry, 59*, 1244-1247. https://doi.org/10.1111/jcpp.12997.

Chodzen, G., Hidalgo, M. A., Chen, D., & Garofalo, R. (2018). Minority stress factors associated with depression and anxiety among transgender and gender-nonconforming youth. *Journal of Adolescent Health, 64*, 467. https://doi.org/10.1016/j.jadohealth.2018.07.006

Clarke, A., Thompson, A. R., Jenkinson, E., Rumsey, N., & Newell, R. (2013). *CBT for appearance anxiety: Psychosocial interventions for anxiety due to visible difference*. West Sussex, UK: John Wiley & Sons.

Cohen-Kettenis, P. T., & Klink, D. (2015). Adolescents with gender dysphoria. *Best Practice & Research Clinical Endocrinology & Metabolism, 29*, 485–495. https://doi.org/10.1016/j.beem.2015.01.004

Cools, M., Nordenström, A., Robeva, R., Hall, J., Westerveld, P., Flück, C., ... Schweizer, K. (2018). Caring for individuals with a difference of sex development (DSD): A consensus statement. *Nature Reviews Endocrinology, 14*, 415–429. https://doi.org/10.1038/s41574-018-0010-8

Day, J. K., Fish, J. N., Perez-Brumer, A., Hatzenbuehler, M. L., & Russell, S. T. (2017). Transgender youth substance use disparities: Results from a population-based sample. *Journal of Adolescent Health, 61*, 729–735. https://doi.org/10.1016/j.jadohealth.2017.06.024

de Vries, A. L., Kreukels, B. P., Steensma, T. D., & McGuire, J. K. (2014). Gender identity development: A biopsychosocial perspective. In B. Kreukels, T. Steensma, & A. de Vries (Eds.), *Gender dysphoria and disorders of sex development* (pp. 53–80). Boston, MA: Springer.

de Vries, A. L., Noens, I. L., Cohen-Kettenis, P. T., van Berckelaer-Onnes, I. A., & Doreleijers, T. A. (2010). Autism spectrum disorders in gender dysphoric children and adolescents. *Journal of Autism and Developmental Disorders, 40*, 930–936. https://doi.org/10.1007/s10803-010-0935-9

Durwood, L., McLaughlin, K. A., & Olson, K. R. (2017). Mental health and self-worth in socially transitioned transgender youth. *Journal of the American Academy of Child & Adolescent Psychiatry, 56*, 116–123. https://doi.org/10.1016/j.jaac.2016.10.016

Eccleston, C., Palermo, T. M., Fisher, E., & Law, E. (2012). Psychological interventions for parents of children and adolescents with chronic illness. *Cochrane Database Systematic Reviews (Online), 8*, CD009660. https://doi.org/10.1002/14651858.CD009660.pub2

Edwards-Leeper, L., Leibowitz, S., & Sangganjanavanich, V. F. (2016). Affirmative practice with transgender and gender nonconforming youth: Expanding the model. *Psychology of Sexual Orientation and Gender Diversity, 3*, 165–172. https://doi.org/10.1037/sgd0000167

Egan, S. K., & Perry, D. G. (2001). Gender identity: A multidimensional analysis with implications for psychosocial adjustment. *Developmental Psychology, 37*, 451–463.

Engberg, H., Strandqvist, A., Nordenstrom, A., Butwicka, A., Nordenskjold, A., Hirschberg, A. L., & Frisen, L. (2017). Increased psychiatric morbidity in women with complete androgen insensitivity syndrome or complete gonadal dysgenesis. *Journal of Psychosomatic Research, 101*, 122–127. https://doi.org/10.1016/j.jpsychores.2017.08.009

Flores, A., Herman, J., Gates, G., & Brown, T. (2016). *How many adults identify as transgender in the United States?* Los Angeles, CA: Williams Institute.

Glidden, D., Bouman, W. P., Jones, B. A., & Arcelus, J. (2016). Gender dysphoria and autism spectrum disorder: A systematic review of the literature. *Sexual Medicine Reviews, 4*, 3–14. https://doi.org/10.1016/j.sxmr.2015.10.003

Hatzenbuehler, M. L., & Pachankis, J. E. (2016). Stigma and minority stress as social determinants of health among lesbian, gay, bisexual, and transgender youth research evidence and clinical implications. *Pediatric Clinics of North America, 63*, 985–997. https://doi.org/10.1016/j.pcl.2016.07.003

Human Rights Watch. (2017). *"I Want to Be Like Nature Made Me": Medically unnecessary surgeries on intersex children in the US*. Retrieved from https://www.hrw.org/report/2017/07/25/i-want-be-nature-made-me/medically-unnecessary-surgeries-intersex-children-us

Hyde, J. S., Bigler, R. S., Joel, D., Tate, C. C., & van Anders, S. M. (2018). The future of sex and gender in psychology: Five challenges to the gender binary. *American Psychologist, 74*, 171. https://doi.org/10.1037/amp0000307

Johns, M. M., Beltran, O., Armstrong, H. L., Jayne, P. E., & Barrios, L. C. (2018). Protective factors among transgender and gender variant youth: A systematic review by socioecological level. *The Journal of Primary Prevention, 39*, 263–301. https://doi.org/10.1007/s10935-018-0508-9

Johnson, E. K., Rosoklija, I., Finlayso, C., Chen, D., Yerkes, E. B., Madonna, M. B., … Cheng, E. Y. (2017). Attitudes towards "disorders of sex development" nomenclature among affected individuals. *Journal of Pediatric Urology, 13*, 608.e601–608.e608. https://doi.org/10.1016/j.jpurol.2017.03.035

Johnson, L. L., Bradley, S. J., Birkenfeld-Adams, A. S., Kuksis, M. A. R., Maing, D. M., Mitchell, J. N., & Zucker, K. J. (2004). A parent-report gender identity questionnaire for children. *Archives of Sexual Behavior, 33*, 105–116.

Jones, B. A., Bouman, W. P., Haycraft, E., & Arcelus, J. (2018). The gender congruence and life satisfaction scale (GCLS): Development and validation of a scale to measure outcomes from transgender health services. *International Journal of Transgenderism, 20*, 1–18. https://doi.org/10.1080/15532739.2018.1453425

Kellogg, T. A., Clements-Nolle, K., Dilley, J., Katz, M. H., & McFarland, W. (2001). Incidence of human immunodeficiency virus among male-to-female transgendered persons in San Francisco. *Journal of Acquired Immune Deficiency Syndromes (1999), 28*, 380–384. https://doi.org/10.1097/00126334-200112010-00012

Klein, A., & Golub, S. A. (2016). Family rejection as a predictor of suicide attempts and substance misuse among transgender and gender nonconforming adults. *LGBT Health, 3*, 193–199. https://doi.org/10.1089/lgbt.2015.0111

Kreukels, B. P., Köhler, B., Nordenström, A., Roehle, R., Thyen, U., Bouvattier, C., … de Vries, A. (2018). Gender dysphoria and gender change in disorders of sex development/intersex conditions: Results from the dsd-LIFE study. *The Journal of Sexual Medicine, 15*, 777–785. https://doi.org/10.1016/j.jsxm.2018.02.021

Lee, P. A., Houk, C. P., Ahmed, S. F., & Hughes, I. A. (2006). Consensus statement on management of intersex disorders. *Pediatrics, 118*, e488–e500. https://doi.org/10.1542/peds.2006-0738

Liao, L. M., & Simmonds, M. (2013). Communicating with clients affected by diverse sex development. In J. Wiggins & A. Middleton (Eds.), *Getting the message across: Communication with diverse populations in clinical genetics* (pp. 42–60). New York: Oxford University Press.

Lindgren, T. W., & Pauly, I. B. (1975). A body image scale for evaluating transsexuals. *Archives of Sexual Behavior, 4*, 639–656.

Martin, C. L., Andrews, N. C., England, D. E., Zosuls, K., & Ruble, D. N. (2017). A dual identity approach for conceptualizing and measuring children's gender identity. *Child Development, 88*, 167–182. https://doi.org/10.1111/cdev.12568

Mendelson, T., Cluxton-Keller, F., Vullo, G. C., Tandon, S. D., & Noazin, S. (2017). NICU-based interventions to reduce maternal depressive and anxiety symptoms: A meta-analysis. *Pediatrics, 139*, e20161870. https://doi.org/10.1542/peds.2016-1870

Meyer-Bahlburg, H. F., Khuri, J., Reyes-Portillo, J., & New, M. I. (2016). Stigma in medical settings as reported retrospectively by women with congenital adrenal hyperplasia (CAH) for their childhood and adolescence. *Journal of Pediatric Psychology, 42*, 496–503. https://doi.org/10.1093/jpepsy/jsw034

Nordenström, A. (2015). Psychosocial factors in disorders of sex development in a long-term perspective: What clinical opportunities are there to intervene? *Hormone and Metabolic Research, 47*, 351–356. https://doi.org/10.1055/s-0034-1398562

Pasterski, V., Mastroyannopoulou, K., Wright, D., Zucker, K. J., & Hughes, I. A. (2014). Predictors of posttraumatic stress in parents of children diagnosed with a disorder of sex development. *Archives of Sexual Behavior, 43*, 369–375. https://doi.org/10.1007/s10508-013-0196-8

Rider, G. N., McMorris, B. J., Gower, A. L., Coleman, E., & Eisenberg, M. E. (2018). Health and care utilization of transgender and gender nonconforming youth: A population-based study. *Pediatrics, 141*, e20171683. https://doi.org/10.1542/peds.2017-1683

Ristori, J., & Steensma, T. D. (2016). Gender dysphoria in childhood. *International Review of Psychiatry, 28*, 13–20. https://doi.org/10.3109/09540261.2015.1115754

Ruble, D. N., Martin, C. L., & Berenbaum, S. A. (2006). Gender Development. In W. Damon, R. Lerner, & N. Eisenberg (Eds.), *Handbook of child psychology: Social, emotional, and personality* (Vol. 3, pp. 858–932). New York: John Wiley & Sons.

Russell, S. T., Pollitt, A. M., Li, G., & Grossman, A. H. (2018). Chosen name use is linked to reduced depressive symptoms, suicidal ideation, and suicidal behavior among transgender youth. *Journal of Adolescent Health, 63*, 503–505. https://doi.org/10.1016/j.jadohealth.2018.02.003

Ryan, C., Russell, S. T., Huebner, D., Diaz, R., & Sanchez, J. (2010). Family acceptance in adolescence and the health of LGBT young adults. *Journal of Child and Adolescent Psychiatric Nursing, 23*, 205–213. https://doi.org/10.1111/j.1744-6171.2010.00246.x

Ryan, C., Toomey, R. B., Diaz, R. M., & Russell, S. T. (2018). Parent-initiated sexual orientation change efforts with LGBT adolescents: Implications for young adult mental health and adjustment. *Journal of Homosexuality*, 1–15. https://doi.org/10.1080/00918369.2018.1538407

Sahler, O. J. Z., Fairclough, D. L., Phipps, S., Mulhern, R. K., Dolgin, M. J., Noll, R. B., … Butler, R. W. (2005). Using problem-solving skills training to reduce negative affectivity in mothers of children with newly diagnosed cancer: Report of a multisite randomized trial. *Journal of Consulting and Clinical Psychology, 73*, 272–283. https://doi.org/10.1037/0022-006x.73.2.272

Sandberg, D. E., Gardner, M., & Cohen-Kettenis, P. T. (2012). Psychological aspects of the treatment of patients with disorders of sex development. *Seminars in Reproductive Medicine, 30*, 443–452. https://doi.org/10.1055/s-0032-1324729

Sax, L. (2002). How common is intersex? A response to Anne Fausto-Sterling. *Journal of Sex Research, 39*, 174–178. https://doi.org/10.1080/00224490209552139

Simons, L., Schrager, S. M., Clark, L. F., Belzer, M., & Olson, J. (2013). Parental support and mental health among transgender adolescents. *Journal of Adolescent Health, 53*, 791–793. https://doi.org/10.1016/j.jadohealth.2013.07.019

Smith, D. S., & Juvonen, J. (2017). Do I fit in? Psychosocial ramifications of low gender typicality in early adolescence. *Journal of Adolescence, 60*, 161–170. https://doi.org/10.1016/j.adolescence.2017.07.014

Steensma, T. D., McGuire, J. K., Kreukels, B. P., Beekman, A. J., & Cohen-Kettenis, P. T. (2013). Factors associated with desistence and persistence of childhood gender dysphoria: A quantitative follow-up study. *Journal of the American Academy of Child & Adolescent Psychiatry, 52*, 582–590. https://doi.org/10.1016/j.jaac.2013.03.016

Tamar-Mattis, A., Baratz, A., Baratz Dalke, K., & Karkazis, K. (2014). Emotionally and cognitively informed consent for clinical care for differences of sex development. *Psychology & Sexuality, 5*, 44–55. https://doi.org/10.1080/19419899.2013.831215

Tishelman, A. C., Shumer, D. E., & Nahata, L. (2017). Disorders of sex development: Pediatric psychology and the genital exam. *Journal of Pediatric Psychology, 42*, 530–543. https://doi.org/10.1093/jpepsy/jsw015

Toomey, R. B., Syvertsen, A. K., & Shramko, M. (2018). Transgender adolescent suicide behavior. *Pediatrics, 142*, e20174218. https://doi.org/10.1542/peds.2017-4218

Trotta, D. (2018, October 9). *New York City creates gender-neutral 'X' option for birth certificates*. Retrieved from https://www.reuters.com/article/us-usa-lgbt-new-york/new-york-city-creates-gender-neutral-x-option-for-birth-certificates-idUSKCN1MJ2OP

Yunger, J. L., Carver, P. R., & Perry, D. G. (2004). Does gender identity influence children's psychological well-being? *Developmental Psychology, 40*, 572–582. https://doi.org/10.1037/0012-1649.40.4.572

Zucker, K. J. (2005). Measurement of psychosexual differentiation. *Archives of Sexual Behavior, 34*, 375–388. https://doi.org/10.1007/s10508-005-4336-7

Zucker, K. J., Bradley, S. J., Sullivan, C. B. L., Kuksis, M., Birkenfeld-Adams, A., & Mitchell, J. N. (1993). A gender identity interview for children. *Journal of Personality Assessment, 61*, 443–456. https://doi.org/10.1207/s15327752jpa6103_2

The Presentation of Child Maltreatment in Healthcare Settings

Kimberly Burkhart and Michele Knox

Introduction

Non-accidental injury is defined as abuse that is deliberately inflicted on a vulnerable person (World Health Organization, 2018). Non-accidental injury perpetrated by a child's caregiver is considered child maltreatment. This chapter focuses on the psychologist's role as a consultant in the hospital setting and in the patient-centered medical home (PCMH), as well as provides an overview of recommended outpatient interventions. The psychologist's role in resident and physician education on child maltreatment prevention and intervention will be explained. Evidence-based interventions to address child maltreatment will be identified.

K. Burkhart (✉)
UH Rainbow Babies and Children's Hospital, Cleveland, OH, USA

Pediatrics and Psychiatry, Case Western Reserve University, Cleveland, OH, USA
e-mail: Kimberly.Burkhart@UHhospitals.org

M. Knox
Department of Psychiatry, University of Toledo College of Medicine and Health Sciences, Toledo, OH, USA

Definition

Child maltreatment refers to abuse and neglect of children under 18 years of age (World Health Organization, 2018). All forms of child maltreatment are considered examples of non-accidental injury. Child abuse involves physical, sexual, and emotional abuse and trauma inflicted upon a child, whereas neglect involves failing to meet the basic needs of the child (Jackson, Kissoon, & Green, 2015). Child physical abuse includes engaging in acts that can inflict harm upon children, including punching, hitting, kicking, beating, biting, pushing, shoving, shaking, burning, and poisoning (Jackson et al., 2015). Child abuse is defined as sexual coercion or exploitation of any child (Child Abuse and Prevention Treatment Act, 2010).

Signs of child sexual abuse are highly variable and may include, among other things, anxiety, fear of being alone, avoidance of certain people or places, bed-wetting or soiling, nonage-typical sexual behavior or knowledge, and/or sexually transmitted disease or pregnancy (Child Abuse and Prevention Treatment Act, 2010).

Emotional abuse is the most difficult type of abuse to identify in the hospital and ambulatory pediatric setting. Examples of emotional abuse include confinement, verbal abuse, exposure to domestic violence, and other parental behaviors that cause the child significant emotional distress

B. D. Carter, K. A. Kullgren (eds.), *Clinical Handbook of Psychological Consultation in Pediatric Medical Settings*, Issues in Clinical Child Psychology, https://doi.org/10.1007/978-3-030-35598-2_34

(Leetch & Woolridge, 2013). Signs of emotional trauma may include, among other things, depression, anxiety, inappropriate fear of caregivers and/or medical personnel, and attachment problems (Leetch, Leipsic, & Woolridge, 2015).

Neglect involves not meeting the emotional, educational, nutritional, supervision, and/or medical needs of the child and is the most common form of child maltreatment (Jackson et al., 2015). Forms of neglect observed in pediatric medical centers often include noncompliance with medical recommendations, delay or failure to seek medical care, inadequate nutrition, non-illness failure to thrive, unmanaged obesity, illicit drug-exposed newborns or childhood ingestions, inadequate nurturance or affection, inadequate clothing, unmet educational needs, abandonment, and homelessness (Jackson et al., 2015). Other forms of neglect include illicit prenatal drug exposure, as well as ingestion of drugs or alcohol by the child. Environmental hazards can also constitute neglect such as access to firearms, inappropriate access to medications, unrestrained children in cars, and exposure to domestic violence and/or exposure to secondhand cigarette smoke for children with pulmonary conditions (Jackson et al., 2015).

Another form of child maltreatment is medical child abuse, also known as factitious disorder imposed on another, or Munchausen syndrome by proxy, in which a caregiver exaggerates or fabricates symptoms the child is experiencing or causes symptoms in the child that result in unnecessary medical care and intervention. More specifically, medical child abuse is a form of physical abuse in which the evaluation or medical intervention serves as the tool for the abuse. Signs of this type of maltreatment include a caregiver-reported history that is inconsistent with the symptom presentation, illness or injury that occurs only when the child is alone with the caregiver, symptoms inconsistent with test results, or repeated or varied illnesses, injuries, or hospitalizations. See Chap. 35 "Munchausen by Proxy and Pediatric Factitious Disorder Imposed on Self" for additional details.

Prevalence

In the United States (USA), three million child abuse cases are reported each year. Based on substantiated cases, 1 in 8 children in the USA has experienced some form of maltreatment. It is estimated that 2–10% of children who present to the ED have medical presentations resulting from abuse and/or neglect (Leetch & Woolridge, 2013). Less than 20% of children who have suspected child abuse reports are placed into the foster care system as Child Service Boards often do not respond by removing children from the home (Child Welfare Information Gateway, 2016). Furthermore, approximately 40% of deaths due to child abuse occur among children who have active or previously investigated child protective service (CPS) cases (Markenson et al., 2007).

National data suggest that half the children evaluated for maltreatment have clinically impairing emotional and behavioral problems, which is 2.5 times greater than the general population (Casanueva et al., 2012). Victimization rates of abuse and neglect are highest among children birth to 3 years of age (Child Maltreatment, 2002). Among this age group, those who are hospitalized related to abuse are more likely to be male and publicly insured (Farst, Ambadwar, King, Bird, & Robbins, 2013). In early childhood, poly-victimization and sexual abuse are most common in 3-year-old girls (Kellogg, 2007), and children who experience maltreatment are more likely than other ED patients to die while hospitalized (King, Farst, Jaeger, Onukwube, & Robbins, 2015). The most common forms of neglect that present in the hospital setting in children ages 0–3 years include tobacco exposure inhalation, second- and third-degree burns of the body, and nonfatal drowning (King et al., 2015).

Children ages 6–8 years have the highest maltreatment rates when considering all forms of abuse (Sedlak, Mettenburg, Basena, et al., 2010). By the age of 18, 1 in 4 females and 1 in 6 males will have experienced sexual abuse (Pulido et al., 2015). Sexual abuse is most often reported when asked by a healthcare professional whether victimization has occurred rather than victims self-initiating disclosure (Schaeffer, Leventhal, & Asnes, 2011).

Protective Factors

Multiple protective factors have been identified that decrease the likelihood of child maltreatment. Protective factors tend to center around the child's family context and include, among others, stable and nurturing relationships with caregivers, social support, clear and developmentally appropriate rules and expectations, and collaborative problem-solving (Centers for Disease Control and Prevention, National Center for Injury Prevention and Control, Division of Violence and Prevention, 2014; Lubell, Lofton, & Singer, 2008).

Risk Factors

Social risk factors are variable and include maternal depression, being a single mother, parental history of child maltreatment, having a nonbiological male caregiver living in the home, being exposed to domestic violence, living in poverty, parent unemployment, social isolation, parental substance abuse, parental incarceration, prior CPS involvement, income inequality, exposure to community violence, poor parental understanding of child development, and being less than 4 years old (Berlin, Dodge, & Reznick, 2013; Centers for Disease Control and Prevention, 2014; Eckenrode, Smith, McCarthy, & Dineen, 2014).

Nonsocial risk factors include inconsistent prenatal care, premature birth, neonatal intensive care stays, a child having special needs or developmental disabilities, immunizations not up-to-date, gas or colic drops, missing well-child checks, more frequent changes in ambulatory care providers, and having no primary care provider (Friedlander, Rubin, Alpern, Mandell, et al., 2008; Keenan, Cook, Olson, Bardsley, & Campbell, 2017; Mason, Schnitzer, Danilack, Elston, & Savitz, 2018). Ethnic characteristics can predict outcomes as well; for example, there is a higher rate of maltreatment and subsequent mortality rate among African American children compared to Caucasian and Hispanic children (Sedlak et al., 2010). Early identification remains one of the most significant challenges for medical professionals, which provides psychologists the opportunity to work collaboratively with other medical professionals to assist with identification of risk factors and promotion of protective factors. Furthermore, to assess and address the myriad possible developmental, emotional, and behavioral outcomes related to child maltreatment, medical providers should be encouraged to consult psychologists when faced with a known or substantiated history of child abuse or neglect.

Reporting Rules

Each US state, as well as American Samoa, the District of Columbia, Guam, the Northern Mariana Islands, Puerto Rico, and the US Virgin Islands, has its own set of laws outlining who must report child maltreatment and what must be reported. Who is mandated to report and under what circumstances mandated reporters must report vary from state to state and territory to territory. Summaries of state laws are available at the Child Welfare Information Gateway (Child Welfare Information Gateway, 2016). Because of these wide variations in state and territory laws, it is imperative that professionals and the public have detailed understanding of these laws and that they update their knowledge whenever they relocate.

Although most states mandate reporting by child educators, mental health and healthcare providers, law enforcement officers, and child care workers, it is important to note that other professions—such as employees at camps, photograph processors, and animal control officers—are mandated in only certain states. In contrast, clergy are expressly not compelled to report suspected maltreatment in certain states.

Some reporting issues relevant to mandated reporting in medical settings are worth noting. First, a mandated reporter cannot delegate or assign his/her duty to report to others. If a mandated reporter knows or suspects abuse, then he or she must make a report. This is the case regardless of whether an attending or another authority instructs otherwise, or whether others on a treatment team were also aware of the abuse. It is also important to note that some individuals who are still in training, such as interns or residents, are mandated reporters in some states.

Usually, mandated reporters are obligated to report when they suspect or have reason to believe that child maltreatment is occurring or has occurred. In some cases, reporting must take place if maltreatment is thought to be likely to occur, or if the child faces a threat of maltreatment in the future. Members of the public in certain jurisdictions must report known maltreatment, but the public in other areas simply have the option to report.

Although most laws require reporting for maltreated individuals under the age of 18, there are some laws mandating reporting for older individuals with impairments or disabilities. Prenatal drug exposure, human trafficking, and involvement in child pornography are reasons for mandated reporting in some, but not all, locations as well.

Reporting is typically made to a CPS or child welfare agency, but various laws state that reporting may be made to sheriff, police, tribal social service, or law enforcement agencies. Toll-free reporting hotlines also are available in many areas. A list of resources by state is available online at the Child Welfare Information Gateway, under "State Child Abuse and Neglect Reporting Numbers."

How to Report Suspected Child Maltreatment

When calling, the reporter should state that they would like to make a report of suspected or known child maltreatment. CPS will typically ask for the following information:

- The name and address of the maltreated child
- The child's age
- The name, contact information, and address of the parent/caregiver
- The reason you know or suspect the child has been or is at risk of being maltreated
- Any other details that may be helpful to the investigation. This may include other indicators of the child's risk or vulnerability, such as impairments, mental health or medical illnesses, or disabilities

A report should be made even if the reporter does not have all, or even most, of these details. Whether the reporter's name must be in the written report also varies by state. Many, but not all, states require the reporter's identity be kept confidential and not released to the public. In some cases, the reporter may not be certain that an incident would be considered maltreatment. In this case, the individual may choose to call CPS and describe the incident without revealing identifying information. CPS staff will sometimes provide feedback as to whether the information is reportable. The clinician should document the call and the feedback in the medical record.

Consultation in the Hospital Setting

Many hospitals utilize child protection teams (CPT) typically comprised of psychologists, social workers, physicians, nurses and other healthcare professionals, and legal professionals. The CPT reviews and addresses cases of suspected child abuse that are identified within the hospital system by healthcare providers. Psychologists on these teams are often in consulting roles, working with team members to differentiate normal from abnormal child behavior and presentations, to identify signs and symptoms of child maltreatment, and to determine if maltreatment needs to be reported and addressed.

In the hospital setting, consulting psychologists should advise physicians that vigilance is recommended, and it may be necessary to inquire about unexplained injuries since skin injuries are the most common physical manifestation of abuse. Studies have found that approximately 27% of abused infants had an injury prior to being identified as being abused with 80% of child injuries being identified by bruising (Bailhache, Leroy, Pillet, & Salmi, 2013). There is no formal screening tool that has been found to be appropriate for detecting abuse; therefore, interviewing about physical abuse should always be conducted when warning signs are present (Bailhache et al., 2013; Sheets et al., 2013).

Providers need to be aware of implicit bias and other factors that may influence or deter the accurate identification of maltreatment (Jenny, Hymel, Ritzen, Reinert, & Hay, 1999; Lane et al., 2002; Laskey, Stump, Perkins, et al., 2012). Physicians are more willing to consider identification of abuse in children with lower socioeconomic status (SES; Laskey et al., 2012). Child abuse is more prevalent in lower SES communities, but considering population-based studies, most families of lower SES do not abuse their children (Sidebothan & Heron, 2006). Social intuition and information obtained through psychosocial interviewing have been associated with deviations in gold standard evaluations, which can result in diagnostic impressions not indicative of abuse (Keenan et al., 2017). In other words, the perception of social risk (e.g., SES and ethnicity) can influence physicians' certainty of abuse resulting in medical diagnoses with an absence of documentation of possible maltreatment if social risk is perceived to be low based on demographics.

In cases in which abuse has been reported or is suspected, child abuse pediatricians will often complete the medical evaluation. When abuse or neglect is being considered, a complete psychosocial assessment also is needed. An appropriate history should be taken with the child interviewed alone if possible. Involvement of a behavioral health consultant can often make the child feel more comfortable. Caregivers should also be interviewed alone. Documentation should include timing, mechanism, proceeding events, and witnesses. In addition to assessing for the type, frequency, and perpetrator of maltreatment, the consultant should assess for parent alcohol and substance abuse, domestic violence, parent psychiatric history, parent incarceration, and prior child protective services involvement (Jenny, 2011). If abuse is suspected, information obtained through medical evaluation and psychosocial interviewing should be provided to CPS and possibly law enforcement, as described above. Law enforcement may come to the location to complete a forensic evaluation (Leetch & Woolridge, 2013).

If child abuse is ruled out as a concern, but the child may be at risk for neglect due to lack of resources, attempts should be made by a behavioral health consultant to connect families with social agencies in the community that assist with providing food and clothing. Some hospitals have medical-legal partnerships in which legal aid can be consulted to assist with obtaining safe housing. When there is noncompliance with medical recommendations, it is advised that the consultant explore with the parent what might be contributing to the noncompliance to assess for stressors and to problem-solve barriers. Reasons for medical neglect often include unemployment, homelessness, difficulty obtaining transportation, illiteracy, intellectual disabilities, and/or language barriers. Within the context of medical neglect, if abuse is not identified, it is recommended that the clinician make reasonable attempts to assist the family with resources needed for medical adherence and to provide education about medical conditions and treatment before reporting to CPS. CPS may also be utilized to access supports for the family. If risks are identified, the behavioral health consultant can work with allied professionals to access needed programming.

Consultation in Patient-Centered Medical Homes

The patient-centered medical home (PCMH) is accountable for meeting both the psychological and mental health needs of the patient including prevention, wellness, and intervention. This type of comprehensive care often includes physicians, advanced nurse practitioners, physician assistants, nutritionists, pharmacists, psychologists, and social workers. Having a PCMH is one of the most promising strategies for providing proactive healthcare and anticipatory guidance (Raney, 2015). A PCMH also allows for the shift from reactive-based care to population-based management and prevention (Aaron & Burtless, 2014). The embedded psychologist is in the unique position to become familiar with families and know their stressors and strengths.

Premature birth and neonatal intensive care stays are risk factors for child maltreatment (Mason et al., 2018). At the point of primary care involvement, psychologists can begin to work with families and track at-risk children's progress. Deviations in normal child development can be more readily identified and may signal the need for screening for child maltreatment. Examples of such deviations include colic, middle of the night awakenings, separation anxiety, poor appetite, problems with toilet training, and developmental disabilities (Schmitt, 1987; Sullivan & Knutson, 1998). For at-risk children, the consulting psychologist can provide brief behavioral intervention related to parent training as well as identify the necessity for further evaluation and referral.

Psychologists can be involved in providing anticipatory guidance about toxic stress within the PCMH. Toxic stress is defined as intense or prolonged activation of the stress response, which can affect brain architecture and physical and mental health (Compton & Shim, 2015). Adverse childhood experiences (ACEs) such as physical, emotional, or sexual abuse, food insecurity, poor housing or education, and exposure to substance use and violence can trigger a toxic stress response resulting in increased cortisol production and changes to the hypothalamic-pituitary-adrenal (HPA) axis (Compton & Shim, 2015). Other areas of anticipatory guidance or brief consultation include topics such as normative child development, positive child behavior management strategies (i.e., assisting with identifying behaviors to reward, ignore, and which should result in consequences), education on privacy and safe/unsafe touches, and connection to support and mutual aid groups to strengthen parents' social supports (Jenny & Crawford-Jakubiak, 2013; Mikton & Butchart, 2009). Psychologists can also be involved in safety planning when a history of maltreatment has been identified.

When there are deviations in normal child development or the presence of ACEs, a psychologist may recommend prevention/intervention programs. Examples of such programs include home visitation programs (e.g., The Nurse-Family Partnership; Olds, Kitzman, Knudtson, et al., 2014) and parent training behavior management programs (e.g., Triple P; Garcia, DeNard, Ohene, Morones, & Connaughton, 2018, Incredible Years; Webster-Stratton & Reid, 2010; ACT Raising Safe Kids Program, Silva, 2011).

The psychologist may be consulted to provide direction to the healthcare provider related to identifying trauma and providing brief intervention or guidance on an external referral. When child maltreatment has occurred, a psychologist can provide brief intervention on behavioral strategies to manage common symptoms associated with trauma such as sleep disturbance, eating disturbance (food refusal, hoarding, and overeating), toileting issues (encopresis, enuresis, constipation), functional abdominal pain, and tension headaches.

Involvement in the Child Advocacy Center

Consulting psychologists can serve as a member of a Child Advocacy Center (CAC) team or can serve as the link between healthcare providers and the CAC. CACs are safe, child-centered facilities for children and adolescents who may have experienced child maltreatment. CAC teams often include healthcare providers, law enforcement, psychologists, and other mental health providers, prosecution teams, child protective services, victim advocates, and other allied professionals. The team works together to promote children's safety and to investigate, manage, and prosecute child maltreatment cases. Interviews are done in a manner that eliminate the need for repeated, potentially stressful questioning of children. The psychologist can assist with the interview, assessment of trauma and mental health problems, and provision or management of needed services. The psychologist can also educate other team members about mental health-related aspects of the case and needs of children and family members. Psychologists who are not

CAC members can link children suspected or known by healthcare providers to be maltreated with needed CAC services.

Education About Physical Punishment and Its Side Effects

Another key role for the psychologist is to serve as the consultant to educate medical professionals about the outcomes of physical punishment and how to advise parents and caregivers about recommended methods for misbehavior/noncompliance. The American Psychological Association has a resolution on physical punishment of children by parents in which it suggests that parents be asked to use alternative forms of discipline.

Consultants are advised to be aware that meta-analyses of the literature substantiate that physical punishment is linked to a variety of negative outcomes or "side effects," including low internalization of parents' morals/values, increased likelihood of childhood aggression, antisocial behavior, externalizing behavior and internalizing problems, mental health problems, negative parent-child relationship, impaired cognitive ability, low self-esteem, abuse victimization, and adult antisocial behavior and mental health problems (Gershoff & Grogan-Kaylor, 2016). In keeping with the research, many healthcare, educational, and other organizations have developed statements against the use of physical punishment. The Gundersen Center for Effective Discipline provides a list online of organizations that have positions against corporal punishment of children. Despite these statements and the research findings, the large majority of US children continue to be subjected to physical punishment in the home (Bender et al., 2007; Regalado, Sareen, Inkelas, Wissow, & Halfon, 2004).

Consultants are urged to help medical professionals use anticipatory guidance and other methods to broach the topic of corporal punishment with families and to teach positive alternatives for shaping behavior. There is some evidence to suggest that anticipatory guidance may be effective in promoting positive, nonviolent parenting practices (Sege, Hatmaker-Flanigan, De Vos, Levin-Goodman, & Spivak, 2006). Anticipatory guidance can be most effective when used before habits develop. In the case of physical punishment, medical professionals should be advised to start addressing the topic in infancy, as by the time US children reach 1 year of age, nearly 25% have been physically punished (Straus & Stewart, 1999).

A recent review has identified a variety of methodologies with research evidence demonstrating some degree of success in reducing physical punishment or attitudes in favor of physical punishment (Gershoff et al., 2017). In one study, a training lasting only 1 h was found to have a significant effect on healthcare providers' attitudes toward physical punishment. However, results indicated that more than one-third of the trainees still had attitudes favorable of physical punishment after training, suggesting a possible need for more or better training. Play Nicely (Scholer, Brokish, Mukherjee, et al., 2008; Burkhart, Knox, & Hunter, 2016) is a program that has been found to be useful with medical trainees and parents alike for decreasing positive attitudes toward corporal punishment. Another program widely used in the hospital setting is The No Hit Zone Program (Gershoff et al., 2017). This program educates hospital staff about physical punishment and has resulted in reduced support of physical punishment and significant increases in the likelihood of intervening in cases of parental physical punishment. The consulting psychologist can have a role in implementation of these programs, as well as in training medical staff about the negative mental and behavioral implications of corporal punishment.

Resident and Physician Education

Consultation and formal training for healthcare providers is a critical component of child maltreatment prevention and intervention. In part, this is due to access. Annual well visits, sporadic sick visits, ED visits, hospital stays, and specialist visits put healthcare providers in more frequent contact with maltreated children than most other mandated professionals. However, a significant proportion of healthcare providers report being underprepared to accurately identify and report suspected child maltreatment (Gunn, Hickson, & Cooper, 2005; Lawrence & Brannen, 2000). Psychologists are in a unique position to provide education and consultation to medical professionals. A thorough curriculum for education about child maltreatment, developed by the American Psychological Association Division 37 Section on Child Maltreatment, provides detailed recommendations and resources for this purpose (Miller-Perrin & Malloy, 2007).

There are also a few existing programs that have at least some evidence or effectiveness in improving mandated reporting skills and maltreatment knowledge. For example, an Internet-based education module about identification and reporting of child maltreatment (Kenny, Lopez-Griman, & Donohue, 2017) addresses maltreatment identification and knowledge and practices. Preliminary research findings indicate that professionals trained using the module had better knowledge of child maltreatment reporting practices and greater ability to identify signs and symptoms of maltreatment compared to a control condition.

Another curriculum was developed and delivered to medical students. The Child Advocacy Studies Training program (CAST) originally was developed by the National Child Protection Training Center and faculty of Winona State University to educate a variety of professionals in diverse fields to successfully prevent, identify, and respond to child maltreatment. The CAST program aims to educate college graduates about child maltreatment and child advocacy (Vieth, 2006). Topics addressed in the CAST curriculum include maltreatment definitions, prevalence, risk and protective factors, role of professionals in addressing maltreatment, reporting suspected maltreatment, physical and mental health indicators of maltreatment, medical perspectives on maltreatment, cycles of family violence, corporal punishment and physical abuse, physician anticipatory guidance for prevention of maltreatment, child and adolescent sexual abuse prevention, advocacy for maltreated children and adolescents, characteristics of sexual offenders and sexual offenses, intimate partner violence, and resources for families affected by maltreatment.

Findings indicate significantly improved perceived preparedness to identify signs of child maltreatment, to report cases of suspected child maltreatment, to recommend or secure needed services for maltreated children, and increased likelihood to report suspected child maltreatment for students who complete CAST (Knox, Pelletier, & Vieth, 2014). Furthermore, compared to students in a control group, CAST students had improved knowledge and intention to report maltreatment, increased commitment to their role in reporting child maltreatment, and reduced concerns that may otherwise prevent reporting (Knox, Pelletier, & Vieth, 2013; Pelletier & Knox, 2016).

Evidence-Based Interventions to Address Child Maltreatment

Trauma-focused interventions for the medical unit are discussed in Chap. 19. When trauma presents as a result of maltreatment, the consulting psychologist can assist with providing an overview of recommended evidence-based treatment interventions. The consulting psychologist will likely refer patients to receive outpatient evidence-based intervention. For younger children, psychologists may refer the family to parent-child interaction therapy (PCIT) or child-parent psychotherapy (CPP). Both interventions focus on improving parent-child interaction and decreasing behavior problems. PCIT has a large evidence base with the focus of intervention on improving interaction through use of a 5-minute special play time with coaching of the PRIDE skills (praise, reflection, imitation, description, and enthusiasm). PCIT is an evidence-based intervention for children who have experienced trauma, diagnosed with an attachment disorder, and/or who are displaying externalizing behavioral problems. CPP is designed for children birth to age 5 and their caregivers. CPP helps the parent-child dyad cope with the loss of a loved one, abuse or violence in the home or community, and for children who have experienced a change in home placement. Older children and adolescents may be referred to receive trauma-focused cognitive behavioral therapy (TF-CBT). This intervention teaches children relaxation techniques, emotion identification, and affect modulation, as well as assists children with developing a trauma narrative (The National Child Stress Traumatic Stress Network, n.d.).

Case Example

A 7-year-old Caucasian female named Sarah presents to her primary care physician (PCP). Sarah's mother reported that over the past 2 months, Sarah has missed school due to complaining of headaches and stomachaches. She has also been quick to anger. During the well-child visit, the PCP observes bruises on Sarah's arms that appear to look like a handprint and finger marks. When asked about how Sarah got the bruises, neither Sarah nor her mother provided an explanation. This caused the PCP to complete a more thorough evaluation, which reveals a bruise on her buttocks. The PCP steps out and consults with the psychologist. The PCP and the psychologist go into the exam room. A complete biopsychosocial interview is completed with the child separated from the parent. Sarah reported that she has recently started staying with her father. She reported that her father hit her. The mother returns to the room and additional information is obtained. The disclosure is discussed and a safety plan is developed. Both the psychologist and the PCP explain that CPS needs to be contacted. Sarah's mother is in agreement. Documentation is made in the Electronic Medical Record (EMR) to document what was observed, the information obtained by Sarah, the discussion with Sarah's mother, and the call made to CPS. The psychologist provides an overview of relaxation strategies to Sarah such as diaphragmatic breathing, progressive muscle relaxation, and guided imagery. Relaxation strategies are addressed because this is a brief intervention that can assist with establishing emotional and behavioral regulation. The psychologist refers Sarah to receive TF-CBT and provides an overview of the treatment. This psychologist will provide short-term intervention until Sarah can receive intervention in an outpatient setting and schedules a follow-up appointment to address emotion identification, affect regulation, and coping strategies to manage physiological symptoms.

Conclusions

Psychologists are in a unique position to work collaboratively with medical professionals to assist with the identification of risk factors and the promotion of protective factors. The psychologist's role in the PCMH offers the opportunity to provide population-based management focused on prevention efforts, assistance with providing anticipatory guidance, early identification of signs of maltreatment, brief intervention, and education of healthcare professionals. Early identification is key, as survivors of abuse have a greater likelihood of having mood disorders, anxiety, and problems with substance abuse (Leetch & Woolridge, 2013).

References

Aaron, H., & Burtless, G. (2014). *Potential effects of the affordable care act on income inequality*. Retrieved from The Brookings Institution website: http://www.brookings.edu/research/papers/2014/01/potential-effects-affordable-care-act-income-inequality-aaron-burtless

Bailhache, M., Leroy, V., Pillet, P., & Salmi, L. R. (2013). Is early detection of abused child possible? A systematic review of the diagnostic accuracy of the identification of abused children. *BMC Pediatrics*. https://doi.org/10.1186/1471-2471-2431-12-202

Bender, H. L., Allen, J. P., McElhaney, K. B., Antonishak, J., Moore, C. M., Kelly, H. O., & Davis, S. M. (2007). Use of harsh physical discipline and developmental outcomes in adolescence. *Development and Psychopathology, 19*, 227–242.

Berlin, L. J., Dodge, K. A., & Reznick, S. (2013). Examining pregnant women's hostile attributions about infants as a predictor of offspring maltreatment. American Medical Association. *JAMA Pediatrics, 167*, 549. http://archpedi.jamanetwork.com

Burkhart, K., Knox, M., & Hunter, K. (2016). Changing healthcare professionals' positive attitudes toward spanking. *Clinical Pediatrics, 55*(11), 1005–1011.

Casanueva, C., Wilson, E., Smith, K., Dolan, M., Ringeisen, H., & Horne, B. (2012). *NSCAW II wave 2 report: Child wELL-being report. OPRE report # 2012-38*. Washington, DC: Office of Planning, Research, and Evaluation, Administration for Children and Families, US Department of Health and Human Services.

Child Abuse and Prevention and Treatment ACT (CAPTA) amended by P.L. 111-320, the CAPTA reauthorization act of 2010.

Child Maltreatment. (2002). *Summary of key study findings. National clearinghouse on child abuse and neglect information: US Department of Health and Human Services Administration for Children and Families*. Retrieved from nccanch.acf.hhs.gov/pubs/factsheets/canstats.cfm

Child Welfare Information Gateway. (2016). *Mandatory reporters of child abuse and neglect*. Washington, DC: U.S. Department of Health and Human Services, Children's Bureau.

Compton, M. T., & Shim, R. S. (2015). *The social determinants of mental health*. Arlington, VA: American Psychiatric Association.

Eckenrode, J., Smith, E. G., McCarthy, M. E., & Dineen, M. (2014). Income inequality and child maltreatment in the United States. *Pediatrics, 133*(3), 454. Retrieved from http://pediatrics.aappublications.org

Farst, K. J., Ambadwar, P. B., King, A. J., Bird, T. M., & Robbins, J. M. (2013). Trends in hospitalization rates and severity of injuries from abuse in young children, 1997-2009. *Pediatrics, 131*, e1796–e1802.

Friedlander, E. Y., Rubin, D. M., Alpern, E. M., Mandell, D. S., et al. (2008). Patterns of health care use that may identify young children who are at risk for maltreatment. *Pediatrics, 116*, 1303–1308.

Garcia, A. R., DeNard, C., Ohene, S., Morones, S. M., & Connaughton, C. (2018). "I am more than past:" parents' attitudes and perceptions of the Positive Parenting Program in child welfare. *Children and Youth Services, 88*, 286–297.

Gershoff, E. T., Font, S. A., Taylor, C. A., Foster, R. H., Garza, A. B., Olson-Dorff, D., & Spector, L. (2017). Effectiveness of a No Hit Zone policy in reducing staff support for and intervention in physical punishment in a hospital setting. *Children and Youth Services Review, 94*, 155–162.

Gershoff, E. T., & Grogan-Kaylor, A. (2016). Spanking and child outcomes: Old controversies and new meta-analyses. *Journal of Family Psychology, 30*(4), 453.

Gunn, V. L., Hickson, G. B., & Cooper, W. O. (2005). Factors affecting pediatricians' reporting of suspected child maltreatment. *Ambulatory Pediatrics, 5*(2), 96–101.

Jackson, A. M., Kissoon, N., & Green, C. (2015). Aspects of abuse: Recognizing and responding to child maltreatment. *Current Problems in Pediatric and Adolescent Health Care, 45*, 58–70.

Jenny, C. (Ed.). (2011). *Child abuse and neglect diagnosis, treatment, and evidence*. St. Louis, MI: Elsevier Saunders.

Jenny, C., & Crawford-Jakubiak, S. E. (2013). The evaluation of children in the primary care setting when sexual abuse is suspected. *Pediatrics, 132*, e558.

Jenny, C., Hymel, K. P., Ritzen, A., Reinert, S. E., & Hay, T. C. (1999). Analysis of missed cases of abusive head trauma. *JAMA, 281*, 621–626.

Keenan, H. T., Cook, L. J., Olson, L. M., Bardsley, T., & Campbell, K. A. (2017). Social intuition and social information in physical child abuse evaluation and diagnosis. *Pediatrics, 140*(5), e20171188. https://doi.org/10.1542/peds.2017-1188

Kellogg, N. D. (2007). Evaluation of suspected child physical abuse. *Pediatrics, 119*(6), 1232–1241.

Kenny, M. C., Lopez-Griman, A. M., & Donohue, B. (2017). Development and initial evaluation of a cost-effective, internet-based program to assist professionals in reporting suspected child maltreatment. *Journal of Child & Adolescent Trauma, 10*(4), 385–393.

King, A. J., Farst, K. J., Jaeger, M. W., Onukwube, J. I., & Robbins, J. M. (2015). Maltreatment-related emergency department visits among children 0 to 3 years old in the United States. *Child Maltreatment, 20*(3), 151–161.

Knox, M., Pelletier, H., & Vieth, V. (2013). Educating medical students about adolescent maltreatment. *International Journal of Adolescent Medicine and Health, 25*, 301–308.

Knox, M. S., Pelletier, H., & Vieth, V. (2014). Effects of medical student training in child advocacy and child abuse prevention and intervention. *Psychological Trauma: Theory, Research, Practice, and Policy, 6*, 129–133.

Lane, W. G., et al. (2002). Racial differences in the evaluation of pediatric fractures for physical abuse. *JAMA, 288*(13), 1603–1609.

Laskey, A. L., Stump, T., Perkins, S. M., et al. (2012). Influence of race and socioeconomic status on the diagnosis of child abuse: A randomized study. *Journal of Pediatrics, 160*(6), 1003–1037.

Lawrence, L. L., & Brannen, S. J. (2000). The impact of physician training on child maltreatment reporting: A multi-specialty study. *Military Medicine, 165*(8), 607–611.

Leetch, A. N., Leipsic, J., & Woolridge, D. P. (2015). Evaluation of child maltreatment in the emergency department setting. *Child and Adolescent Psychiatric Clinics of North America, 24, 41*.

Leetch, A. N., & Woolridge, D. (2013). Emergency department evaluation of child abuse. *Emergency Medicine Clinics North America, 31*, 853–873.

Lubell, K. M., Lofton, T., & Singer, H. H. (2008). *Promoting health parenting practice across cultural groups: A CDC research brief.* U.S. Department of Health and Human Services. Centers for Disease Control and Prevention.

Markenson, D., Tunik, M., Cooper, A., Olson, L., Cook, L., et al. (2007). A national assessment of knowledge, attitudes, and confidence of prehospital providers in the assessment and management of child maltreatment. *Pediatrics, 119*(1), e103. https://doi.org/10.1542/peds.2005-2121

Mason, S. M., Schnitzer, P. G., Danilack, V. A., Elston, B., & Savitz, D. A. (2018). Risk factors for maltreatment-related infant hospitalizations in New York City, 1995–2004. *Annals of Epidemiology, 28*(9), 590–596.

Mikton, C., & Butchart, A. (2009). Child maltreatment prevention: A systematic review of reviews. *Bulletin World Health Organization, 87*, 353–361.

Miller-Perrin, C., & Malloy, L. C. (2007). Curriculum guide for instruction in child maltreatment. Section on Child Maltreatment Division, 37.

Olds, D. L., Kitzman, H., Knudtson, M., et al. (2014). Effect of home visiting by nurses on maternal and child mortality results of two-decade follow-up of a randomized clinical trial. *JAMA Pediatrics, 168*(9), 800–806.

Pelletier, H., & Knox, M. (2016). Incorporating child maltreatment training into medical school curricula. *Journal of Child & Adolescent Trauma, 10*, 267–274.

Pulido, M. L., Dauber, S., Tully, B. A., Hamilton, P., Smith, M. J., & Freeman, K. (2015). Knowledge gains following a child sexual abuse prevention program among urban students: A cluster-randomized evaluation. *American Journal of Public Health, 105*(7), 1344–1352.

Raney, L. E. (Ed.). (2015). *Integrated care*. Arlington, VA: American Psychiatric Association.

Regalado, M., Sareen, H., Inkelas, M., Wissow, L. S., & Halfon, N. (2004). Parents' discipline of young children: Results from the National Survey of Early Childhood Health. *Pediatrics, 113*, 1952–1958.

Schaeffer, P., Leventhal, J. M., & Asnes, G. (2011). Children's disclosures of sexual abuse: Learning from direct inquiry. *Child Abuse & Neglect: The International Journal, 35*(5), 343–352.

Schmitt, B. D. (1987). Seven deadly signs of childhood: Advising parents about difficult developmental phases. *Child Abuse and Neglect, 11*(3), 421–432.

Scholer, S., Brokish, P. A., Mukherjee, M. D., et al. (2008). A violence prevention program helps teach medical students and pediatric residents about childhood aggression. *Clinical Pediatrics, 47*(9), 891–900.

Sedlak, A. J., Mettenburg, J., Basena, M., Petta, I., McPherson, K., Creene, A., & Li, S. (2010). *Fourth National Incidence Study of Child Abuse and Neglect (NIS-4)*. Washington, DC: US Department of Health and Human Services. Retrieved from http://www.acf.hhs.gov/programs.opre/research/project/national-incidence-study-of-child-abuse-and-neglect-nis-4-2004-2009

Sege, R. D., Hatmaker-Flanigan, E., De Vos, E., Levin-Goodman, R., & Spivak, H. (2006). Anticipatory guidance and violence prevention: Results from family and pediatrician focus groups. *Pediatrics, 117*(2), 455–463.

Sheets, L. K., Leach, M. E., Koszewski, I. J., Lessmeier, A. M., Nugent, M., & Simpson, P. (2013). Sentinel injuries in infants evaluated for child physical abuse. *Pediatrics, 131*(4), 701–707.

Sidebothan, P., & Heron, J. (2006). Child maltreatment in the "children of the nineties:" A cohort study of risk factors. *Child Abuse & Neglect, 30*(5), 497–522.

Silva, J. (2011). *ACT facilitator manual: ACT raising safe kids program*. Washington, DC: American Psychological Association.

Straus, M. A., & Stewart, J. H. (1999). Corporal punishment by American parents: National data on prevalence, chronicity, and duration, in relation to child and family characteristics. *Clinical Child and Family Psychology Review, 2*, 55–70.

Sullivan, P. M., & Knutson, J. F. (1998). The association between child maltreatment and disabilities in a hospital-based epidemiological study. *Child Abuse and Neglect, 22*(4), 271–288.

The Centers for Disease Control and Prevention. (2014). Retrieved from https://www.cdc.gov

The National Child Traumatic Stress Network. (n.d.). Retrieved from https://www.nctsn.org

Vieth, V. I. (2006). Unto the third generation: A call to end child abuse in the United States within 120 years (revised and expanded). *Hamline Journal of Public Law and Policy, 28*, 1.

Webster-Stratton, C., & Reid, J. (2010). Adapting the incredible years an evidence-based parenting programme for families involved in the child welfare system. *Journal of Children's Services, 5*(1), 25–42.

World Health Organization. (2018, October 10). *Child maltreatment*. Retrieved from http://www.who.int/news-room/fact-sheets/detail/child-maltreatment

Munchausen by Proxy and Pediatric Factitious Disorder Imposed on Self

Natacha D. Emerson and Brenda Bursch

Munchausen by proxy (MBP) is the most widely recognized term to describe abuse and/or neglect by a caregiver who falsifies an illness or condition in another due to *factitious disorder imposed on another* psychopathology (American Professional Society of the Abuse of Children [APSAC], 2018). Not a formal diagnosis, MBP refers to both the abuse of the victim and to the psychopathology of the abuser. Children, adults, and pets can be MBP victims.

Many terms have been proposed to describe child abuse and neglect based on the overreporting or induction of symptoms/disability in a child. Within the United States, three related terms have been used. *Abuse by pediatric condition falsification* (APCF) is defined as "a form of child maltreatment in which an adult falsifies physical and/or psychological signs and/or symptoms in a victim, causing the victim to be regarded as more ill or impaired than is objectively true" (APSAC, 2018; Ayoub et al., 2002). The term *medical child abuse* (MCA) is a related term used by many pediatricians when a "child receives unnecessary and harmful, or potentially harmful, medical care at the instigation of a caregiver" (Roesler & Jenny, 2009). MCA does not include falsified symptoms, distress, or disability that are presented to professionals outside of medical settings, such as false depressive symptoms presented to a psychologist, acute suicidality reported to a police officer, or learning problems presented to a teacher. *Caregiver-fabricated illness in a child* (CFIC) is the term recommended by the American Academy of Pediatrics (AAP; Flaherty & MacMillan, 2013). Within the United Kingdom, the term *fabricated or induced illness by carers* (FII) is used, defined as "deliberate production or fabrication of physical or psychological symptoms in a child by a parent or carer" (Royal College of Paediatrics and Child Health, 2009).

Factitious disorder imposed on another (FDIA) is the psychopathology of MBP abusers

N. D. Emerson
UCLA Mattel Children's Hospital,
Los Angeles, CA, USA

Jane and Terry Semel Institute for Neuroscience and Human Behavior, Los Angeles, CA, USA

Department of Psychiatry and Biobehavioral Sciences, David Geffen School of Medicine at UCLA, Los Angeles, CA, USA

B. Bursch (✉)
UCLA Mattel Children's Hospital,
Los Angeles, CA, USA

Jane and Terry Semel Institute for Neuroscience and Human Behavior, Los Angeles, CA, USA

Department of Psychiatry and Biobehavioral Sciences, David Geffen School of Medicine at UCLA, Los Angeles, CA, USA

Department of Pediatrics, David Geffen School of Medicine at UCLA, Los Angeles, CA, USA
e-mail: bbursch@mednet.ucla.edu

B. D. Carter, K. A. Kullgren (eds.), *Clinical Handbook of Psychological Consultation in Pediatric Medical Settings*, Issues in Clinical Child Psychology, https://doi.org/10.1007/978-3-030-35598-2_35

(American Psychiatric Association, 2013). Abusers falsify or induce physical, psychological, or developmental signs or symptoms in another individual and present the victim to others as more ill, impaired, or injured than they would be without the abusive interference. *Factitious disorder imposed on self* (FDIS) has been identified in both children and adults (American Psychiatric Association, 2013). The criteria are the same as in FDIA except that the focus of the falsification is on the self rather than on another. The diagnosis of FDIA/FDIS requires that the individual engaged in intentional deception, differentiating it from anxiety, psychosis, or other psychiatric disorders. While malingering can be comorbid, FDIA/FDIS is diagnosed when external rewards do not fully account for the falsification behavior. The underlying goal of an individual with FDIA/FDIS is to satisfy a psychological need. Those with FDIA/FDIS, similar to those with a substance abuse disorder or pedophilia, ignore the needs and well-being of others in order to satisfy their own needs. The individual may provide false information, fail to report or deny clinically relevant data, induce or worsen illness, neglect medical protocols and regimens, and/or simulate symptoms. They may coach victims and others into corroborating false claims (Yorker, Alexander, & Sanders, 2018).

It is important for psychologists to be aware of FDIA/FDIS because they may (1) encounter patients they come to suspect as being victims or perpetrators of MBP or to have FDIS, (2) be asked to assist in a clinical or forensic evaluation, and/or (3) receive requests for treatment referrals.

Etiology

Like other forms of child abuse and psychopathology, condition falsification behavior does not appear to have one etiology. With very limited available data, no brain defect or dysfunction has been consistently identified to explain falsification behavior. Case study data from the neurological and neuropsychological assessment of a small number of pathological liars (including those who falsify illness) suggest the possibility that prefrontal impairment (Fenelon, Mahieux, Roullet, & Guillard, 1991; Yang et al., 2005) and/or right hemispheric central nervous system dysfunction (Modell, Mountz, & Ford, 1992; Mountz et al., 1996; Pankratz & Lezak, 1987) might increase risk for this behavior.

History of trauma, abuse, or neglect can be a risk factor. Those with FDIA and/or FDIS may continue an intergenerational chain of abuse by recreating trauma they survived (APSAC Taskforce, 2018). Inducing or falsifying illness may be an attempt to correct trauma experienced when younger (Carlson, 1984). For MBP abusers, the goal is to prove themselves to be attentive, attuned parents, unlike that of their own family of origin. The behavior may also be a way to seek comfort and support from others or to relieve isolation by propelling the family into a system of care that responds to their emotional needs (Carlson, 1984). Every family history and dynamic is unique.

Individuals with FDIA are overwhelmingly identified as adult females. The majority have unexplained symptoms themselves (including somatic symptom disorders and FDIS), and, when carefully evaluated, nearly all have a comorbid cluster B personality disorder (Bass & Jones, 2011; Bools, Neale, & Meadow, 1994). Substance misuse and learning disorders are also detected, with less frequency (>30%; Bools, Neale, and Meadow, 1994). Some abusers do not appear to suffer from any comorbid psychopathology. Among those with a history of trauma or caregiver abandonment, sick-role behavior may be a compensatory response. For example, condition falsification behaviors can be a way of establishing or stabilizing one's sense of self, of maintaining relationships with others, and of garnering acceptance, sympathy, importance, prescribed roles, and a sense of belonging. The behavior can start after a psychologically reinforcing experience with an injury, disability, or illness (in oneself or another), may start in childhood or adulthood, and/or may develop in reaction to lifelong MBP victimization.

Adults with FDIS generally have the same demographic and comorbid psychopathology as those with FDIA (Bass & Halligan, 2014; Eisendrath, 1994). An analysis of posts in an online support group for those with a self-identified factitious disorder revealed that "receiving affection" was the most frequently cited motivation for occupying the sick role (Lawlor & Kirakowski, 2014). The experiences and behaviors of those with FDIS are often congruent with those of addicts (including the presence of cravings that increase during times of stress and the inability to consider the needs of others when cravings are present). While youth as young as 8 years old have been identified has having FDIS (Libow, 2000), children as young as 3 have been found to participate in deceitful reporting of false symptoms. Based on 42 published cases (with an average age of 13.9 years old), the older the child with FDIS, the more likely the child was female (Libow, 2000).

Many with FDIA or FDIS are excellent impostors, adeptly misleading experts on a regular basis (Libow, 2000; Sheridan, 2003). They are at risk of escalating the deceitful and dangerous behavior over time, underscoring the need for early identification and intervention even if the falsification first appears to be mild or benign (Yorker et al., 2018). Moreover, remission of falsification is not necessarily associated with permanent relief as the individual may stop the behavior for a period of time only to reinitiate it again later (APSAC Taskforce, 2018).

Prevalence

Like all forms of child abuse and neglect, accurate prevalence estimates of MBP are difficult to establish due to under-identification. The AAP estimates the incidence to be from 0.5 to 2.0 per 100,000 children younger than 16 years (Flaherty & MacMillan, 2013). Sheridan (2003) identified induction (creating symptoms or conditions, such as via poisoning) in more than half of cases, with about half of all induction episodes occurring while the child was hospitalized. MBP is not constrained by culture, race, or socioeconomic status and has been documented in 24 countries (Bass & Glaser, 2014).

MBP is often comorbid with a verified condition, making identification even more difficult (Levin & Sheridan, 1995). In this subset of victims, symptoms of the genuine condition may be exacerbated, exaggerated, or falsely described. MBP may be specific to one caregiver-child dyad or may pervade an entire family. Caregivers may abuse the youngest child, the child with special needs, the child that is most difficult to parent, or they may abuse all children in the household at one time or sequentially (APSAC Taskforce, 2018). In addition to medical setting presentations, MBP in school and mental health settings have been identified (Schreier & Bursch, 2018). Finally, as mentioned earlier, adults and pets may also be targeted, though prevalence rates are unknown.

Rates of FDIS are even more difficult to estimate as under-reporting is not augmented by mandated reports to legal agencies. Preliminary attempts suggest prevalence rates to be 1% among hospitalized adults (Fliege et al., 2007; Reich & Gottfried, 1983; Sansone, Wiederman, Sansone, & Mehnert-Kay, 1997) and up to 9.3% among adults with unexplained symptoms (Krahn, Li, & O'Connor, 2003; Poole, 2010). The prevalence rate of youth with FDIS is unknown.

Assessment Techniques

Diagnosticians rely heavily on patient and caregiver report of history, symptoms, distress, and disability. Even the keenest diagnostician is vulnerable to the fabrications of a seemingly earnest individual. It is not possible for any professional, including mental health professionals or law enforcement, to reliably detect deception by clinical interview (ten Brinke, Stimson, & Carney, 2014). Moreover, individuals with FDIA/FDIS often study the conditions they are falsifying, misleading clinicians by reporting the exact symptoms to match the desired diagnosis. They have also been known to falsely report that prior clinicians confirmed a diagnosis or condition. Thus, assessing for MBP and/or for a factitious disorder requires a heavy reliance on collateral sources.

Review of Records

The gold standard and backbone of a thorough evaluation is an exhaustive and systematic behavioral analysis based on medical and other records. As detailed by Bursch, Emerson & Sanders (2019), who write about the recommended evaluation process for forensic psychologists, the evaluation must commence with requesting all available medical records *directly from* medical centers and/or other facilities. This is also true if the evaluation is completed by a psychologist in a clinical consultant role. The evaluator must never trust that records provided by the family are accurate reflections of history. Instead, the evaluator may be aided by signed releases of information or by a court order for records. Separate requests are needed for records from emergency medical services, home health services, outpatient visits, emergency department visits, and inpatient stays. Likewise, requesting records from nearby health facilities may prove useful, as families may hospital hop and not be forthright in listing all health encounters. The evaluator may also review online social media content and, if permitted, records of other family members for additional evidence of falsification. Finally, school records, child protective records, police reports, and other sources of observations may be solicited.

The data contained in the records are best analyzed with the use of a chronological table to summarize each visit's date and location, claims made by the parent (or patient), exam and test data, and resulting diagnoses/treatments. Signs of neglect, such as missed appointments, and threats of hospital discharges *against medical advice* are important to include. Importantly, the table must explicitly delineate objective data from caregiver or patient-reported information. See Fig. 1 for an example.

Once the records are summarized within the table, the goal is to determine whether there is evidence of symptom induction or falsification. Induction of symptoms may be documented in records in the form of abnormal test results (such as toxic levels of a substance that explains symptoms) or by those who directly observe tampering (such as a nurse seeing a parent smothering a child, contaminating a central line, or discarding needed medications). Simulation of a condition can be detected with documentation of tampering with assessments to cause the results to appear pathological (such as by moving the depth of a pH probe or changing a teacher's answers on a behavioral checklist) or by presenting false evidence of illness (such as falsely claiming a contaminated urine sample came from the patient). Simulation can also come in the form of images, labs, or reports downloaded from the Internet and falsely attributed to the patient. An example of this might include showing a photo of a rash discovered online as belonging to the child. Falsifying, or lying, includes misrepresenting clinical history, family history, and/or the presence of symptoms, distress, or disability. Exaggerating includes overstating the frequency or severity of genuine symptoms, distress, or disability (American Psychiatric Association, 2013; APSAC Taskforce, 2018).

The logic behind the symptom or disability presentation must be considered. For example, abusers may present their children as having a variety of unrelated conditions (e.g., having neurologic, psychiatric, gastrointestinal, and cardiac symptoms) without a unifying diagnosis or hypothesis to explain the multisystemic nature of the symptoms. Occasionally, symptom or disability reports defy common sense. An example is a parent who reported that her son has explosive diarrhea only when he eats tuna sandwiches in California. Any condition, illness, or symptom can be falsified. Thus, it is important to avoid ruling out conditions, disabilities, or symptoms that are difficult to feign, such as cancer. Kelly and Wang (2018) provide a summary of simulation and induction presentations across bodily systems.

Separation

When a suspected MBP victim is protected from the alleged abuser, it can be helpful to observe the impact of the separation on the clinical status of the child. In the hospital, the suspected abuser may be asked to voluntarily refrain from caregiving

Date	Patient/ BIB	Health care contact	Subjective caregiver reports	Objective findings	Diagnosis/ recommendations	Others
9/17/18	Amy BIB mom	Dr. Rockwood, Emergency Medicine, Memorial Hospital ER	Mom reports constipation and sleeping difficulty since birth. Reports 8 days of severe vomiting and food refusal. Called Peds GI who advised her to go to ER	No apparent distress. Exam benign. Labs and vitals WNL. KUB WNL. Took 3 oz. of formula from bottle. No emesis in ER	AGE suspected Provided IVF and told to return if symptoms persist	Mom accurately summarized all guidance and agreed to plan. However, she did not remember the name of her GI doctor
9/18/18	Amy BIB mom	Dr. Berg Emergency Medicine, Children's Hospital ER	Mom reports constipation and apnea since birth. Reports 2 weeks of severe vomiting and food refusal	No apparent distress. Exam benign. Labs and vitals WNL. No emesis in ER. Mild diaper rash noted	Admit for evaluation of GI symptoms and apnea	Mom mentioned Amy was born at 36 weeks, but review of record suggests 39 weeks

Abbreviations:
AGE – acute gastroenteritis
BIB – brought in by
IVF – intravenous fluids
KUB – abdominal x-ray, including images of the kidneys, ureters, and bladder
WNL– within normal limits

Fig. 1 Example template for chronological behavioral record analysis

duties or from visiting the child in the hospital for a period of time. However, a court order may be required if the suspected abusers refuse to allow separation. Skilled and careful clinical observers can be assigned to sit in the patient room to determine if the reported symptoms or concerning behaviors occur. However, this approach is not foolproof, as abusers have successfully poisoned or otherwise harmed their children in the presence of a sitter. Additionally, some sitters are befriended and misled by the suspected abuser. Stringent abuser visitation rules may be required to ensure protection from induction and from interpersonal pressure upon the victim to conform to the abuser's story of illness or disability (see APSAC, 2018 for recommended visitation guidelines). Likewise, efforts exerted by the abuser to leverage others to influence the victim must also be monitored, including the provision of hidden messages or routes of poisoning. Finally, consideration must be given to the nature of the alleged problems in order to determine what might be expected if the abuser lost the ability to perpetuate the false narrative. For example, if an abuser reports that a baby has episodes of severe apnea several times each night, it will take one night to determine if this is accurate. If an abuser reports an episode every 2–3 weeks, it will take longer to assess accuracy. If the child is suffering from medication side effects, such as lethargy from high levels of sedating medication, one would not expect a change until the medication is adjusted. Likewise, disruption in the functioning of the intestinal tract via starvation might take time to resolve and could require feeding therapy if the child has developed an oral aversion. Nevertheless, a careful analysis of such changes in an alleged victim can provide powerful evidence of MBP abuse and neglect.

Overt or Covert Videotape

Overt or covert video recordings can be helpful when it is expected that a suspected abuser can be caught inducing (e.g., suffocating, poisoning, or tampering with lines) or falsely reporting symptoms (e.g., apnea or seizures). In such situations, continuous monitoring is strongly recommended so that staff can immediately intervene to protect the child, if needed (APSAC, 2018).

In the United States, video surveillance of the child in the hospital room may be permissible to (1) protect the child, (2) assist in diagnostic evaluations, and (3) protect medical center employees from negligence allegations. Case law suggests that a hospital room is not a location with constitutionally protected privacy. To increase protection from liability, medical staff may obtain a court-ordered warrant, include permission for video surveillance in admission paperwork, explicitly request permission separately, focus the camera only on the child's bed, and/or use audio recording only when needed to capture conversations (Yorker, 1995).

Video surveillance does require caution as it runs the risk of exposing the child to further abuse by prolonging the evaluation. Additionally, video surveillance evidence can be misleading or prohibited from being admitted into evidence. Thus, if used, it is recommended that video surveillance evidence be presented to child abuse or legal authorities as one component of a larger set of data that was obtained via careful evaluation.

Psychological Evaluation of MBP Abusers and Co-caregivers

The psychological evaluation of the identified or suspected abuser and, separately, of the co-parent/caregiver can be helpful. While the record analysis may be completed by any knowledgeable professional during a hospitalization or ongoing outpatient care of the child, comprehensive psychological evaluations of the caregivers are typically conducted by court-ordered mental health experts. Nevertheless, some initial efforts by the consulting psychologist to understand the suspected abuser's motives and family dynamics can be helpful in the pediatric setting.

Clinical evaluations allow the evaluator to hear firsthand what these individuals say about the history and current well-being of the identified or suspected child victim, to test their ability and/or willingness to consider an alternate view, to determine if there are additional aspects to the case that warrant further review, to develop hypotheses about the potential contributors to the abusive behavior, and to identify comorbid psychopathology that needs to be incorporated into a treatment plan. Collateral interviews, especially with individuals from the family of origin of the abuser, can be very informative in the verification of trauma histories and other facts, in obtaining developmental and functional history, in determining if the alleged abusers are known to falsify information (health-related or other topics), and in the evaluation of personality disorders.

Caregivers with FDIA often seem appropriately concerned and knowledgeable about their children's conditions. Few have criminal histories and many are known to be helpful and caring toward other families and children in their communities, making the detection of manipulative and deceitful behaviors difficult (Weber, 2018). As in other forms of abuse, psychological testing can result in a normative profile. Thus it is a clinical error to rely on a caregiver's "normal" clinical presentation or testing to be evidence of safe caregiving.

Psychological evaluations are best used to rule out important differential diagnoses including psychotic and anxiety disorders (Bursch et al., 2019). Individuals with health-related delusions may present similarly to those with FDIA/FDIS in their adamancy that something is wrong. Likewise, highly anxious, somatically focused individuals may advocate for over-medicalization to quell their own worries of a "missed diagnosis." While these behaviors might result in abusive over-medicalization that warrants intervention, those with anxiety or a delusional disorder alone do not routinely, deliberately falsify medical information (Bursch et al., 2019).

Evaluation of caregivers who participate in caring for the MBP victim but not identified as the primary abuser, such as spouses or extended family members, is also helpful (Sanders & Ayoub, 2018). One, the evaluator should strive to understand how the adult(s) failed to protect the child within the family dynamic at the time of the abuse. For example, was the individual aware of the abuse or neglect? Did the individual observe the reported symptoms or disabilities of the victim? Did the individual (knowingly or unknowingly) repeat the false story of symptoms or disability or participate in the deception in other ways? Are they fearful of the abuser? Two, the adult(s) must be assessed to determine if they are safe to serve as caregivers. This requires evaluation of disorders and/or deficits that contributed to poor parenting, to abuse or neglect, or to lack of awareness of the abuse. Awareness of the MBP abuse in the co-parent/co-caregiver can range from complete unawareness to knowing denial to active participation in the deception (Sanders, 1995). Even among those who are aware of the abuse, it can be exceedingly difficult to stand up to an abuser to protect a victim, akin to standing up to stop the behavior of a severe substance abuser.

Psychological Evaluation of the Child

The psychological evaluation of the MBP victim can be conducted in any setting and has two main purposes. The first goal is to determine if the child is suffering from any psychological or behavioral problems, reported or unreported by the abuser. Particular attention should be paid to correctly detecting signs and symptoms of attachment disorders and psychological trauma caused by medical evaluations or treatments. Due to the unreliability of caregiver report, observational approaches, objective testing, and input from teachers can be very helpful. However, it is important to note that children can be coached to perform poorly on formal evaluations and they can appear delayed due to deprivation. Thus, findings must be interpreted with the knowledge that performance might improve with remediation.

The second goal is to obtain an understanding of the child's history, functional ability, adaptive skills, and daily life in order to corroborate the information provided by the abuser. Most victims of MBP abuse appear to be unaware of their victimization and will corroborate much of the history provided by the abuser as they are used to repeating important clinical and social information they have heard their caregiver report to professionals. Nevertheless, they do sometimes provide helpful information. A 6-year-old may, for example, report that she can eat, even though her parent reports that she is unable to eat. Or, she might report that she is only allowed to eat macaroni and cheese on days she goes to the emergency room for imaging of her belly, not realizing she has revealed how her abuser perpetuated the false story of chronic constipation. Due to their own distorted perceptions, assessment measures used to evaluate "faking bad" in children cannot be relied upon to rule out MBP or to differentiate FDIA from FDIS.

Case reports and reviews provide a picture of MBP victims (Sheridan, 2003). Boys and girls appear to be equally abused. While the literature suggests that a large majority of MBP victims are younger than 3 years of age (Flaherty & Macmillan, 2013), older children are also abused, typically without their knowledge. The harm inflicted on MBP victims can be profound. In addition to both temporary and permanent physical harm, victims are also vulnerable to severe psychological harm. Physical harm has included exposure to unnecessary painful procedures, medications, and radiation, altered gut functioning, surgical removal or alteration of body parts, placement of unnecessary medical devices, impairment of sensory organs, brain damage, and death. Psychological harm due to MBP has resulted in disturbed attachments, severe reality confusion (especially about one's health, abilities, and relationships), post-traumatic stress disorder, depression, anxiety, disordered eating, highly passive and compliant behavior, aggression, and adoption of self-falsification or somaticizing behaviors. It is typical that MBP victims are also thwarted in achieving appropriate developmental milestones via removal from school, excessive school accommodations, overcontrol of normative social experiences, restriction of activity, and other MBP behaviors. MBP victims may not have had a safe place to retreat from the false stories perpetuated by their abuser. Extended family members, school personnel, community members, and friends of the family may have all been misled by the abuser, thus unwittingly participated in reinforcing the sick role for the child victim.

It is important that the evaluator maintains a neutral and curious stance. As with other forms of abuse, suspected victims should not be evaluated in the presence of the suspected abuser or other collusive individuals. It is typically clinically unhelpful, and will not help rapport, to suggest to an unsuspecting child that they have been victimized. MBP victims are often highly dependent and enmeshed with their abusers and extremely fearful of separation from them. In the exceedingly rare instance in which abuse might be revealed to the evaluator, it is important to recognize that such a revelation might not equate to a desire to escape the abusive situation due to the uncertainty of an unknown future. Also, presuming the child has not been victimized, by expressing strong belief in the false story of the abusing caregiver, can problematically reinforce the child's distorted perceptions and helplessness. Thus, evaluators are encouraged to carefully modulate their reactions to information provided to them by the child in order to be optimally supportive. Other abuse and neglect, including physical or sexual, can be present (or falsely reported by the abuser).

Finally, evaluators must be aware that FDIS can be responsible for unexplained symptoms or disability in youth with or without the co-occurrence of MBP. Among some MBP victims, FDIS can be a conscious or unconscious attempt to take control of an abusive situation.

Role of the Psychologist

Consulting psychologists may encounter patients they suspect of having FDIS or of being a victim or perpetrator of MBP, they may be asked to assist in a clinical or forensic evaluation, and/or they might receive a request for treatment referrals. It is strongly recommended that the psychologist strive to avoid serving in dual roles, such as court expert and therapist.

Warning Signs and Clinical Management Recommendations

Psychologists working in inpatient or outpatient settings might develop a concern regarding condition falsification by a child or caregiver. Warning signs of condition falsification appear in Table 1. Suspicions of child abuse or neglect must be reported to child abuse authorities, consistent with local reporting laws. When making a report, the details driving the concern are helpful to share with the reporting agency so they can appropriately follow up.

When confronted with an unclear situation, as is often the case, the steps recommended in Table 2 can clarify if condition falsification appears more or less likely.

Working Within a Multidisciplinary Team

The role of the psychologist within a multidisciplinary team can vary, based on the skills and experience of the psychologist and other team members. Potential roles include serving as expert consultants within the team, participating in evaluations (including record-based behavioral analyses and clinical evaluations), providing sup-

Table 1 Warning signs of condition falsification

• The individual reports symptoms/impairments incongruent with objective evaluations/observations
• The individual provides clinical/social history that is incongruent with records or collateral data
• Careful and appropriate evaluations fail to identify a reasonable explanation for the reported problems
• The timing of symptoms or impairments is suspicious, such as only occurring in certain settings or in the presence of specific individual(s)
• Laboratory findings do not make sense, are clinically unlikely, or reveal the presence of unexpected chemicals, medications, or contaminants
• Other individuals or pets in the home currently have or have a history of unusual or unexplained illnesses or conditions
• The individual tries to prevent clinicians from obtaining past records and/or making contact with other providers or family members for collateral information
• A family member or provider expresses concern about possible falsification or high-healthcare utilization
• Observations of falsification, simulation, or induction of symptoms

Table 2 Clinical management recommendations

• Obtain prior records and consider making contact with prior providers
• Discuss suspicions of condition falsification with other providers, if appropriate
• Attempt to contact and regularly communicate with both parents/caregivers, even if one is reportedly not involved or not reachable
• Provide ongoing education and feedback about normal development and functioning, assessment findings, and recommendations to all caregivers and, when appropriate, other involved providers
• Ensure understanding of education and recommendations by asking the patient and caregivers to repeat back the information
• Document important details, including information related to discussions with collateral contacts, all education and recommendations provided, and the understanding and emotional responses displayed by the patient and caregivers
• Systematically and objectively challenge suspected false claims using careful evaluations and/or a rehabilitation treatment approach
• Accept verbal reports of symptoms or impairments with appropriate caution, with increased reliance on objective assessments and direct observations
• Consider ways in which induction or simulation might be present and develop an evaluation plan to assess, which might require close inpatient observation
• Agree only to school or other accommodations that are objectively supported
• Consider consultation with a MBP expert, if needed

port to children and/or caregivers, supporting team members impacted by efforts by the suspected MBP abuser to pit team members against each other, and serving as therapists or consultants to address falsification.

The vast majority of pediatricians, and even those specializing in the field of child abuse, have not received comprehensive training on the topic of condition falsification. Adopting a stance of appropriate suspicion is extremely challenging, especially with a well-liked family. Many incorrectly assume the presence of a genuine condition or disability rules out FDIS or MBP abuse and neglect. Others wrongly believe a mandated report is required only if MBP induction is clearly detected. Some pediatricians have the necessary MBP knowledge and experience, but may be as likely to appropriately evaluate as they are to want to avoid the time-consuming, unreimbursed, and frequently litigious task of conducting a proper evaluation. Therefore, pediatricians may rely upon the psychologist to assess for or validate their concerns about condition falsification, they might request the psychologist intervene with a child or caregiver who has engaged in falsification, or they may be unaware they are being misled and inadvertently perpetuating condition falsification. Finally, even when pediatricians (or others) suspect condition falsification, they may not inform the psychologist of these concerns due to uncertainty or a desire to avoid the need to respond to suspected abuse.

Perhaps the most challenging scenario is when the psychologist suspects falsification, but the medical team does not share this concern or wish to further evaluate. In such situations, it is necessary to gather relevant facts, consider what elements might be required for a reasonable evaluation plan, weigh the relative risks of evaluating or deferring an evaluation, and determine the best way to communicate concerns to receptive team members. When considering which team members to approach first, it may be beneficial to consider factors such as who is knowledgeable on this topic and who may have been successfully misled by the family. In addition to sharing concerns with team members, obtaining consultation from a MBP expert, a hospital-based suspected child abuse team, or an ethicist may be helpful. Consider if the team first needs improved education before attempting an evaluation. The APSAC practice guidelines (2018) and companion papers may be used when education is needed. See Sanders (1999) for a hospital-based evaluation protocol.

When overuse of health services is present (either as reportable child abuse or not), some institutions have adopted the practice of alerting other professionals via verbal discussion, through documenting the concern in clinical notes, and/or by adding a flag to the electronic medical record to alert clinicians to contact the primary pediatrician and/or to exert caution when recommending evaluations, accommodations, or interventions, especially those that are based on verbal reports alone. If suspected child abuse or neglect is documented in the record, documentation of the completed mandated report to legal authorities is also indicated.

Informing Patients or Caregivers About Concerns

Following efforts to alter behaviors with ongoing education and feedback, the next intervention typically consists of informing the patient (in cases of suspected FDIS) and caregivers (in cases of suspected FDIS, FDIA, or MBP) of the falsification concerns. It is recommended that parents/caregivers be provided with data to support these concerns. Family members are rarely receptive to such information; it is also common for there to be a surprising lack of anger or obvious distress when concerns are shared. It is recommended the team maintain a nonjudgmental stance and communicate the desire to help the family regardless of the underlying problem. A rehabilitation approach to remediate the condition can also be helpful to suggest to a family. As long as it is safe for the child, caregivers should be informed that a mandated report will be or has been made. While not the norm, there are cases in the literature of suicidal ideation, psychiatric decompensation, and attempts to flee care by the person engaged in falsification (Vennemann et al., 2006; Yorker & Kahan, 1991). Thus, psychological support and a safety plan should be in place prior to disclosing such information. Both nursing and security should be aware and prepared to assist, if needed.

Referrals for Therapy for Victims, MBP Abusers, and Co-caregivers

Therapists are as vulnerable to being misled by those with FDIA or FDIS as any other individual. It is not appropriate to refer an abuser and/or victim to a therapist as the only solution to ongoing MBP abuse or neglect. Careful consideration is needed when making therapy referrals. Sanders and Bursch (2019) have published a paper on treatment approaches for victims, MBP abusers and other involved individuals.

Therapy with MBP Victims

Children may not believe they were victimized and, thus, may be confused about the purpose of treatment and/or the reason for removal from their home. Therapists can provide a safe and nonjudgmental opportunity for children to independently review and sometimes reformulate their past experiences (Bursch, 1999). In some situations, it is only with the passage of time and lack of ongoing clinical problems and impairments that the child slowly begins to notice a change in their health status and wonder about the reasons for improvement.

Evidence-based approaches are recommended to treat post-traumatic stress reactions, attachment disorders, feeding or eating disorders, somatic symptom disorders, anxiety disorders, falsification behavior (even in young children), and other problems developed by children who have been abused or neglected. Overall, a behavioral rehabilitation approach is encouraged for all spheres of the child's life (social, academic, health, etc.), with increasing independent functioning to support appropriate self-perceptions of health and abilities. Youth capable of abstract thought can benefit from a narrative approach, including a review of their own pertinent records that they may compare to their memories of the events in question (Bursch, 1999).

Therapy for MBP Abusers and Co-caregivers

Treatment successes can occur and are most frequent among those rare MBP abusers who admit the details of their role in the abuse and neglect, demonstrate genuine empathy for their victim(s), have the ability and motivation to learn parenting and coping skills that will reduce the stress that exacerbates the motivation to falsify, and demonstrate the ability and motivation to use those skills over time rather than relapse into falsification behaviors (Sanders & Bursch, 2019).

Psychotherapy is less effective among caregivers with severe personality disorders and/or who have engaged in induction (such as smothering or poisoning; Davis et al., 1998; Jones, 1987).

Thus, psychotherapy should include a focus on the caregiver taking full responsibility for their MBP behaviors and developing more effective parenting and coping strategies (Bursch et al., 2019).

Narrative therapy can be helpful to understand family history and to create a healthier vision for the future (Sanders, 1996). Evidence-based therapies designed to address comorbidities, such as psychotropic medications, parent-child interaction therapy (PCIT), dialectical behavioral therapy, and trauma-focused cognitive behavioral therapy, may be effective (APSAC, 2018). Relapse prevention and monitoring strategies are also needed (APSAC, 2018). See Bursch (2018) for guidance on evaluating progress in therapy.

Some consider the other parent/co-caregiver to be a non-offending participant. However, it is crucial to remember that other involved adults fail to protect for a variety of reasons. Identification of the factors and dynamics that contributed to the inability of other adults to protect the child (or children) needs to be incorporated into treatment plans for these individuals.

Therapy for Youth with FDIS

Little is known about treatment with youth with FDIS; however the general treatment approaches and evidence-based therapies described above are likely to be relevant.

Summary

Psychologists may suspect one of their patients of having FDIS or of being a victim or perpetrator of MBP, they may be asked to conduct an evaluation, and/or they might receive requests for treatment referrals. Thus, psychologists in medical settings must be aware of this complex and challenging condition and be willing to work with team members and individuals in the community to provide safe and effective interventions.

References

American Psychiatric Association. (2013). *Diagnostic and statistical manual of mental disorders* (5th ed.). Washington, DC: American Psychiatric Association.

APSAC Taskforce. (2018). Munchausen by proxy: Clinical and case management guidance. *The APSAC Advisor, 30*(1), 8–32.

Ayoub, C. C., Alexander, R., Beck, D., Bursch, B., Feldman, K. W., Libow, J. ... Yorker, B. (2002). Position paper: Definitional issues in Munchausen by proxy. Child Maltreatment, 7(2), 105–111.

Bass, C., & Glaser, D. (2014). Early recognition and management of fabricated or induced illness in children. *The Lancet, 383*(9926), 1412–1421.

Bass, C., & Halligan, P. (2014). Factitious disorders and malingering: Challenges for clinical assessment and management. *Lancet, 383*(9926), 1422–1432.

Bass, C., & Jones, D. (2011). Psychopathology of perpetrators of fabricated or induced illness in children: Case series. *The British Journal of Psychiatry, 199*(2), 113–118.

Bools, C. N., Neale, B. A., & Meadow, S. R. (1994). Munchausen syndrome by proxy: A study of psychopathology. *Child Abuse & Neglect, 18*, 773–788.

Bursch, B. (1999, October). Individual psychotherapy with child victims. In H. Schreier (Chair), *Munchausen by proxy: Psychiatric presentations, treatment findings, what to do when a new child is born*. Symposium meeting of the American Academy of Child & Adolescent Psychiatry, Chicago.

Bursch, B. (2018). Child Protective Services management of cases of suspected child abuse/neglect due to factitious disorder imposed on another. *APSAC Advisor, 30*(1), 76–82.

Bursch, B., Emerson, N. D. & Sanders, M. J. (2019). Evaluation and Management of Factitious Disorder Imposed on Another. Journal of Clinical Psychology in Medical Settings. Published online Oct 14, 2019, pp 1–11. https://doi.org/10.1007/s10880-019-09668-6

Carlson, R. J. (1984). Factitious psychiatric disorders: Diagnostic and etiologic considerations. *Psychiatric Medicine, 2*(4), 383.

Davis, P., McClure, R. J., Rolfe, K., Chessman, N., Pearson, S., Sibert, J. R., & Meadow, R. (1998). Procedures, placement, and risks of further abuse after Munchausen syndrome by proxy, non-accidental poisoning, and non-accidental suffocation. *Archives of Diseases in Childhood, 78*, 217–221.

Eisendrath, S. J. (1994). Factitious physical disorders. *Western Journal of Medicine, 160*(2), 177–179.

Fenelon, G., Mahieux, F., Roullet, E., & Guillard, A. (1991). Munchausen's syndrome and abnormalities on magnetic resonance imaging of the brain. *British Medical Journal, 302*(6783), 996–997.

Flaherty, E. G., & Macmillan, H. L. (2013). Caregiver-fabricated illness in a child: A manifestation of child maltreatment. *Pediatrics, 132*(3), 590–597.

Fliege, H., Grimm, A., Eckhardt-Henn, A., Gieler, U., Martin, K., & Klapp, B. F. (2007). Frequency of ICD-10 factitious disorder: Survey of senior hospital consultants and physicians in private practice. *Psychosomatics, 48*(1), 60–64.

Jones, D. P. H. (1987). The untreatable family. *Child Abuse & Neglect, 11*, 409–420.

Kelly, M., & Wang, C. (2018). Diagnostic aid to identify simulation and/or induction: Abuse by pediatric condition falsification/caregiver-fabricated illness in a child/medical child abuse. *APSAC Advisor, 30*(1), 32–52.

Krahn, L. E., Li, H., & O'Connor, M. K. (2003). Patients who strive to be ill: Factitious disorder with physical symptoms. *American Journal of Psychiatry, 160*(6), 1163–1168.

Lawlor, A., & Kirakowski, J. (2014). When the lie is the truth: Grounded theory analysis of an online support group for factitious disorder. *Psychiatry Research, 218*(1–2), 209–218.

Levin, A. V., & Sheridan, M. S. (Eds.). (1995). *Munchausen syndrome by proxy: Issues in diagnosis and treatment*. San Francisco, CA: Jossey-Bass.

Libow, J. A. (2000). Child and adolescent illness falsification. *Pediatrics, 105*(2), 336–342.

Modell, J. G., Mountz, J. M., & Ford, C. V. (1992). Pathological lying associated with thalamic dysfunction demonstrated by [99mTc] HMPAO SPECT. *Journal of Neuropsychiatry and Clinical Neuroscience, 4*(4), 442–446.

Mountz, J. M., Parker, P. E., Liu, H. G., Bentley, T. W., Lill, D. W., & Deutsch, G. (1996). Tc-99m HMPAO brain SPECT scanning in Munchausen syndrome. *Journal of Psychiatry & Neuroscience, 21*(1), 49–52.

Pankratz, L., & Lezak, M. D. (1987). Cerebral dysfunction in the Munchausen syndrome. *Hillside Journal of Clinical Psychiatry, 9*(2), 195–206.

Poole, C. J. (2010). Illness deception and work: Incidence, manifestations and detection. *Occupational Medicine (London), 60*(2), 127–132.

Reich, P., & Gottfried, L. A. (1983). Factitious disorders in a teaching hospital. *Annals of Internal Medicine, 99*(2), 240–247.

Roesler, T. A., & Jenny, C. (2009). *Medical child abuse: Beyond Munchausen syndrome by proxy (1st edition)*. American Academy of Pediatrics, Elk Grove Village. Retrieved from http://reader.aappublications.org/medical-child-abuse/1

Royal College of Paediatrics and Child Health. (2009). Fabricated or induced illness by carers (FII): A practical guide for paediatricians. https://www.rcpch.ac.uk/resources/fabricated-or-induced-illness-fii-carers-practical-guide-paediatricians, https://www.rcpch.ac.uk/sites/default/files/Fabricated_or_Induced_Illness_by_Carers_A_Practical_Guide_for_Paediatricians_2009.pdf

Sanders, M. J. (1995). Symptom coaching: Factitious disorder by proxy with older children. *Clinical Psychology Review, 15*(5), 423–442.

Sanders, M. J. (1996). Narrative family therapy with Munchausen by proxy: A successful treatment case. *Family, Systems, and Health, 14*(2), 315–329.

Sanders, M. J. (1999). Hospital protocol for the evaluation of Munchausen by proxy. *Clinical Child Psychology & Psychiatry, 4*(3), 379–391.

Sanders, M. J., & Ayoub, C. (2018). Munchausen by proxy: Risk assessment, support and treatment of spouses and other family caregivers. *APSAC Advisor, 30*(1), 66–75.

Sanders, M. J. & Bursch, B. (2019). Psychological Treatment of Factitious Disorder Imposed on Another/Munchausen by Proxy Abuse. Journal of Clinical Psychology in Medical Settings. Published online May 14, 2019, pp 1–11. https://doi.org/10.1007/s10880-019-09630-65.

Sansone, R. A., Wiederman, M. W., Sansone, L. A., & Mehnert-Kay, S. (1997). Sabotaging one's own medical care. Prevalence in a primary care setting. *Archives of Family Medicine, 6*(6), 583–586.

Schreier, H. A., & Bursch, B. (2018). Munchausen by proxy in educational and mental health settings. *APSAC Advisor, 30*(1), 61–65.

Sheridan, M. S. (2003). The deceit continues: An updated literature review of Munchausen syndrome by proxy. *Child Abuse & Neglect, 27*(4), 431–451.

ten Brinke, L., Stimson, D., & Carney, D. R. (2014). Some evidence for unconscious lie detection. *Psychological Science, 25*(5), 1098–1105.

Thomas, R., & Zimmer-Gembeck, M. J. (2012). Parent–child interaction therapy: An evidence-based treatment for child maltreatment. *Child Maltreatment, 17*, 253–266.

Vennemann, B., Perdekamp, M. G., Weinmann, W., Faller-Marquardt, M., Pollak, S., & Brandis, M. (2006). A case of Munchausen syndrome by proxy with subsequent suicide of the mother. *Forensic Science International, 158*(2), 195–199.

Weber, M. (2018). Investigation of factitious disorder imposed on another or medical child abuse. *APSAC Advisor, 30*(1), 53–60.

Yang, Y., Raine, A., Lencz, T., Bihrle, S., Lacasse, L., & Colletti, P. (2005). Prefrontal white matter in pathological liars. *British Journal of Psychiatry, 187*, 320–325.

Yorker, B., Alexander, R., & Sanders, M. (2018). Introduction to the special issue: Munchausen by proxy: Abuse by pediatric condition falsification, caregiver-fabricated illness in a child, or medical child abuse due to factitious disorder imposed on another. *The APSAC Advisor, 30*(1), 4–7.

Yorker, B. C. (1995). Covert video surveillance of Munchausen syndrome by proxy: The exigent circumstances exception. *Health Matrix (Cleveland, Ohio), 5*(2), 325–346.

Yorker, B. C., & Kahan, B. B. (1991). The Munchausen syndrome by proxy variant of child abuse in the family courts. *Juvenile and Family Court Journal, 42*(3), 51–58.

Pediatric Palliative Care

Michelle R. Brown and Barbara Sourkes

The goal is to add life to the child's years, not simply years to the child's life.
(American Academy of Pediatrics [AAP], 2000)
Food, toys and love are what we need to live!
6-year-old child (Sourkes, 1995, p. 112)

Introduction

Pediatric palliative care is a new interdisciplinary frontier in the comprehensive care of children living with serious medical conditions. Over the last two decades, an integrated vision toward their optimal care has begun to emerge (Association for Children with Life-threatening and Terminal Conditions and their Families and the Royal College of Paediatrics and Child Health, 2003; Institute of Medicine, 2003). Broadly defined:

> Palliative care for children and young people with [complex chronic], life-limiting or life-threatening conditions is an active and total approach to care, from the point of diagnosis or recognition throughout the child's life and death. It embraces physical, emotional, social and spiritual elements, and focuses on enhancement of quality of life for the child/young person, support for the family, [decision-making and the establishment of goals of care for the child]. It includes the management of distressing symptoms, provision for respite, and care through death and bereavement. [Palliative care may extend over many years.] (Together for Short Lives, 2018, p. 9)

"Life-threatening" includes illnesses for which cure is possible, although the threat of death remains. Such an illness may convert into a life-limiting condition when curative options no longer exist. "Life-limiting conditions" include those for which there is no reasonable chance of cure from the outset; even if children survive years and decades, they will not live out a normal life expectancy. The inclusion of "complex chronic" conditions is recent and attests to the fragility of children living with incurable diseases even when the diagnosis does not portend premature death. As is evident, end-of-life and hospice care are not synonymous with palliative care; rather, they are components of this very broad spectrum of care.

Traditionally, palliative care was only initiated late in the course of an illness, once all curative options were exhausted. Disease-directed therapy and palliative care were considered mutually exclusive. Today, the emerging model is of *concurrent care*, whereby disease-directed therapy (curative/life-prolonging) and palliative care (symptom management, decision-making, quality-of-life considerations) coexist throughout the illness trajectory, although their emphasis may shift at different stages of the illness.

M. R. Brown (✉)
Lucile Packard Children's Hospital Stanford, Palo Alto, CA, USA

Department of Psychiatry, Stanford University School of Medicine, Stanford, CA, USA
e-mail: brownmi@stanford.edu

B. Sourkes
Lucile Packard Children's Hospital Stanford, Palo Alto, CA, USA

Department of Pediatrics, Stanford University School of Medicine, Stanford, CA, USA

B. D. Carter, K. A. Kullgren (eds.), *Clinical Handbook of Psychological Consultation in Pediatric Medical Settings*, Issues in Clinical Child Psychology, https://doi.org/10.1007/978-3-030-35598-2_36

Pediatric palliative care encompasses a broad range of ages and disease-related conditions. With over half of all childhood deaths occurring under 1 year of age, most often related to congenital disorders and chromosomal abnormalities potentially detectable during the perinatal period (Heron, 2018), palliative care may be initiated even before a child's birth. The spectrum of disease-related conditions across the age span can be conceptualized to fall within one of four categories (Association for Children with Life-threatening and Terminal Conditions and their Families, National Council for Hospice and Specialist Palliative Care Services, Scottish Partnership Agency for Palliative and Cancer Care, 2001):

1. Life-threatening conditions for which curative treatment may be feasible but can fail (e.g., cancer).
2. Conditions in which premature death is anticipated but intensive treatment may prolong life and improve quality of life (e.g., cystic fibrosis).
3. Progressive diseases for which treatment is exclusively palliative and may extend over years (e.g., Duchenne muscular dystrophy).
4. Irreversible but nonprogressive conditions causing severe disability that lead to susceptibility to health complications and likelihood of premature death (e.g., severe cerebral palsy).

Impact of Pediatric Palliative Care

While the science of pediatric palliative care is emerging, the majority of the evidence base consists of retrospective cohort studies and qualitative or descriptive case studies, rather than randomized controlled trials. Systematic review is complicated by the fact that the practice of pediatric palliative care is broad, where a comprehensive set of services are provided to a wide age range of children across a number of disease groups at various points along the illness trajectory, while the evidence regarding impact is often narrowly focused on a specific outcome in a particular patient population. Yet, among the existent literature, integration of pediatric palliative care services appears to improve outcomes, including improved pain and symptom management (Wolfe et al., 2008) and quality of life (Friedrichsdorf et al., 2015), reduced length of stay in the pediatric intensive care unit and emergency department visits (Ananth, Melvin, Feudtner, Wolfe, & Berry, 2015), fewer invasive interventions and deaths in the ICU (Keele, Keenan, Sheetz, & Bratton, 2013), and improved end-of-life communications with children and families (Kassam, Skiadaresis, Alexander, & Wolfe, 2015).

The Team in Pediatric Palliative Care

Pediatric palliative care requires an interdisciplinary team to deliver optimal care. Whether the team is a formally defined set of professionals, or a group of individuals who come together as needed to design and provide palliative care interventions, integration of care is crucial. While each member of the team brings a unique specialization and perspective, a certain overlap in knowledge and skills is also evident. An overarching challenge for an interdisciplinary team is to promote a unified approach toward care, while respecting and building on each profession's contribution (Friebert, Chrastek, & Brown, 2011; Papadatou, Bluebond-Langner, & Goldman, 2011; Sourkes et al., 2005). Virtually all pediatric palliative care teams function as *consultants* to the primary team; that is, they do not take over primary care of the child. Continuity of care across treatment setting is emphasized and, when possible, palliative care teams meet with children and families on both an inpatient and outpatient basis, in addition to coordinating care with community providers.

Teams vary in composition depending on many factors, including the readiness of the institution to embrace palliative care, the availability of expertise in different disciplines, and financial support. Most programs function with a core team (or even just one "core" individual)—often a physician and/or nurse—who partners with the primary team and ancillary services who are already involved in the patient's care. Psychologists less often have time formally allocated to pediatric palliative care teams (Feudtner et al., 2013). Rather, psychologists who care for patients with chronic, complex, life-threatening conditions through either an inpatient consultation-liaison service or an outpatient medical subspecialty may collaborate with the palliative care team to formulate a comprehensive, interdisciplinary treatment plan. Among the care providers, open communication and flexible boundaries are key in delineating roles, which will vary by case and throughout a patient's course of treatment.

Pediatric Palliative Care Consultation: Children and Families

Reasons for referral of a child and family to the pediatric palliative care team fall into the following overlapping categories.

Symptom Management

Children who live with a complex chronic or life-threatening illness face extraordinary physical and psychological challenges. Whether children are receiving disease-oriented or palliative treatment—or both concurrently—enhancing their comfort and minimizing their distress is an ongoing challenge. While many physical symptoms are a predictable manifestation of an underlying disease or disorder, the intensity and frequency of their occurrence can be highly variable. Psychological symptoms are often not as predictable and, as a result, may take longer to identify and address. Common symptoms include pain, nausea and vomiting, fatigue, weakness, depression, and anxiety. To varying degrees, these symptoms can comprise both physical and psychological components; social and cultural or religious factors may all impact how children experience and interpret symptoms.

While it is important not to overemphasize psychopathology in the medically ill child, there is also a risk failing to recognize or minimizing important symptoms. Although sadness and anxiety are typical and expected reactions to prolonged illness and treatment, under sustained stress, such responses may progress to clinical disorders that necessitate psychotherapy and/or psychotropic medication. This is especially true in the child with preexistent vulnerabilities, or when there is a prior psychiatric history in the child or a family member. Differential diagnosis may be difficult since normal emotions of sadness and grief overlap with the symptoms of a clinical depression (e.g., crying, changes in appetite, sleep difficulties, and decreased concentration). Somatic symptoms of depression and anxiety also overlap considerably with the physical effects of illness and its treatment. The presence of anhedonia, feelings of worthlessness, or self-blame may help to differentiate psychological symptoms from the illness process and/or treatment. As physical effects of illness and treatment significantly impact mood and anxiety (e.g., sleep deprivation, pain), it is also critical to assess and treat such symptoms (Muriel, Case, & Sourkes, 2011; Sourkes et al., 2005).

Decision-Making and Establishing Goals of Care

Uncertainty and hope coexist throughout the trajectory of a child's life-threatening condition. Palliative care offers children and families an opportunity to consider goals for their care in light of what is known about the prognosis, treatment options, and available means for enhancing their quality of life (Kasl-Godley, King, & Quill, 2014). Direct and compassionate communication, whereby families feel respected and supported, facilitates their partnership with the team in developing an overarching plan. These discussions are especially critical when curative or life-prolonging treatment options are diminished or no longer exist. Asking about what the child and family are hoping for is the first step in defining goals. Whereas an initial response may speak to the hope for their child's survival, query about *additional* hopes often reveals families' values and their concerns about quality of life. For example, some families define hope as exhausting all possible treatment options. They may elect to proceed with highly experimental therapies that necessitate hospitalization and procedures, even with little likelihood of long-term survival. Other families may choose to focus on comfort and minimizing suffering as a priority, with the hope that the child can spend as much time as possible outside of the hospital. These discussions should be revisited as changes occur in the child's condition or new clinical information becomes available—or simply because hope is a dynamic entity and thus goals can shift over time.

The establishment of goals of care guides how the medical team presents treatment options and how families choose a pathway for their child. Historically, the paternalistic culture of western medicine meant that treatments were decided by the physician with little input from the patient and family. More recently, with a focus on autonomy, families are often asked to choose among treatment options that are offered. Families with no medical training or overall context can be overwhelmed by the responsibility of making such critical decisions. Palliative care providers are instrumental in helping families examine the benefits (the likelihood of success) and burdens inherent in the treatment. Burdens include not only pain and suffering per se, but the broader impact on children and their families' quality of life. The palliative care team can also guide the primary providers in *recommending* the option that seems most aligned with medical reality and with the values of the family. Any recommendation, of course, is counterbalanced by the reassurance to families that the team will continue to care for the child regardless of the option they choose. Expected "waypoints" should also be identified to prepare the family for developments or events that lend themselves to reevaluation of the appropriateness of the treatment plan (Macauley, 2018).

There are instances when disagreements arise between the medical team and families around what is "best" for the child. In some instances, the family wants to continue or pursue additional disease-directed treatment regimens, when the medical team no longer sees their value; the converse can also occur. An important role of the palliative care team can be to meet separately with the team and the family, listen carefully to their viewpoints, and then facilitate discussions between them to arrive at a compromise, if possible. These interventions can be critical in preventing the escalation of polarization and conflict.

In most instances, parents are tasked with making treatment decisions that are in the child's best interests. However, to varying degrees, children and adolescents may be involved in such discussions. Although very young children cannot participate meaningfully in medical decision-making, as children reach school age, many understand the realities and implications of their condition. Some children and adolescents may be hesitant to express their thoughts about treatment options, particularly when their wishes or goals differ from those of the parents and medical providers. At these critical junctures, the palliative care psychologist can be an important liaison, by bringing the child's voice (either by encouraging the child to speak directly or by report) into the discussion toward a common goal.

Advance Care Planning

Advance care planning enables patients to express their goals and values for future eventualities in case they lose their decision-making capacity at some point during the illness. Specific treatment that they wish to receive or decline (including intubation and cardiopulmonary resuscitation) can be documented in a legally binding advance care directive. Much of the literature on pediatric advance care planning has focused on the parents, since they have legal decision-making authority for their children. Parents are encouraged to clarify and document their wishes for their child proactively, so that they are not forced to make critical decisions in the extreme stress of a life-threatening crisis. Although preferences may change in the moment, research has shown that parents typically adhere to previously expressed decisions when such situations present themselves (Hammes, Klevan, Kempf, & Williams, 2005).

There is increasing belief that children and adolescents should also have a role in decision-making for their end-of-life care (American Academy of Pediatrics, 2000; Hinds et al., 2005) and many adolescents express the desire to be included (Lyon, McCabe, Patel, & D'Angelo, 2004). Research has shown that, as a result of being involved in advance care planning discussions, adolescents were better informed about end-of-life decisions and were more likely to limit disease-oriented treatments (Lyon, Jacobs, Briggs, Cheng, & Wang, 2013). Whereas advance care planning enables providers and families to understand and honor the adolescents' wishes, providers (Davies et al., 2008; Feudtner, 2007) and parents (Steele & Davies, 2006) report difficulty initiating such discussions. Advance care planning tools such as Voicing My CHOiCES (Zadeh, Pao, & Wiener, 2015) and My Wishes (Aging with Dignity, 2018) may be helpful in fostering such conversations using a developmentally appropriate approach and language. Of course, even in the absence of a written document, the process of communication may foster collaborative decision-making and articulation of a clear treatment plan.

Planning for Care at the End of Life

Palliative care providers can assist families in anticipating and preparing for the time when death is certain and imminent and care shifts toward the optimization of the child's comfort. Care can be provided in a variety of settings. The majority of children (~56%) die in the hospital (of these, more than 85% in the intensive care unit) (Carroll, Wright, & Frankel, 2011), the home (with or without home hospice support), and, infrequently, in freestanding hospices for children or long-term care facilities. When there is the possibility to plan for the setting, some families choose to stay in (or return to) the hospital for the child's death. Reasons include strong relationships with their hospital "family," inadequate resources at home, or cultural or religious beliefs that limit the use of hospice care. Other families wish for their children to be cared for away from the confines of the hospital, opting for hospice services at home. While hospice can refer to a physical place, more commonly, it refers to a health-care system providing palliative care in a home environment. It is crucial that the staff respect the family's choice and reassure them that they can change course at any time. Recent studies have shown that families' opportunity to plan for the child's death in their *preferred* location may be a more important variable than the actual location of death; it was associated with parental perceptions of high-quality end-of-life care (Dussel et al., 2009).

Psychological Guidance, Assessment, and Treatment

As the field of pediatric palliative care develops, there is a window of opportunity to define the parameters of optimal psychological care for these children. Ideally, the psychological status of each child who is referred to palliative care should be evaluated in the same way as medical and nursing assessments are performed. The specific contribution of the psychologist (and other mental health professionals) include evaluation of the child's psychological status, diagnosis of psychological/psychiatric symptoms and disturbance, psychotherapy and recommendations for psychotropic medication, and guidance for the family and team.

Within the framework of psychotherapy—through words, drawings, and play—children may confront the exigencies of living with life-threatening illness, express the ebb and flow of anticipatory grief and hope, and, at times, find their voice in the decision-making process (Muriel et al., 2011; Sourkes et al., 2005). While the evidence base for psychotherapeutic approaches with children and adolescents in palliative care is not yet developed, many best practices can be extrapolated from the broader literature in child clinical (Weisz & Kazdin, 2017) and pediatric psychology (Carter, 2014). Cognitive-behavioral therapy, motivational interviewing, and acceptance and commitment therapy all provide interventions relevant to the concerns that present in children with life-threatening disease. Self-help techniques such as relaxation, guided imagery, and hypnosis may be integrated into the process. The psychotherapeutic relationship itself can be a profound intervention in managing children's distress, as it affords a space wherein emotions can be expressed freely, without fear of others' reactions. On its own or in combination with the child's individual psychotherapy, family therapy can open lines of communication and play a pivotal role in sustaining and strengthening coping resources for each member. Healthy siblings, who have lived through the illness experience with the same intensity as the child and parents, should be included in the care.

There are two caveats to bear in mind with regard to psychological intervention in pediatric palliative care. First is that the availability of psychological consultation is often limited. Under these circumstances, other team members can provide thoughtful emotional support for the child in a carefully planned manner, ideally in consultation with a mental health professional. While it is true that psychological treatment is not universally necessary, the ability to identify "high-risk" children and intervene in a timely fashion is extremely important. A second caveat is that many children in pediatric palliative care have diagnoses with cognitive as well as physical manifestations. The spectrum includes children with mild/moderate limitations to those with severe global developmental deficits and minimal awareness of the world around them. In addition are children who, although cognitively unaffected, may not be able to communicate effectively during certain phases of the illness. Thus, traditional modes of assessment and intervention may not be appropriate at all, or, at the least, must be adapted.

Bereavement Follow-Up

Bereavement follow-up by the professional team is an intrinsic component of comprehensive pediatric palliative care. Families often express the sense of a double loss: first and foremost is the loss of their child, and second, compounding their grief, they mourn the loss of their "professional family"—the treatment team whom they have known and trusted, often over years (Contro, Larson, Scofield, Sourkes, & Cohen, 2002). Contact from a team member after the child's death not only assuages the family's sense of abandonment, but it can also serve a crucial preventive role in identifying families at heightened risk for serious psychological, social, emotional, and physical sequelae. The palliative care team, in conjunction with community providers, may assess the needs of bereaved families and either provide the necessary follow-up or advocate for and engage appropriate resources for them (Contro, Kreicbergs, Reichard, & Sourkes, 2011; Contro & Sourkes, 2012).

Pediatric Palliative Care Consultation: Trainees and Staff

Consultation and support for staff and trainees is also a vital role for the palliative care team. These interventions may take the form of individual (confidential) meetings, team debriefings, or educational sessions. In addition to the request to discuss palliative care management of a specific child, themes across all these formats include the impact of working with seriously ill children and their families on one's personal and professional life, distress when one's own values are not congruent with those of a family or one's team, conflict within a team or between the team and family, the impact of a child's death and the toll of cumulative loss, and preserving resilience over the "long haul."

Crosscutting Considerations

Culture

From its inception, the field of palliative care has been attentive to culturally determined aspects of care, beginning at the most basic level with the impact of language barriers, including nonverbal communication (Strada, 2018). How families communicate with their child about diagnosis and prognosis, from an open approach to one of limiting information with the goal of protection, may derive from their cultural background more than from their "psychology." The locus of decision-making may depend on how "collectively" family is defined—and determine whether the parents defer to an authority figure in the family or to a larger group of extended family. Gender differences, particularly the role of women in the family, can be significant. Cultural meanings of illness and death can affect the experience and tolerance of pain (Wiener, McConnell, Latella, & Ludi, 2013), openness to discuss treatment preferences at the end of life, and attitudes toward hospice care (Macauley, 2018; Strada, 2018).

Given the many ways that cultural differences can influence children's and families' experience of life-threatening illness, asking about their background is a critical part of an overall assessment. Medical interpreters play an invaluable role in interpreting not only words, but also styles of communication and culture. Culturally competent palliative care requires patience and respect from the team in creating a therapeutic alliance.

Spirituality/Religion

Many families identify spirituality and religion as important in the face of illness and death: from making sense of and ascribing meaning to the experience to finding and defining hope, to providing guidance in decision-making, to giving emotional sustenance. In one study, 73% of parents reported that spirituality or religion was what helped them the most during the last stages of their child's illness (Robinson, Thiel, Backus, & Meyer, 2006). Yet many health-care professionals lack training (and comfort) in discussing these issues with families. Newly published guidelines have recognized the need to focus on spiritual care as a central domain in palliative care (National Consensus Project for Quality Palliative Care, 2018).

Ethics

Ethical issues in palliative care arise when the personal, cultural, and institutional values involved in decision-making conflict, whether among family members, between patient and family, patient/family and provider, or among professionals. Determining "the right thing to do" in emotionally laden life and death situations involving children is a huge challenge, for families and for medical teams alike. Consultation with an institution's ethics team can help to delineate the concerns and offer recommendations based upon identified ethical principles and precedent. Following are the key ethical dilemmas that arise most commonly in pediatric palliative care (Macauley, 2018):

- Requests for nondisclosure. In the desire to protect their child from overwhelming emotion, parents may ask the medical team not to share information related to their illness. This request often causes significant distress for medical teams who value open communication and access to information.
- Nonbeneficial care. Significant advances in medicine have contributed to the false assumption that every sick child can be cured. When are interventions "medically futile"?
- Refusal of medical treatment. While the standard for pediatric decision-making is consent of the parents and assent of the child, there are times when either the family rejects the "best" treatment option for their child or the child or adolescent's goals for treatment differ from those of the parents and medical team.
- Withholding or withdrawing life-sustaining medical intervention. Who makes that decision for the child? What are the criteria? How is quality of life defined for this child?

Barriers to Optimal Pediatric Palliative Care

There are many medical, psychosocial cultural, and financial barriers to the ideal delivery of comprehensive pediatric palliative care. Perhaps the greatest barrier is the still prevalent view that curative and palliative care are mutually exclusive. As a result, in the face of prognostic uncertainty, both medical teams and families may perceive palliative treatment as "giving up." Physicians may wait to initiate palliative care until they are absolutely certain that curative options no longer exist and that death is inevitable. In so doing, the provision of valuable services may be delayed, and opportunities to support quality of life for the child throughout the course of treatment, as well for the family, may be missed. One of the foremost goals of the field is to initiate palliative care for children proactively, early in the illness trajectory. An uncertain prognosis should be a signal to initiate, rather than to delay, palliative care (Sourkes et al., 2005).

Misconceptions and fear around the use of opioids for pain and symptom management are another barrier (Collins, Berde, & Frost, 2011). Many professionals are not comfortable in prescribing the appropriate escalating dosages necessary for optimal symptom management, often because they have not been educated in the principles of their administration. Both families and professionals may harbor fears about whether these drugs will cause addiction or immediately hasten the death of a child. These factors may lead to the imposition of limits on the very medications that would otherwise contribute to the child's comfort and potentially enhance quality of life over an extended period—not just in the last phases of the illness.

At the hospital level, staffing issues often serve as barriers to optimal palliative care. Physicians typically rotate off-service on a weekly or biweekly basis and primary nursing care is often not available. These frequent changes in the treatment team may contribute to miscommunication and confusion around the child's treatment plan. An incoming team may lack clarity about the rationale for a family's goals or care and/or may disagree with a previous team's direction or decisions. Varying levels of experience with palliative care generally, and understanding of the model of concurrent care specifically, may also cause confusion among providers.

Community barriers include the paucity of hospice and other health-care professionals familiar with pediatric symptom management. Children and their families typically become intensely dependent on the specialists in their tertiary care center for all aspects of their care. As a result, community professionals, including their primary pediatrician, often miss opportunities to gain expertise in pediatric palliative care. There continues to be a concerted effort to educate community practitioners both through didactic training and through discussions to address their concerns about working with seriously ill and dying children and their families.

Reimbursement issues are another major hindrance in developing comprehensive palliative care services (Harris, 2004). For many years, children with life-threatening illnesses were not eligible for palliative services while receiving curative or life-prolonging care. More recent legislation such as the Concurrent Care for Children Requirement of the Affordable Care Act (2010) has enabled children who are eligible for hospice to receive all other services related to the treatment of their condition, including those deemed life-prolonging such as blood transfusions and palliative chemotherapy.

Pediatric Palliative Care Consultation: Case Studies

Sarah was a 17-year-old girl diagnosed with a brain tumor at the age of 15. She had undergone three surgeries together with chemotherapy and radiation. She had one remission (disease-free period) of 9 months' duration. Following relapse and subsequent hospitalization, the palliative care team was consulted to discuss goals of care with Sarah and her family. In a series of care conferences, in which the palliative care team was present, the oncology team explained that any remaining treatment options were of uncertain benefit and could cause serious complications, or even shorten her life. The team presented "comfort only" measures as an equally acceptable option. Over the next days, Sarah and her parents weighed the benefits and burdens of various interventions, in discussions among themselves and with members of the palliative care team. Ultimately, they elected to pursue the route of palliative care at home, where Sarah received excellent symptom management from a community hospice. She died peacefully 4 months later.

Sarah's story illustrates the traditional model in which disease-directed care transitioned to palliative measures once cure was no longer an attainable goal. The illness course had a somewhat predictable timeframe and symptom management was relatively straightforward, allowing her to preserve good quality of life until her death.

Role of psychologist: Sarah was followed in psychotherapy beginning 1 year after her diagnosis. (The referral to the palliative care psychologist actually served as a point of entry for the entire palliative care team.) Major themes of discussion included awareness of her poor prognosis and how she would know when she had had "enough," concern for her parents and her 12-year-old brother and the pain of witnessing their suffering, deciding which meetings with the medical team she wanted to attend—and which she just wanted her parents to "report back" on, and the "what if's," in particular her wish that her parents make any decisions for her if she were not no longer competent. Through her intensifying anticipatory grief, Sarah articulated her emerging goals of care: if her time were limited, she wanted to be home with her family. The psychologist also met several times with Sarah's brother (as well as maintaining contact with his school counselor) to ensure that his concerns were addressed. After Sarah's death, the psychologist provided follow-up for her brother and referred the parents to a couple's therapist in the community who was experienced in bereavement.

Carlos was an infant in whom heart failure and neurologic anomalies had been identified prenatally by ultrasound. However, the diagnosis of a complex genetic syndrome was not confirmed until he was a month old. Because neither the diagnosis nor the prognosis were yet certain, parents expressed a desire to pursue all interventions that would give him the best chance for long-term survival. The neonatology and cardiology services consulted the palliative care team at this juncture. In his first week of life, Carlos was evaluated for potential listing for a heart transplant. He then underwent placement of a biventricular assist device (BiVAD)—an artificial heart—to support his heart function while he awaited a donor organ. While he initially responded favorably to the BiVAD, over the subsequent weeks, he developed serious complications including excessive blood clotting, a septic event causing pulmonary hemorrhage, followed by a stroke resulting in significant neurological injury. Given the parents' concerns about both his immediate suffering and longer-term quality of life, they requested that the BiVAD be discontinued. At the age of 8 weeks, he was disconnected from the BiVAD, extubated, and died in his parents' arms.

Carlos's care exemplified the way which intensive medical intervention and palliative care can be provided concurrently, with each predominating at different points along his treatment course. Carlos's parents faced several critical junctures of decision-making after uncertain prenatal ultrasounds: to initiate heart transplant evaluation and place onto a BiVAD, to continue with intensive care following a number of complications, and then to remove all intensive care measures. At each decision point, his parents carefully reexamined their goals of care, balancing their hopes to prolong his life with their desire to minimize his suffering.

Role of psychologist: The palliative psychologist initially met the parents during transplant evaluation and remained available throughout Carolos's life. The sessions were a forum for the parents to articulate their thinking, both individually and as a couple, and to provide guidance about explaining Carlos' illness and death to their 4-year-old son. When the parents' brought up their fear for any future pregnancies, the psychologist introduced them to a genetic counselor who would be available to meet with them in the future. The parents welcomed a referral to an organization focused on bereavement after neonatal death and maintained occasional telephone contact with the psychologist. The hospital team requested a debriefing after Carlos's death; they had become very attached to this family and wanted to understand better the concurrence of intensive intervention coupled with palliative care and how the family had negotiated this duality.

Future Directions

The field of pediatric palliative care offers unique opportunities for pediatric psychologists to participate in enhancing the quality of life of our most vulnerable children and families. Although psychological services have been integrated into medical settings, they remain on the periphery in pediatric palliative care (Feudtner et al., 2013), limiting opportunities for clinical exposure and training. A number of resources exist that provide education in palliative care more broadly including the *Clinical Practice Guidelines for Quality Palliative Care, Fourth Edition* (National Consensus Project for Quality Palliative Care, 2018), and programs through Education in Palliative and End-of Life Care (EPEC; http://www.epec.net) and the End-of-Life Nursing Education Consortium (ELNEC; http://www.aacn.nche.edu/elnec). Pediatric specific materials are available through the National Hospice and Palliative Care Organization (NHPCO; http://www.nhpco.org/palliative-care-resources-series).

Formal training programs or certification options are not yet available for psychologists. Specific knowledge and skills necessary for psychologists to engage in effective palliative care recently have been proposed (Kasl-Godley et al., 2014; Strada, 2018). Future development of practice guidelines and standardized training curriculum will promote increased integration of psychology into pediatric palliative care as the field continues to evolve.

References

Aging with Dignity. (2018). My Wishes.

American Academy of Pediatrics. (2000). Palliative care for children. *Pediatrics, 106*(2 Pt 1), 351–357.

Ananth, P., Melvin, P., Feudtner, C., Wolfe, J., & Berry, J. G. (2015). Hospital use in the last year of life for children with life-threatening complex chronic conditions. *Pediatrics, 136*(5), 938–946. https://doi.org/10.1542/peds.2015-0260

Association for Children with Life-threatening and Terminal Conditions and their Families and the Royal College of Paediatrics and Child Health. (2003). *A guide to the development of children's palliative care services*. Bristol.

Association for Children with Life-threatening and Terminal Conditions and their Families, National Council for Hospice and Specialist Palliative Care Services, Scottish Partnership Agency for Palliative and Cancer Care. (2001). *Palliative care for young people ages 13–24*. London.

Carroll, J. M., Wright, J., L., & Frankel, L. R. (2011). Settings of care. In J. Wolfe, P. S. Hinds, & B. M. Sourkes (Eds.), *Textbook of interdisciplinary pediatric palliative care* (pp. 64–73). Philadelphia: Elsevier/Saunders.

Carter, B. (2014). Introduction to the CPPP special issue on evidence-based interventions in pediatric psychology. *Clinical Practice in Pediatric Psychology, 2*(3), 207–211.

Collins, J. J., Berde, C. B., & Frost, J. A. (2011). Pain assessment and management. In J. Wolfe, P. S. Hinds, & B. M. Sourkes (Eds.), *Textbook of interdisciplinary pediatric palliative care* (pp. 284–299). Philadelphia: Elsevier/Saunders.

Contro, N., Kreicbergs, U., Reichard, W., & Sourkes, B. M. (2011). Anticipatory grief and bereavement. In J. Wolfe, P. S. Hinds, & B. M. Sourkes (Eds.), *Textbook of interdisciplinary pediatric palliative care* (pp. 41–54). Philadelphia: Elsevier/Saunders.

Contro, N., Larson, J., Scofield, S., Sourkes, B., & Cohen, H. (2002). Family perspectives on the quality of pediatric palliative care. *Archives of Pediatrics & Adolescent Medicine, 156*(1), 14–19.

Contro, N., & Sourkes, B. M. (2012). Opportunities for quality improvement in bereavement care at a children's hospital: Assessment of interdisciplinary staff perspectives. *Journal of Palliative Care, 28*(1), 28–35.

Davies, B., Sehring, S. A., Partridge, J. C., Cooper, B. A., Hughes, A., Philp, J. C., ... Kramer, R. F. (2008). Barriers to palliative care for children: Perceptions of pediatric health care providers. *Pediatrics, 121*(2), 282–288. https://doi.org/10.1542/peds.2006-3153

Dussel, V., Kreicbergs, U., Hilden, J. M., Watterson, J., Moore, C., Turner, B. G., ... Wolfe, J. (2009). Looking beyond where children die: Determinants and effects of planning a child's location of death. *Journal of Pain and Symptom Management, 37*(1), 33–43. https://doi.org/10.1016/j.jpainsymman.2007.12.017

Feudtner, C. (2007). Collaborative communication in pediatric palliative care: A foundation for problem-solving and decision-making. *Pediatric Clinics of North America, 54*(5), 583–607,. ix. https://doi.org/10.1016/j.pcl.2007.07.008

Feudtner, C., Womer, J., Augustin, R., Remke, S., Wolfe, J., Friebert, S., & Weissman, D. (2013). Pediatric palliative care programs in children's hospitals: A cross-sectional national survey. *Pediatrics, 132*(6), 1063–1070. https://doi.org/10.1542/peds.2013-1286

Friebert, S., Chrastek, J., & Brown, M. R. (2011). Team relationships. In J. Wolfe, P. S. Hinds, & B. M. Sourkes (Eds.), *Textbook of interdisciplinary pediatric palliative care* (pp. 148–158). Philadelphia: Elsevier/Saunders.

Friedrichsdorf, S. J., Postier, A., Dreyfus, J., Osenga, K., Sencer, S., & Wolfe, J. (2015). Improved quality of life at end of life related to home-based palliative care in children with cancer. *Journal of Palliative Medicine, 18*(2), 143–150. https://doi.org/10.1089/jpm.2014.0285

Hammes, B. J., Klevan, J., Kempf, M., & Williams, M. S. (2005). Pediatric advance care planning. *Journal of Palliative Medicine, 8*(4), 766–773. https://doi.org/10.1089/jpm.2005.8.766

Harris, M. B. (2004). Palliative care in children with cancer: Which child and when? *Journal of the National Cancer Institute. Monographs, 2004*(32), 144–149. https://doi.org/10.1093/jncimonographs/lgh007

Heron, M. (2018). *Deaths: Leading causes for 2016. National vital statistics reports, 67*(6). Hyattsville, MD: National Center for Health Statistics.

Hinds, P. S., Drew, D., Oakes, L. L., Fouladi, M., Spunt, S. L., Church, C., & Furman, W. L. (2005). End-of-life care preferences of pediatric patients with cancer. *Journal of Clinical Oncology, 23*(36), 9146–9154. https://doi.org/10.1200/JCO.2005.10.538

Institute of Medicine. (2003). *When children die: Improving palliative and end-of-life care for children and their families*. Washington, DC: The National Academies Press. https://doi.org/10.17226/10390

Kasl-Godley, J. E., King, D. A., & Quill, T. E. (2014). Opportunities for psychologists in palliative care: Working with patients and families across the disease continuum. *The American Psychologist, 69*(4), 364–376. https://doi.org/10.1037/a0036735

Kassam, A., Skiadaresis, J., Alexander, S., & Wolfe, J. (2015). Differences in end-of-life communication for children with advanced cancer who were referred to a palliative care team. *Pediatric Blood & Cancer, 62*(8), 1409–1413. https://doi.org/10.1002/pbc.25530

Keele, L., Keenan, H. T., Sheetz, J., & Bratton, S. L. (2013). Differences in characteristics of dying children who receive and do not receive palliative care. *Pediatrics, 132*(1), 72–78. https://doi.org/10.1542/peds.2013-0470

Lyon, M. E., Jacobs, S., Briggs, L., Cheng, Y. I., & Wang, J. (2013). Family-centered advance care planning for teens with cancer. *JAMA Pediatrics, 167*(5), 460–467. https://doi.org/10.1001/jamapediatrics.2013.943

Lyon, M. E., McCabe, M. A., Patel, K. M., & D'Angelo, L. J. (2004). What do adolescents want? An exploratory study regarding end-of-life decision-making. *Journal of Adolescent Health, 35*(6), 529.e521–529.e526. https://doi.org/10.1016/j.jadohealth.2004.02.009

Macauley, R. C. (2018). *Ethics in palliative care: A complete guide*. New York, NY: Oxford University Press.

Muriel, A. C., Case, C., & Sourkes, B. M. (2011). Children's voices: The experiences of patients and their siblings. In J. Wolfe, P. S. Hinds, & B. M. Sourkes (Eds.), *Textbook of interdisciplinary pediatric palliative care* (pp. 18–29). Philadelphia: Elsevier/Saunders.

National Consensus Project for Quality Palliative Care. (2018). *Clinical practice guidelines for quality palliative care* (4th ed.) Richmond, VA: National Coalition for Hospice and Palliative Care. Retrieved from https://www.nationalcoalitionhpc.org/ncp

Papadatou, D., Bluebond-Langner, M., & Goldman, A. (2011). The team. In J. Wolfe, P. S. Hinds, & B. M. Sourkes (Eds.), *Textbook of interdisciplinary pediatric palliative care* (pp. 55–63). Philadelphia: Elsevier/Saunders.

Robinson, M. R., Thiel, M. M., Backus, M. M., & Meyer, E. C. (2006). Matters of spirituality at the end of life in the pediatric intensive care unit. *Pediatrics, 118*(3), e719–e729. https://doi.org/10.1542/peds.2005-2298

Sourkes, B. (1995). Armfuls of time: The psychological experience of the child with a life-threatening illness. Pittsburgh, PA: University of Pittsburgh Press.

Sourkes, B., Frankel, L., Brown, M., Contro, N., Benitz, W., Case, C., … Sunde, C. (2005). Food, toys, and love: Pediatric palliative care. *Current Problems in Pediatric and Adolescent Health Care, 35*(9), 350–386. https://doi.org/10.1016/j.cppeds.2005.09.002

Steele, R., & Davies, B. (2006). Impact on parents when a child has a progressive, life-threatening illness. *International Journal of Palliative Nursing, 12*(12), 576–585. https://doi.org/10.12968/ijpn.2006.12.12.22544

Strada, E. A. (2018). *Palliative psychology: Clinical perspectives on an emerging subspecialty*. New York, NY: Oxford University Press.

Together for Short Lives. (2018). A guide to children's palliative care. Bristol: Together for Short Lives

Weisz, J. R., & Kazdin, A. E. (2017). *Evidence-based psychotherapies for children and adolescents* (3rd ed.). New York: The Guilford Press.

Wiener, L., McConnell, D. G., Latella, L., & Ludi, E. (2013). Cultural and religious considerations in pediatric palliative care. *Palliative & Supportive Care, 11*(1), 47–67. https://doi.org/10.1017/S1478951511001027

Wolfe, J., Hammel, J. F., Edwards, K. E., Duncan, J., Comeau, M., Breyer, J., … Weeks, J. C. (2008). Easing of suffering in children with cancer at the end of life: Is care changing? *Journal of Clinical Oncology, 26*(10), 1717–1723. https://doi.org/10.1200/JCO.2007.14.0277

Zadeh, S., Pao, M., & Wiener, L. (2015). Opening end-of-life discussions: How to introduce Voicing My CHOiCES™, an advance care planning guide for adolescents and young adults. *Palliative & Supportive Care, 13*(3), 591–599. https://doi.org/10.1017/S1478951514000005

Technological Innovations in Pediatric Psychological Consultation

Ethan Benore, Eric L. Scott, and Erin Webster

To best serve our patients, pediatric psychologists must adapt to the rapid technological "upgrades" and advances in the field. Most hospital systems now use electronic medical records to optimize patient care (e.g., documentation, care coordination, appointment scheduling, patient-provider communication) (Chaudhry et al., 2006; Jamal, McKenzie, & Clark, 2009), with future advances in telehealth bringing even more options for patient care (Balkhi et al., 2015; Reynolds & Maughan, 2015; Trnka et al., 2015). This generation of children and families that psychologists serve has also evolved. "Generation Z" (children born between 1995 and 2012) is growing up in a highly sophisticated media and computer environment, resulting in increasingly tech-savvy youth. Up to 95% of youth have direct access to a smartphone (Perrin & Duggan, 2015) and almost half (44%) say they go online multiple times a day. As a result of the increases in electronic exposure, attention spans may be shorter, youth may lack the requisite skill in multitasking, and media can produce a generational divide between clinician and patient. This changing landscape will undoubtedly force clinicians to identify ways to engage children that have ready access to self-help interventions, audiovisual distractions, and social media outlets at their fingertips.

Due to this changing landscape, children and families stand to benefit from increased access to digital information and resources previously unavailable, particularly in underserved populations. Given the severe limitations in pediatric access to mental health care (Cuellar, 2015), it has been essential to leverage technology to expand the reach of services. While technology advances may lead to increased access and improvements in care, it is not entirely without drawbacks. The rapid changes in technology lead to a gap in the evidence base for new technological features. This chapter serves to highlight the current use of technology for psychological consultation-liaison services as well as outpatient psychological treatment for the medically ill child. We then address necessary considerations to further our knowledge and evidence-based practice in this field.

E. Benore (✉)
Center for Pediatric Behavioral Health, Cleveland Clinic Children's, Cleveland, OH, USA

Clinical Assistant Professor at Cleveland Clinic Lerner College of Medicine, Cleveland OH, USA
e-mail: benoree@ccf.org

E. L. Scott
Department of Pediatrics, C.S. Mott Children's Hospital, University of Michigan Medical School, Ann Arbor, MI, USA

Department of Anesthesiology, C.S. Mott Children's Hospital, University of Michigan School of Medicine, Ann Arbor, MI, USA

E. Webster
Department of Psychology, Dayton Children's Hospital, Dayton, OH, USA
e-mail: webstere@childrensdayton.org

B. D. Carter, K. A. Kullgren (eds.), *Clinical Handbook of Psychological Consultation in Pediatric Medical Settings*, Issues in Clinical Child Psychology, https://doi.org/10.1007/978-3-030-35598-2_37

Current Status of Technological Applications in Psychological Treatment

Like nearly all professional fields, pediatric psychology is being increasingly molded and shaped by the rapid advances in technology, changing the acquisition and implementation of the psychological principles and knowledge in dramatic ways. Clinicians now have at their disposal a variety of innovative ways to collect and evaluate psychological data about patient's mental, physical, and emotional states while also providing engaging and novel ways to disseminate behavioral interventions.

Current technology-based interventions have been used to implement change strategies include self-assessment and self-monitoring, psychoeducation, goal setting, skill building, and feedback. These interventions share a number of commonalities with face-to-face interventions—predominately, empirically based theories of behavior change (Wu, Steele, Connelly, Palermo, & Ritterband, 2014). There are several current examples supporting digital interventions. First, online treatment (with minimal therapist involvement) has demonstrated significantly better results than traditional face-to-face CBT for youth with anxiety (Kendall, Khanna, Edson, Cummings, & Harris, 2011). Similarly, standalone online CBT programs have been shown to be more effective compared to traditional CBT (Pajovic et al., 2011) and online CBT superior to waitlist control (March, Spence, & Donovan, 2009). Similar results were published for the use of online CBT for depression. An RCT in New Zealand tested a computerized CBT to a psychoeducation component, which demonstrated a significant reduction on child depression rating scales—although remission rates were not statistically different (Stasiak, Hatcher, Frampton, & Merry, 2014). In a related study, online CBT resulted in 78% of adolescents achieving remission of depressive symptoms (Fleming, Dixon, Frampton, & Merry, 2012). A recent meta-analysis further supports the benefit of technologically delivered mental health interventions to children (Grist, Croker, Denne, & Stallard, 2019).

Systematic reviews of technology-based psychological services highlight key factors which may optimize therapeutic benefit for children. For example, communication via telephone is an effective medium for delivering psychological care, provides the same benefits to patients, and can reduce dropouts by reducing barriers to care (Mohr, Burns, Schueller, Clarke, & Klinkman, 2013). Additionally, psychotherapy provided via instant messaging systems produces results similar to face-to-face services (Mohr et al., 2013). Mobile technologies are also amenable to intervention strategies consistent with evidence-based treatment such as appointment reminders, mobile therapy, mobile symptoms tracking, and virtual reality exposure therapy. Compliance to appointments was 64% (compared to 50% receiving no reminder) when utilizing a mobile appointment reminder (Aboujaoude & Salame, 2016). Providers may find these digital platforms allow for a *more* (not less) engaged patient who utilizes technology on a daily basis (Richardson, Stallard, & Velleman, 2010).

Technological Applications in the Inpatient Pediatric Medical Setting

One of the first applications of the use of technology in the pediatric hospital setting was to facilitate the child's psychological adjustment to the hospital, his/her medical condition, and to noxious procedures. Historically, medical care has benefited from psychologically based interventions such as the tell-show-do method (e.g., Farhat-McHayleh, Harfouche, & Souaid (2009)), art and recreational therapies (e.g., Ortiz et al. (2017)) to create a child-friendly environment (e.g., Pinquart, Skolaude, Zaplinski, & Maier (2011)), and modifying procedures by providing information or increasing child choice to reduce anxiety (Farkas et al., 2015). Books such as those published by Magination Press (http://www.apa.org/pubs/magination/) provide a source of materials intended to improve the child's understanding of the hospital experience, medical conditions, and medical procedures in efforts to reduce distress and improve coping. However, in the last two decades, newer tech-savvy delivery methods to promote adjustment have emerged. Examples include an interactive computer program where children can actively author and share their stories through interactive storytellers—or develop virtual environments (Bers et al., 2002). Mossman (2004) demonstrated the benefit of walkie-talkies to reduce children's separation anxiety prior to surgery. Philanthropic missions have also increased access to coping and adjustment resources for hospitalized children. As one example, Seacrest Studios (Ryan Seacrest Foundation) provides children opportunities to participate in interviews and live performances with artists and celebrities, to host live radio shows, and to create music videos or shows. Hospital-based pediatric psychologists, along with other services such as Child Life, are often in a position to advocate with their hospitals for the acquisition of appropriate technologies for their patients and can help developers construct effective platforms that positively influence psychosocial functioning in the medically ill child.

Video-Based Modalities

Technology has also provided a means to increase children's knowledge of medical procedures, and familiarity with hospital experiences, thereby fostering mastery and confidence in the hospital. The Coping Club (http://copingclub.com/) is a website developed by and for children to learn about specific medical conditions, hospital procedures, coping with hospitalization, and more general information like dealing with getting an IV, talking to others about their illness, or taking medications. An accompanying mobile "Coping Cart" (at Norton Children's Hospital in Louisville) has helped generate much of the video footage available on the Coping Club website. The "Coping Cart" is a mobile device packed with a large iMac computer display, a video camera for generation of digital recordings, biofeedback devices, and online access to videos, all designed to give easy patient/family access to the videos generated by other patients and also facilitate their generating material that other patients can use (Novotney, 2010). It capitalizes on principles from social learning theory, understanding that current patients can learn from the experiences of previous patients coping with similar concerns or challenges.

CL psychologists increasingly rely on resources like YouTube and Vimeo to build digital toolkits and repertoires to share child and family-friendly materials (most are 2–5 min long) providing sufficient information in a child-friendly manner. Illustrative examples include:

"It doesn't have to hurt." (https://www.youtube.com/watch?v=KgBwVSYqfps)
"Understanding pain in 10 minutes." (https://www.youtube.com/watch?v=C_3phB93rvI)
Paul and the dragon video about cancer. (https://www.acco.org/paulandthedragon/)
What is diabetes? (https://www.youtube.com/watch?v=4EEtubB74lM)
Going to the hospital. (https://www.youtube.com/watch?v=FpT02esukOI)
What to expect at a sleep study. (https://www.youtube.com/watch?v=H1359kRK6mk)
A guide to a children's MRI scan (https://www.youtube.com/watch?v=HVp3uV0RAgc)
SPPsychology. (https://www.societyofpediatricpsychology.org/consultation)

As an example of the efforts to assess the benefit (and limits) of these types of videos, Farkas et al. (2015) reviewed 25 educational videos on needle pain. They concluded that while most videos were accurate and created by a trustworthy source, none directly address techniques specific to treating a diagnosis of needle phobia. As is the case with other videos, while broad-based content may increase the number of "clicks" on a video, it may fall short of meeting the child's specific need. Further research is needed to examine the acceptability and impact of multimedia education as an effective intervention.

Online Informational/Educational Documents

Kidshealth.org (www.kidshealth.org) provides a broad wealth of information which can be read aloud to the child. Readily searchable topics range from child-friendly anatomy and physiology to illnesses and injuries and coping with difficult emotions. There are also a number of conditions for which groups have created specific educational material—as one example, Headache Relief Guide (http://www.headachereliefguide.com/) provides excellent child-friendly information about headaches and headache treatments. Other condition-specific resources are introduced and updated regularly.

For pediatric psychologists in a medical setting CL role, it is beneficial to develop a repertoire of easily accessed clinically useful resource materials including website links, YouTube videos, interactive online environments, appropriate chat rooms, etc. When building such a toolkit, the psychologist should consider the following themes for a child: (1) What is my medical condition? (2) What happens to me at the hospital? (3) What are my medications and side effects? (4) What happens in a procedure? (5) What do I need to know going home from the hospital? (6) How can I best communicate with nurses, doctors, and surgeons as part of my health care team?

Clinical Biofeedback

There has been a growing use of biofeedback within the pediatric field and strong consideration should be given to their use by CL psychologists for several reasons. First, user-friendly equipment allows patients to access biofeedback devices with as little as a smartphone or tablet and, if needed, a peripheral sensor. The familiarity of smartphones and simplicity of handheld devices/stand-alone machines make them less intimidating for CL psychologists and patients alike, often reducing initial fear of adoption. Ease of adoption also increases patient buy-in and sets the stage for outpatient intervention upon discharge. Second, devices that are highly responsive to patient behavior and effort (e.g., heart rate variability, HRV; galvanic skin response, GSR; and respiration rate, RR) can offer a "wow factor" and increase the connection between the patient's cognitions, emotions, and physiologic state. These characteristics help to increase initial engagement—especially when the patient is new to the technology. Once the patient and family understand the rationale and have "seen it with their own eyes," they may be more likely to engage in follow-up care, both in the hospital and upon discharge.

For these reasons and for budgetary constraints, starting with small handheld thermometers used to teach thermal biofeedback, mood rings, biodots, or GSR stand-alone machines makes sense. Their high portability, single use to reduce cross contamination and risk of infection, low cost, and wide availability to the public increase their appeal. Other low-cost/high-impact models include the respErate abdominal stretch monitor, the Heartmath Inner Balance sensor (HRV), the Alive for EmWave (HRV), or a GSR monitor. Many of these devices are affordable at <$500, portable (usually handheld), and simple enough to show patients immediately. While the consulting psychologist should ultimately seek to educate themselves on the psychophysiology and theoretical underpinnings of biofeedback-based modalities, these devices have immediate clinical utility and require a modicum of training or special knowledge.

Biofeedback continues to show promise in brief interventions studies in children. As one example, Knox et al. (2011) demonstrated a significant reduction in depression and anxiety symptoms using cognitive-behavioral intervention enhanced with user-friendly models of biofeedback: freeze frame and/or Wild Divine. (It should be noted that these programs have since been enhanced, but upgraded models are available through heartmath.com, unite.com, and somaticvision.com.) In a second study incorporating the Wild Divine program for biofeedback-assisted relaxation training, hospitalized children receiving less than two sessions of biofeedback on average during their admission reported improvements in pain and anxiety (McKenna, Gallagher, Forbes, & Ibeziako, 2015). While there are obvious limitations in research methodologies on an ever-changing inpatient unit, there is promise for biofeedback as a readily available, user-friendly, and efficient tool to modify target variables and children's experience during their hospitalization.

Smartphone Apps

There are an exponentially growing number of smartphone apps which have been used to facilitate relaxation training, mindfulness, implementation of cognitive-behavioral therapy, and tracking and monitoring of specific behaviors. The BrightHearts app has shown promise in the management of procedural pain and anxiety (Morrow, Burton, Watanabe, Cloyd, & Khut, 2018). Other potential apps include Healing Buddies Comfort Kit and Pain Tricks. The What's Up app gives specific info on CBT techniques; Headspace and Breathe2Relax offer elements of breath training and mindfulness training. Unfortunately, little research has been conducted on the inexpensive apps most available to children. Also, many apps are discontinued to the cost to the developer of maintaining the technology.

Application in Outpatient Integrated Subspecialty and Primary Care Settings

While much of the technology options presented above can also be used in an outpatient setting, regular follow-up with patients over a longer period of time while they are not hospitalized provides additional opportunities for technology-assisted psychological interventions and continuity between in-hospital and outpatient care.

Clinical Biofeedback

The bulk of data supporting biofeedback as an effective tech-savvy procedure has been established in outpatient medical settings. Several companies such as Heartmath, Somatic Vision, Zukor, and Wild Divine (among others) have created engaging software platforms to learn self-regulation skills. Additionally, many apps on tablet and smartphone devices, some with peripheral attachments and some without, which are virtual "plug-and-play" methods to perform some variant of a biofeedback procedure, are being continually developed and becoming increasingly affordable.

There have been empirical studies touting the benefits of biofeedback therapies to treat several pediatric conditions including chronic pain (Fahrenkamp & Benore, 2019; Roers, Curwick, O'connor, Canny, & Harbeck-Weber, 2016), IBS (Stern, Guiles, & Gevirtz, 2014), migraine (Stubberud, Varkey, McCrory, Pedersen, & Linde, 2016), elimination disorders (Santos, Lopes, & Koyle, 2017), and anxiety (Goessl, Curtiss, & Hofmann, 2017). Additionally, Tan and colleagues (2016) have specifically summarized data supporting various forms of biofeedback technology for 40 separate conditions (e.g., ADHD, diabetes, epilepsy, incontinence, PTSD, traumatic brain injury). While multiple meta-analyses have been performed on adult populations, there are some meta-analyses or reviews that specifically examine effectiveness of biofeedback for pediatric conditions (e.g., Cortese et al., 2016; Darling, Benore, & Webster, 2019; Fazeli et al., 2015; Stubberud et al., 2016). In all studies, however, researchers cite limitations in standardized methodology necessary to improve the evidence base (see also Strout & Burton, 2004).

Smartphone Apps

The use of mobile health apps has seen a dramatic rise in terms of application and integration for health behavior change. As an example, Bauer, de Niet, Timman, and Kordy (2010) used computer-generated text messages as part of a weight loss program for children (Bauer et al., 2010). Others have demonstrated the benefit of text messaging for medication adherence (Badawy & Kuhns, 2016). Newer models are emerging for treating pain with mobile apps or Internet delivery systems (Hedman-Lagerlof et al., 2018; Palermo, de la Vega, Dudeney, Murray, & Law, 2018). However, a limitation has been cited in the development of these apps—limited engagement between technology developers, clinicians, and the end user may prevent these apps from truly benefiting children (Brannon & Cushing, 2015; Reynoldson et al., 2014). There is often a lag between popular games, technologies, and direct applications for psychological interventions and an additional lag time to complete research that evaluates the effectiveness of the technology on a problem of interest.

Wearables

Wearable sensors have also given psychologists increased opportunities to record relevant clinical data and use this for specific behavior change. Devices such as the popular FitBit have demonstrated the potential to increase physical activity with active monitoring and embedded reinforcements (Amresh, Lyles, Small, & Gary, 2017; Hooke, Gilchrist, Tanner, Hart, & Withycombe, 2016). However, there are concerns raised with the quality of the data (Meltzer, Hiruma, Avis, Montgomery-Downs, & Valentin, 2015; Toon et al., 2016; Meltzer et al., 2015; Toon et al., 2016). According to a recent review (Peake, Kerr, & Sullivan, 2018), many of these sensors and applications have not been fully validated for clinical research use. More strongly validated devices like the ProDiary (https://www.camntech.com/products/pro-diary/pro-diary-overview) have been validated for research purposes, but are not always practical for clinical use due to their undesirable look, fragility, and expense. In other words, while wearables may promote behavior change, the actual data gathered may be insufficient to truly assess patient functioning.

Adaptation

To best capitalize on the use of digital technology for clinical practice in an in-hospital or outpatient medical setting, clinicians may need to identify and respond to (1) the widespread availability of digital technology and (2) the rapid change in technology. By the time a particular technology-based intervention undergoes sufficient testing (e.g., RCT), that technology may have become obsolete. Additionally, rapid changes in digital technologies may lead to boredom or nonadherence to outdated programs, even if scientifically sound (Wu et al., 2014). Thus, clinicians may need to be flexible in their adoption of technology into clinical practice and stick to the up-to-date technologies available that are consistent with evidence-based treatments. Psychologists should also use digital technologies that reach across disciplines such as recreational therapy, art therapy, music therapy, and child life to develop collaborative innovative programs for hospitalized children. This will strengthen child-friendly and family-friendly education, distraction and coping activities, compliance with medical procedures, psychological skill development and application, and behavior modification.

For the practicing psychologist, technology is well suited to supporting novel interventions that reach children at the right time, in the right context, and in a convenient, engaging way. Clinicians can capitalize on the flexibility of technology used by children to derive the active ingredients from evidence-based treatments. For instance, smartphone apps exist to self-monitor, provide feedback, earn rewards for identifiable behaviors, facilitate relaxation, and challenge automatic and negative thoughts. Research on new technologically enhanced interventions can be supported by single case experiments (Dallery, Cassidy, & Raiff, 2013), as well as studies which target the active ingredients of interventions as opposed to intervention packages (BinDhim & Trevena, 2015; Ritterband, Thorndike, Cox, Kovatchev, & Gonder-Frederick, 2009), allowing for tailoring over time to adapt to the ever-changing digital technology world.

Psychologists should also attend to leaders in the field of digital technology, who note both far-reaching potential and the hurdles this field must overcome to expand evidence-based medicine in a technologically advancing society (Riley et al., 2011). Michie, Yardley, West, Patrick, and Greaves (2017) thoroughly highlight the pros and cons of developing evidence-based treatments in a rapidly growing technological age under the six following themes: (1) achieving rapid and efficient development, (2) understanding and promoting engagement, (3) advancing models and theories, (4) evaluating effectiveness, (5) evaluating cost-effectiveness, and (6) ensuring regulatory, ethical, and information governance. Psychologists interested in further developing technology to assist with psychological care should review and adhere to these recommendations in their research. There is value in identifying how the digital technology approach creates a model of development and hypothesis testing. Therefore, while few intervention packages are readily available in technological formats, digital technology as an adjunct or mechanism for intervention delivery is an essential step forward for psychological care in an inpatient hospital setting.

The use of digital technologies also comes with barriers and challenges including language barriers, access to technology, and user error. Many digital or technological interventions developed to date target primarily English- and Spanish-speaking families, thereby limiting the benefit of these interventions to non-English-speaking families. Historically, socioeconomic status, race, and ethnicity have been barriers to technological adoption; this gap has fortunately narrowed over the last 15 years, but not enough. Recent statistics from PEW Internet survey indicate those with college educations are more likely than those who do not have high school diplomas to use the Internet. Similarly, those households earning more than $75,000 are more likely to be Internet users (Perrin & Duggan, 2015). Adoption of Internet usage has improved in minorities to narrow the gap with 78% of blacks and 81% of Hispanics using the Internet, compared with 84% of whites and 97% of English-speaking Asian Americans. Moreover, those who live in rural areas are less likely than those in the suburbs and urban areas to use the Internet, although 78% of rural residents are online (Perrin & Duggan, 2015). This may be particularly problematic if patients are dependent on the use of the device for practice or learning and lack access to continued use of the intervention strategies and generalization. Finally, there is real concern for user error in utilizing digital technologies, which may limit use of the technology or increase harm to patients. Poorly designed interactions between humans and technology can negatively affect medical decision-making and create hazards or errors leading to patient harm (Magrabi et al., 2016; Sciences, 2011). It is imperative that clinicians understand and appropriately utilize technology to support patient safety and confidentiality.

Available Resources and Support

Examples of existing technology-based applications are provided in Fig. 1. However, it should be noted that, given the rate of technological advancement and deployment of resources, newer applications are likely available and some existing applications listed above may not be updated. The best places to learn about new technologies may be at conferences (e.g., Society for Pediatric Psychology Annual Conference, International Association for the Study of Pain, American Psychological Association, Society for Behavioral Medicine, and Association for Applied Psychophysiology and Biofeedback) where most professionals come together to share innovative ideas and initial data at poster sessions and symposia. These conferences also provide an informal forum to discuss innovations and ideas with colleagues who may be doing the innovative work of clinical adaptation, hospital applications, and novel uses of digital technology. In some cases (e.g., AAPB, APA), technology vendors also attend the meeting to discuss future products and projects. Additionally, start-up companies and smaller labs driving innovation are reaching out to hospitals for opportunities—psychologists should speak with their hospital representatives about accessing these technologies and working with innovators to develop effective clinical programs that will enhance their practice.

Psychological Application	Technology Modality	Example
Education	Website	www.kidshealth.com www.headachereliefguide.com YouTube "What to expect at a sleep study" YouTube "A guide to a children's MRI scan"
	Apps	What's Up Pain Tricks
Adjustment	Website	www.kidsshealth.com
	Apps	What's up
	Other	Virtual environments Seacrest studios
Skill development	Website	Coping Cart / Coping Club Camp Cope-a-lot
	Apps	Breathing Zone Breath2Relax Calm Smiling Mind Headspace Moodnotes Pacifica SuperBetter Happify
	Biofeedback	RespErate (www.resperate.com) Inner Balance (https://store.heartmath.com/innerbalance) Alive (http://www.somaticvision.com/products/aliveclinical) Nexus 4, Nexus 10 (https://www.mindmedia.com/) ProComp Infiniti (http://thoughttechnology.com/index.php/)
Compliance	Website	Coping Cart / Coping Club
	Apps	BrightHearts Simple Habit Waterminder Plant Nanny Drink water aquarium My Therapy: Medication Reminder
	Virtual Reality	Distraction during wound dressing changes Assisting mobility therapy in rehabilitation
	Other	Text messaging reminders

Fig. 1 Examples of technology-based applications to support pediatric psychologists (it should be noted that, given the rate of technological advancement and deployment of resources, newer applications are likely available and existing applications listed above may not be updated)

A Case Example

Sofia was a 10-year-old initially diagnosed with a malignant brain tumor whose treatment required multiple tests and prolonged hospitalization. A virtual reality headset provided Sofia with an interactive "playground" she could employ for distraction to minimize the stress and anxiety with multiple venipuncture procedures. Sofia also watched videos to educate herself about anatomy, body functions, cancer cells, and hospital procedures to help her better understand and anticipate events in the hospital. Sofia worked with an art and music therapist using an interactive iPad program to create a narrative of what was happening to her in the hospital and the coping strategies she found useful. She shared this video with her teacher and friends at school to minimize their concerns for her and enhance a sense of community and connection while she was away. She was also able to connect with her friends at school using a web portal. Online schooling for the 6-month duration of her treatment helped Sofia stay up on her schoolwork and normalize her day with structured activities, including working on group projects. Clinical biofeedback, utilizing both respiration and heart rate variability modalities, helped her relax, improved her sleep, and seemed to give her some relief from the stress of confinement in the hospital. Sofia was even able to teach her parents some of her stress management skills which had a soothing effect on them as well. Given her lack of appetite and minimal hydration at times during treatment, a smartphone app was employed which reinforced her daily caloric intake and hydration. After discharge from inpatient treatment, Sofia remained connected with her medical care team via Telehealth visits. She and her family also maintained a supportive network with a web-based cancer support group. Now, several years posttreatment, Sofia is cancer-free, but still requires periodic checkups. Physicians are now utilizing technology to teach Sofia how to monitor her own medical status and adhere to medication regimen as she transitions to young adult care.

References

Aboujaoude, E., & Salame, W. (2016). Technology at the service of Pediatric Mental Health: Review and assessment. *Journal of Pediatrics, 171*, 20–24. https://doi.org/10.1016/j.jpeds.2015.12.009

Amresh, A., Lyles, A., Small, L., & Gary, K. (2017). FitBit Garden: A mobile game designed to increase physical activity in children. Paper presented at the Proceeding of the 2017 international conference on digital health, London, UK, July 02–05, 2017

Badawy, S. M., & Kuhns, L. M. (2016). Economic evaluation of text-messaging and smartphone-based interventions to improve medication adherence in adolescents with chronic health conditions: A systematic review. *JMIR mHealth and uHealth, 4*(4), e121.. v4i4e121 [pii]. https://doi.org/10.2196/mhealth.6425

Balkhi, A. M., Reid, A. M., Westen, S. C., Olsen, B., Janicke, D. M., & Geffken, G. R. (2015). Telehealth interventions to reduce management complications in type 1 diabetes: A review. *World Journal of Diabetes, 6*(3), 371–379. https://doi.org/10.4239/wjd.v6.i3.371

Bauer, S., de Niet, J., Timman, R., & Kordy, H. (2010). Enhancement of care through self-monitoring and tailored feedback via text messaging and their use in the treatment of childhood overweight. *Patient Education and Counseling, 79*(3), 315–319.

Bers, M. U., Gonzalez-Heydrich, J., & DeMaso, D. R. (2002). Future of technology to augment patient support in hospitals. *Stud Health Technol Inform, 80*, 231–244.

BinDhim, N. F., & Trevena, L. (2015). Health-related smartphone apps: Regulations, safety, privacy and quality. *BMJ Innov, 1*, 1–3. https://doi.org/10.1136/bmjinnov-2014-000019

Brannon, E. E., & Cushing, C. C. (2015). A systematic review: Is there an app for that? Translational science of pediatric behavior change for physical activity and dietary interventions. *Journal of Pediatric Psychology, 40*(4), 373–384. https://doi.org/10.1093/jpepsy/jsu108. jsu108 [pii].

Chaudhry, B., Wang, J., Wu, S., Maglione, M., Mojica, W., Roth, E., … Shekelle, P. G. (2006). Systematic review: Impact of health information technology on quality, efficiency, and costs of medical care. *Annals of Internal Medicine, 144*(10), 742–752. 0000605-200605160-00125 [pii].

Cuellar, A. (2015). Preventing and treating child mental health problems. *The Future of Children: Policies to Promote Chid Health, 25*(1), 111–134.

Cuthbert, J. P., Staniszewski, K., Hays, K., Gerber, D., Natale, A., & O'Dell, D. (2014). Virtual reality-based therapy for the treatment of balance deficits in patients receiving inpatient rehabilitation for traumatic brain injury. *Brain Injury, 28*(2), 181–188. https://doi.org/10.3109/02699052.2013.860475

Cortese, D., Ferrin, M., Brandeis, D., Holtmann, M., Aggensteiner, P., Daley, D., … Sonuga-Barke, R. J. (2016). Neurofeedback for attention deficit/hyperactivity disorder: Meta-analysis of clinical and neuropsychological outcomes for randomized controlled trials. *Journal of the American Academy of Child and Adolescent Psychiatry, 55*, 444–455.

Dallery, J., Cassidy, R. N., & Raiff, B. R. (2013). Single-case experimental designs to evaluate novel technology-based health interventions. *Journal of Medical Internet Research, 15*(2), e22. https://doi.org/10.2196/jmir.2227. v15i2e22 [pii].

Darling, K. D., Benore, E. R., & Webster, E.E. (2019). Biofeedback in pediatric populations; a systematic review and meta-analysis of treatment outcomes. Translational Behavioral Medicine, ibz124, https://doi.org/10.1093/tbm/ibz124.

Dascal, J., Reid, M., IsHak, W. W., Spiegel, B., Recacho, J., Rosen, B., & Danovitch, I. (2017). Virtual reality and medical inpatients: A systematic review of ran-

domized, controlled trials. *Innovations in Clinical Neuroscience, 14*(1–2), 14–21.
Fahrenkamp, A., & Benore, E. (2019). The role of heart rate variability biofeedback in pediatric chronic pain rehabilitation: A case series design. *Clinical Practice in Pediatric Psychology*, 7(4), 358–370. https://doi.org/10.1037/cpp0000259.
Farhat-McHayleh, N., Harfouche, A., & Souaid, P. (2009). Techniques for managing behaviour in pediatric dentistry: Comparative study of live modelling and tell-show-do based on children's heart rates during treatment. *Journal of the Canadian Dental Association, 75*(4), 283.
Farkas, C., Solodiuk, L., Taddio, A., Franck, L., Berberich, F. R., LoChiatto, J., & Solodiuk, J. C. (2015). Publicly available online educational videos regarding pediatric needle pain: A scoping review. *The Clinical Journal of Pain, 31*(6), 591–598. https://doi.org/10.1097/AJP.0000000000000197
Fazeli, M. S., Lin, Y., Nikoo, N., Jaggumantri, S., Collet, J. P., & Afshar, K. (2015). Biofeedback for non-neuropathic daytime voiding disorders in children: A systematic review and meta-analysis of randomized controlled trials. *The Journal of Urology, 193*, 247–280.
Fleming, T., Dixon, R., Frampton, C., & Merry, S. (2012). A pragmatic randomized controlled trial of computerized CBT (SPARX) for symptoms of depression among adolescents excluded from mainstream education. *Behavioural and Cognitive Psychotherapy, 40*(5), 529–541. https://doi.org/10.1017/S1352465811000695. S1352465811000695 [pii].
Goessl, V. C., Curtiss, J. E., & Hofmann, S. G. (2017). The effect of heart rate variability biofeedback training on stress and anxiety: A meta-analysis. *Psychological Medicine, 47*(15), 2578–2586. https://doi.org/10.1017/S0033291717001003. S0033291717001003 [pii].
Grist, R., Croker, A., Denne, M., & Stallard, P. (2019). Technology delivered interventions for depression and anxiety in children and adolescents: A systematic review and meta-analysis. *Clinical Child and Family Psychology Review, 22*(2), 147–171. https://doi.org/10.1007/s10567-018-0271-8
Guo, C., Deng, H., & Yang, J. (2015). Effect of virtual reality distraction on pain among patients with hand injury undergoing dressing change. *Journal of Clinical Nursing, 24*(1–2), 115–120. https://doi.org/10.1111/jocn.12626
Hedman-Lagerlof, M., Hedman-Lagerlof, E., Axelsson, E., Ljotsson, B., Engelbrektsson, J., Hultkrantz, S., ... Andersson, E. (2018). Internet-delivered exposure therapy for fibromyalgia: A randomized controlled trial. *The Clinical Journal of Pain, 34*(6), 532–542. https://doi.org/10.1097/AJP.0000000000000566
Hooke, M. C., Gilchrist, L., Tanner, L., Hart, N., & Withycombe, J. S. (2016). Use of a fitness tracker to promote physical activity in children with acute lymphoblastic leukemia. *Pediatric Blood & Cancer, 63*(4), 684–689. https://doi.org/10.1002/pbc.25860
Hua, Y., Qiu, R., Yao, W. Y., Zhang, Q., & Chen, X. L. (2015). The effect of virtual reality distraction on pain relief during dressing changes in children with chronic wounds on lower limbs. *Pain Management Nursing, 16*(5), 685–691. https://doi.org/10.1016/j.pmn.2015.03.001
Jamal, A., McKenzie, K., & Clark, M. (2009). The impact of health information technology on the quality of medical and health care: A systematic review. *Health Information Management, 38*(3), 26–37.
Jeffs, D., Dorman, D., Brown, S., Files, A., Graves, T., Kirk, E., ... Swearingen, C. J. (2014). Effect of virtual reality on adolescent pain during burn wound care. *Journal of Burn Care & Research, 35*(5), 395–408. https://doi.org/10.1097/BCR.0000000000000019
Kendall, P. C., Khanna, M. S., Edson, A., Cummings, C., & Harris, M. S. (2011). Computers and psychosocial treatment for child anxiety: Recent advances and ongoing efforts. *Depression and Anxiety, 28*(1), 58–66. https://doi.org/10.1002/da.20757
Knox, M., Lentini, J., Cummings, T., McGrady, A., Whearty, K., & Sancrant, L. (2011). Game-based biofeedback for paediatric anxiety and depression. *Mental Health in Family Medicine, 8*(3), 195–203.
Koller, D., & Goldman, R. D. (2012). Distraction techniques for children undergoing procedures: A critical review of pediatric research. *Journal of Pediatric Nursing, 27*(6), 652–681. https://doi.org/10.1016/j.pedn.2011.08.001. S0882-5963(11)00575-6 [pii].
Magrabi, F., Liaw, S. T., Arachi, D., Runciman, W., Coiera, E., & Kidd, M. R. (2016). Identifying patient safety problems associated with information technology in general practice: An analysis of incident reports. *BMJ Quality and Safety, 25*(11), 870–880. https://doi.org/10.1136/bmjqs-2015-004323. bmjqs-2015-004323 [pii].
Malloy, K. M., & Milling, L. S. (2010). The effectiveness of virtual reality distraction for pain reduction: A systematic review. *Clinical Psychology Review, 30*(8), 1011–1018. https://doi.org/10.1016/j.cpr.2010.07.001
March, S., Spence, S. H., & Donovan, C. L. (2009). The efficacy of an internet-based cognitive-behavioral therapy intervention for child anxiety disorders. *Journal of Pediatric Psychology, 34*(5), 474–487. https://doi.org/10.1093/jpepsy/jsn099. jsn099 [pii].
McKenna, K., Gallagher, K. A., Forbes, P. W., & Ibeziako, P. (2015). Ready, set, relax: Biofeedback-assisted relaxation training (BART) in a pediatric psychiatry consultation service. *Psychosomatics, 56*(4), 381–389. https://doi.org/10.1016/j.psym.2014.06.003
Meltzer, L. J., Hiruma, L. S., Avis, K., Montgomery-Downs, H., & Valentin, J. (2015). Comparison of a commercial accelerometer with Polysomnography and Actigraphy in children and adolescents. *Sleep, 38*(8), 1323–1330. https://doi.org/10.5665/sleep.4918. sp-00501-14 [pii].
Michie, S., Yardley, L., West, R., Patrick, K., & Greaves, F. (2017). Developing and evaluating digital interventions to promote behavior change in health and health care: Recommendations resulting from an

international workshop. *Journal of Medical Internet Research, 19*(6), e232. https://doi.org/10.2196/jmir.7126. v19i6e232 [pii].

Mohr, D. C., Burns, M. N., Schueller, S. M., Clarke, G., & Klinkman, M. (2013). Behavioral intervention technologies: Evidence review and recommendations for future research in mental health. *General Hospital Psychiatry, 35*(4), 332–338. https://doi.org/10.1016/j.genhosppsych.2013.03.008. S0163-8343(13)00069-8 [pii].

Morrow, A. M., Burton, K. L. O., Watanabe, M. M., Cloyd, B. H., & Khut, G. P. (2018). Developing BrightHearts: A pediatric biofeedback-mediated relaxation app to manage procedural pain and anxiety. *Pain Practice, 18*(6), 698–708. https://doi.org/10.1111/papr.12655

Mossman, B. A. (2004). Using walkie talkies to overcome the fear of separation in children having surgery. *ORL Head Neck Nurs, 22*(2), 21-22.

National Academy of Sciences. (2011). *Health IT and patient safety*. Washinton, DC: National Academies Press. Retrieved from http://www.ncbi.nlm.nih.gov/pubmed/24600741

Novotney, A. (2010). Lights, camera, action! Children with chronic illness star in their own self-help videos, thanks to this pediatric psychologist. *Monitor on Psychology, 41(7)*, 58–60.

Ortiz, G. S., O'Connor, T., Carey, J., Vella, A., Paul, A., Rode, D., & Weinberg, A. (2017). Impact of a child life and music therapy procedural support intervention on parental perception of their Child's distress during intravenous placement. *Pediatric Emergency Care, 35*, 498. https://doi.org/10.1097/PEC.0000000000001065

Pajovic, S., Corson, T. W., Spencer, C., Dimaras, H., Orlic-Milacic, M., Marchong, M. N., ... Gallie, B. L. (2011). The TAg-RB murine retinoblastoma cell of origin has immunohistochemical features of differentiated Muller glia with progenitor properties. *Investigative Ophthalmology & Visual Science, 52*(10), 7618–7624. https://doi.org/10.1167/iovs.11-7989. iovs.11-7989 [pii].

Palermo, T. M., de la Vega, R., Dudeney, J., Murray, C., & Law, E. (2018). Mobile health intervention for self-management of adolescent chronic pain (WebMAP mobile): Protocol for a hybrid effectiveness-implementation cluster randomized controlled trial. *Contemporary Clinical Trials*. S1551-7144(18)30328-8 [pii], *74*, 55. https://doi.org/10.1016/j.cct.2018.10.003

Peake, J. M., Kerr, G., & Sullivan, J. P. (2018). A critical review of consumer Wearables, Mobile applications, and equipment for providing biofeedback, monitoring stress, and sleep in physically active populations. *Frontiers in Physiology, 9*, 743. https://doi.org/10.3389/fphys.2018.00743

Perrin, A., Duggan, M. (2015). *Americans' Internet Access: 2000–2015*. Retrieved October 27, 2018, from http://www.pewinternet.org/2015/06/26/americans-internet-access-2000-2015/

Pinquart, M., Skolaude, D., Zaplinski, K., & Maier, R. F. (2011). Do clown visits improve psychological and sense of physical well-being of hospitalized pediatric patients? A randomized-controlled trial. *Klinische Pädiatrie, 223*(2), 74–78. https://doi.org/10.1055/s-0030-1267932

Reynolds, C. A., & Maughan, E. D. (2015). Telehealth in the school setting: An integrative review. *The Journal of School Nursing, 31*(1), 44–53. https://doi.org/10.1177/1059840514540534

Reynoldson, C., Stones, C., Allsop, M., Gardner, P., Bennett, M. I., Closs, S. J., ... Knapp, P. (2014). Assessing the quality and usability of smartphone apps for pain self-management. *Pain Medicine, 15*(6), 898–909. https://doi.org/10.1111/pme.12327

Richardson, T., Stallard, P., & Velleman, S. (2010). Computerised cognitive behavioural therapy for the prevention and treatment of depression and anxiety in children and adolescents: A systematic review. *Clinical Child and Family Psychology Review, 13*(3), 275–290. https://doi.org/10.1007/s10567-010-0069-9

Riley, W. T., Rivera, D. E., Atienza, A. A., Nilsen, W., Allison, S. M., & Mermelstein, R. (2011). Health behavior models in the age of mobile interventions: Are our theories up to the task? *Translational Behavioral Medicine, 1*(1), 53–71. https://doi.org/10.1007/s13142-011-0021-7

Ritterband, L. M., Thorndike, F. P., Cox, D. J., Kovatchev, B. P., & Gonder-Frederick, L. A. (2009). A behavior change model for internet interventions. *Annals of Behavioral Medicine, 38*(1), 18–27. https://doi.org/10.1007/s12160-009-9133-4

Roers, L., Curwick, K., O'connor, J., Canny, M., & Harbeck-Weber, C. (2016). Emphasis of functioning in biofeedback intervention for pediatric patients with chronic pain. *Pain Medicine, 17*(2), 436.

Santos, J. D., Lopes, R. I., & Koyle, M. A. (2017). Bladder and bowel dysfunction in children: An update on the diagnosis and treatment of a common, but underdiagnosed pediatric problem. *Canadian Urological Association Journal, 11*((1–2 Suppl 1), S64–S72. https://doi.org/10.5489/cuaj.4411

Schmitt, Y. S., Hoffman, H. G., Blough, D. K., Patterson, D. R., Jensen, M. P., Soltani, M., ... Sharar, S. R. (2011). A randomized, controlled trial of immersive virtual reality analgesia, during physical therapy for pediatric burns. *Burns, 37*(1), 61–68. https://doi.org/10.1016/j.burns.2010.07.007. S0305-4179(10)00183-X [pii].

Schwartz, M. S., & Andrasik, F. (Eds.). (2016). *Biofeedback: A practitioner's guide* (4th ed.). New York: Guilford Press.

Stasiak, K., Hatcher, S., Frampton, C., & Merry, S. N. (2014). A pilot double blind randomized placebo controlled trial of a prototype computer-based cognitive behavioural therapy program for adolescents with symptoms of depression. *Behavioural and Cognitive Psychotherapy, 42*(4), 385–401. https://doi.org/10.1017/S1352465812001087. S1352465812001087 [pii].

Stern, M. J., Guiles, R. A., & Gevirtz, R. (2014). HRV biofeedback for pediatric irritable bowel syndrome and functional abdominal pain: A clinical replication series. *Applied Psychophysiology and Biofeedback, 39*(3–4), 287–291. https://doi.org/10.1007/s10484-014-9261-x

Strout, T. D., & Burton, J. H. (2004). Clinically significant change in physician-assigned numeric pain rating scale scores. *The American Journal of Emergency Medicine, 22*(3), 243–245. S0735675704000750 [pii].

Stubberud, A., Varkey, E., McCrory, D. C., Pedersen, S. A., & Linde, M. (2016). Biofeedback as prophylaxis for pediatric migraine: A meta-analysis. *Pediatrics, 138*(2), e20160675. https://doi.org/10.1542/peds.2016-0675. e20160675 [pii].

Sveistrup, H., McComas, J., Thornton, M., Marshall, S., Finestone, H., McCormick, A., … Mayhew, A. (2003). Experimental studies of virtual reality-delivered compared to conventional exercise programs for rehabilitation. *Cyberpsychology & Behavior, 6*(3), 245–249. https://doi.org/10.1089/109493103322011524

Tan, G., Shaffer, F., Lyle, R., & Teo, I. (2016). Evidence-based Practice in Biofeedback and Neurofeedback: 3rd Edition. Wheat Ridge, CO: Association for Applied Psychophysiology and Biofeedback.

Toon, E., Davey, M. J., Hollis, S. L., Nixon, G. M., Horne, R. S., & Biggs, S. N. (2016). Comparison of commercial wrist-based and smartphone accelerometers, Actigraphy, and PSG in a clinical cohort of children and adolescents. *Journal of Clinical Sleep Medicine, 12*(3), 343–350. https://doi.org/10.5664/jcsm.5580. jc-00211-15 [pii].

Triberti, S., Repetto, C., & Riva, G. (2014). Psychological factors influencing the effectiveness of virtual reality-based analgesia: A systematic review. *Cyberpsychology, Behavior and Social Networking, 17*(6), 335–345. https://doi.org/10.1089/cyber.2014.0054

Trnka, P., White, M. M., Renton, W. D., McTaggart, S. J., Burke, J. R., & Smith, A. C. (2015). A retrospective review of telehealth services for children referred to a paediatric nephrologist. *BMC Nephrology, 16*, 125. https://doi.org/10.1186/s12882-015-0127-0

Wiederhold, B. K., Gao, K., Sulea, C., & Wiederhold, M. D. (2014). Virtual reality as a distraction technique in chronic pain patients. *Cyberpsychology, Behavior and Social Networking, 17*(6), 346–352. https://doi.org/10.1089/cyber.2014.0207

Wu, Y. P., Steele, R. G., Connelly, M. A., Palermo, T. M., & Ritterband, L. M. (2014). Commentary: Pediatric eHealth interventions: Common challenges during development, implementation, and dissemination. *Journal of Pediatric Psychology, 39*(6), 612–623. https://doi.org/10.1093/jpepsy/jsu022. jsu022 [pii].

Advocacy in Pediatric Psychological Consultation

Elaine A. T. Gilbert and Kristie V. Schultz

"It should be our aim to discover neglected problems and, so far as in our power, to correct evil and introduce reform."
Isaac Abt, First President of American Academy of Pediatrics (AAP, 2009, p. viii)

A growing body of the literature in clinical pediatrics has focused on the issue of child advocacy (Paulson, 2001), necessitating a corresponding response within pediatric psychology as well. Brown and Roberts (2000) note that it has long been a goal of pediatric psychology to support both the psychological and physiological aspects of a child in order to fully engage in preventative efforts. However, possibly due to a gap in the training of pediatric psychologists, such prevention efforts have yet to come to fruition, leading to the call for the development of evidence-based advocacy strategies and interventions to be addressed within pediatric psychology (Palermo et al., 2014).

Traditional Model of Advocacy

Advocacy can be seen as occurring at four system levels: federal, state, community, and individual (AAP, 2009). Advocacy efforts at the federal and state levels are typically focused on the creation of legislation, often in the form of health-care reform. Pediatricians have long been involved in legislative efforts to inform change focused on ensuring the health, safety, and welfare of children. For example, pediatricians in Tennessee advocated for seat belt restraint laws to ensure the safety of children (Sanders & Dan, 1984). This initiative led to national and even global changes in enforcement of vehicle restraint mechanisms which have reduced injuries and saved thousands of lives. Community-level advocacy frequently targets regional and local needs of at-risk populations based on geographic location, cultural identity, or systemic factors that affect access to resources. Advocacy at the individual level most often targets the provision of direct individual patient care (Paulson, 2001). Individual advocacy is considered part of standard patient care, but specific roles and strategies for advocacy have been poorly defined and delineated (Drotar, 2004; Lequerica, 1993; Paulson, 2001). While much of this chapter will focus on advocacy at the micro-system level (i.e., efforts focused on the individual patient/caregiver level), macro-system-level interventions (i.e., efforts focused on community-based or administration levels) will also be addressed. Advocacy efforts can be considered to fall along a continuum as conceptualized in Fig. 1.

E. A. T. Gilbert (✉)
Departments of Psychiatry and Pediatrics, Riley Hospital for Children, Indiana University School of Medicine, Indianapolis, IN, USA

K. V. Schultz
Department of Pediatrics, Norton Children's Hospital, University of Louisville School of Medicine, Louisville, KY, USA

B. D. Carter, K. A. Kullgren (eds.), *Clinical Handbook of Psychological Consultation in Pediatric Medical Settings*, Issues in Clinical Child Psychology, https://doi.org/10.1007/978-3-030-35598-2_38

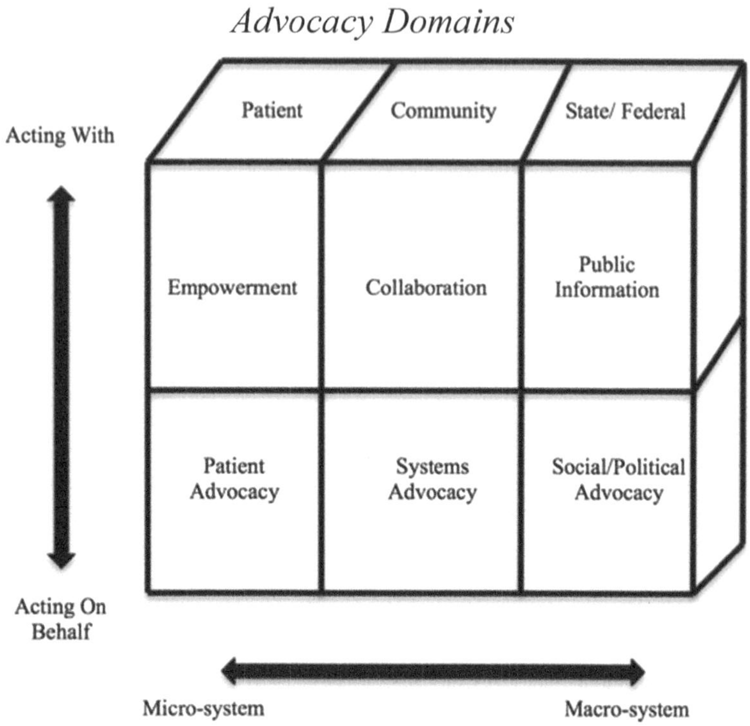

Fig. 1 Advocacy domains depicting multisystem efforts at micro-system and macro-system advocacy, when acting with and/or behalf of the patient. Adapted from "Advocacy Competencies" by J. Lewis, M. Arnold, R. House, and R. Toporek, 2003, American Counseling Association

Advocacy as an Extension of Psychological Consultation

With the ever-expanding scope of pediatric psychological practice, advocacy has increasingly become an integral part of comprehensive clinical and consultative work. At the most basic level, advocacy involves collaborative efforts concerning such activities as establishing communication with other health-care providers participating in a mutual patient's care. However, the pace of busy interdisciplinary clinical practice presents challenges in advocating for patients and their families due to the often time-intensive efforts needed that extend well beyond direct (i.e., billable) patient care efforts. However, as Drotar (2013) noted, reimbursable services per se seldom define the value or worth of the important work being done on behalf of the patient and their family.

The role of the pediatric psychologist has been created out of necessity in order to better address the unmet needs of children, adolescents, and their families within pediatric health-care settings and is characterized by a blending of behavioral medicine and health psychology to provide comprehensive services. The theoretical Integrated Comprehensive Consultation-Liaison Model (ICCLM; Carter et al., 2017) incorporates Bronfenbrenner's Bioecological Systems Framework (BST; Bronfenbrenner, 1979) and Kazak's Pediatric Psychosocial Preventative Health Model (PPPHM; Kazak, 2006), all within the context of the emerging role of the pediatric psychologist conceptualized as the "six Cs of consultation" (i.e., crisis, coping, compliance/adherence, communication, collaboration, and changing systems). The ICCLM addresses the multiple system-level practice areas in which a pediatric psychologist may intervene in order to impact child and family health, welfare, and development while extending awareness of prevention and intervention (Carter et al., 2017). However, the pediatric psychologist's role often goes beyond the delineated and longstanding "six Cs of consultation." There is an increasing role for pediatric psychology in *advocating,* or *championing*, for children and families at the individual, family, community, health-care system, and larger system levels in order to better meet the health-care needs of some of the most vulnerable in need of services in our health-care system. In fact, it is proposed that "championing" be added to the alliterative Cs of consultation as the seventh C of consultation.

Advocacy is becoming increasingly important in addressing some of the most pressing societal issues affecting the health and welfare of youth. For example, from 2000 to 2014, the death rate from drug overdoses doubled (Rudd, Aleshire, Zibbell, & Gladden, 2016), and most recent statistics show a continued increase in opioid-related deaths (Scholl, Seth, Kariisa, Wilson, & Baldwin, 2019), often dramatically impacting the family dynamics and living arrangements for many children. Children are facing higher rates of adverse childhood experiences (ACE), with increased exposure to physical and psychological abuse, neglect, and negative household events, which put them at a greater risk for developing psychological and physical health concerns into adulthood (Felitti et al., 1998). Early intervention and prevention are needed to address these challenges, often requiring advocacy efforts for the creation and maintenance of more comprehensive resources and services for these children and families. The systems perspective often inherent in pediatric psychology training and practice (see Chap. 3, this volume) place our subspecialty in a particularly pivotal position in advocating for children and their families who are navigating a complicated and rapidly changing health-care system.

Advocacy in Inpatient Pediatric Medical Settings

Within the inpatient pediatric hospital setting, the primary objective of advocacy is to address the health and safety needs of the patient, while ensuring ethical treatment and considering the patient's overall welfare and individual rights. Communication and collaboration are the building blocks of advocacy within inpatient settings, not only between providers but between the providers and patients as well, requiring pediatric psychologists to serve as bidirectional liaisons between families and the other multidisciplinary team members in forming a biopsychosocial approach to care that acknowledges the interplay between medical and psychosocial factors (Shaw & DeMaso, 2006). Family functioning is directly related to psychological adjustment of children with chronic medical conditions, further underlining the importance of uniting and joining with the family in order to identify areas for advocacy and remove barriers to change. Joining with the family and patient is a critical tool for building rapport and trust, which is not only essential to patient care but to advocacy as well (Drotar, 1997; Kazak, 1997).

Mechanisms of Advocacy in Inpatient Settings

The consulting psychologist has regular access to two primary mechanisms for advocacy in the inpatient medical setting: the electronic medical record (EMR) and care conferences.

Electronic Medical Record (EMR)

EMR documentation may be one of the most accessible and basic mechanisms for advocacy in the inpatient setting, providing a method for regular communication with all providers on a specific patient to inform coordinated comprehensive care and treatment. In approaching the creation of EMR entries, the psychologist's documentation should strive to be inclusive of important information for guiding care, while still being concise and avoiding unnecessary patient disclosures that may jeopardize confidentiality essential to establishing and maintaining rapport with the patient and family. Attentive clinical judgment is needed in determining what information should be included and excluded (Nielsen, Baum, & Soares, 2013). Notes should be detailed enough to inform other providers and should include conceptualizations which integrate both medical and psychosocial domains. Shaw and DeMaso (2006) also suggest documenting the strengths of a patient and family, rather than just focusing on areas of difficulty or need for growth, to fully inform other providers with a comprehensive view of the patient and family.

EMR documentation should always include specific treatment recommendations and the rationale behind them in order to demystify psychological interventions and to allow transparency in collaboration in the treatment approach. It is acceptable to use recommendations to advocate for evidence-based interventions in the inpatient medical setting; for example, the consulting psychologist may advocate for extended hospitalization in order to implement necessary intensive behavioral protocols (e.g., such as for eating/feeding conditions, choking phobias, complex somatization disorders, concerns for factitious-disorder-by-proxy dynamics). Advocacy often goes beyond the EMR and may necessitate such actions as the petitioning of hospital administration to justify an extended hospital admission for purposes of observation, safety, and/or intensive interventions.

In addition to documentation in the patient's chart, it is important to supplement documentation through verbal communication with collaborating colleagues. In the often fast-paced inpatient medical setting, especially in the role of consultant, it is essential that the pediatric psychologist cultivate communication styles and timelines that are compatible with those of their medical colleagues (Haley et al., 1998). This includes developing a working mastery of the medical conditions, diagnostic procedures, treatments, and terminology (see Chap. 7, this volume) related to the different specialties with which one works. Lengthy, depth-oriented psychological analyses and speculations without practical concrete recommendations are taxing for busy inpatient physicians and hospital staff, and such EMR entries likely go unread and thus have minimal impact on patient care. Clear, concise communication has been shown to result in more equitable distribution of inpatient resources, more fully supporting the patient and family through diagnosis and treatment (Winters, Hanson, & Stoyanova, 2007).

Care Conferences

While many consultation situations in the hospital can be resolved with a brief evaluation and concrete recommendations for the medical team to address, there are times when a cursory consultation is inadequate, due in part to the involvement of multiple medical specialists on the case. In such situations, confusion can occur when specialists give conflicting information to the patient/family and/or hospital staff. Metaphorically, this is often referred to as the blind men describing the elephant (i.e., each person basing their description on the one part of the elephant they are touching rather than seeing the elephant in totality). In these situations, it is often the psychologist or a member of the psychosocial consultation team who may suggest that all the major providers involved with the case have a collaborative team meeting that is followed by what is typically referred to as a care conference. Care conferences, which are meetings among key providers involved in a patient's care in order to more effectively meet the informational and emotional needs of the patient and family, can be one of the most effective modalities for patient advocacy in the inpatient medical setting. While there are various formats for conducting a care conference, it is essential for the multidisciplinary team to develop their own framework with the goal of improving communication (between team members, as well as between providers and the patient/family) and care coordination (Eggly et al., 2011). Hospital settings may vary as to who has the privilege to request a care conference; in many children's hospitals, it is common for pediatric psychologists to take on the role of initiating and facilitating these multidisciplinary meetings with the patient and/or family, often in coordination with the medical social worker for the unit/team. It is important to determine who to invite (e.g., medical specialists, nurse coordinators, residents, social workers, art/expressive therapists, physical therapists, child life specialists, palliative care, hospital administration, ethics team members, forensics team members) and whether or not the patient and/or family should be in attendance and in what order or combination. Attendees should be predetermined, and their presence requested. Special considerations may be needed to accommodate other nonmedical professionals (e.g., Child Protective Services (CPS), school personnel), as needed.

Decisions should also be made about the location and duration of the care conference, aiming for maximum availability and convenience for all involved. Timing becomes an essential factor in the effectiveness and success of a care conference; key issues and concerns must be covered while also respecting the valuable time for each professional in attendance, which is why following an agenda is most beneficial. During the allotted time, it is helpful to review the patient's history from both a physical/medical and psychosocial perspective. The focus of the care conference should be on active problem-solving and ideally result in improved communication and understanding, with the end product being some agreed-upon goals and procedures. All communication should be respectful; the patient and family members should be addressed by name to emphasize the personal and empathetic needs of all involved in providing the most appropriate care for the patient. While coordination of care conferences can be challenging, having all providers in one room can streamline discussions and empower the patient (and family) by fully addressing comprehensive care and informing the treatment plan.

Consulting psychologists are often put in a difficult role of advocating for patient and family needs while balancing medical recommendations with institutional constraints. Moral distress can occur when providers recognize an ethical dilemma, and due to external constraints (e.g., time, lack of resources, power differentials, institutional policy, legal considerations), the "right" course cannot be or is not pursued (Dudzinski, 2016). A form of psychological disequilibrium often ensues for providers resulting in moral and ethical conflict between, as well as within, teams, families, and institutions. As an advocate, the pediatric psychologist can lead and encourage process-oriented discussions of difficult cases. Structured tools can be helpful in shaping such dialogues. Dudzinski (2016) has proposed the moral distress map (see Appendix) to help care teams and families openly discuss and explore feelings and experiences that can potentially inform change at multiple levels (e.g., communication, protocols, resources, hospital policy).

Challenges Associated with Length of Hospital Stay

Within inpatient medical settings, while short hospital stays are increasingly more common, both short and extended hospital stays present unique challenges. Short hospital stays vary in length, but may range from under 24 h to a few days, with psychological consultations often being requested in the midst of many other specialty consultations. There are times when the pediatric psychologist may see the patient and family only once before a discharge occurs. Thus, that single consultation meeting may serve as an intake/assessment, intervention, and termination session. In the case of short hospital stays, advocating for referrals and appropriate follow-up care is extremely important and often crucial to addressing the consultation referral request.

Extended hospital stays, on the other hand, may last for weeks or months and present notable challenges. Lengthy hospital stays, and their associated multiple stressors, create conditions for interpersonal conflicts for even the most emotionally healthy patients and families, making it essential to promote parental and patient self-care. Conflicts may arise due to a variety of factors, including poor communication, contrasting views for the best patient care, differentials in medical knowledge/understanding, distrust of medical providers, or parental unavailability (Studdert et al., 2003). In these instances, the consulting psychologist may advocate for a meeting of key providers, a care conference with the patient/family, increased structure for the patient/family through daily schedules, behavioral plans, continued involvement of other ancillary services (e.g., physical therapy, art/expressive therapy), or administrative support. If unaddressed, such conflicts can result in disruptions to the patient's inpatient medical care and management, as well as increase emotional and psychological distress for the patient, family, and medical team members.

Advocacy in Outpatient Pediatric Medical Settings

The consulting pediatric psychologist will often experience the need to engage in advocacy when practicing in primary and specialty outpatient settings, particularly in matters impacting the continuity of care for the pediatric patient. When the psychologist is able to engage with both the patient and family during the child's inpatient hospitalization and also in their follow-up care in the outpatient clinic setting, the potential for continuity of care is greatly increased (as is the ability to document and address nonadherence to follow-up appointments and treatment). In such conditions the consulting psychologist is better able to provide continuity in advocating for the academic needs of patients (e.g., recommending comprehensive psychological or neurocognitive assessments or requesting accommodations under a 504 plan or individualized education programs (IEP)) and social involvement (e.g., increasing activity to counter social isolation through peer support services, community involvement, or extracurricular activities). Efforts to get families to implement such changes often extend beyond writing a letter or making a telephone call and may include the psychologist attending school conferences/meetings or going to court to advocate for a patient's safety.

The psychologist's involvement in advocacy can often be time-intensive, while at the same time nonreimbursable. However, in many situations it may be the most effective route to meaningful and sustained treatment gain for the patient, both medically and psychosocially. This often presents a dilemma for the consulting psychologist, where productivity requirements may be based on billable direct-care hours. When practicing with high-risk populations, it is important to factor in and develop institutionally supported mechanisms to build in time for advocacy-related activity, as well as support personnel (e.g., medical social workers, discharge planners) and structures (e.g., teleconferencing capabilities to avoid travel time to engage in advocacy) that allow advocacy to become a part of comprehensive pediatric health care.

Advocacy at the Macro-System Level

While much of the advocacy work of a pediatric psychologist may be at the individual patient/family level, these efforts are often most effective when they extend beyond the micro-system level as well. Advocacy at the macro-system level can encompass such activities as engaging in health-care reform efforts, addressing health-care disparities, social justice, human rights, and violence prevention (APA, n.d.). The American Psychological Association (APA) has suggested that psychologists need to advocate at a larger level (e.g., state and federal) by applying their expertise to raise awareness of the value of the skill set of our profession in addressing population level health and mental health needs, advancing the principles and ethics of the field of psychology, and championing for the funding of these efforts on a national level (APA, n.d.). While federal and state level advocacy efforts (such as reaching out to lawmakers and lobbyists through written or spoken word) may seem daunting to some, local level efforts may actually be more feasible and get quicker results. Such advocacy could include things such as speaking with public officials to encourage more funding and support for local and regional general and specialized mental health and substance abuse services, writing an opinion article in a local newspaper or magazine, and supporting advocacy by involving students or trainees (DeAngelis, 2018). Pediatric psychologists can also engage in community-based advocacy by providing psychoeducation to various groups on mental health issues and their impact on overall health/well-being and quality of life, creating and disseminating resources (e.g., brochures, lists of community resources), and personally serving as a resource presence at health and mental health fairs in their communities.

As many pediatric psychologists are employed within pediatric hospitals and/or academic medical center settings, system-level advocacy almost inevitably becomes an essential aspect of the psychologist's role. As a pediatric psychologist advances though their career, there may be increasingly more opportunities to take on administrative roles and serve on committees and boards that are involved in planning, decision-making, and policy-making. At the system level, advocacy efforts may take the form of championing with medical colleagues and/or hospital administration for increased funding for integrated psychological services at all levels (e.g., inpatient, outpatient primary, and specialty clinics) or providing additional training opportunities within medical residency and fellowship programs for exposure to the work of psychological consultation to medical patients. Advocacy for system-level changes can promote and impact future patient care, such as requesting administration to change hospital policy regarding when to engage bedside sitters for unattended children admitted to the hospital. While barriers may exist for change at the system level, relying on medical colleagues as allies, using diplomatic communication, and trusting one's own expertise can be impactful in championing for change.

Adapting Advocacy to Patient and Family Needs

Advocacy must be tailored to each patient and family, with consideration of cultural needs and health disparities. Pediatric psychologists are trained to treat patients with both flexibility and fidelity to treatment modalities, which necessitates adaptation.

Cultural Awareness, Competency, and Humility

Cultural competence is defined as the ability to provide appropriate and effective services to minority group members while taking into consideration language, histories, traditions, and values (Betancourt, Green, Carrillo, & Ananeh-Firempong, 2003). Cultural and associated demographic factors may include, but are not limited to, race/ethnicity, religion, socioeconomic status, identity associated with sexual orientation, geographic location, immigrant or refugee status, age, sex/gender, or health status (see Chap. 33, this volume). Cultural factors have the potential to impact multiple aspects of pediatric health care, including access to care, adherence to medical treatment, and communication about appropriate care (Flores, Abreu, Schwartz, & Hill, 2000). It is the responsibility of the pediatric psychologist to be aware of potential culturally related barriers to competent health care and increase the awareness of all providers to those cultural factors that may adversely impact the effective provision of services. In fact, there are many aspects of culture that arise in the context of medical care, including language differences and culturally based explanations of illness, as well as parental and patient beliefs about illness and treatment. To illustrate, some cultures may be dutiful and unconditionally accepting of the advice of experts (e.g., physicians), while patients and families from other cultures may be cautious and even skeptical of medical care and strongly rejecting of any form of psychosocial services (Perloff, Bonder, Ray, Ray, & Siminoff, 2006). Psychologists and all medical providers must also be aware of their own cultural values, as well as the culture of their patients, and work to acquire the skills and knowledge to provide culturally sensitive and effective treatment (Beach et al., 2005; Flores, 2000; Tucker, 2002).

When language barriers between patients/families and providers are identified, it is important to advocate for appropriate translation services. Asking patients or family members to serve as a translator is inappropriate due to ethical considerations. Interpreter services (in person or via digital devices) are essential when communicating verbally (e.g., in the office visit or via telephone) with a patient and/or family when providers are not conversant in the identified spoken language. Competent interpreters should be able to translate language bidirectionally; when in medical settings, the interpreter needs to be familiar with medical terminology, in addition to the identified language spoken. Translators, on the other hand, translate language in written materials and typically only translate unidirectionally; translators may be beneficial when providers use written assessment tools and handouts (Phelan & Parkman, 1995). It is crucial for providers to focus on cultural inclusiveness when providing comprehensive patient care.

Cultural humility extends beyond cultural competence, focusing on the continual process of learning. Cultural humility is the recognition of the power imbalances in practitioner-patient relationships and emphasizes being open to learning about and from patients and their experiences. Often the consulting psychologist may be faced with the need to advocate for other providers to go beyond what is known and comfortable to them. Cultural humility is not static, but rather challenges practitioners, regardless of discipline, to be humble and open when working with diverse populations (Tervalon & Murray-Garcia, 1998).

Advocacy and Health Disparities

Health disparities refer to inequalities in disease occurrence or survival rates of disadvantaged populations as compared to the more advantaged population. Racial and ethnic minorities, individuals of lower socioeconomic status, and residents of rural geographic regions are currently designated as populations likely to experience health disparities (National Institutes of Health, 2009). Health disparities are considered to be preventable and caused by systemic policies and practices that limit access to care (APA, n.d.). Advocacy efforts employed by pediatric psychologists are intended to further educate medical providers, administrators, and government officials about such inequalities to ensure sensitive, comprehensive care and champion for the elimination of these social inequities.

The ways in which pediatric psychologists can advocate for reducing health disparities can include dissemination of culturally sensitive health education materials (e.g., having materials that can be easily understood by individuals not familiar with medical procedures or terminology, offering materials with pictorial descriptions/instructions for individuals who are not literate or have language barriers). Additionally, as many recommendations may include the use of technology in care (e.g., access to cell phones or the Internet, electronic patient portals for communications), pediatric psychologists must be sensitive to barriers for patient access due to economic status, or even objections to the use of technology for personal/cultural reasons. It is important to tailor treatment recommendations in consideration of these potential barriers and be willing to have discussions centered around such topics, which can also model for other providers strategies for identifying and overcoming existing health disparities.

Legal Considerations in Advocacy

Knowledge of applicable state and federal law is imperative to the consulting pediatric psychologist's work in championing for patients in the health-care system. Pertinent laws include those regarding the age of consent, assent for medical care, types of abuse or neglect, patient privilege, and involuntary holds and hospitalization. Institutional and hospital policies include matters of confidentiality, limits on parental involvement, limits on visitor engagement, and discharge criteria. Awareness of abuse and neglect reporting guidelines is paramount, as they may vary from state to state. Reports are often made to the Department of Health and Human Services; division titles may vary by state, but are commonly referred to as Child Protective Services (CPS), Department of Child Services (DCS), or Children in Need of Services (CHINS). Time constraints on filing a report and specifying to whom the report is to be made are also important. Common information requested when reporting includes the instance and timeline of abuse or neglect, patient's name and date of birth, current physical address, contact information, the alleged perpetrator and their address, any other affected children, and if there are safety concerns in the home that may be a potential danger to workers who go to the home (e.g., firearms, dogs). The reporter may also need to provide education to the intake recorder or CPS worker, who are non-medical professionals, about the severity of potential implications of the patient's medical condition on safety (e.g., nonadherence resulting in serious health complications or death).

Advocacy in Practice: Case Vignette

Josh is an 8-year-old Black male with developmental delay awaiting heart transplant in the hospital. The medical team consulted pediatric psychology for a psychosocial risk assessment due to concerns of nonadherence. Josh lived with his mother and siblings and had limited contact with his father. Historically, Josh has had multiple no shows to clinic visits, at times being lost to follow up with limited communication about his health status; drug assays also showed that Josh was not taking his medication as prescribed. The cardiology team indicated a history of social work and CPS involvement due to medical neglect. The psychology consultation team witnessed conflictual communication and interactions between Josh's mother and extended family members while he was in the hospital. Josh himself was observed to be combative with nursing staff and other members of his medical team (e.g., biting, kicking, shouting obscenities). The psychosocial pre-transplant evaluation determined high level of risk for continued future nonadherence; despite this behavioral risk, the consulting psychology team recommended that Josh still be favorably considered for heart transplant with the strong recommendation psychological intervention be provided to address the observed concerns that could compromise his posttransplant adherence and health.

Weeks after Josh was listed for a heart transplant (status 1A, requiring hospitalization until transplant), the medical team reported that Josh's disruptive behaviors in the hospital had increased, leading to concerns for cooperation (and ultimately safety) during and after necessary procedures. Josh's mother was typically not present at bedside to aid in dealing with Josh's behaviors, resulting in Josh's increased anxiety regarding separation and further behavioral regression. The consulting psychology team created an age-appropriate behavior plan and advocated for nursing involvement to ensure consistent intervention across shifts. The medical team was provided psychoeducation to help encourage empathy and use of positive reinforcement for more appropriate behaviors by Josh. Hospital policy dictated that if a parent was present, even minimally, a sitter was not required. The pediatric psychology team appealed to hospital administration and strongly advocated for an around-the-clock sitter for Josh to reduce his social isolation and ensure safety. As Josh's hospitalization stay lengthened, it became increasingly concerning that he had had no academic instruction for several months due to frequency of hospitalization prior to listing and multiple moves. The pediatric psychology team advocated for in-hospital homebound teacher in order for Josh to have access to academic instruction at bedside and provide more structure and distractions during the day as well as for brief psychological testing necessary to implement a future IEP. Such a request centered around academic needs was unusual for a medically hospitalized child, since the cardiology team was most focused on ensuring Josh's physical health and survival; however, the medical team was supportive when the psychology team explained the developmental importance of addressing Josh's in-hospital behavior issues for his quality of life and adherence to treatment, both while in the hospital and posttransplant. Figure 2 illustrates the complex network of services involved in Josh's care while in the hospital.

During the course of Josh's hospital stay, pediatric psychology implemented weekly care conferences to facilitate communication, comprehensive care, and support among providers. Unfortunately, despite repeated efforts from multiple care team members, Josh's mother was absent from these meetings. The team became increasingly concerned as to whether or not Josh's mother would be able to provide appropriate post-transplant care, especially given that she was also not adequately caring for herself at this time (e.g., refusal to comply with medical and mental health recommendations for herself despite assistance

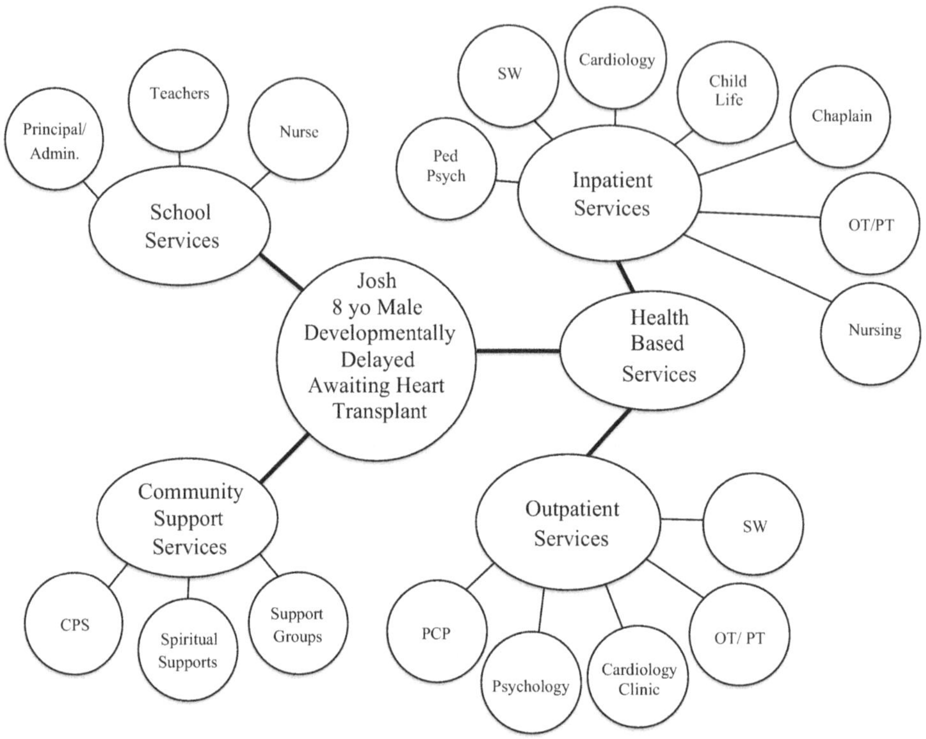

Fig. 2 Service network diagrams depict areas of a patient's life impacted by advocacy, illustrating comprehensive patient care. Adapted from "Continuity of care for children with complex chronic health conditions" by A. R. Miller, C. J. Condin, W. H. McKellin, N. Shaw, A. F. Klassen, & S. Sheps, 2009, BMC Health Services Research, 9, p. 242

from hospital social work). The team collectively decided to re-engage CPS and made a new report of medical neglect. The CPS worker was hesitant to take the case, stating that once Josh received a heart, his medical prognosis would improve. The psychology consultation team advocated for Josh, educating the CPS worker on the realities of life after transplant and that if a guardian was not present and actively engaged in Josh's medical care and follow-up (e.g., ensuring Josh took medications at exact times twice per day), it would be life-threatening for Josh. A CPS case worker was assigned to Josh's case and began attending the weekly care conferences, either in person or via conference call.

Josh ultimately received a heart transplant, but his mother became less and less involved, eventually leading to abandonment. Thus, the cardiology attending joined with the psychology consultant to petition CPS and the court to place Josh in a medically fragile foster home at discharge from the hospital.

Support for the Advocate

While engaging in advocacy on behalf of medically fragile children and their families can be very rewarding, outcomes can vary and there is always the risk for burnout, making self-care essential. Burnout is defined as "a state of physical, emotional, and mental exhaustion caused by long-term involvement in situations that are emotionally demanding" (Pines & Aronson, 1988, p. 9). Advocacy often necessitates a repeated emotional investment by the pediatric psychologist and, as such, puts one at risk for burnout. The American Psychological

Association (APA) Practice Organization reported that burnout is one of the top three problems most likely to impact the functioning of a psychologist, with 54% endorsing burnout. Potential warning signs for burnout include loss of empathy (both professionally and personally), increased negative thoughts and emotions, and feelings of hopelessness (APA, 2009).

In the highly demanding health-care work environment, there are often unrealistic time constraints and competing work expectations that result in the psychologist having to become an advocate for themselves in setting realistic expectations. Work-life balance is vital to professional longevity and maintaining one's ability to empathize with and care for their patients. Simply put, one must take care of themselves in order to continue to care for others. At times, this may require saying "no" to additional requests, educating medical colleagues on the risk of burnout and need for self-care, and becoming comfortable with setting limits, including time limitations and obligations to other aspects of one's life and seeking out interests and sources of stimulation and fulfillment outside of the work environment.

Pediatric psychologists, while working on a multidisciplinary team, can also be isolated as the only mental health practitioner, especially when advocating for holistic and culturally sensitive care. Therefore, it becomes vital to develop an external support network, both within the institution and beyond (e.g., regional and national organizations). Consultation with colleagues within one's professional specialty can be extremely beneficial and provide support and additional perspective; pediatric psychologists should know when to ask for help from colleagues and be comfortable in initiating support (Carter, 2014). While pediatric psychologists often encourage their patients to ask for help when needed, it may be difficult for the pediatric psychologist to acknowledge that they may need help and assistance. However, additional support can help them feel more supported and less isolated.

Additionally, engaging in regular self-care will aid in ensuring one's own mental and physical health. Such self-care practices may include regular physical activity or exercise, engaging in preferred activities or hobbies, adaptive sleep hygiene techniques, and spending time with family and friends (APA, 2009). It may also involve activities with colleagues at work, such as taking the time to have lunch or socializing. While self-care is often the first thing to be neglected by the busy consulting psychologist, it is essential for professional and personal survival and growth, as well as ensuring continued support and advocacy for those who cannot advocate for themselves.

Appendix: Moral Distress Mapping Tool (Dudzinski, 2016)

	Emotions	Source(s)	Constraints	Conflicting responsibilities	Possible actions	Final action
Case	What emotions are you experiencing? (i.e., sadness, anger)	What precisely is the source of the moral distress? (i.e., inadequate staffing; disagree with decision)	Internal and external constraints to taking action (i.e., fears my concerns will be ignored; but patient does not qualify for needed services)	Fill in X and Y Value/ responsibility X conflicts with value/ responsibility Y	What actions *could* you take? – To improve outcome for the patient(s) – To cope with own moral distress	What action(s) *should* you take?

From "Navigating moral distress using the moral distress map" by D. M. Dudzinski, 2016, *Journal of Medical Ethics, 42*, p. 323

References

American Academy of Pediatrics (AAP). (2009). *Advocacy Guide*. Grassroots Solutions. Retrieved from www.aap.org/en-us/advocacy-and-policy/state-advocacy/Documents/AdvocacyGuide.pdf

American Psychological Association (APA). (n.d.). Retrieved from www.apa.org/advocacy/guide

American Psychological Association (APA) Practice Organization. (2009). *An action plan for self-care*. Good Practice, pp. 16–17.

Beach, M. C., Price, E. G., Gary, T. L., Robinson, K. A., Gozu, A., Palacio, A., … Cooper, L. A. (2005). Cultural competency: A systematic review of health care provider educational interventions. *Medical Care, 43*(4), 356–373.

Betancourt, J. R., Green, A. R., Carrillo, J. E., & Ananeh-Firempong, O. (2003). Defining cultural competence: A practical framework for addressing racial/ethnic disparities in health and health care. *Public Health Reports, 118*, 293–302.

Bronfenbrenner, U. (1979). *The ecology of human development: Experiments by nature and design*. Cambridge, MA: Harvard University Press.

Brown, K. J., & Roberts, M. C. (2000). Future issues in pediatric psychology: Delphic survey. *Journal of Clinical Psychology in Medical Settings, 7*(1), 5–15.

Carter, B. D. (2014). Carolyn S. Schroeder Award for Outstanding Clinical Practice: Creativity and innovation in the practice of pediatric psychology. *Clinical Practice in Pediatric Psychology, 2*(4), 378–383. https://doi.org/10.1037/cpp0000079

Carter, B. D., Kronenberger, W. G., Scott, E. L., Kullgren, K. A., Piazza-Waggoner, C., & Brady, C. E. (2017). Inpatient pediatric consultation-liaison. In M. C. Roberts & R. G. Steele (Eds.), *Handbook of pediatric psychology* (5th ed., pp. 105–118). New York, NY: Guilford Press.

DeAngelis, T. (2018). 8 ways to advocate for psychology. *Monitor on Psychology, 49*(3), 34.

Drotar, D. (1997). Relating parent and family functioning to the psychological adjustment of children with chronic health conditions. What have we learned? What do we need to know? *Journal of Pediatric Psychology, 22*, 149–165.

Drotar, D. (2004). Commentary: We can make our own dime or two, help children and their families, and advance science while doing so. *Journal of Pediatric Psychology, 29*(1), 61–63. https://doi.org/10.1093/jpepsy/jsh009

Drotar, D. (2013). Reflections on clinical practice in pediatric psychology and implications for the field. *Clinical Practice in Pediatric Psychology, 1*(2), 95–105. https://doi.org/10.1037/cpp0000017

Dudzinski, D. M. (2016). Navigating moral distress using the moral distress map. *Journal of Medical Ethics, 42*(5), 321–324.

Eggly, S., Meert, K. L., Berger, J., Zimmerman, J., Anand, K. J., Newth, C. J., … & The Eunice Kennedy Shriver National Institute of Child Health and Human Development Collaborative Pediatric Critical Care Research Network. (2011). A framework for conducting follow-up meetings with parents after a child's death in the pediatric intensive care unit. *Pediatric Critical Care Medicine, 12*(2), 147–152. https://doi.org/10.1097/PCC.0b013e3181e8b40c.

Felitti, V. J., Anda, R. F., Nordenberg, D., Williamson, D. F., Spitz, A. M., Edwards, V., … Marks, J. S. (1998). Relationship of childhood abuse and household dysfunction to many of the leading causes of death in adults: The adverse childhood experiences (ACE) study. *American Journal of Preventive Medicine, 14*, 245–258.

Flores, G. (2000). Culture and the patient-physician relationship: Achieving cultural competency in health care. *The Journal of Pediatrics, 136*(1), 14–23.

Flores, G., Abreu, M., Schwartz, I., & Hill, M. (2000). The importance of language and culture in pediatric care: Case studies from the Latino community. *The Journal of Pediatrics, 137*(6), 842–848. https://doi.org/10.1067/mpd.2000.109150

Haley, W. E., McDaniel, S. H., Bray, J. H., Frank, R. G., Heldring, M., Johnson, S. B., … & Wiggins, J. G. (1998). Psychological practice in primary care settings: Practical tips for clinicians. *Professional Psychology: Research and Practice, 29*(3), 237–244.

Kazak, A. (1997). A contextual family/systems approach to pediatric psychology: Introduction to the special issue. *Journal of Pediatric Psychology, 22*(2), 141–148.

Kazak, A. (2006). Pediatric psychosocial preventative health model (PPPHM): Research, practice, and collaboration in pediatric family systems medicine. *Families, Systems & Health, 24*, 381–395.

Lequerica, M. (1993). Stress in immigrant families with handicapped children: A child advocacy approach. *American Journal of Orthopsychiatry, 63*(4), 545–552. https://doi.org/10.1037/h0079472

Lewis, J., Arnold, M. S., House, R., & Toporek, R. (2003). Advocacy competencies: American Counseling Association task force on advocacy competencies. Retrieved from www.counseling.org/Resources/Competencies/Advocacy_Competencies.pdf.

Miller, A. R., Condin, C. J., McKellin, W. H., Shaw, N., Klassen, A. F., & Sheps, S. (2009). Continuity of care for children with complex chronic health conditions: Parents' perspectives. *BMC Health Services Research, 9*(1), 242. https://doi.org/10.1186/1472-6963-9-242

National Institutes of Health (NIH). (2009). *NIH health disparities strategic plan and budget, fiscal years 2009–2013*. Retrieved from www.nimhd.nih.gov/docs/2009-2013nih_health_disparities_strategic_plan_and_budget.pdf

Nielsen, B. A., Baum, R. A., & Soares, N. S. (2013). Navigating ethical issues with electronic health records in developmental-behavioral pediatric practice. *Journal of Developmental & Behavioral Pediatrics, 34*(1), 45–51.

Palermo, T. M., Janicke, D. M., McQuaid, E. L., Mullins, L. L., Robins, P. M., & Wu, Y. P. (2014). Recommendations for training in pediatric psychology: Defining core competencies across training levels. *Journal of Pediatric Psychology, 39*(9), 965–984. https://doi.org/10.1093/jpepsy/jsuo15

Paulson, J. A. (2001). Pediatric advocacy. *Pediatric Clinics of North America, 48*(5), 1307–1318.

Perloff, R. M., Bonder, B., Ray, G. B., Ray, E. B., & Siminoff, L. A. (2006). Doctor-patient communication, cultural competence, and minority health: Theoretical and empirical perspectives. *American Behavioral Scientist, 49*(6), 835–852.

Phelan, M., & Parkman, S. (1995). How to work with an interpreter. *British Medical Journal, 311*(7004), 555.

Pines, A., & Aronson, E. (1988). *Career burnout: Causes and cures*. New York: Free Press.

Rudd, R. A., Aleshire, N., Zibbell, J. E., & Gladden, R. M. (2016). Increases in drug and opioid overdose deaths—United States, 2000–2014. *Morbidity and Mortality Weekly Report, 64*(50), 1378–1382.

Sanders, R. S., & Dan, B. B. (1984). Bless the seats and the children: The physician and the legislative process. *JAMA, 252*(18), 2613–2614. https://doi.org/10.1001/jama.1984.03350180067035

Scholl, L., Seth, P., Kariisa, M., Wilson, N., & Baldwin, G. (2019). Drug and opioid-involved overdose deaths—United States, 2013–2017. *Morbidity and Mortality Weekly Report, 67*, 1419–1427.

Shaw, R. J., & DeMaso, D. R. (2006). *Clinical manual of pediatric psychosomatic medicine: Mental health consultation with physically ill children and adolescents*. Washington, DC: American Psychiatric Publishing, Incorporated.

Studdert, D. M., Burns, J. P., Mello, M. M., Puopolo, A. L., Truog, R. D., & Brennan, T. A. (2003). Nature of conflict in the care of pediatric intensive care patients with prolonged stay. *Pediatrics, 112*(3), 553–558. https://doi.org/10.1542/peds.112.3.553

Tervalon, M., & Murray-Garcia, J. (1998). Cultural humility versus cultural competence: A critical distinction in defining physician training outcomes in multicultural education. *Journal of Health Care for the Poor and Underserved, 9*(2), 117–125.

Tucker, C. M. (2002). Expanding pediatric psychology beyond hospital walls to meet the health care needs of ethnic minority children. *Journal of Pediatric Psychology, 27*(4), 315–323.

Winters, N. C., Hanson, G., & Stoyanova, V. (2007). The case formulation in child and adolescent psychiatry. *Child and Adolescent Psychiatric Clinics, 16*(1), 111–132.

Index

B. D. Carter, K. A. Kullgren (eds.), *Clinical Handbook of Psychological Consultation in Pediatric Medical Settings*, Issues in Clinical Child Psychology, https://doi.org/10.1007/978-3-030-35598-2

Y

The manufacturer's authorised representative in the EU is Springer Nature Customer Service Centre GmbH, Europaplatz 3, 69115 Heidelberg, Germany. If you have any concerns regarding our products, please contact ProductSafety@springernature.com

Printed and bound by CPI Group (UK) Ltd, Croydon, CR0 4YY
30/09/2026
02225556-0020